Applications of Biophotonics and Nanobiomaterials in Biomedical Engineering

Applications of Biophotonics and Nanobiomaterials in Biomedical Engineering

Mohammad E. Khosroshahi

Amirkabir University of Technology
Faculty of Biomedical Engineering
Biomaterial Group
Tehran-Iran

MIS-Electronics
Nanobiophotonics and Biomedical R&D Center
Toronto, ON
Canada

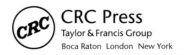

CRC Press
Taylor & Francis Group
Boca Raton London New York

CRC Press is an imprint of the
Taylor & Francis Group, an **informa** business

A SCIENCE PUBLISHERS BOOK

Cover credit:

The figure used on the cover is original and taken from the author's research paper published in Journal of Nanomedicine Nanotechnology by OMICS publisher.

CRC Press
Taylor & Francis Group
6000 Broken Sound Parkway NW, Suite 300
Boca Raton, FL 33487-2742

First issued in paperback 2020

ISBN-13: 978-1-4987-4848-3 (hbk)
ISBN-13: 978-0-367-78176-7 (pbk)

Library of Congress Cataloging-in-Publication Data

Names: Khosroshahi, Mohammad E., author.
Title: Applications of biophotonics and nanobiomaterials in biomedical
    engineering / Mohammad E. Khosroshahi, Department of Mechanical
    Engineering, University of Toronto, Toronto, ON, Canada.
Description: Boca Raton, FL : CRC Press, 2017. | "A Science Publishers book."
    | Includes bibliographical references and index.
Identifiers: LCCN 2017026613| ISBN 9781498748483 (hardback : alk. paper) |
    ISBN 9781498748490 (e-book : alk. paper)
Subjects: LCSH: Biomedical engineering. | Imaging systems in medicine. |
    Nanostructured materials.
Classification: LCC R856 .K52 2017 | DDC 610.28--dc23
LC record available at https://lccn.loc.gov/2017026613

Visit the Taylor & Francis Web site at
http://www.taylorandfrancis.com

and the CRC Press Web site at
http://www.crcpress.com

Preface

During the last decade, the different branches of science (physics, chemistry and biology), engineering (material) and nanotechnology have evolved so much, that their interaction in many fields is almost unavoidable and has truly become an interdisciplinary subject. The key roles played by each of these subjects in the various areas of biomedical and clinical engineering such as cancer diagnosis, therapy, bioimaging and drug delivery are indisputable. On one hand, nanomaterials with unique optical, thermal, and magnetic properties mainly consisting of a significant area to volume ratio, tunable optical emission, superb magnetic behaviour and others are being designed and fabricated on a molecular and biological material scale in the form of antibodies and protein ligands, which facilitates their possible medical applications, on the other hand, biophotonics, while expanding its province of dominance in biomedical optics, has long reached the inevitable concurrence with nanotechnology in many applications.

Despite such fruitful combinations, there are, however, some issues and problems which are worth discussing when it comes to the applications where all the different kinds of disciplines are playing their respective roles in a common game. The question that I am interested in and for which I intend to raise perhaps more than the final correct answer itself is the participation percentage of each field and the effects they may have on the final result. In a typical biomedical example, one may be dealing with the chaotic nature of coherent laser light, thermodynamically unstable cancerous cells, targeted or untargeted nanoparticles inside a cell where they are likely polydispersed and distributed homogenously or inhomogenously. How important is the nanoparticle displacement under the action of a laser-intense electric field within the cell? Does the rate of energy dissipation and therefore, the propagation of emitted dipole radiation due to the harmonic oscillation of localized surfaced plasmon resonance affect the intercellular mechanisms? Should one care about the static changes of polydispersed ensemble within the cell? After all the nanoparticles collapse in the domain under the van der Waals attraction force up to a full contact of their surfaces, hence the change in the interparticle gap will cause a red shift of domain absorption spectrum maximum. In the case of dynamic changes, however, the heating and melting of the nanoparticle core increases the electron relaxation constant and thus reduces the quality factor, i.e., degrades the quality of the nanosystem. Can these questions play a part in the quality of imaging, detection and therapy? This book is an introduction to the above questions and one may consider it as a textbook. It is based on the graduate courses on nanomaterials and nanobiotechnology that I have delivered over the years at the Amirkabir University of Technology and my collection of papers. The book is divided into four sections: (I) Light and Matter, (II) Nanobiophotonics: biophotonics and nanotechnology, (III) Nanobiomaterials, (IV) Nanomedicine: applications of biophotonics and nanobiomaterials. Most chapters end with a few related research works of my PhD students. The main goal is to make a comprehensive prospective available to the readers who are interested in learning, practicing and teaching the subject. Although, the collection of articles presented here addresses the numerous scientific and technical challenges ahead, the future of nanomedicine is undoubtedly bright and its apparent technical limitations will probably be resolved by taking different views of the problems and devising an innovative approach. Finally, it is important for me to express my appreciation and thanks to my family for being patient and for their continuous support during the time of preparation of this book. Also, I wish to thank every single student who worked hard to carry out the research according to the schedule and for their discussions and feedback.

Contents

Part III: Nanobiomaterials

Part V: Nanomedicine: Applications of Biophotonics and Nanobiomaterials

Part I
Light and Matter

1

Basics of Quantum Physics

1.1 Language and knowledge

Let us suppose that two people are interested in discussing a problem. The first possible obstacle they may confront is language, which is basically the ability to achieve and use complex systems of communication and it relies on social convention and learning. Let us assume for the sake of simplicity that the communication language is the same, however, the subject of debate is not ordinary but more technical. Now, there are a number of possibilities that they can face, either both have a preconception of the subject, neither of them has any idea about the subject or one may possibly have an advantage over the other in terms of technical knowledge. Also, we should remember that the more the discussion tends to cover the details, the more they have to strive to establish a mutual understanding in order to keep the conversation going due to the use of different terminologies and concepts. So, the first question which arises is their subconscious awareness about their possible divergence from the main point of discussion and again being optimistic, we assume that such divergence is not necessarily because of the intentional disagreement but due to the nature of the conclusion drawn, based on their understanding of terms, definitions and vocabularies. Therefore, in order to have a relatively comfortable flowing discussion, there must be at least one or two common points from which it can grow more systematically. Speaking of knowledge, as mentioned above, it can have different meanings depending on how one defines and looks at it. For empiricists, it is acquired by sensibility, hence the '*experience*', whereas for rationalists, it is achievable through reasoning, hence '*understanding*'. Through the former, objects are given to us and through the latter, the objects are thought and understood.

In simple terms, the two main interdependent functions of a language are the description of phenomena and the communication of experiences. However, if a particular phenomenon is to be communicated to another person who has no knowledge of any kind, the description becomes totally nonsense and must transcend the case in question. In other words it would be like describing the rainbow to a person who is born blind, the person cannot possibly imagine or understand the concept of a rainbow since he has no experience of the sensibility of colors nor the thought through understanding the phenomenon. Concepts in ordinary language are roughly speaking fixed classifications of phenomena and experiences forming the basis from which concepts on the higher levels of abstraction evolve. Beyond doubt, a keen layman who is interested in delving into the quantum world expects to encounter some fairly unusual phenomena, namely paradoxical (Polkinighorne 1984). This is because of both the lack of knowledge of any kind about the subject and also due to the inherent unusual nature of the quantum world. He will encounter the paradoxical and will miss it unless it is pointed out to him by a compassionate professional friend. There is no dissent regarding the quantum theory success on the small-scale structure of the world but there is equally an open subject of debate about its interpretation. The latter revolves around two major issues: the nature of reality and the nature of measurement.

1.2 Causality and chance

It is well-known that nothing including organic and inorganic materials remains unaltered in nature and that it is subject to a continuous change of states: motion, transformation, evolution, degradation, etc. Perhaps more intriguing than causality itself is that nothing in nature just disappears out of the blue without a reason and trace. Apparently, the events go hand-in-hand to complete a mission or serve a purpose which in scientific jargon is referred to as a '*cycle*' such as those of biological and biochemical processes. When we scrutinize the events, we are confronted with a seemingly simple fact that amidst all the complexity of change there exists a relationship between the individual events as a part of the whole system. A process by which one thing or an event appears out of other thing and systematically holds constant relationships within a wide variety of transformations is by no means accidental. These relationships are called '*necessary*' meaning that it could not be otherwise, since they are inevitable part of the natural law. The relationships between objects, events and conditions at a defined time and those at later times are called '*causal laws*' (Bohm 1957). Thus, according to Newton's laws of motion, an object thrown up will fall down due to the gravitational force. But, there could be some cases where the change in conditions, i.e., contingencies may impose some changes in the occurrence of the event, for example, ordinarily one expects snowflakes, like the stone, to fall on the ground but on the contrary if they are subjected to strong winds, they will go even higher due to the fluctuation in air conditions. These contingencies result in '*chance*' where the events under certain conditions do not follow the physical laws. Therefore, the necessity of a law of nature is conceived as '*conditional*' because it only applies when these contingencies are neglected. But, this does not imply that they are not important and should be ignored in all real conditions, particularly in cases where one cannot completely isolate the system from its surrounding environment to study it. In fact, there is no such system in the external world which is completely independent of its surrounding medium. One such situation is a biological system which is constantly under internal and external influences.

1.3 Fundamentals of classical mechanics

Classical mechanics is undoubtedly one of the most fundamental, old and familiar branches of physics. Its basic concepts revolve around important parameters of mass, force, acceleration and others. The two complementary approaches to the theory of mechanics: equilibrium (statics) and motion (dynamics) can be traced back to the Antiquity era where early works on the former were established by Archimedes and the latter by Aristotle. Then, the work was continued by many great natural philosophers until the seventeenth century when a breakthrough was achieved by Newton who formulated and reformulated all his principles around the three axioms of motion documented in the '*Principia*' (1713). Since then, the restless caravan has been on move until now with many fundamental developments, perhaps with the exception of Einstein's achievement in the early years of the twentieth century, when he introduced his theory of relativity and completely shattered the old vision of time-space concept.

Nonetheless, it is worth noticing that no matter how impressive and well-established these laws appear to be, we can never claim a universal validity for them. We can only be confident that they provide an acceptable description of a particular phenomenon for which their predictions have been sufficiently tested. For example, on the ordinary scale, Euclid's axioms are absolutely valid and satisfactory. However, we are not allowed to assume that they would work either on a cosmological or a sub-microscopic scale. In fact, they have been well-modified by Einstein's theory of gravitation (general relativity). By the same argument, the laws of classical mechanics are no exception. Newton's laws of motion have been uniquely valid in many aspects such as moving satellites around the earth but they have equally failed in two areas: atomic microscopic scale and nuclear physics, that is to say, moving electrons around an atom cannot be modelled or thought of as moving satellites around the earth. This does not mean that classical mechanics has lost its value. Both quantum mechanics and the theory of relativity are indeed extensions of classical mechanics, that is, they reproduce their results in other appropriate limiting cases. Finally, it should be noticed that the most important, basic and fundamental assumption of classical physics is that space and time are continuous, i.e., the geometry of space is Eclidian and that there is no limit to the accuracy with which we can measure positions and velocities. These assumptions are abandoned at the microscopic scale by quantum mechanics as we will see shortly.

Now let us continue briefly with the position and velocity of a particle as this will form a part of our main body of discussion throughout this chapter. In simple language it is not possible to give an accurate description of the interdependence between the position and velocity quantities. But when the concepts are transformed into ideal mathematical equations then the problem can be easily defined. If a particle moves in 3-D Euclidian space and the trajectory is continuous and has a differential curve, it is possible to set up for example a Cartesian system (X,Y,Z) in which the position of the particle is given by three differential functions of time: x(t), y(t), z(t). The corresponding velocity of the particle is then given by $\left[\dfrac{dx}{dt}, \dfrac{dy}{dt}, \dfrac{dz}{dt}\right]$. Therefore, we can say that at any instant of time t, a material particle has an exact position of x(t), y(t), z(t) and an exact defined velocity $\left[\dfrac{dx}{dt}, \dfrac{dy}{dt}, \dfrac{dz}{dt}\right]$. Introducing the concept of linear momentum, P which is the product of mass, m and the velocity, v of the particle, we get

$$\left[m\frac{dx}{dt}, m\frac{dy}{dt}, m\frac{dx}{dt}\right] \tag{1.1}$$

Thus, at any given time t, a material particle has an exactly defined position x(t), y(t), z(t) and momentum. According to Newton's laws of motion the acceleration of a body is directly proportional to the force acting on it and inversely proportional to its mass and is expressed by a differential equation,

$$F = m\frac{d^2x}{dt^2} \tag{1.2}$$

where x is the position vector of the body and F is the force acting on it. Newton's laws of motion imply that the future behaviour of a body is determined completely and accurately for all time in terms of the initial positions, velocities and the forces acting on it. These forces can be both external, which arise outside of the system under consideration, or internal due to the interaction between the various particles that form the system. Let us consider an isolated system comprising N particles (or bodies), which we label by an index i = 1,2,....N. So, when we say that the system is isolated, it means that all other particles are sufficiently remote to have a negligible influence on it. Each of the particles is assumed to be small enough to be treated as a point particle. The position of the ith particle with respect to a given inertial frame will be denoted by $r_i(t)$. Its velocity and acceleration are,

$$V_i(t) = \dot{r}_i(t)$$

$$a_i(t) = V_i(t) = \ddot{r}_i(t) \tag{1.3}$$

where the dots denote the differentiation with respect to the time t. No particle is ever characterized by a scalar constant, its mass m_i. The momentum of the particle P_i is defined by the product of mass and its velocity:

$$P_i = m_i V_i \tag{1.4}$$

Newton's second law of motion shows how the particle will move

$$F_i = m_i a_i = \dot{P}_i(t) \tag{1.5}$$

where F_i is the total force acting on the particle. In a more realistic situation, this force is composed of a sum of forces due to the other particles in the system. Hence, the force on the ith particle due to the jth particle by F_{ij} is:

$$F_i = F_{ij} + F_{12} + \ldots F_{iN} = \sum_{j=1}^{N} F_{ij} \tag{1.6}$$

where $F_{ij} = 0$ since there is no force on the ith particle due to itself. Note that F_{ij} is a function of the positions, velocities and internal structures of the ith and jth particles but is unaffected by the other particles. The two-particle forces must satisfy Newton's third law, which states that 'action and reaction' are equal and opposite, $F_{ij} = -F_{ij}$. But because of the relativity principle it can depend on the relative position,

$$r_{ij} = r_i - r_j \qquad (1.7)$$

and the relative velocity,

$$v_{ij} = \dot{r}_{ij} = \dot{r}_i - \dot{r}_j \qquad (1.8).$$

Now, if forces are known as the functions of positions and velocities, then from (1.4), the future motions of the particles can be predicted. In systems or bodies with structure, two types of internal forces that are central and conservative between their constituent parts can give rise to other forces which are still conservative, i.e., independent of velocity but are not central, i.e., not directed along the line joining the particles. The forces can have the form,

$$F_{ij} = \hat{r}_{ij} \, f(r_{ij}) \qquad (1.9)$$

where $\hat{r}_{ij}$ is the unit vector in the direction of r_{ij} and $f(r_{ij})$ is a scalar function of the relative distance r_{ij}. If $f(r_{ij})$ is positive, the force F_{ij} is a repulsive force directed outwards along the line joining the bodies; if, however, $f(r_{ij})$ is negative then it is an attractive force directed inwards.

According to Newton's law of universal gravitation which *states that the force between two particles (or bodies such as moon and earth) is inversely proportional to the square of the distance between them,*

$$f\left(r_{ij}\right) = \frac{Gm_i m_j}{r_{ij}^{\,2}} \qquad (1.10)$$

where $G = 6.67 \times 10^{-11}$ Nm² kg⁻² is the gravitational constant. Since, the masses are always positive, this force is always attractive. Similarly, according to Coulomb's law for two electrically charged particles we have,

$$f(r_{ij}) = \frac{q_i q_j}{4\pi\varepsilon_0 r_r r_j^{\,2}} \qquad (1.11)$$

where q_i and q_j are their electric charges and $\varepsilon_0 = 8.85 \times 10^{-12}$ Fm⁻¹ is another constant known as the permittivity of free space. Note that the analogue of Newton's constant G is,

$1/4\pi\varepsilon_0 = 8.99 \times 10^9$ N m² C⁻². Electric charges can be either positive or negative and therefore, the electrostatic forces can be either attractive or repulsive depending on the sign. Going back to our earlier point: in many cases, the external forces can be so small that they are neglected, while the internal forces can be entirely considered in terms of the positions and velocities of the centers of mass of the constituent particles. This for example, applies well the in case of the planets' motion around the sun where Newton's laws of motion determine the future motions of the bodies solely in terms of the positions and velocities of the bodies at a given instance of time. Thus, there exist a set of causal relationships, i.e., for a given set of causes (initial position and velocity of each body), there are a set of effects (later position and velocity of each body).

Based on this mechanistic conception of the external world, Laplace went one step further by supposing that the entire universe consisted of literally nothing but bodies which underwent defined motions through a vast space according to Newton's laws. To him everything was clearly written and predetermined, that is once the positions and velocities of all heavenly bodies are known at a given time, then the future behaviour of everything in the entire universe can be determined for all times. For him all this was possible because he believed in a superior being out there who had all the knowledge required for such precise prediction and control of future events in the universe. Having said all that, even within this notion, no system of bodies is really completely isolated in the sense that there exist absolutely no other external influential forces acting upon each other. Distant stars have some effects on others, comets entering the solar system can deflect the orbit of a planet considerably, tidal effects on planets' motion and so on. Therefore, for a complete causal determination of future motions one must consider the various other forces, both internal and external as well as the information regarding the initial positions and velocities of the bodies. In summary, despite central and conservative forces, we cannot, however, conclude that everything can be explained simply in terms of them. As we will see shortly, the concepts of classical mechanics cannot really be applied to the small-scale structures of matter and for that we need a different approach, i.e., quantum mechanics. Quantum mechanics provides a new set of laws and a method of description of microscopic systems that has been very successful. The next section will discuss some of the fundamental principles of this highly controversial subject. At this point it must be emphasized that the interpretation of an external world including the universe itself in terms of quantum mechanics in not the intension of the book nor is it inclined to reflect such an impression and the interested readers can refer to many basic and advanced technical and philosophical texts written in this area that are easily available.

1.4 Conceptual quantum physics

Let us start by questioning why quantum mechanics seems to be so hard for newcomers to learn and understand. Intuition from everyday experience is helpless and sometimes even misleading. There are two major reasons: conceptual and technical. In the preceding section we said that in classical physics one can accurately know where a particle such as an electron is and what it is doing, which in technical terms means that both the position and the velocity of the particle can be known. But as we shall see shortly, Heisenberg abolished such an easy notion. In quantum physics, it is difficult to uphold a sharp distinction between the object and the observer. For any measurement of a physical quantity, the measuring instrument must interact with the object under investigation. In simple language, for example, to monitor or measure the path of a particle which is not observable with the naked eye using a microscope, light is need to see it. But, the interaction of the light beam with the particle causes it to be deflected slightly away from its original path. If the light intensity is reduced greatly to avoid such a deviation then we will not be able to see the object anyway. It is very hard to decide precisely whether the localized position of the particle by microscope represents the particle before, during or after the measurement. The theory of quantum mechanics has led to many applications: laser, the electron microscope, tunneling diodes, silicon chip and many other technological devices.

1.4.1 A bit of history

Although, Newton had a corpuscular notion about light, the modern perception of quantum all began on Dec. 14, 1900 when Max Planck presented his historical paper "On the Theory of the Energy Distribution Law of the Normal Spectrum" at the meeting of the German Physical Society. His life taking milestone research intended to explain the problem encountered by Rayleigh and Jean when they studied black body radiation a few years before him. Their experiment showed that the energy density always remains finite and that it becomes zero at high frequencies. This in physics is known as "*Ultraviolet Catastrophe*". What eventually appears to have convinced him of the correctness and deep significance of his quantum hypothesis was its support of the statistical concept of entropy and third law of thermodynamics. It was in that meeting, that for first time Planck introduced a fundamental constant h, after his name which has a value of 6.66×10^{-34} Js. This on the scale of everyday life experience is an extremely small quantity and that is why the quantum theory was not comprehended very well until it was developed to a stage where tiny systems of atomic and subatomic dimensions were investigated and probed.

Prior to the discovery of h, electromagnetic energy was regarded as continuous but now it comes in packets, i.e., just as a heap of sand is composed of many individual grains, so does the electromagnetic radiation come in lumps. The discrete lumps or quanta of light are called photons. The discrete nature of radiation manifests itself in the processes of absorption or emission by matter, which occurs only in multiple units of these energy packets. The photon energy, E_p is different for different wavelengths, λ or frequencies, v and is defined by the relation:

$$E_p = hv = hc/\lambda \tag{1.12}$$

where $c = 3.8 \times 10^8\, ms^{-1}$ is the speed of light in vacuum. Note that the shorter the wavelength (or higher the frequency), the more energetic the photons are. So, a light with $v = 10^{15}$ Hz has an energy of 10^{-19} J which is very small at the macroscopic scale but very effective at the microscopic level. Young Einstein whose deep insight into electromagnetism and statistical mechanics was perhaps unchallengeable by anyone at that time, found out, as a result of Planck's work, that it was time for sweeping change in classical statistics and electromagnetism. He advanced predictions of many physical phenomena which were strongly confirmed by experiment.

In 1924, Louis de Broglie had suggested that atomic particles might have a wave-like aspect to their behaviour. He connected the momentum of the particle to the wavelength of 'matter waves' by

$$P = h/\lambda \tag{1.13}$$

The relation (1.13) shows that as the mass (hence p) becomes large, λ becomes very small and the length scale over which wave-like behaviour can be discerned diminishes correspondingly. For example, at room temperature an average atom of oxygen has a de Broglie wavelength of 4×10^{-11} m and for a DNA molecule $\approx 10^{-14}$ m.

1.4.2 Heisenberg's principle of uncertainty

So far we have talked about position and momentum. They are just examples of what in dynamics are called the co-ordinate q and its conjugate momentum p. These quantities are always related physically by the fact that their combined dimensions are those of actions, i.e., the product of q . p can always be assigned to a value in units of Planck's constant $\hbar = h/2\pi$. Also, we have mentioned that, a physical observation implies a mutual interaction between the object under investigation and the instrument of observation. This interaction occurs via a field of force such as an electric field, a magnetic field, elastic forces and so on, which can be a part of the measuring instrument. Visual observation of a material particle implies that the particle emits or reflects light, meaning that the particle has to interact with an electromagnetic field. Supposing F is the field force through which observation takes place and δt is a small time interval during the observation, so according to Newton's second law of motion we have,

$$F = \frac{\delta p}{\delta t} \tag{1.14}$$

where δp is the exchange of momentum between the particle and the field of force during δt. If δs is the spatial displacement of the particle in the time δt, then the exchange of energy δE between the particle and F becomes

$$\delta E = F . \delta s = \delta p/\delta t . \delta s$$

or $\delta E\, \delta t = \delta p . \delta s$ \hfill (1.15).

In a Cartesian system of coordinates, we have $\delta s = (\delta x, \delta y, \delta z)$ and similarly, $\delta p = (\delta p_x, \delta p_y, \delta p_z)$

So, the Eq. (1.15) can be written as:

$$\delta E\, \delta t = (\delta p_x \delta x, \delta p_y \delta y, \delta p_z \delta z) \tag{1.16}.$$

Every term in relation (1.16) has the same dimension and represents the same physical quantity, which is called '*Action*'. Therefore, the dimension of an action can be expressed both in terms of energy × time and as linear momentum × distance. The punch line is that, each term of relation (1.16) shows an interaction between the particle and the measuring or observing instrument. Thus, the only time that an observation of the particle can occur is when the action-terms in Eq. (1.16) do not all vanish. Combining this concept with the previous concept expressed in relation (1.12), we then have the following highly probable postulate:

"*A physical observation implies that manifestation of an action which is an integral multiple of h*". \hfill (1.17)

This principle is fundamental to quantum theory.

Now, according to the principle (1.17), the smallest possible interaction is

$$\left| \delta p_x' \, \delta x' \right| = h \tag{1.18}.$$

The quantities $\delta p_x'$ and $\delta x'$ cannot be separately taken into account because any attempt to measure these quantities would mean introducing new indeterminate quantities $\delta p_x''$ and $\delta x''$ satisfying a similar equation. So, we can conclude that at any instant of time, p_x and x are subject to indeterminacies $\Delta p_x \geq \left| \delta p_x' \right|$ and $\Delta x \geq \left| \delta x' \right|$. Substituting this into Eq. (1.18), we get

$$\Delta p_x \, \Delta x \geq h \tag{1.19a}.$$

Therefore, a determination of the momentum component p_x with indeterminacy Δp_x introduces a fundamental indeterminacy $h/\Delta p_x$ in the position coordinate x and similarly vice versa that is, indeterminacy ($h/\Delta x$ in p_x). Generally, this argument can be applied to other relations $\delta p_y \, \delta y$, $\delta p_z \, \delta z$, and $\delta E \, \delta t$ and we get:

$$\Delta p_y \, \Delta y \geq h \tag{1.19b}$$

$$\Delta p_z \, \Delta z \geq h \tag{1.19c}$$

$$\Delta E \, \Delta t \geq h \tag{1.19d}.$$

The inequality (1.19d) states that a measurement of the energy of the particle with indeterminacy ΔE introduces a fundamental indeterminacy $h/\Delta E$ in the time coordination of the particle. Conversely, a time determination of the particle with indeterminacy Δt introduces a fundamental indeterminacy $h/\Delta t$ in the energy. Indeed, Heisenberg's indeterminacy relations seem to affect all of classical mechanics. But, because of extremely small quantum action, these indeterminacy relations do not manifest themselves when the classical, i.e., large objects are considered. I have always tried to give a kind of naive but practical and comprehensible analogous example to my students in helping them to get a vague idea about the subject, though at the beginning I admit that this is not strictly speaking a true reflection of the truth, but nonetheless it might do the trick.

Imagine on a warm summer night in the park you are interested in capturing on video the mosquitoes buzzing around the light. If you are asked how many mosquitoes are there, you may come up with any number but let us say 10. But when the video is played in slow motion, you will find out that there were only 5. In other words, the objects are so small and moving around so fast in a small space that there appear to be so many of them, i.e., one mosquito appears to be in more than one place. So, a smaller mass with higher velocity increases the indeterminacy of the mosquitoes' positions. Thus, it appears to the observer that there are so many of them but we know that it is not true. In quantum physics, the appearance of a single particle or point as a continuous line or curve is referred to as 'wave function' and is frequently used in wave-matter discussion. Now, let us take another example, consider a particle with a mass of 1gram and very precisely determined velocity, with indeterminacies,

$$\Delta v_x \approx \Delta v_y \approx \Delta v_z \approx 10^{-6} \, \mathrm{ms^{-1}}$$

assuming that the mass of the particle is precisely determined and from inequalities (1.19) we see that the indeterminacies in the position become

$$\Delta x \approx \Delta y \approx \Delta z \approx 6.66 \times 10^{-34} \, (\mathrm{Js})/10^{-3} \, (\mathrm{kg}) \times 10^{-6} \, (\mathrm{ms^{-1}}) = 6 \times 10^{-25} \, \mathrm{m}.$$

It is therefore, theoretically possible to determine the position of the particle with this high accuracy, which is well beyond the resolving power of any measuring instrument. Now if we consider an electron with a known velocity and indeterminacy, we get

$$\Delta x \approx \Delta y \approx \Delta z \approx 6.66 \times 10^{-34} \, (\mathrm{Js})/9 \times 10^{-31} \, (\mathrm{kg}) \, 10^{-6} \approx 700 \, \mathrm{m}.$$

Where the mass of the electron is 9×10^{-31} (kg). This demonstrates our complete lack of knowledge about the electron's position.

No doubt Niels Bohr whom Heisenberg was collaborating with had an immense influence on the establishment of the modern quantum theory, particularly when he introduced his *principle of complementarity* which states that: a complete knowledge of phenomena on atomic dimensions requires a description of both wave and particle properties. It is impossible to observe both the wave and particle aspects simultaneously (Eisberg and Resnick 1985). In effect, the complementarity principle implies that phenomena on the atomic and subatomic scale are not strictly like large-scale particles or waves (e.g., billiard balls and water waves). Such particle and wave characteristics in the same large-scale phenomenon are incompatible rather than complementary. Knowledge of a small-scale phenomenon, however, is essentially incomplete until both these aspects are known. Consider the puzzling problem of the relation of biology to physics. Living systems certainly have physical components but one has to be a very thorough reductionist to feel comfortable with the notion that biology is nothing but physics. Bohr points out that if we tear a living system apart into its component atoms hoping that we will get more information, we are completely mistaken because we have already killed it. There is a complementarity between life and atomic physics. This is one aspect of my debate, that how much research really takes this point seriously. In relation to physics-biology, our understanding is less complementary and is becoming more of a descriptive than an interpretive principle. Among scientists, biophysicists are certainly more capable of scrutinizing the processes occurring within living cells. Anyhow, we should know that with an uncertainty principle we are not going to have determinate dynamics in which position and momentum are known simultaneously. This aspect of quantum mechanics has proved to be very distasteful to many scientists including the great notorious men themselves who had a share in creating it in the first place. I would like to end this section by referring to some of the quotes made by these scientists.

1.4.3 Quantum physics in simple language

I think we all agree that converting or translating the preceding issues and questions into simple, ordinary and everyday language is an almost impossible task and as was mentioned earlier, this difficulty is not just due to the lack of knowledge of the person about the subject but also due to the paradoxes that he is facing. This difficulty gets even worse when one attempts to move from scientific language to ordinary language and of course sometimes the converse is true too. The shift of the main body of communication in either direction is done through mathematical language and terminologies which are an inherent part of the scientific methodology. So, the description of something as an object which cannot be observed directly by measuring sensory devices requires a new set of terminology because objects of such kind do not belong to our everyday life experiences. On the other hand, while trying to keep the logic of the ordinary language and the unambiguity, which is the scientific requirement, during description, you will confront yet another paradox as both of these requirements are strangers and do not make any sense in the realm of the quantum world. But let us try it.

By definition, a microscope is an observing device which is meant to look at (scope) objects at small (micro) scales so as to meet and serve particular scientific demands. Some examples of microscopes are: optical, acoustic, electron (both scanning-SEM and transmission-TEM), scanning probe, confocal, atomic force microscopy (AFM) and so on. The first fact is that the interpretation of the object-image observed under a microscope strongly depends on the specimen preparation method. During this procedure, materials undergo significant changes particularly mechanical and chemical if not other types before they are placed under a microscope. These changes in turn affect the sample's structural properties. So, the interpretation of the image must take this point into account. Secondly, in ultra microscopes for example, where high magnification is required, the image is almost distorted due to inevitable lens aberration and diffraction effects. In a simple low magnification microscopes, however, these effects are not a major issue.

Figure 1.1 shows the resolving power of a microscope. There is an upper limit for the magnification which can be used. The limit of resolution, $\Delta\Theta$ is

$$\Delta\Theta = \frac{\lambda}{2n\sin\theta} = \frac{\lambda}{N.A.} \qquad (1.20)$$

where n is the refractive index of the material used beneath the objective and α is the half-angle subtended by the objective at the object and N.A. is the numerical aperture, which is the ability of light collection. The limit of resolution for the best optical microscope is ≈ 200 nm. The eye can only resolve ≈ 0.01 cm (or 100 μm).

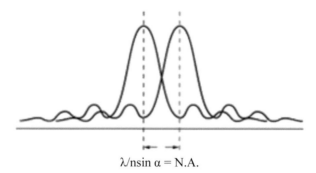

$$\lambda/n\sin\alpha = N.A.$$

Figure 1.1. Rayleigh's criteria for just resolvable diffraction pattern.

However, the resolving power can be improved significantly by using shorter wavelengths, UV or X-ray but at the expense of renouncing observation of the object directly through the microscope. Further still, the higher magnification can be enhanced by using an electron beam or e-beam (SEM or TEM). Once, the specimen is coated suitably with, e.g., gold, it is placed inside a vacuum chamber where it is irradiated by the e-beam thereby producing a magnified shadow picture on a screen or a photographic plate. The structure of many molecules composed of a large number of atoms has been observed by this instrument. The regular structure arrangement of atoms or ions in a crystal lattice acts as a grating which under appropriate optical condition, the diffracted x-ray or e-beam will form an interference pattern on the screen, see Fig. 1.2. The pattern can be studied via Bragg's relation,

$$2d = n\sin\theta \qquad (1.21)$$

where d is the crystal plate spacing, n is the order of diffraction and θ is the angle of beam incidence.

So, if the crystal lattice of NaCl is irradiated by an x-ray with a wavelength of 0.150×10^{-9} m and assuming that the first order of diffraction is observed at 15.8° then d = 277×10^{-12} (277 pm). This is

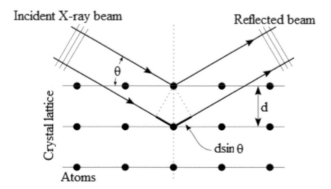

Figure 1.2. X-ray reflection (Bragg) from a crystal atomic planes.

obviously far away from the direct observation of a single atom. The object directly observed is the interference pattern, and its correlation with the spatial distribution of indivitual atoms involves atomic theory itself. Whenever, the intention is to depict the structure of molecules, we are very close to the limitation of geometrical picturing due to the quantum action that we have previously discussed in section 1.4.2. Therefore, regardless of the type of microscope, a large number of the atomic constituents of the radiation must participate in the picturing process. If a beam of electrons traverse through a single atom, a diffuse spot will be observed on the image screen under correct conditions due to the electrons' deviation from their initial direction and scattering by the atom. Now, this is a key point to notice, that if an electron is supposed to contribute in creating the picture then it must have interaction with the atom's internal constituents. But any such interaction would imply a change in the atomic state because of transition from the initial state to a new state caused by the actions of a few quanta. But there is no such open escape door, a large number of interactions are needed to build up the picture and that would change the state of the atom among many others. So, microscopic picturing appears to be an inherently impossible task prevented by quantum action but it is not very disappointing if we look at it differently that is, observational situations in quantum physics prove the limitation of the spatial structure.

According to quantum theory, experiments monitoring the structure of an atom will have an essentially statistical character. Even when a large number of identical atoms interact with the observing instrument to produce a more accurate picture of an atom, it still will have a statistical nature. This statistical element can be verified by spectroscopy where scientists attain their extensive and detailed knowledge of atomic structures by analysing the atomic line spectra. The statistical element in the measuring instrument is evident in for example the spectral line on the photographic plate as a result of the interaction of many photons with the plate. Thus, the observation technique in quantum physics which enables the recording of an elementary atomic object is never meant to use give the actual picture of the object but instead a coordination of the object as a whole in the system of reference given by the macroscopic instruments of observation. This can be seen as a spot in a photographic film produced by x-rays and photons, which provides some information regarding the atomic structure or tracking subatomic particles in a bubble chamber and many other examples.

Of course there are many physicists that maintain that the elementary atomic objects are essentially classical objects and that the entire statistical quantum mechanics is regarded as the result of an observational hurdle caused by the quantum of actions. However, it is also claimed that in order to observe an atomic object it is necessary to disturb it and the quantum of action is the least possible perturbation that will strongly affect the object's state caused by observation. Therefore, an inherently statistical description is unavoidable. For quantum physics, the question of how objectivity is presented and maintained is far more significant than what kind of reality might be ascribed to atomic objects. The interdependence between the act of observation and the description of quantum quantal phenomena makes it impossible to use the same perception of objectivity in the ordinary and classical sense in quantum physics.

Since, to preserve an unperturbed state of an atom and to apply governing classical laws while observing it is something that will never happen in quantum physics unless for some extraordinary reasons, the disturbance caused by the action observation is exceedingly small or somehow compensated for in the description of phenomena. Therefore, it is seen that the describability of an observed phenomena in an ordinary language is a vital element of physical objectivity (Bergstein 1972). Under no circumstances can atomic objects be conceived within ordinary language but the objectivity of quantal experiments eventually relies on ordinary language. The basic significance of ordinary language in physical science is mainly seen in the *corresponding principle* which states that classical physics must be a limiting case of quantum physics. When the quantum of action is vanishingly small as compared to the actions in a physical experiment, quantal phenomena will not be observed and the conceptual frame of classical physics can be consistently applied. In short, quantum mechanics regards the interactions of the object and the observer as the ultimate reality. It uses the language of physical relations and processes rather than that of physical qualities and properties. It rejects as meaningless and useless the notion that behind our perception there exists a hidden objective; instead it confines itself to the description of the relations among perceptions.

Quotation Marks

Among the most profound critics of Bohr-Heisenberg's view of a fundamental indeterminacy in physics were Einstein, Schrodinger, de Broglie and Bohm.

> *"Light and matter are both single entities, and the apparent duality arises in the limitations of our language."* **(Werner Heisenberg)**

> *"Isolated material particles are abstractions, their properties being definable and observable only through their interaction with other systems."* **(Niels Bohr)**

> *"I think that matter must have a separate reality independent of the measurements. That is an electron has spin, location and so forth even when it is not being measured. I like to think that the moon is there even if I am not looking at it."* **(Albert Einstein)**

> *"I don't like it, and I'm sorry I ever had anything to do with it."* **(Erwin Schrodinger)**

> *"We can reasonably accept that the attitude adopted for nearly 30 years by theoretical quantum physicists is, at least in appearance, the exact counterpart of information which experiment has given us of the atomic world. At the level now reached by research in microphysics it is certain that the methods of measurement do not allow us to determine simultaneously all the magnitudes which would be necessary to obtain a picture of the classical type of corpuscles and that the perturbation introduced by the measurements, which are impossible to eliminate, prevent us in general from predicting precisely the result which it will produce and allow only statistical predictions. The construction of purely probabilistic formulae that all theoreticians use today was thus completely justified. However, the majority of them, often under the influence of preconceived ideas derived from positivist doctrine, have thought that they could go further and assert that the uncertain and incomplete character of the knowledge that experiment at its present stage gives us about what happens in microphysics is the result of a real indeterminacy of the physical states and of their evolution. Such an extrapolation does not appear in any way to be justified… .This teaches us, in effect that the actual state of our knowledge is always provisional and that there must be, beyond what is actually known, immense new regions to discover"* **(de Broglie)**—(From Causality and Chance in Modern Physics by David Bohm, 1957, Routledge & Kegan Paul).

> *"It is safe to say that nobody understands quantum mechanics."* **(Richard Feynman)**

Keywords: Classical physics, Ultraviolet catastrophe, Quantum mechanics, Bohr, Planck, Constant, Quantum physics, Heisenberg's principles of uncertaintity, Knowledge, Chance, Causality, Principle of complementarity.

References

Bergstein, T. 1972. Quantum Physics and Ordinary Language. The Macmillan Press, New York.

Bohm, D. 1957. Causality and Chance in Modern Physics. Routledge & Kegan Paul Press, London.

Eisberg, R. and R. Resnick. 1985. Quantum Physics of a Atoms and Molecules, Solids, Nuclei and Particles. John Wiley & Sons Press, New York.

Polkinghorne, J.C. 1984. The Quantum World. Longman Press, London.

2

Ordinary Light

2.1 Review of the nature and properties of light

The study of light is one of the oldest scientific subjects. The earliest scientific theories of the nature of light were proposed around the end of the 17th century. In 1690, Christian Huygens proposed a theory that explained light as a wave phenomenon. However, a rival theory was offered by Isaac Newton in 1704. Newton, who had discovered the visible spectrum in 1666, stated that light is composed of tiny particles, or corpuscles, emitted by luminous bodies. By combining this corpuscular theory with his laws of mechanics, he was able to explain many optical phenomena. However, important experiments were performed on the diffraction and interference of light by Thomas Young (1801) and Fresnel (1814) that could only be interpreted in terms of the wave theory. The polarization of light was another phenomenon that could only be explained by the wave theory. Thus, in the 19th century the wave theory became the dominant theory of the nature of light. The wave theory received additional support from the electromagnetic theory of Maxwell (1864), who showed that electric and magnetic fields were propagated together and that their speed was identical to the speed of light. It thus became clear that visible light was a form of electromagnetic radiation, constituting only a small part of the electromagnetic spectrum. Maxwell's theory was confirmed experimentally with the discovery of radio waves by Hertz in 1886.

At this stage two issues remained to be solved: (i) the luminiferous ether, a hypothetical medium suggested as the carrier of light waves, just as air or water carries sound waves, (ii) the photoelectric effect, which involved the interaction of light with matter. Einstein extended the quantum theory of thermal radiation proposed by Planck in 1900 to cover not only the vibrations of the source of radiation but also the vibrations of the radiation itself. He thus suggested that light travels as tiny bundles of energy called light quanta, or photons. The energy of each photon is directly proportional to its frequency,

$$E_p = \frac{hc}{\lambda} \tag{2.1}$$

where E_p is the energy of photon, λ is the light wavelength, h is the Planck constant, and c is the speed of light. With the development of the quantum theory of atomic and molecular structure by Bohr and others, it became clear that light and other forms of electromagnetic radiation are emitted and absorbed in connection with the energy transitions of the particles of the substance radiating or absorbing the light. In these processes, the quantum or particle nature of light is more important than its wave nature. When the transmission of light is under consideration, however, the wave nature dominates over the particle nature. In 1924, Louis de Broglie showed that an analogous picture holds for particle behaviour, with moving particles having certain wave-like properties that govern their motion, so that there exists a complementarity between particles and waves known as *particle-wave duality*. The quantum theory of light has successfully explained all aspects of the behaviour of light. Figure 2.1 is a simplistic schematic, which compares the wave and particle nature of light where the former is thought of as a continuous drink and the latter as an encapsulated amount of juice.

Wave is continuous amount of energy

Classical
(Analogue)

Photon is quantized amount of energy package

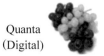
Quanta
(Digital)

Figure 2.1. Analogous comparison of wave and particle nature of light.

Figure 2.2 represents an electromagnetic spectrum where the frequency is inversely proportional to wavelength. Most of the interactions between light and biological matter as molecular media involve electronic polarization of the molecule subjected to an electric field. Therefore, the description of a light wave focuses on the nature of the oscillating electric field E, which has both a direction and amplitude (the value corresponding to maxima and minima of the wave). The direction of the electric field E, for a plane wave traveling in one direction is always perpendicular (i.e., orthogonal) both to the direction of propagation and to the oscillating magnetic field B. However, it can be linearly polarized, when the electric field of each point is in the same direction. When the electric field is distributed equally in a plane perpendicular to the direction of propagation, it is called circularly polarized. The propagation of light in the z direction with its oscillating electric field E(z,t) is described mathematically as:

$$F(z,t) = E_0 \cos(\omega t - kz) \tag{2.2}$$

and

$$k^2 = \frac{\varepsilon \omega^2}{c^2} \tag{2.3}$$

where E_0 defines the amplitude of the initial electric field, $\omega = 2\pi v$ is the angular frequency, $k = 2\pi/\lambda$ is the wave number and ε is called the dielectric constant. The Eq. 2.4 characterizes the phase of the optical wave with respect to a reference point ($z = 0$); thus, kz describes the relative phase shift with respect to the reference point. The speed, v of an optical wave (light) is described by the propagation of waves in a medium. This propagation is characterized by two velocities: phase velocity which describes the travel of phase front and group velocity which describes the travel of wave packet. The ratio of the two speeds c and v is called the refractive index, n, of the medium. In other words, n = c/v. Therefore, n can be viewed as the resistance offered by the medium towards the propagation of light. The higher the refractive index the lower the speed. In summary, the classical-type wave energy can be imagined as an analogue-type and as a continuous quantity such as a water flow whereas the quantized wave energy can be imagined as the digital-type (an integer and no decimals) with defined discrete units or a package like grapes. The properties of an ordinary light can be briefly summarized as follows:

1. Photons are polychromatic, i.e., they have different colors due to different atomic optical transitions
2. Photons are multi-wavelengths
3. Photons are emitted randomly in all directions as unpolarized light
4. Photons are incoherent, i.e., they are out of phase and travel in different directions, Fig. 2.3. This aspect is similar to people walking everyday in the street in different directions. By some chance, a few people could be walking in the same direction with some lagging (i.e., out of phase) in their steps.

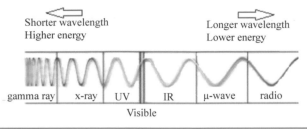

Type of radiation	Wavelength	Frequency (Hz)	Quantum energy (eV)
Radio waves	100 km	3×10^3	1.2×10^{-11}
Microwaves	300 mm	10^9	4×10^{-6}
Infrared	0.3 mm	10^{12}	4×10^{-3}
Visible	$0.7\ \mu m$	4.3×10^{14}	1.8
Ultraviolet	$0.4\ \mu m$	7.5×10^{14}	3.1
X rays	$0.03\ \mu m$	10^{16}	40
γ rays	0.1 nm	3×10^{18}	1.2×10^4
	1.0 pm	3×10^{20}	1.2×10^6

Figure 2.2. Electromagnetic spectrum.

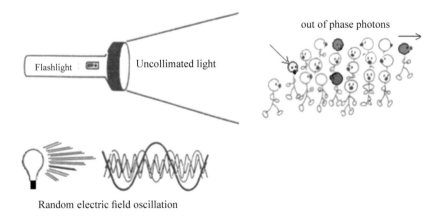

Figure 2.3. Schematic illustration of fluctuating electric field of incoherent photons emitted from a flash light as an ordinary source.

2.2 Properties of chaotic light

As was discussed in the previous sections, according to Newton's law of motion, if the forces between particles and their initial positions and velocities are known then one can predict the future of the particles' motion. On the other hand, such exactness at the microscopic level is prohibited by Heisenberg's principle of uncertainty in favour of knowing either the position or velocity of the particle. A term which has not been introduced so far is *Chaos* in a dynamical system, i.e., a system whose state is time-dependent and consists of some variables or dynamical equations. Chaos is a fundamental property that posses nonlinearity and a sensitive dependence on *initial conditions*, i.e., each point in a chaotic system is arbitrarily closely approximated by other points with significantly different future paths, or trajectories. Sensitivity to initial conditions is commonly known as the "*butterfly effect*", called so because of the title of a paper given by Edward Lorenz in 1972. Thus, an arbitrarily small change, or perturbation, of the current trajectory may lead to significantly different future behaviour. Because of the nonlinearity in a chaotic system it becomes very difficult to make accurate predictions about the system over a given time interval. The knowledge of these variables indeed determines the state of the system at a given time. Of course, many researchers were aware of the complex dynamics from the early 1900s. It was the prominent French mathematician, Poincaré who first noted the sensitivity to initial conditions in the dynamical systems. As he believed that small differences in the initial conditions produce very great ones, hence, the significant amount of error in the final phenomena. As a result of which a precise prediction of the phenomena's future becomes impossible.

Chaos is the phenomena of irregular variations of a system's outputs derived from models that are suitably described by a set of deterministic equations and is different from "*random*" events. Chaos is generated in accordance with the deterministic order and the chaotic dynamics refer to deterministic development with chaotic results. The present system evolves in a deterministic way and its current state depends very much in a deterministic way on the previous one, i.e., there is causal connection whereas in the case of a random system, there is no such connection. Despite the deterministic models, the future of the output is not foreseeable, since chaos is very sensitive to the initial conditions. It should be noted that chaos always has some degree of nonlinearity implying that the values of properties in the system depend on the conditions of earlier state. The term *phase space* indicates the set of all possible states of the system. If we imagine that the state of the system is a one point in phase space, then as time proceeds, the point moves in phase space. By using the dynamical equations we can determine how this points moves and hence calculate its state at an instance of time. Therefore, the entire picture of such motion from the beginning to the instant that we are interested in knowing in the phase space is called *trajectory*. Figure 2.4 tends to represent this concept by illustrating the trajectory motion of planets (points) in space (phase space).

A motion can be: (i) quasiperiodic (or integrable) or (ii) non-quasiperiodic (non-integrable). In the first case, the Fourier transformation of any coordinate consists of sharp peaks, as shown in Fig. 2.5a and in the second case; systems have a broadband, continuous component in their spectra as indicated in Fig. 2.5b. Another property of a chaotic system is the loss of information about initial conditions (Milonni et al. 1987).

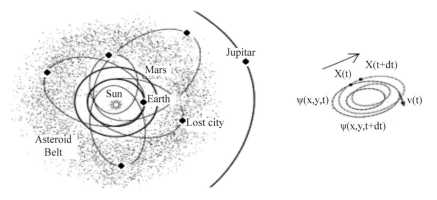

Figure 2.4. An example of trajectory path in phase space where a point has moved from x(t) to x(t+dt).

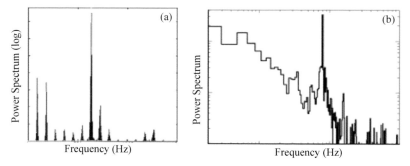

Figure 2.5. (a) Typical example of frequency spectrum of some coordinates of a quasiperiodic system and (b) a chaotic system.

If the system is chaotic, then the uncertainty of $\Delta x \Delta v$ of a given particle in phase space grows in time from high certainty with low space occupied to low certainty with high space occupied shown by say, divided space represented by the number of boxes N(t). Thus, the growth in uncertainty is (Moon 2004),

$$N(T) = N_0(t) \, e^{\lambda_i t} \qquad (2.4)$$

where λ_i is related to the concept of entropy in information theory and is called positive *Lyapunov exponent*. The fact that the Lyapunov exponent λ_i is positive means that an arbitrarily small initial difference between two points on the attractor grows exponentially to a considerable value. This sensitive dependence on the initial conditions is called *deterministic chaos* whereas a negative or zero exponent means a quasiperiodicity. Deterministic chaos happens even though these systems are deterministic, meaning that their future behaviour is completely determined by their initial conditions, with no random elements involved. In other words, the deterministic nature of these systems does not make them predictable.

There is a difference between random and chaotic motions. In the former case, we really do not know about input forces and only some statistical information is available to us. The latter case, however, is used for deterministic problems where there are no random or unpredictable parameters. By definition, chaotic is a term which is used to indicate the class of motions in a deterministic physical and mathematical system whose time history has a strong dependence on initial conditions. The ways by which a system can make the transition from regular, quasiperiodic behaviour to chaotic are called *routes*, for example; fluids, lasers, and semiconductor devices. It is important to distinguish between two types of light sources: (i) conventional light source where the different atoms are excited and emitted independently of one another and with characteristics mentioned for ordinary light in §2.1. This type of light source is chaotic and has a similar statistical description, (ii) The second type is laser which has different statistical properties. Chaos can be observed in various fields including engineering, physics, chemistry, biology and economics. Nonlinear systems can be observed in optics, optical materials and optical devices such as laser. For example the areas, which have benefited from *chaotic* phenomena are: turbulence such as weather (Fig. 2.6a), pattern of a peacock feather (Fig. 2.6b), snail's shell (Fig. 2.6c) and many others including a rising column of smoke, eddy currents behind a boat or aircraft wing, traffic forecasting, and economic models, etc.

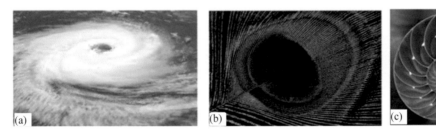

Figure 2.6. Examples of chaotic phenomena: (a) weather turbulence, (b) peacock feather and (c) snail's shell.

2.3 A brief review of Fourier analysis

When a number of harmonic waves of the same frequency even with different amplitudes and phases are added together, the result is a harmonic wave of the given frequency again. However, if the added or superposed waves are also different in frequency, then the result will be anharmonic and may possess an arbitrary shape. An infinite number of such shapes can be made in this way. The inverse process of decomposition of a given waveform into its harmonic components is called *Fourier analysis* which is readily done by the *theorem of Dirichlet*. Let us suppose that f(t) is a bounded function of period T with a finite number of maxima and minima or discontinuities in a period, then the Fourier series

$$f(t) = \frac{a_0}{2} \sum_{m=1}^{\infty} a_m \cos m\omega t \sum_{m=1}^{\infty} b_m \sin m\omega t \qquad (2.5)$$

converges to f(t) at all points where f(t) is continuous. In Eq. (2.5), m is an integer and $\omega = 2\pi f = 2\pi/T$, the sine and cosine terms can be interpreted as harmonic waves with amplitudes of a_m and b_m, respectively, and frequencies of $m\omega$. The magnitudes of the coefficients or amplitudes determine the contribution of each harmonic wave in producing the resultant anharmonic waveform. Now, if the Eq. 2.5 is multiplied by dt and integrated over one period T, the sine and cosine integrals vanish and we get,

$$a_0 = \frac{2}{T} \int\limits_{t_0}^{t_0+T} f(t)dt \tag{2.6}$$

multiplying the Eq. 2.5 by cos $n\omega t$, where n is any integer and integrating over a period one finds

$$a_m = \frac{2}{T} \int\limits_{t_0}^{t_0+T} f(t) \cos m\omega t \, dt \tag{2.7}$$

$$b_m = \frac{2}{T} \int\limits_{t_0}^{t_0+T} f(t) \sin m\omega t \, dt \tag{2.8}.$$

Thus, once f(t) is known, each of the coefficients a_0, a_m, b_m can be calculated, and the analysis is complete. Equation (2.5) can be expressed in a complex form as

$$f(t) = \sum_{n=-\infty}^{+\infty} c_n e^{in\omega t} \tag{2.9}$$

where

$$c_n = \int\limits_{t_0}^{t_0+T} f(t) \, e^{in\omega t} d \tag{2.10}.$$

If we wish to represent a nonperiodic function as a periodic function whose period T approaches infinity, it is done by expressing the Fourier series as *Fourier integral.* So, a single pulse which is a nonperiodic function can be thought of as periodic extending from $t = -\infty$ to $t = +\infty$.

$$f(t) = \int\limits_{-\infty}^{+\infty} g(\omega)e^{-i\omega t}d\omega \tag{2.11}$$

$$g(\omega) = \frac{1}{2\pi} \int\limits_{-\infty}^{+\infty} f(t)e^{i\omega t}dt \tag{2.12}$$

Equations (2.11) and (2.12) are known as the *Fourier-transform pair (FTP)* where (2.11) is the Fourier transform that transforms a signal or system in the time domain (TD) into frequency domain (FD) and (2.12) is the inverse FT, i.e., from FD to TD. Therefore, instead of a discrete spectrum of frequencies given by Fourier series in Eq. (2.10), we have a continuous spectrum or continuous distribution of the frequency components defined by Eq. (2.12). Now, a *power spectrum* of a TD signal is a representation of that signal in the FD. The frequency spectrum can be generated by FT of the signal, and the results are shown in terms of amplitude and phase, both plotted versus frequency. The frequency spectrum g (ω) can be calculated from Eq. (2.12).

$$g(\omega) = \frac{1}{2\pi} \int\limits_{-\infty}^{+\infty} f(t)e^{i\omega t}dt = \frac{1}{2\pi} \int\limits_{-\tau_{0/2}}^{\tau_0/2} e^{i(\omega-\omega_0)t}dt \tag{2.13}$$

Integrating the Eq. (2.15) and using the identity $e^{ix} - e^{-ix} \equiv 2i \sin x$,

$$g(\omega) = \frac{\sin[(\tau_0/2)(\omega-\omega_0)]}{\pi(\omega-\omega_0)} = \frac{\tau_0}{2\pi}\left[\frac{\sin[(\tau_0/2)(\omega-\omega_0)]}{[\tau_0/2(\omega-\omega_0)]}\right] \tag{2.14}$$

if $u = (\tau_0/2)(\omega-\omega_0)$, we have $g(\omega) = (\tau_0/2\pi)[(\sin u)/u]$,

when the sinc function $(\sin u)/u$ vanishes whenever $\sin u = 0$ except at $u = 0$, and $g(\omega) = 0$ when $\omega = \omega_0 \pm 2\pi n/\tau_0$. As ω increases or decreases from ω_0 then, $g(\omega)$ passes periodically through zero. The increase in the amplitude of u or the denominator of Eq. (2.16) gradually decreases the amplitude of harmonic variation. When the amplitude is squared, the resulting curve is the power spectrum, see the example in Fig. 2.5.

2.4 Fourier analysis and chaotic light

A comprehensive and detailed account on the quantum theory of light is given by (Loudon 1983) for those who are interested in this field. Here, we only intend to investigate the spectrum of a fluctuating light beam. Let us suppose that in an experiment a beam of light passes a fixed observation point where the time dependence of its electric field is measured. The frequency spectrum of the light at the observation point is defined by the Fourier components of the electric field,

$$E(\omega) = \frac{1}{2\pi} \int_{-\infty}^{\infty} E(t)e^{i\omega t}dt \qquad (2.15).$$

The average intensity of the light frequency ω is proportional to

$$\left|E(\omega)\right|^2 = (\frac{1}{4\pi^2}) \int_{-\infty}^{\infty} \int_{-\infty}^{\infty} E_1(t)E_2^*(t')e^{i\omega(t'-t)}dt\,dt' \qquad (2.16)$$

$$\left|E(\omega)\right|^2 = (\frac{1}{4\pi^2}) \int_{-\infty}^{\infty} \int_{-\infty}^{\infty} E_1(t)E_2^*(t+\tau)e^{i\omega\tau}dt\,d\tau \qquad (2.17)$$

$$\tau = t'-t \qquad (2.18).$$

Since, in a practical experiment the integration never goes to infinity so we replace the t integration by a large but finite time T. The first-order electric field correlation function is defined as:

$$\langle E_1(t)E_2^*(t+\tau)\rangle = \frac{1}{T}\int_T E_1(t)E_2^*(t+\tau)dt \qquad (2.19).$$

The cross-correlation function is a measure of the similarity of two waveforms as a function of a time-lag applied to one of them and contains only the frequencies that are common to both the waveforms. In other words, it describes how the value of the electric field at time t affects the probability of its various possible values at a later time $t + \tau$.

If the parameters that influence the fluctuation statistics are assumed constant that is, the statistical properties are stationary, then the average in Eq. (2.19) does not depend on the particular starting time of the period T provided the characteristic time scale of the fluctuations is much smaller than T. The time averaging in Eq. (2.19) can sample all the electric field values permitted by the statistical properties of the source and their relative probabilities. It should be noted that the experimental determination of the correlation function is possible on the right of the Eq. (2.19) but the function is determined by a statistical average over all values of the field at time t and $t + \tau$. The intensity (2.14) at frequency ω becomes

$$\left|E(\omega)\right|^2 = (\frac{T}{4\pi^2}) \int_{-\infty}^{\infty} \langle E_1(t)E_2^*(t+\tau)e^{i\omega\tau}d\tau \qquad (2.20).$$

The Eq. (2.20) provides the frequency-dependent spectrum of the light as measured by ordinary spectroscopy. The integrated intensity is:

$$\int_{-\infty}^{\infty}\left|E(\omega)\right|^2 = (T/2\pi)\langle E_1(t)E_2^*(t)\rangle \qquad (2.21).$$

The normalized spectral distribution function is defined as:

$$F(\omega) = |E(\omega)|^2 / \int\limits_{-\infty}^{\infty} |E(\omega)|^2 \, d\omega \qquad (2.22).$$

$$= (\frac{1}{2\pi}) \int\limits_{-\infty}^{\infty} \Gamma^{(1)}(\tau) e^{(i\omega t)} d\tau$$

So, the degree of first-order temporal coherence of the light is defined as:

$$\Gamma^{(1)}(\tau) = \frac{\langle E_1(t) E_2^*(t+\tau) \rangle}{\langle E_1(t) E_2(t) \rangle} \qquad (2.23).$$

The relation between the results of spectroscopic experiments (spectrum of light) and those of the time-dependent fluctuation properties of light (first-order correlation function) is given by Wiener-Khintchine theorem. But, we know from Eq. (2.19) that the correlation function depends solely on the time-lag between two field measurements, hence we can write:

$$\Gamma^{(1)}(-\tau) = \frac{\langle E_1(t) E_2^*(t-\tau) \rangle}{\langle E_1(t) E_2^*(t) \rangle} = \frac{\langle E_1(t) E_2^*(t+\tau) \rangle}{\langle E_1(t) E_2^*(t) \rangle} = \Gamma^{(1)}(\tau)^* \qquad (2.24)$$

$$F(\omega) = (\frac{1}{\pi}) \mathrm{Re} \int\limits_{-\infty}^{\infty} \Gamma^{(1)}(\tau) \, e^{(i\omega t)} dt \qquad (2.25)$$

that is, the normalized spectrum distribution function is proportional to the normalized first-order correlation function. We will use this concept in defining the complete and incomplete coherence in Chapter 3. According to Lyapunov exponents, chaos implies that there is no stable periodic cycle and clearly, spectral analysis is an essential tool in characterizing the temporal behaviour of a system. The temporal behaviour of a function f(t) is quasiperiodic if its FT consists of sharp peaks. Since quasiperodicity implies order, it follows that chaos implies non-quasiperiodic motion. Therefore, chaotic motion does not have a purely discrete Fourier spectrum but must have broadband and continuous components in its spectrum as was shown in Fig. 2.5.

2.5 Spontaneous emission

Another name for this process is natural emission where it implies the natural decay of the excited atoms from upper state (E_2) to lower or the ground level (E_1) without any external excitation. Assuming from a classical point of view that an electric dipole oscillates at frequency ω_0, if the positive charge is fixed at the center then the position of the negative charge with respect to the center is:

$$\mathbf{r} = \mathbf{r_0} \cos(\omega_0 t + \phi) = \mathrm{Re}(r_0' e^{i\omega_0 t}) \qquad (2.26)$$

where Re is the real part and $\mathbf{r_0}' = \mathbf{r_0} e^{i\phi}$. We know from Maxwell's equations that the accelerated electric charge during its oscillatory motion emits an e.m.w. with a power P_r proportional to the square of the acceleration and is given as:

$$P_r = \frac{n\mu^2 \omega_0^4}{12\pi\varepsilon_0 c_0^3} \qquad (2.27)$$

where $\mu = e \, r_0 = e |r_0'|$ is the amplitude of the electric dipole moment, e is the charge of electron, n is the refractive index of the medium surrounding the dipole, and c_0 is the velocity of light in vacuo. The average total energy of the oscillating electron is given by the sum of the kinetic and potential energies.

$$\langle E \rangle = 1/2m \left(\frac{\mu \omega_0}{e} \right)^2 \tag{2.28}$$

where m is the mass of the electron and the amount of energy loss dE in the time dt is $dE = P_r \, dt$

$$dE = -\frac{E}{\tau_c} dt \tag{2.29}$$

where the characteristic lifetime of the oscillating dipole is defined as:

$$\tau_c = -\frac{E}{P_r} = \frac{6\pi\varepsilon_0 mc_0{}^3}{ne^2\omega_0{}^2} \tag{2.30}.$$

Therefore, when a dipole radiates, both the initial amplitudes of oscillation r_0 and the electric dipole moment μ decrease in time. In the simplest case, the wave functions ψ(r,t) for an unperturbed eigenfunction of levels 1 and 2 of an atom can be written:

$$\psi_1 = A_1 e^{iE_1 t / \hbar} \tag{2.31a}$$

$$\psi_2 = A_2 e^{-iE_2 t / \hbar} \tag{2.31b}.$$

Now let us suppose that the atom now decays from state 2 to state 1, so ψ(r,t) during the transition can be written as:

$$\psi(r,t) = z_1(t)\, \psi_1 + z_2(t)\, \psi_2 \tag{2.32}$$

where z_1 and z_2 are time-dependent complex numbers. It is known from quantum mechanics that the coefficients $|z_1|^2$ and $|z_2|^2$ represent the probability of finding the atom in either state 1 or 2 at a given time and

$$|z_1|^2 + |z_2|^2 = 1, \tag{2.33}$$

and the electric dipole moment is:

$$\mu = \int re |\psi|^2 \, dV \tag{2.34}$$

substituting (2.34) in (2.36) we get:

$$\mu_{21} = \mathrm{Re}\,[(e^{i\omega_0 t})2z_1 z^*_2 \mu_{21}] \tag{2.35}$$

where * stands for the complex conjugate and $\omega_0 = (E_2 - E_1)/\hbar$. The relation (2.35) shows that an oscillating dipole moment which emits radiation with power p_r is the cause of spontaneous emission. The rate of change per unit time of $|z_2|^2$ is obtained from the energy balance

$$-P_r = \hbar\omega_0 = \frac{d|z_2|^2}{dt} \tag{2.36}$$

P_r can be obtained from Eq. (2.24) and

$$\frac{d|z_2|^2}{dt} = -\frac{1}{\tau_s}\,(1 - |z_2|^2)|z_2|^2 \tag{2.37}$$

where τ_s is called the spontaneous emission lifetime of state 2.

$$\tau_s = \frac{3\pi\hbar\varepsilon_0 c_0{}^3}{\omega_0{}^3 n |\mu|^2} \tag{2.38}$$

The solution for the Eq. (2.37) is

$$|z_2|^2 = \frac{1}{2}\left[1 - \tanh\left(\frac{t-t_0}{2\tau_s}\right)\right] \tag{2.39}$$

where t_0 can be found from the initial condition. Note that as soon as the atomic collision occurs, the wavefunctions will no longer have the same phase with respect to the incident e.m.w. Thus, after each collision the initial conditions and the relative phase between atoms will be subject to change and the incident e.m.w. suffers a random jump. The dependence on the initial condition is a main feature of chaotic behaviour and the $|z_2(t)|^2$ can be approximated by an exponential law as $|z_2(t)|^2 = z_2(0)|^2 e^{-(t/\tau_s)}$.

Keywords: Corpuscule, Complementarity principle, Wave-particle duality, Chaos, Phase change, Trajectory, Lyapunov exponent, Fourier analysis, Spontaneous emission.

References

Lorenz, E.N. 1972. Predictability: does the flap of a butterfly's wings in Brazil set off a tornado in Texas?. Proc. 139th Annual Meeting of the American Association for the Advancement of Science 139: 195–204.

Milonni, P., M. Shih and J. Ackerhaly. 1987. Chaos in Laser-Matter Interaction. World Scientific Press, Singapore.

Moon, F. 2004. Chaotic Vibrations. Wiley Intersciennce, New York.

3

Laser Basics

3.1 Introduction

The history of laser goes back to early 1917 when Einstein first predicted a new radiative process known as stimulated emission. However, his theoretical work largely remained unattended and unexploited until Townes and Schawlow in 1958 employed the idea and developed a **M**icrowave **A**mplifier based on the concept of the **S**timulated **E**mission of **R**adiation using ammonia gas as the medium. This device was called MASER. Shortly after that they were able to shift the excitation spectrum into the visible region and the first solid state laser (Ruby) at 964.3 nm was invented by Maiman in 1960. It was shortly after this discovery that Javan in 1961 was able to invent the first gas (He-Ne) laser operating at two wavelengths of infrared (IR) at 1.15 μm and visible at 632.8 nm. Lasers were able to establish their scientific and technological position, and importance followed by the discovery of other types of lasers. Undoubtedly, with the invention of optical fibers and semiconductor optoelectronic devices as two major technological advancements, laser as a unique source of intense and coherent light has revolutionized optics and today it is an inevitable part of the scientific, industrial, medical and military world.

3.2 Quantum theory of radiation

According to Einstein's theory, the interactive process of radiation with matter takes place in three distinct steps characterized by the so-called *Einstein's coefficients*: spontaneous emission (A_{21}), stimulated absorption (B_{12}) and stimulated emission (B_{210}), where the indices represent the direction of the transition of the atom, i.e., from level 1 to 2 or vice versa. The importance of the quantum theory of radiation and the operation of the laser lies in the meaning of these coefficients. The processes are illustrated in Fig. 3.1, where for the sake of simplicity we have assumed a two-level system.

Basically, the energy of the emitted photon during natural decay is given by the difference between the higher (E_2) and the lower (E_1) energy levels ($\Delta E = E_2 - E_1$). This energy determines the wavelength of light, which in fact is its color. When many atoms in a medium undergo spontaneous (natural) orbital decay, the process is known as spontaneous emission defined by A_{21}, Fig. 3.1a. If, however, we imagine that the atoms are initially at the ground state and are required to be excited in such a way so as to achieve a coherent output, it is done via stimulated absorption defined by B_{12}, Fig. 3.2b. Following the atomic transition, it leads to the corresponding emission of coherent photons defined by B_{21}, Fig. 3.1c. Unlike the atoms emitting radiation by spontaneous emission transitions, which occur randomly in time, atoms undergoing stimulated emission radiate their quanta of energy in phase with the stimulating radiation. This means that if an atom is stimulated to emit light energy by a propagating wave, the additional quantum of energy liberated in the process adds to that wave on a constructive basis, increasing its amplitude.

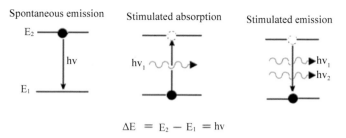

Figure 3.1. Energy-state-transition diagram differentiating between stimulated absorption, spontaneous emission, and stimulated emission. A black dot indicates the state of the atom before and after the transition takes place. In the stimulated emission process, energy is added to the stimulating wave during the transition; in the absorption process, energy is extracted from the wave.

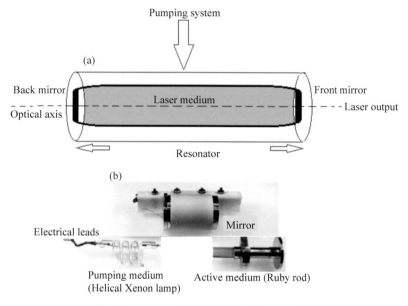

Figure 3.2. Basic arrangement of a typical laser.

Einstein Relations

It was shown by Einstein that the rates of the above processes are related mathematically. The reciprocal of A_{12} is the time for the $(2 \rightarrow 1)$ transition to occur and therefore, the spontaneous lifetime of the state is given by

$$(\tau_{12} = 1/A_{12}) \tag{3.1}.$$

If there are N_1 atoms in the collection with energy E_1, the number of atoms per second that undergo spontaneous emission (i.e., rate of transition) is proportional to the population at any time (Fig. 3.1a).

$$\left(\frac{dN_2}{dt}\right)_{sp} = -A_{21}N_2 \tag{3.2}$$

so,

$$N_2(t) = N_{20}e^{-iA_{21}t} \tag{3.3}$$

where N_{20} is the initial number of atoms in level 2.

Similarly, the rate at which N_1 atoms are raised from energy level E_1 to E_2 (Fig. 3.1b) is given by:

$$\left(\frac{dN_1}{dt}\right)_{abs} = -B_{12}N_1\rho(\upsilon) \qquad (3.4).$$

The photon density is expressed as a function of frequency by $\rho(\upsilon)$ (joule–sec/m^3), and the constant of proportionality, B_{12}, is the Einstein coefficient of stimulated absorption.
For the stimulated emission we have,

$$\left(\frac{dN_2}{dt}\right)_{ste} = -B_{21}N_2\rho(\upsilon) \qquad (3.5)$$

where B_{21} is the Einstein coefficient of stimulated emission. It turns out that the coefficients B_{12} and B_{21} are closely related and are equal under the conditions of *non-degeneracy* of the quantum states that correspond to energy levels E_1 and E_2. Degeneracy levels are those in which two or more states have the same energy. Assuming that the radiation field $\rho(\upsilon)$ has the spectral distribution characteristics of a blackbody at temperature T and that the atom population densities N_1 and N_2 at energy levels E_1 and E_2, respectively, are distributed according to the Boltzmann distribution at that temperature then,

$$\frac{dN_2}{dt} = 0 = -A_{21}N_2 - B_{21}N_2\rho(\upsilon) - B_{12}N_1\rho(\upsilon) \qquad (3.6)$$

$$\rho(\upsilon) = \frac{8\pi h\upsilon^3}{c^3}\frac{1}{e^{h\upsilon/k_BT}-1} \qquad (3.7)$$

where k_B is the Boltzmann constant and for the Boltzmann distribution of atoms between the two energy levels,

$$\frac{N_2}{N_1} = e^{-(E_2-E_1)/k_BT} = e^{-h\upsilon/k_BT} \qquad (3.8)$$

$$\frac{A_{21}N_2}{B_{21}N_2\rho(\upsilon)} = \frac{8\pi h\upsilon^3}{c^3} \qquad (3.9)$$

substituting (3.6) we get

$$R = \frac{A_{21}}{B_{21}} = e^{h\upsilon/k_BT} - 1 \qquad (3.10).$$

Thus, if the conditions of thermal equilibrium are assumed, $B_{12} = B_{21}$, the relation (3.9) states that the ratio of the probability of spontaneous emission to the probability of stimulated emission for a given pair of energy levels is proportional to the cube of the frequency of the transition radiation. This cubic dependency on v accounts for the principal difficulty in achieving laser action at x-ray wavelengths, where v is of the order of 10^{16} Hz. At this frequency, spontaneous emission occurs so rapidly for a high-energy transition that light amplification by the stimulated emission process is not easily achieved. Fortunately, this is not a great problem for most lasers at visible wavelengths.

3.3 Structure and principles

Figure 3.2 illustrates the three main components of any laser device which include:

 i) the gain (or active) medium
 ii) the pumping source, and
 iii) the optical resonator.

The active medium consists of a collection of atoms, molecules, or ions (in solid, liquid, or gaseous forms), which acts as an amplifier for light waves. For amplification, the medium has to be kept in a state of population inversion, i.e., in a state in which the number of atoms in the upper energy level is greater than the number of atoms in the lower energy level. The pumping mechanism enables obtaining such a state of population inversion between a pair of energy levels of the atomic system. When the active medium is placed inside an optical resonator the system acts as an oscillator. An optical resonator is the distance between the front and back mirrors of the laser. As such, it is analogous to the electrical positive feedback oscillators where a certain amount of the output is fed back in phase with the input, resulting in oscillation at some frequency characteristic of the circuit. In effect, the oscillator selects a frequency component from the noise always present from biasing, amplifies it, and oscillates at that frequency. The laser does essentially the same thing except that an optical oscillator can operate in many allowed modes (natural resonator frequencies).

Active (or gain) medium

The type of active medium infact represents the type of corresponding laser and the various types of lasers are mainly classed as:

(1) Solid, (2) Liquid Dye, (3) Gas (atomic, ion and molecular), (4) Semiconductor and (5) Free electron

Pumping mechanisms

1. Electrical: mainly used for gas and solid state lasers
2. Optical: solid state and dye lasers
3. Chemical: some molecular lasers

Resonator configurations

1. Plane-Parallel (or Fabry-Perot)
2. Concentric (or spherical)
3. Confocal
4. Combined Plane and Spherical

Note that all the above resonators are examples of two spherical mirrors of different radii of curvature, i.e., positive or negative separated by a defined distance. These resonators are generally divided into two broad categories of *stable* and *unstable* resonators. In the former case, the ray remains bounded whereas in the latter case, it will bounce back and forth between the two mirrors, and hence diverge indefinitely away from the optical resonator axis. The optical resonator, because of its geometrical configuration, provides for a highly unidirectional output and at the same time, through the feedback process, for sufficient stimulated radiation in the laser to ensure that most transitions are stimulated. The phenomenon of stimulated emission, in turn, produces a highly monochromatic, highly coherent output. The combined action of the resonator and stimulated emission produces an extremely bright light source even for lasers of relatively low power output. When a plane wave with an intensity corresponding to a photon flux F is propagating along z-direction within the gain medium, as shown in Fig. 3.2, an elemental change of F due to both absorption and stimulated emission is given by:

$$dF = \sigma_t F (N_2 - N_1) \, dz \qquad (3.11)$$

where σ_t is called the transition cross-section. According to Eq. (3.11), there can be different conditions.

i) If, $N_2 < N_1$, which is a thermal condition, the gain medium acts an absorber,
ii) If, however, $N_2 > N_1$ (i.e., dF/F > 0) which is a non-equilibrium condition, then it acts as an amplifier.

The former case is described by:

$$\frac{N_2}{N_1} = e^{\left[-\frac{E_2 - E_1}{k_B T} \right]} \qquad (3.12).$$

The latter case is referred to as the *population inversion* process. All laser action begins with the establishment of a population inversion by the excitation process. Photons traveling through the active medium can stimulate excited atoms or molecules to undergo radiative transitions when the photons pass near the atoms or molecules. This factor in itself is unimportant except that the stimulated and stimulating photons are in phase, travel in the same direction, and have the same polarization. This phenomenon provides for the possibility of gain or amplification. Only those photons traveling nearly parallel to the axis of the resonator will pass through a substantial portion of the active medium. A percentage of these photons will be fed back (reflected) into the active region, thus ensuring a large buildup of stimulated radiation, which is much more than the spontaneous radiation at the same frequency. Lasing will continue as long as the population inversion is maintained above a certain threshold level.

It is, however, important to realize that in order for a laser to lase, a certain threshold condition which is known as *critical inversion* must be reached. According to Eq. (3.11), the gain per pass in the active medium (i.e., the ratio of output to input photon flux) is given by the term $\exp[\sigma_t(N_2-N_1)l] = 1$, where l is the length of the medium. If only the losses due to transmission are present inside the resonator, then the critical inversion is shown to be:

$$N_2-N_1 = \frac{\ln(R_1R_2)}{2\sigma_t l} \tag{3.13}$$

where R_1 and R_2 are respectively, the percentage of light reflected from the mirror surface. But the first problem that we will encounter is the fact that we are not able to achieve a lasing action for a 2-level system at the condition of thermal equilibrium. This is so, because under this condition, $B_{12} = B_{21}$ so, the population inversion is not possible, in other words when $N_2 = N_1$ and we wish to obtain $N_2 > N_1$, the maximum percentage of atoms that can be excited is 50% and thereafter the decay will prevent further pumping. For this reason the lasers are based on 3-level and 4-level systems where now it is possible to obtain stable, self-sustained lasing action, though the action of population inversion in the latter case is easier than the former.

Assuming, that a laser has now reached an operational condition, one last point which remains to be noted is that of the *laser modes*. These are the discrete frequency components covering a large spectral range which refers to the way light wavelengths oscillate and propagate inside the laser cavity to replicate themselves after two reflections in order and the electric fields are added in phase. The two main allowed modes are:

i) Longitudinal (axial) where the modes are formed by plane waves traveling exactly along the laser axis joining the centers of the cavity mirrors. The allowed modes of the cavity Þ are those where the mirror separation distance L is equal to an exact multiple of half the wavelength, λ shown in Fig. 3.3.

$$L = Þ\, \lambda/2 \tag{3.14}$$

If for example, L = 0.3 m and λ = 600 nm (red), then Þ is about 1×10^6 and the therefore, $\Delta v = 500$ MHz.

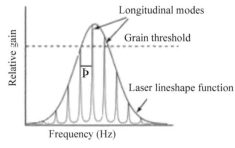

Figure 3.3. The lineshape function of longitudinal cavity modes.

ii) Transverse modes are modes where the direction of the oscillations is perpendicular to the cavity optical axis. These modes are normally known as Transverse Electro Magnetic or TEMqr modes. The integer q gives the number of minima as the beam is scanned horizontally and r the number of minima as it is scanned vertically. Hence, TEM$_{00}$ (Gaussian mode) implies uniphase mode, since all parts of the propagating wavefront are in phase, consequently it represents the greatest spectral purity, and degree of coherence.

3.4 Properties of laser light

Laser light is characterized by a number of key optical properties, most of which play an important role in the interaction with various materials. The major optical properties are:

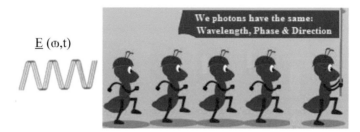

$\underline{E}(\omega, t)$

We photons have the same: Wavelength, Phase & Direction

Figure 3.4. An illustration of coherent beam where the waves are in perfect phase and incoherent beam where waves become out of phase.

(a) Monochromaticity, (b) Coherence, (c) Directionality, (d) High intensity and (e) Brightness. The cartoon sketch in Fig. 3.4 tends to summarize these properties under one flag.

Monochromaticity

The term implies a 'single color'. However, light from sources other than lasers covers a range of frequencies. True single-frequency operation of a gas laser can be achieved by careful design. Although it is more difficult, such a laser can be constructed to have frequency stability at constant temperature better than one part in 10^{10}. Multimode operation of course reduces the monochromaticity of laser. A small helium-neon laser generally has three or four longitudinal modes excited with a spacing of a few hundred megahertz, depending on the cavity length. This still gives a bandwidth of a few parts in 10^{6}. Solid state lasers tend to have rather larger frequency spreads.

Coherence

This is a measure of the degree of phase correlation that exists in the radiation field of a laser at different locations and times; that is, when the stimulated wave is in phase with the stimulating wave, the spatial and temporal variation of the electric field of the two waves is the same. Figure 3.5 illustrates that two points P_1 and P_2 with corresponding electric fields E_1 and E_2 at time $t = 0$ lie on the same wavefront. The phase difference is, $\Delta\phi = 0$ at $t = 0$. If this condition remains the same for $t > 0$, it is said to have a perfect coherence. If, however, $\Delta\phi > 0$ for $t > 0$, then it begins to deviate from perfect coherency which is called *partial coherence* until it reaches its maximum value of $\Delta\phi = 1$, i.e., maximum out of phase. Thus in a 'perfect' laser one expects the electric field to vary with time in an identical fashion for every point on the beam cross section. Such a beam would have perfect *spatial* coherence. Another related property is the *temporal* coherence, where we consider the electric field E of the wave at a given point P at two different times of t and $t + \tau_d$. If, for a given time delay τ_d, the phase difference between two field values remains constant for any time t, it is said there is temporal coherence over time τ_d. If the phase changes uniformly

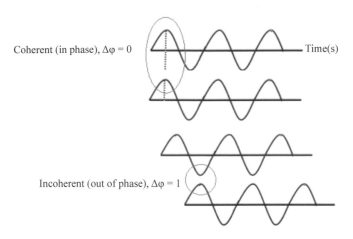

Coherent (in phase), $\Delta\varphi = 0$ — Time(s)

Incoherent (out of phase), $\Delta\varphi = 1$

Figure 3.5. An illustration showing a laser photons properties.

with time then the beam is said to show perfect temporal coherence which is a measure of the degree of monochromaticity of light.

Two useful quantities that are related to temporal coherence are the coherence time, t_c and the coherence distance, ℓ_c. An approximate expression for the distance traveled by a light ray before it loses coherence, known as the coherence distance, is given by:

$$\ell_c = c/\delta v$$
$$= \lambda^2/\delta\lambda \tag{3.15}$$

where λ is the wavelength, $\delta\lambda$ and δv are the spread in wavelength and frequency respectively. The coherence time of a laser may then be defined as the time taken for the wave trains to travel a coherence distance before they become out of phase or incoherent. In other words, is a measure of the average time interval over which one can continue to predict the correct phase of the laser beam at a given point in space. Thus,

$$t_c = \ell_c/c \tag{3.16}$$

where c is the velocity of light. It can be shown that t_c is related to the line width of the emission (Δv) via the equations,

$$t_c = \frac{1}{\Delta v}$$

and

$$\delta\lambda = \frac{\lambda^2}{\ell_c} \tag{3.17}$$

The relation (3.17) is infact a statement of the Heisenberg principle of uncertainty in quantum mechanics which was discussed in § 1.4.2 where a wave pulse is used to represent, an electron. The line width of spectral sources can be measured and the average coherence times and coherence distance can be approximately calculated. For example, a white light covers roughly between 400–700 nm, so it has a line width of around 300 nm and taking the average wavelength at 550 nm, using Eq. (3.15) we obtain:

$$\delta\lambda = \frac{550^2}{300} \approx 1000 \text{ nm} \approx 2\lambda_a$$

which is a very small value for coherency indeed, about 1 mm. If the source is replace by a green line of mercury at 546 nm with a line width of 0.025 nm, it would give $\ell_c \approx 1.2$ cm and similarly, for a single mode He-Ne laser at 632 nm stabilized to 1 MHz, gives $\ell_c \approx 300$ m. The coherence lengths of some typical lasers are given in Table 3.1.

Table 3.1. Summary of coherence distance of some common lasers.

Laser	Typical coherence length (m)
He-Ne single transverse, single longitudinal mode	Up to 1000
He-Ne multimode	0.1 to 0.2
Argon multimode	0.02
Nd:YAG	10^{-2}
Nd:glass	2×10^{-4}
GaAs	1×10^{-3}
Ruby	10^{-2}

Divergence

The amazing degree of directionality of a laser beam is due to the design of the laser cavity, and the monochromatic and coherent nature of the stimulated emission of light. This is a very useful feature for a number of applications since it means that it is very easy to collect the emitted radiation and focus it onto a small area using a fairly simple lens system. By contrast conventional sources emit radiation nearly isotropically over a solid angle of 4π sr, and only a small fraction of it can be collected and focused. However, even in the case of a laser, the beam will after traveling a definite distance suffer from divergence and reduction of parallelism. This is not because of some fault in the laser design but is due to the diffraction caused by the wave nature of light. This is schematically shown in Fig. 3.6 where a monochromatic beam of light of 'infinite' extent passes through a circular aperture of diameter D. The light beam is perfectly collimated for a short distance known as the near field. However, the beam will now diverge or spread in the far field by an amount dependent on the size of D. The beam-spread angle φ is given by the relationship:

$$\varphi = \frac{1.27\lambda}{D} \tag{3.18}.$$

Therefore, for a He-Ne laser at 632 nm with a beam waist of diameter 0.5 mm, it yields a value of $\varphi = 1.6 \times 10^{-3}$ radians (or 1.6 mrad).

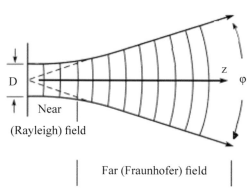

Figure 3.6. Beam divergence from a circular aperture.

High intensity

This is perhaps the property for which lasers are best known outside the field of optics. Although the optical power output from a small He-Ne laser may only be say 2 mW, a beam diameter of 0.5 mm leads to a power density of about 1 W cm^{-2}. Such a beam can readily be focused by a simple lens to a spot of 0.05 mm diameter because it is monochromatic and coherent. The incident power density is then 100 Wcm^{-2}. A high-power carbon dioxide laser can be obtained which is able to deliver a substantial fraction of 1 kWcm^{-2} without focusing. Focusing optics produces a beam of sufficient intensity to melt, cut or weld structural materials. Plasma and ablation require incident power densities in excess of 10 MWcm^{-2}. Such high-power densities are impossible to attain by conventional light sources. Pulsed lasers which incorporate a Q switch, routinely produce beams of these intensities and for higher periods of a few tens of nanoseconds. The limiting factor is not the power that is available from commercial lasers, but rather the threshold for damage in the irradiated sample. Indeed, many pulsed lasers are too powerful and must be used at reduced power if the lasers are to be used appropriately for material processing and modification.

Brightness

Brightness is defined as the power emitted per unit area per unit solid angle (the SI units of brightness are thus Wm^{-2}sr^{-1}). Sometimes the term specific brightness is used and this is the brightness per unit wavelength range. The divergence of a laser beam is generally very small when compared to the more conventional sources. Thus, although similar amounts of optical power may be involved, the small solid angle into which the laser beam is emitted ensures a correspondingly high brightness. High brightness is essential for the delivery of high power per unit area to a target. In this context the size of the spot to which the beam can be focused is also important. It is interesting, from a safety point of view, to note that the sun has a brightness of 1.5×10^5 lumens/cm^2-sterad. The average spectral brightness of the sun is its luminance divided by its bandwidth which is about 300 nm. Thus, the average brightness is $\dfrac{1.5 \times 10^5}{300 \text{ nm}} \approx 500$ lumens/cm^2-st-nm. On the other hand 1 mW He-Ne laser with 0.2 nm bandwidth gives a brightness of $\dfrac{2 \times 10^7}{0.2 \text{ nm}} \approx 10^8$ lumens/cm^2-st-nm. Therefore, one must consider the safety issues such as using suitable goggles during laser operation.

3.5 Line broadening mechanisms

It is known that the line broadening processes in the source can cause the electric field and intensity of the beam to fluctuate about their mean values on a time-scale inversely proportional to the frequency band of the light. The temporal variance and the frequency spread represent the identical physical properties of the radiating atoms which constitute the light source. Thus, fluctuations of light sources can be better understood by applying the broadening mechanisms. But what exactly is meant by line broadening? In many situations such as in cases with optical or electrical devices, the output is represented by a signal which is displaced in terms of frequency or wavelength. Ideally, the output is desired to be a single line without a width indicating the system's high gain. However, in the real world, this is not possible as there are many factors causing some deviation from having a sharp line output and hence, there is some degree of spread. The width of the line shape is called frequency bandwidth. A typical example of line shape is shown in Fig. 3.7.

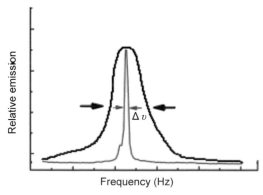

Figure 3.7. The emission curve for transition between E2 and E1. The exact form of the line shape depends on the spectral broadening mechanisms.

The precise shape of the curve is given by the line shape function, which represents the frequency distribution of the radiation in a given spectral line. There are two types of broadenings: (i) Homogeneous, where the line shape of the individual atom and hence the whole system is broadened in similar way (e.g., collision and spontaneous broadening in gas or solid state lasers), (ii) Inhomogeneous where the resonance frequencies of the atoms are distributed giving a broadened line for the system as a whole without broadening the line of each atom (e.g., Doppler broadening in gas lasers).

As far as the fluctuation of light is concerned, collision broadening is the most dominant mechanism. Imagine that a wave train of e.m.w. is steadily emanating from the atom until it collides with the other atoms. During the collision, the energy levels of the radiating atom are shifted by the interaction forces between the two colliding atoms. This physically implies an interruption in the radiating wave train. Once the wave of frequency ω_0 returns to its position after the collision, it will have the same identical parameters except that the phase of the wave is now changed. If the duration of collision is sufficiently short then it is possible to ignore any secondary effects such as radiation emitted during the collision while the frequency is shifted from ω_0. The spread in the emitted frequencies is mainly due to fact that the waves are interrupted and divided in finite sections whose Fourier decomposition includes frequencies other than ω_0. The field amplitude of the wave train emitted by a single atom can be written as:

$$E(t) = E_0 e^{-i\omega_0 t + i\phi(t)} \tag{3.19}.$$

The frequency ω_0 and the amplitude E_0 are the same for any period. If there are a large number of such atoms, the total electric field amplitude is:

$$E(t) = E_1(t) + E_2(t) + \dots E_n(t) \tag{3.20a}$$

$$E(t) = E_0 e^{-i\omega_0 t B(t)} e^{i\varphi(t)} \tag{3.20b}$$

where φ indicates the sum of ϕ_1, ϕ_2,.... ϕ_n each with different random variations, the amplitude B and phase $\varphi(t)$ are different at different instants of time. The Fourier decomposition of the modulated wave contains some information related to the frequencies spread about ω_0, which is controlled by the collision-broadened lineshape. The average of beam intensity in free space is:

$$\langle I \rangle (t) = \frac{1}{2}\varepsilon_0 c |E(t)|^2 = \frac{1}{2}\varepsilon_0 c E_0^2 B(t)^2 \tag{3.21}.$$

The intensity (t) contains the time-dependence resulting from the random amplitude modulation B (t).

3.6 Origin of chaotic properties of laser light

The fundamental concepts of chaos were covered in §2.4 and an area where they are strongly relevant is the field of the laser light properties. Chaos is always related to nonlinearity and the presence of nonlinearity in a system implies the dependence of the measured values on the initial conditions. One such optical system is the laser where it is characterized by variables like the electromagnetic field, polarization of matter and population inversion. The fields of laser physics and chaos theory were developed independently by Haken in 1975, when he discovered an analogy between the Lorenz equations of fluid convection and the Maxwell-Bloch equations used for the light-matter interaction modelling. The nonlinear interaction between wave propagation in the laser cavity and radiative recombination producing macroscopic polarization produced similar dynamical instabilities as those found in the Lorenz equations. The early experimental results of laser chaos were obtained in a CO_2 laser by Arecchi et al. (1982) and Midavaine et al. (1985). Lorenz-Haken chaos in a free-running laser was later achieved in an 81.5 μm-NH_3 laser by Weiss and others (Weiss et al. 1988), in which low pressure and long wavelength combined to reduce the secondary laser threshold. Areechi and Meucci (2008) investigated the laser system using the characteristic relaxation times of the above variables and divided the lasers into three distinct categories:

a) Class A: $\gamma_\perp \approx \gamma_{\text{II}} \gg k$, e.g., He-Ne, Ar, Kr, Dye lasers,
b) Class B: $\gamma_\perp \approx \gamma_{\text{II}} \geq k$, e.g., Ruby, Nd:YAG, most Diode lasers,
c) Class C: $\gamma_\perp \approx \gamma_{\text{II}} \approx k$, e.g., Far IR lasers,

where $\gamma_\perp$ and γ_{II} are the dissipation rates for the polarization and population inversion respectively, and $k = n\pi/L$ is the cavity loss mode, n is an integer and L is the distance between mirrors. Classes A and B can exhibit chaotic dynamics when one or more modes or degrees of freedom are introduced to the laser. Class B lasers such as solid state and CO_2 lasers are characterized by the rate equations for field and population inversion and are readily destabilized by an extra mode acting as an external perturbation. Class C are the only lasers, which have rate equations with three variables and show chaotic dynamics. Multimode lasers can easily become chaotic when they posses at least three modes and they are coupled by nonlinearities.

Understanding the importance of instabilities and the statistical properties of chaotic light has practical applications in accurate predictions of the emitted irradiance of the laser, in characterizing and detecting chaos in optical systems, and in laser light interaction with materials. As was discussed, the emission of a laser is affected by chaos due to feedback in the system. Feedback originates from the reflections in the optical cavity of the laser and is amplified through multiple reflections and emissions. This feedback becomes chaotic as it leaves the optical cavity and enters the external cavity of the laser where a time delay takes place. Hence, the intensity of the emitted beam may be modelled by the chaotic properties of the external feedback. Therefore, the chaos theory should be applied when considering the laser's intensity over a given time. However, a parameter which should be taken into account during this time interval is stability. A system is considered to be stable when a condition converges toward a single point within a set range. On the other hand, a system becomes unstable when conditions diverge from a fixed point and depart from this range. Furthermore, when the system diverges and splits, i.e., the locations where this occurs are known as *bifurcation* points and a more complicated situation is created. As the system progresses with time it exponentially develops more bifurcation points. These points are related to the chaotic behaviour of two synchronized laser systems. It is not our intention to go through every working mathematical detail, but just outlining some of the main steps may hopefully will lead to an understanding of how a change in a laser parameter such as current can lead to chaotic output behaviour due to inherent fluctuation or perturbation in the complex amplitude.

Stability of the intensity system

Let us consider a semiconductor laser, for example, a diode laser, which is one of the major types of lasers in clinical use. The basic operation of the laser may be described by the following coupled differential equations, which relate the complex amplitude and carrier density (N) as functions of time given by:

$$\frac{dE}{dt} = -\alpha_i E + k[(N-1) - i\alpha N]\, E \tag{3.22}$$

$$\frac{dN}{dt} = J - \gamma N - 2k(N-1)|E|^2 \tag{3.23}$$

where,

E	:	Electric field envelop	$-\gamma N$	:	Loss of carriers
N	:	Carrier density	J	:	Pumping (current)
$-i\alpha^* E$	:	Loss	$k[(N-1)]E$	:	Gain from stimulated emission
$-i\alpha N$	:	Change of refractive index (carrier density dependent)	$-2k(N-1)|E|^2$	:	Consumption of carriers from stimulated emission.

This set of equations which characterizes the behaviour of the semiconductor lasers is called a *Complex Amplitude System*. A steady point is obtained when,

$$\frac{dE}{dt} = 0, \quad \frac{dN}{dt} = 0 \tag{3.24}$$

The Eq. (3.22) can be transformed into a differential equation for intensity (I) by using the relation,

$$I = |E|^2 = E^*E$$

$$\frac{dI}{dt} = \frac{d(E^*E)}{dt}$$

$$= E^* \frac{dE}{dt} + E \frac{dE^*}{dt}$$

$$= E^*E\{-\alpha_i - \alpha_i + k\,[(N-1) - i\alpha N] + k\,[(N-1) + i\alpha N]\}$$

$$= 2I\,[-\alpha_i + k(N-1)] \tag{3.25}$$

Since Eq. (3.22) contains the intensity term, there is no need for manipulation. Hence, the Intensity System is:

$$\frac{dI}{dt} = 2I\,[-\alpha_i + k\,(N-1)] \tag{3.26}$$

$$\frac{dN}{dt} = J - \gamma N - 2k\,(N-1)I \tag{3.27}$$

Physically, the fixed point of interest is when the laser is emitting a coherent beam of light. In this case, the complex amplitude may be said to be coherent with respect to time and for a fixed point this condition further implies the same form of Eq. (3.24). In solving (3.24), (3.26) has the form:

$$\alpha_i I = k\,(N-1)I \Rightarrow I = 0, \ N = \frac{\alpha_i}{k} + 1 \tag{3.28}$$

The solution on the left-hand side represents the condition when the laser is "off", which is our interest. For an "on" fixed point, we use the second solution on the right-hand side and use in the zero solution of Eq. (3.27) and after some manipulation we get:

$$J = \gamma N - 2k\,(N-1)I$$

$$\Rightarrow I = \frac{1}{2}\left(\frac{J - \gamma}{\alpha_i} - \frac{\gamma}{k}\right) \tag{3.29}$$

In summary, the fixed point, i.e., "on" is defined by:

$$-(I_0, N_o) = \left(\frac{1}{2}\left(\frac{J-\gamma}{\alpha_i} - \frac{\gamma}{k}\right), \frac{\alpha_i}{k} + 1\right) \tag{3.30}$$

A set of numerical values towards which a system tends to evolve for a wide variety of starting conditions of the system is termed *Attractor*. Since, a fixed point may be defined as a point that possesses attractors about an orbit, it follows that small deviations from this point will be stable if they return to the fixed point. It is these deviations which are considered to be perturbations in the system of differential equations. To test the stability of this fixed point, a linearization can be performed with perturbation variables χ and η on I_0 and N_0, respectively. So that,

$I_0 \rightarrow I_0 + \chi$, $N_0 \rightarrow N_0 + \eta$, $\ni \chi$, $\eta \ll 1$, $\chi \in \mathbb{C}$, $\eta \in \mathbb{R}$, where $\mathbb{C}$ and $\mathbb{R}$ are complex and real number sets, respectively. Substituting these new values of I_0 and N_0 into the *Intensity System* and performing linearization after some simplifications gives:

$$\frac{d\chi}{dt} = [2(k\,(N_0-1) - \alpha_i)]\,\chi + (2I_0 k)\,\eta \tag{3.31}$$

$$\frac{d\eta}{dt} = (1-N_0)\,\chi - (\gamma + I_0)\,\eta \tag{3.32}$$

The Eqs. (3.31) and (3.32) represent a linear system of differential equations, which can be expressed in matrix form,

$$\frac{d}{dt}\begin{pmatrix} \chi \\ \eta \end{pmatrix} = \begin{pmatrix} w & x \\ y & z \end{pmatrix}\begin{pmatrix} \chi \\ \eta \end{pmatrix} \tag{3.33}$$

where, $w = 2[-\alpha_i + k(N_0-1)]$ and $x = 2I_0 k$, $y = 1$, and $z = -\gamma - I_0$.

The solution to this exponential growth equation as a perturbed system is in the form of matrix **A**;

$$\begin{pmatrix} \chi \\ \eta \end{pmatrix}(t) = \mathbf{C}e^{\mathbf{A}t} \tag{3.34}$$

where C is a 2×1 matrix, A is a square matrix with two linearly independent eigenvalues, $[\lambda_1, \lambda_2] \in \mathbf{P}$ and $e^{\mathbf{A}t}$ is the invertible matrix exponential, which plays a key role in solving linear differential equations and is defined as:

$$e^A = \sum_{n=1}^{\infty} \frac{A^n}{n!} = \frac{1}{1!}A + \frac{1}{2!}A^2 + \frac{1}{3!}A^3 + \dots \frac{1}{(n-1)!}A^{n-1} = \mathbf{PDP^{-1}} \tag{3.35}$$

where D is a diagonal matrix with elements e^{λ_i}. When the real parts of the eigenvalues of A are less than zero, then the "on" fixed point for the Intensity System will be stable. To find these eigenvalues, we set $\det(\mathbf{A} - \lambda\mathbf{I}) = 0$ which yields,

$$\lambda = \frac{-(\gamma + I_0) \pm \sqrt{(\gamma + I_0)^2 + 8\,[I_0(1-N_0)]}}{2} \tag{3.36}$$

The critical points occur; $I_0 = 0$ and $N_0 = 1$. By applying these conditions to Eq. (3.30), it is revealed that the Intensity System will be stable as long as the current $(J) < \gamma\left(\dfrac{\alpha_i}{k} + 1\right)$ and $\dfrac{\alpha_i}{k} > 0$.

Stability of the complex amplitude system

In order to develop a relationship between the electric field and the carrier density, the stability of the complex amplitude should be established. Since the complex amplitude is exponential, therefore, the solution for the phase must be negative in order to be stable. The complex amplitude equation is,

$$E_0 = A_0\,e^{-i\alpha N_0 t} \tag{3.37}$$

where A_0 is the amplitude and $-\alpha N_0 t$ is the phase.

$$A_0 = \sqrt{I_0} = \sqrt{\frac{1}{2}\left(\frac{J-\gamma}{\alpha_i}\frac{\gamma}{k}\right)} \tag{3.38}$$

Similar to the preceding work, the perturbation variables e and n are defined for the complex amplitude and carrier density, respectively.

$E_0 \rightarrow E_0 + e$, $N_0 \rightarrow N_0 + n$, $\ni e, n \ll 1$, $e \in \mathbb{C}, n \in \mathbb{R}$, hence, the perturbed complex amplitude is

$$\left|E_0 + e\right|^2 = (E_0 + e)(E_0{}^* + e^*) \tag{3.39}$$

In order to solve the eigenvalues for the Eq. (3.39), first a 3×3 matrix is formed, then by substituting and simplifying, three linear equations are obtained. The matrix is dependent upon e, e* and n:

$$\frac{d}{dt}\begin{pmatrix} e \\ e^* \\ n \end{pmatrix} = \begin{pmatrix} -ki\alpha_0 N_0 & 0 & kE_0(1-i\alpha) \\ 0 & -ki\alpha N_0 & kE_0{}^*(1-i\alpha) \\ -kE_0{}^*(N_0-1) & -2kE_0(N_0-1) & -(2k|A_0|^2+\gamma) \end{pmatrix}\begin{pmatrix} e \\ e^* \\ n \end{pmatrix} \tag{3.40}$$

By substituting the values in (3.30) and (3.38), in (3.40) the values for the laser pumping current obtained. These effects can be observed by, for example, a graphical analysis using appropriate values for k, γ, α, α_i and MATLAB to solve the above eigenvalues, which are independent of time. Without going through the details, we can treat the feedback effect which is added to the original complex amplitude system's electric field in a similar manner. In this case, the reflection term (r), phase component (φ) and time delay (τ) are added. The three differential equations comprise the feedback system and perturbation parameters. It is suggested to use Laplace Transform in analysing these equations due to the presence of delay time. For those who are interested in following the subject in more detail, they can refer to Glendinning (1994), Arluke et al. (1998) and Juang et al. (2005).

Statistical properties of chaotic laser light

Without going through vigorous treatment regarding the analysis of the statistical properties of laser, some of the analysis outcomes, which may be helpful because of their practical applications in studying, characterizing and detecting chaos in optical systems, are briefly addressed. An extensive and detailed analysis can be found in Loudon (1986). For example, let us consider the quantum efficiency of a detector, η_q

$$\eta_q = \eta_q c\hbar\omega T/V \tag{3.41}$$

where c is the velocity of light, ω is the angular frequency, T is the counting time and V is the volume of the active medium. Also, let us suppose, p(t) is the probability that the light beam causes an atom in the detector to emit electrons and record a signal count on the display unit during the time interval between t and t + τ.

$$p(t) = \eta_q \langle I \rangle(t)\, dt \tag{3.42}$$

where $\langle I \rangle$ is the cycled-average intensity and it fluctuates between one period and the next for chaotic light and the measured photon-count distribution $P_m(T)$ is an average of $P_m(t,T)$ over a large number of different starting times t.

$$P_m(T) = \frac{\langle m \rangle^m}{m!} e^{-\langle m \rangle} \tag{3.43}$$

where $\langle m \rangle = \eta_q \langle I \rangle T$ is the mean number of counted photons. The size of the fluctuations in the photon count about the mean is given by the root-mean square deviation Δm of distribution.

$$(\Delta m)^2 = \langle m \rangle \tag{3.44}$$

The fluctuations, Δm, that occur for a beam of light with constant intensity are referred to as *particle fluctuations* and $\Delta m \propto \sqrt{I}$. As we know, the photon rate equations can be used to investigate the effect of the atomic absorption and emission processes on the statistical properties of an incident laser photon distribution. If the beam during the interaction with a material is attenuated and the number of atoms in ground state is higher than the number in the upper level ($N_1 > N_2$), then the beam is said to be weakened. If, however, $N_2 > N_1$, then the beam is said to be amplified. The occurrence of photon absorption and emission causes the number of photons in each mode of the radiation field in the cavity to fluctuate. According to the *ergodic theory* of statistical mechanics, which is concerned with the behaviour of a dynamical system when it is allowed to run for a long time, for the certain systems the time average of their properties is equal to the average over the entire space. In other words, time averages are equivalent to averages taken over a large number of similar systems. Each cavity in the ensemble (i.e., the supposed collection of similar systems) has a certain defined number of photons. The fraction of cavity modes that contains n photons is determined by the probability function or thermal distribution P_n,

$$P_n = \frac{\langle n \rangle^n}{(1 + \langle n \rangle)^{1+n}} \text{ for chaotic light} \tag{3.45}$$

$$P_n = \frac{\langle n \rangle^n}{n!} e^{-\langle n \rangle} \text{ for coherent light} \tag{3.46}$$

where $\langle n \rangle$ is the mean number of photons which is defined by the Planck thermal excitation function,

$$\langle n \rangle = \frac{1}{e^{\hbar \omega / k_B} - 1} \tag{3.47}$$

where $k_B = 1.38 \times 10^{-23}$ JK^{-1} is the Boltzmann constant. Figure 3.8 illustrates the probability distribution of photons for a chaotic and coherent light source, respectively.

It is helpful to characterize the distribution by its fractional moments, defined as:

$$\overline{n(n - 1(n - 2)...(n - r + 1))} = \sum_n n \ (n-1)(n-2)...(n-r+1)P_n \tag{3.48}$$

where r is a positive integer. Now, the size of the fluctuation in photon-number is characterized by the root-mean square deviation Δn of the distribution.

$$(\Delta n)^2 = \sum_n (n - \langle n \rangle)^2 \ P_n = \langle n^2 \rangle - \langle n \rangle^2 \tag{3.49}$$

The second factorial moment obtained from Eq. (3.48) yields,

$$\langle n \rangle^2 - \langle n \rangle = 2\langle n \rangle^2 \tag{3.50}$$

Hence,

$$\Delta n = \left\{ \langle n \rangle^2 + \langle n \rangle \right\}^{1/2} \tag{3.51}$$

Clearly, the magnitude of the fluctuation in n is always larger than the mean value $\langle n \rangle$. For larger $\langle n \rangle$, the Eq. (3.51) becomes:

$$\Delta n = \langle n \rangle + 1/2 \text{ and } \langle n \rangle \gg 1 \tag{3.52}.$$

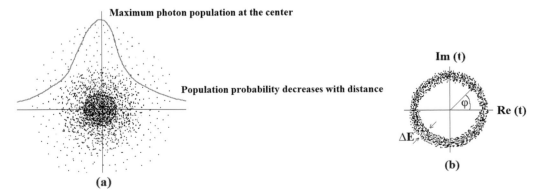

Figure 3.8. Probability distribution of photons in (a) chaotic and (b) laser source.

At larger times, the statistical properties of the light depend on the relative magnitudes of initial mean photons n_o and $\dfrac{N_2}{(N_2-N_1)}$.

When $\langle n_0 \rangle (N_2-N_1) \ll N_2$, the spontaneous emission dominates the stimulated emission and it applies to a chaotic light source. If, however, $\langle n_0 \rangle (N_2-N_1) \gg N_2$, the reverse happens, which is applied to a coherent light source. It is often convenient to divide $\langle n_0 \rangle$ into its contributing parts:

$$\langle n_0 \rangle = \langle n_c \rangle + \langle n_i \rangle \tag{3.53}$$

where $\langle n_c \rangle$ and $\langle n_i \rangle$ represent, respectively, the mean photon number in the cavity mode and the initial mean photon number when $\langle n_0 \rangle = 0$. On a longer time scale, the ratio of coherent to chaotic photon number is:

$$\frac{\langle n_c \rangle}{\langle n_i \rangle} = \frac{\langle n_0 \rangle (N_2-N_1)}{N_2} \tag{3.54}$$

and

$$(N_2-N_1)\Upsilon t \gg 1 \tag{3.55}$$

where $\Upsilon = \dfrac{2\pi c^3 \gamma_r}{\gamma'}$ is the rate of spontaneous emission into the particular cavity mode, $\gamma' = \gamma_r + \gamma_c$ is the total linewidth of atomic transition, and r and c stand for the radiative and collisional parts, respectively. It can be seen that stimulated emission by a number of atoms tends to preserve the coherent properties of the stimulating light. Thus, more coherent light is produced by stimulating coherent light and more chaotic light is produced by stimulating chaotic light. As far as the quantum theory of lasers is concerned, the number of photons in a cavity is not a determined quantity. The photon-number fluctuations are governed by three key parameters: vacuum fluctuations, spontaneous emission and pump noise. Quantum theory predicts a decrease of the photon-number fluctuations in one laser mode above the lasing threshold. In other words, as the generated field intensity increases, the photon number satisfies changes. Near the lasing threshold the emission has Bose-Einstein statistics;

$$\langle \Delta n^2 \rangle = n_0^2 + n_0 \tag{3.56}$$

and above the threshold the photons tend to Poison statistics with a variance;

$$\langle \Delta n^2 \rangle \rightarrow n_0 \tag{3.57}$$

i.e., the intensity becomes stabilized. Photon statistics distribution of the light field can be characterized quatitatively with H_2-factor introduced by Haken (1983).

$$H_2 = \frac{\langle n^2 \rangle - \langle n \rangle}{\langle n^2 \rangle} - 1 \tag{3.58}$$

It is well-known that for light from thermal sources, the distribution of photon number shows Bose-Einstein statistics, i.e.,

$$\langle n^2 \rangle = \langle n \rangle + 2 \langle n \rangle^2 \tag{3.59}$$

According to the Eq. (3.58), $H_2 = 1$ for light from a thermal source. The ideal laser light is the one which exhibits a Poisson distribution, i.e.,

$$\langle n^2 \rangle = \langle n \rangle + \langle n \rangle^2 \tag{3.60}$$

and we get $H_2 = 0$. In order to obtain the H_2-factor, one needs to determine the ensemble averages of n and n^2. A value between 0 and 1 indicates that a chaotic laser light has a light field with super-Poisson statistical distribution, in other words, between Poisson distribution and Bose-Einstein distribution. Peitgen et al. (1992), and Korsch and Jodle (1998) found that chaotic motion is ergodic, i.e., the ensemble average of any measurable quantity of the system is equivalent to its infinite-time average given by,

$$\langle x \rangle = \lim_{T \to \infty} \frac{1}{T} \int_{-T/2}^{T/2} x(t)\, dt \qquad\qquad (3.61)$$

where $\langle x \rangle$ is the ensemble average of the measurable quantity x, $x(t)$ represents the time evolution of x for sample. Therefore, one can replace the ensemble average with the average performed over a long time period, i.e., the time average. Thus, one can follow the time evolution of a sample and calculate the long time average of the photon-number and its square during the evolution, which according to Eq. (3.61), can be considered as the approximated values of the corresponding ensemble averages. Thus, a cavity which produces photons at a shorter wavelength (i.e., higher frequency) at constant energy would produce lower $\langle n \rangle$ as compared to a cavity at longer wavelength at the same energy. For example, if $\langle n \rangle = 10^{16}$ (at UV), $\langle n \rangle^2 = 10^{32}$ while for $\langle n \rangle = 10^{22}$ (at IR), $\langle n \rangle^2 = 10^{44}$.

3.7 Table of some laser systems

Some common lasers with their specifications for particular industrial and biomedical applications are listed in Tables (3.2) and (3.3).

Table 3.2. Some laser systems.

Laser type	Wavelength	Typical pulse duration
Argon ion	488/514 nm	CW
Krypton ion	531/568/647 nm	CW
He-Ne	633 nm	CW
CO_2	10.6 μs	CW or pulsed
Dye laser	450–900 nm	CW or pulsed
Diode laser	670–900 nm	CW or pulsed
Ruby	694 nm	1–250 μs
Nd:YLF	1053 nm	100 ns–250 μs
Nd:YAG	1064 nm	100 ns–250 μs
Ho:YAG	2120 nm	100 ns–250 μs
Er:YSGG	2780 nm	100 ns–250 μs
Er:YAG	2940 nm	100 ns–250 μs
Alexandrite	720–800 nm	50 ns–100 μs
XeCl	308 nm	20–300 ns
XeF	351 nm	10–20 ns
KrF	248 nm	10–20 ns
ArF	193 nm	10–20 ns
Nd:YLF	1053 nm	30–100 ps
Nd:YAG	1064 nm	30–100 ps
Free electron laser	800–6000 nm	2–10 ps
Ti:Sapphire	700–1000 nm	10 fs–100 ps

Table 3.3. Wavelengths and photon energies of selected laser systems.

Laser type	Wavelength (nm)	Photon energy (eV)
ArF	193	6.4
KrF	248	5.0
Nd:YLF (4ω)	263	4.7
XeCl	308	4.0
XeF	351	3.5
Argon ion	514	2.4
Nd:YLF (2ω)	526.5	2.4
He-Ne	633	2.0
Diode	810	1.56
Nd:YLF	1053	1.2
Nd:YAG	1064	1.2
Ho:YAG	2120	0.6
Er:YAG	2940	0.4
CO_2	10600	0.1

Keywords: Spontaneous emission, Stimulated absorption, Stimulated emission, Maser, Einstein's coefficients, Einstein relations, Degeneracy, Active medium, Resonator, Population inversion, Las modes, Monochromaticity, Coherence, Divergence, Line broadening, Chaos.

References

Arecchi, F.T., R.M. Meucci, G. Puccioni and J. Tredicce. 1982. Experimental evidence of subharmonic bifurcations, multistability, and turbulence in a Q-switched gas laser. Phys. Rev. Lett. 49: 1217–1220.

Arecchi, T.F. and R. Meucci. 2008. Chaos in lasers. Scholarpedia 3: 7066–7077.

Arluke, A., T. Bergevin and T. Cadwallader. 1998. Dynamical Systems, Chaos and Control. The University of Arizona.

Glendinning, P. 1994. Stability, Instability, and Chaos: An Introduction to the Theory of Non-Linear Differential Equations. Cambridge University Press, NY.

Haken, H. 1975. Analogies between higher instabilities in fluids and lasers. Phys. Lett. A 53: 77–78.

Haken, H. 1983. Laser Theory. Springer-Verlag, Berlin.

Javan, A., W. Bennett and D. Herriott. 1961. Population inversion and continuous optical maser oscillation in a gas discharge containing a He-Ne mixture. Phys. Rev. Lett. 6: 85–88.

Juang, C.S., Chang, N. Hu and C. Lee. 2005. Laser chaos induced by delayed feedback and external modulation. Jap. J. Appl. Phys. 44: 1–4.

Korsch, H. and H. Jodle. 1998. A Program Collection for the PC. Springer-Verlag, Berlin.

Loudon, R. 1986. The Quantum Theory of Light. Clarendon Press, Oxford.

Maiman, T.H. 1960. Optical and microwave—optical experiments in ruby. Phys. Rev. Lett. 4: 564–66.

Midavaine, T., D. Dangoisse and P. Glorieux. 1985. Observation of chaos in a frequency-modulated CO_2 laser. Phys. Rev. Lett. 55: 1989–1992.

Peitgen, H., H. Jurgens and D. Saupe. 1992. Chaos and Fractals: New Frontiers of Science. Springer-Verlag, New York.

Schawlow, A. and C.H. Townes. 1958. Infrared and optical masers. Phys. Rev. 112: 1940–1944.

Weiss, C.O., N. Abraham and U. Hubner. 1988. Homoclinic and heteroclinic chaos in a single-mode laser. Phys. Rev. Lett. 61: 1587–1590.

4

Matter

4.1 The structure and properties of matter

Let us start with the definition of a substance which is a distinct form of matter. The amount of substance, n in a sample is reported in terms of a unit called a mole where 1 mol is the amount of substance that contains as many as entities (molecules, atoms,...) as there are in exactly 12 g of carbon-12. This number is called the Avogadro constant, $N_A = 6.02 \times 10^{23}$. Thus, if a sample contains N entities, the amount of substance it contains is n = N/N_A. An extensive property is one which depends on the amount of substance in the sample such as mass and volume. An intensive property on the other hand, is independent of the amount of substance such as temperature, pressure and mass density. By studying the properties of matter, forces, energy and their various interactions, scientists can have a better understanding regarding the behaviour of solids, liquids and gases—the three main phases of matter.

4.1.1 Molecules: The building components of matter

Experimental evidence supports the idea that matter in all the three phases is composed of tiny particles called molecules which are continuously in motion. For any given single substance, the molecules are identical in mass, structure and other properties. They range in size from 10^{-10} m (0.1 nm) to about 10^{-6} m (1 μm). Molecules consists of groups of atoms, which themselves consist of electrons and nuclei. As the molecules are forced together, the electrons belonging to the various atoms that make up the molecules interact, repelling each other. This repulsion is a very short-range force, and predominates when the distance between the molecules is only about 10^{-10} m. The attraction between molecules, however, is of a longer range, and is called the van der Waals force. Its origin is complicated, but again depends on the electrical interaction between molecules. In solids and liquids, the molecules move relatively slowly (have relatively low kinetic energies) and they, therefore, interact fairly strongly. However, in the case of gases, the molecular force can often be neglected because the molecules are, on average, widely-separated and they interact relatively briefly. For this reason, a simple analysis of the behaviour of gases is much easier than that of solids and liquids. There are two principal quantum mechanical theories of molecular electronic structure: (a) *Valence-bond theory*, where the main point is the concept of the shared electronic pair and that how the theory introduces the concepts of σ and π bonds and hybridization, (b) *Molecular orbital theory*, where the concept of atomic orbital is extended to that of the molecular orbital, which is a wavefunction that spreads over all the atoms in a molecule. This theory can help us to describe the electromagnetic properties of solids, and to explain electrical conduction and semiconduction.

The energies of a diatomic molecule are so different that can produce rotations and vibrations independently. Using the Born-Openheimer first approximation, the total energy of a diatomic molecule is given by,

$$E_T = E_I + E_J + E_V + E_{e^-} \tag{4.1}$$

where E_1, E_j, E_v, E_e are respectively, the linear, rotational, vibrational and electronic energies. The rotational energy is defined as:

$$E_j = \frac{h^2}{8\pi^2 I} J(J+1) \quad \text{(Joules)} \qquad \text{where } J = 0,1,2,... \tag{4.2}$$

$$I = \frac{m_1 + m_1}{m_1 m_2} r_0^2 = \mu_r \ r_0^2 \tag{4.3}.$$

Here h is Planck's constant, I is the moment of inertia, r_0 is the equilibrium distance and μ_r is called the reduced mass of the system with m_1 and m_2 respectively. Expressing in terms of wavenumber,

$$\varepsilon_j = \frac{h^2}{8\pi^2 Ic} J(J+1) \quad (cm^{-1}) \tag{4.4}$$

$$\varepsilon_j = BJ \ (J+1)$$

where $B = \dfrac{h}{8\pi^2 Ic}$ is the rotational constant measured in (cm^{-1}) and c is the velocity of light.

4.1.2 The simple harmonic oscillator

Figure 4.1 illustrates the curve for the energy of a diatomic molecule undergoing compression and stretching motion, exhibiting a simple harmonic oscillation varying with the internuclear distance. At the minimum the internuclear distance is referred to as the equilibrium distance r_0 or the bond strength.

The compression and extension of a bond may be modelled to the behaviour of spring which obeys Hook's law.

$$F = -\kappa(r - r_0) \tag{4.5}$$

Where F is the restoring force, κ is the spring constant, and r the internuclear distance. An elastic bond, like a spring has a certain vibration frequency dependent upon the mass of the system and then force constant but independent of the amount of distortion. The oscillation frequency is given as:

$$\upsilon_0 = \frac{1}{2\pi} \sqrt{\frac{\kappa}{\mu_r}} \quad \text{Hz} \tag{4.6}.$$

In terms of spectroscopy, we must divide the relation (4.2) by the velocity of light c, obtaining

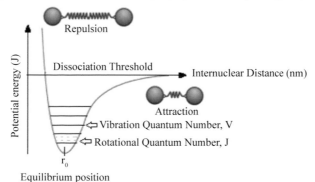

Figure 4.1. The Morse curve of a diatomic molecule indicating the potential energy change with interatomic separation between the molecules. The parabolic potential leads to harmonic oscillations and at high excitation energies it undergoes anharmonic compressions and extensions.

$$\upsilon_0 = \frac{1}{2\pi c} \sqrt{\frac{\kappa}{\mu_r}} \quad cm^{-1} \tag{4.7}.$$

Vibrational energies like all other molecular energies are quantized. For the simple harmonic oscillator we have,

$$E_v = (V + \frac{1}{2}) h\upsilon_0, \qquad (V = 0,1,2,..) \tag{4.8}$$

where V is called the vibrational quantum number. At the lowest vibrational energy, V = 0, the Eq. (4.4) becomes:

$$E_v = \frac{1}{2} h\upsilon_0 \tag{4.9}$$

which is known as the *zero point energy*. This is the basic difference between the classical and the quantum mechanical wave prediction of molecular vibration, i.e., in the former case, there is no objection for a molecule to have no vibration whereas in the latter case, it must always vibrate to some extent. Based on the Schrodinger equation and the *selective rule*, the change in vibrational quantum number for the hamonic oscillator undergoing vibrational changes, is $\Delta V = \pm 1$. The vibration energy changes will result in an observable spectrum if the vibration can interact with radiation and that vibration involves a change in the dipole moment of the molecule. Therefore, the vibrational spectra are expected to be observed only for hetronuclear diatomic molecules since homonuclear molecules have no dipole moment. However, the molecules do not exactly obey the laws of simple harmonic motion but rather exhibit a deviation which is referred to as *anharmonic oscillator.* Despite some degree of compression and stretching, the bond is considered to be elastic but at larger amplitudes the bond between atoms is stretched and at a certain limiting point the molecule dissociates into atoms.

4.1.3 Atoms: The building components of molecules

Atoms are the basic building blocks of ordinary matter with typical diameter sizes of about 0.1 to 0.5 nanometers (1 nm is one-billionth of a meter). They can join together to form molecules, which in turn form most of the objects around us. Just as substances can be broken down into molecules, molecules can themselves be broken down into atoms. Atoms in molecules are bound together in various ways, although all of these interatomic forces arise basically from interactions between electrons in the atoms. In some molecules, for example, loosely-bound atomic electrons are shared between adjacent atoms. An atom is the smallest particle that can represent a particular chemical element. There are three types of particles that can, in a simple description, be considered as making up a typical atom. The central nucleus, with a diameter of around 1×10^{-14} m, i.e., about 10,000 times smaller that of the whole atom, is comprised of neutrons and protons. (The hydrogen nucleus is unique in having no neutron, only a single proton.) The neutron is a particle with no electrical charge, whereas the proton has a single positive charge. Both have roughly the same mass. Circulating about this central region, held in orbit under the influence of the protons' positive charge, are the electrons. These are subatomic particles, each with a single negative charge and an extremely small mass: 1/1836 that of a proton.

Each chemical element is characterized—and identified—by its atomic number, Z, which is the number of protons in the nucleus. Since an electrically neutral atom must contain an equal number of protons and electrons, Z also equals the number of electrons orbiting the nucleus. The mass number A of an atom is the sum of the number of protons and neutrons in the nucleus (thus A–Z is the number of neutrons). As an example, consider the element helium, which has an atomic number (Z) of 2 and a mass number (A) of 4, written as $^4_2$He. It has two protons (and hence two electrons) and two neutrons. Electrons of an atom are attracted to the protons in an atomic nucleus by this electromagnetic force. The protons and neutrons in the nucleus are attracted to each other by a different force, the nuclear force, which is usually stronger than the electromagnetic force repelling the positively charged protons from one another.

Atomic interaction

The atoms in crystalline solids are arranged in neat and ordered structures, but the forces which hold the atoms together are different. Consider, first, the general situation of two identical atoms in their ground states being brought together from an infinite separation. The points of interest are the natures of the forces which come into play, whether these forces are attractive or repulsive and the energy of the interaction of the atoms. Initially, the energy of their interaction is zero. As the atoms approach, the attractive forces increase and the energy increases in a negative sense (the energy of attraction is negative since the atoms do the work, while that of repulsion is positive as work has to be done on atoms to bring them closer together). In ionic systems, the attractive force arises from the electrostatic charge and the repulsive force from the electron shells, which act as a sort of tough elastic sphere resisting further compression. The repulsion may be described as arising from two effects. First, the penetration of one electron shell by the other, which means that the nuclear charges are no longer completely screened and therefore, tend to repel one another. The other effect arises from the Pauli exclusion principle which states that two electrons of the same energy cannot occupy the same element of space. For them to be in the same space (overlapping). the energy of one must be increased—this is equivalent to a force of repulsion.

At a separation of a few atomic radii, repulsive forces begin to assert themselves, and the atoms reach an equilibrium separation r_0 at which the repulsive and attractive forces are equal and the mutual potential energy is a minimum. The situation is shown in Fig. 4.2. The repulsive forces have a much shorter range than the attractive forces and are partly due to the electrostatic repulsion of like charges and partly to the non-violation of the Pauli exclusion principle. As the atoms come closer together, the Pauli principle would be violated unless some of the electrons move to higher energy states; the system therefore gains energy, a situation that is equivalent to the action of an interelectron repulsive force.

In general, the total potential energy can be written as:

$$E(r) = -E_{att} + E_{rep} \tag{4.10}$$

where E_{att} can be written as a small index power law,

$$E_{att} = \frac{-A}{r^n} \tag{4.11}$$

and E_{rep} as a high index power law or an exponential,

$$E_{rep} = B/r^m \qquad \text{or} \qquad B \exp\left(\frac{-r}{\Re}\right) \tag{4.12}.$$

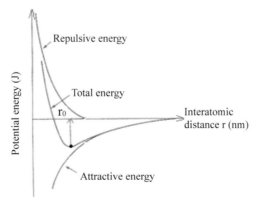

Figure 4.2. Potential energy curves for two atoms/molecules as a function of separation. There is a long-range attractive and a short range repulsive force which operates only when the molecules approach too close together.

Substituting (4.11) and (4.12) in (4.10) we get:

$$E(r) = -A/r^n + Be^{-r/\Re} \qquad\qquad (4.13)$$

where $\Re$ is a characteristic length that governs the rate at which the repulsive energy falls with distance. The values of the constants, A and B, the indices n and m and $\Re$ are governed by the actual nature of the bonding between the atoms, which is related to the charge distributions in the atoms making up the solid. However, in all cases, the interaction provides the cohesive energy that brings the atoms of the solid together, which can be thought of as the difference between the atomic energy in the crystal and the energy of the free atoms.

4.1.4 The nature of the electron

As was discussed in Chapter 1, the electrons are considered as point electric charges but sometimes, they appear to behave like hard spheres (for example, in collisions with other particles) whereas in other respects—such as electron diffraction—they behave as if they were waves. This wave-particles' duality of electrons was recognized in de Broglie's relationship ($\lambda = h/mv$), which assigns a wavelength to any particle of known mass and velocity. According to the theory of wave mechanics, electrons orbiting a nucleus are not particles moving in orbits, but standing waves that can be represented mathematically by what is called a wave function (which measures the probability of an electron being at a particular point in space). Peak values of this function can be taken to represent the orbits of the electrons. There is only a high probability—not a certainty—that the electrons will be found on the orbits; the certainty of the old theory has been replaced by a statistical probability measured by the wave function.

According to Heisenberg's uncertainty principle ($\Delta x \Delta p \geq h$), which arises from wave-particle duality, it is impossible to measure simultaneously both the position and momentum of a particle within certain limits. It can also be shown that it is similarly impossible to measure the total energy and lifetime of a particle ($\Delta E \Delta T \geq h$) simultaneously and with limitless accuracy. Although, the seemingly totally accurate and certain theories of classical physics have been replaced by the probability arguments and uncertainties of the quantum theory, it turns out that concepts such as Heisenberg's uncertainty principle predict new, hitherto unexpected phenomena. Finally, electrons play a major role in determining the properties of the various elements. At the turn of the century, physicists spent much effort in trying to derive all the observed phenomena related to the elements from a mathematical model of the atom. One key phenomenon was the production of spectral lines by atoms on being heated: each element has its own unique atomic spectrum. In trying to explain the generation and appearance of atomic spectra, physicists found that they had to introduce one of the basic concepts of modern physics: the quantum.

4.2 Mesoscopic forces

The fundamental forces that drive the interactions between the various forms of matter are electrostatics, gravity and magnetism. However, there are other subtle natural forces that in combination with geometric and dynamic effects determine the interactions of biological molecules. These include: cohesive forces (van der Waals), hydrogen bonding, electrostatics, steric forces, fluctuation forces, depletion forces and hydrodynamic interactions.

4.2.1 van der Waals forces (Cohesive forces)

As it was seen in Fig. 4.1, the van der Waals forces include attraction and repulsion between atoms, molecules, and surfaces, as well as other intermolecular forces (Pauli exclusion principle, electrostatic interaction, polarization and London dispersion). They are different from covalent and ionic bonding in that they are caused by correlations in the fluctuating polarizations of the nearby particles. In the limit of close-approach, the spheres are sufficiently large as compared to the distance between them; i.e., $r \ll R_1$ or R_2. The van der Waals force (F_w) between two spheres of constant radii R_1 and R_2 is given by,

$$F_w = -\frac{AR_1R_2}{(R_1+R_2)\,6r^2} \qquad (4.14)$$

It is seen from the Eq. (4.14), that the van der Waals force decreases with the decreasing size of bodies (R) and the increasing intermolecular distance (r). Consequently, the van der Waals forces become dominant for collections of very small particles such as very fine-grained dry powders even though the force of attraction is smaller in magnitude than it is for larger particles of the same substance. It is well-known that van der Waals interaction is the most dominant cohesion force between matter with a relatively weak bond strength of about 1 kJmol^{-1}. The origin of this force is an attractive force that acts between two molecules due to the interaction between two dipoles. The potential $V_{12}(r)$ which gives rise to the dispersive van der Waals force between molecules 1 and 2 can be defined as:

$$V_{12}(r) = -\frac{A_{12}}{r^6} \qquad (4.15)$$

where A_{12} is the Hamaker constant whose value depends on the type of molecule considered and the distance r. The cohesive forces are sometimes called dispersion interaction, because the same parameters determine both of the optical properties of the molecules, i.e., the dispersion of light and the forces between them. The van der Waals forces are long range and can be effective at large distances (> 10 nm) down to interatomic spacing (< 0.1 nm). In molecular dynamics, the energy of interactions E(r) between biomolecules is normally shown by the Lennard-Jons potential,

$$E(r) = E_c\left[\left(\frac{r_0}{r}\right)^{12} - 2\left(\frac{r_0}{r}\right)^6\right] \qquad (4.16)$$

where E_c is the characteristic energetic constant. The attractive (negative) term corresponds to the van der Waals force for a point particle and the repulsive (positive) term is the hard sphere force. The van der Waals forces exist between all atoms and molecules, whatever other forces may also be involved. We may divide van der Waals forces into three groups: (i) Dipole–dipole forces, (ii) Dipole-induced dipole forces and (ii) Dispersion forces.

4.2.2 Hydrogen bonding

This is an important effect in a wide range of hydrogenated polar molecules and determines their different molecular shapes. Hydrogen bonds are typically stronger than van der Waals forces and have energies in the range of 10–40 kmol^{-1} but are weaker than ionic or covalent interactions by an order of magnitude. Hydrogen bonding plays a key role in molecular self-assembly processes such as micelle formation, biological membrane structure and the determination of protein conformation.

4.2.3 Electrostatics

The magnitude of the electrostatic force of interaction between two point charges q_1 and q_2 is directly proportional to the scalar multiplication of the magnitudes of the charges and is inversely proportional to the square of the distance between them. The force F is along the straight line, joining them, see Fig. 4.2. If the two charges have the same sign, the electrostatic force between them is repulsive; if they have opposite signs, the force between them is attractive.

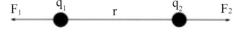

Figure 4.3. The interaction forces between two charges at a distance.

Coulomb's law can be stated as the scalar and vector forms. The magnitude of force between the charges is given by,

$$|F| = K_c \frac{|q_1 q_2|}{r^2} \tag{4.17}$$

where K_c is the coulomb's constant ($8.987 \times 10^9 \, Nm^2C^{-2}$) and the scalar r is the distance between the charges. Coulomb's law, ion-dipole and dipole-dipole interactions are needed for calculating the electrostatic interaction between biomolecules. Also, Coulomb's law for the interaction energy E_i between two point charges is given by,

$$E_i = \frac{q_1 q_2}{4\pi\varepsilon_r\varepsilon_0 r} \tag{4.18}$$

where ε_r and ε_0 are the relative dielectric permittivity and permittivity of free space, respectively. The next important electrostatic interactions experienced are those between ions and dipoles. The energy interaction E_i' between a dipole p and a point charge q is given by,

$$E_i' = -\frac{p^2 q^2}{(4\pi\varepsilon_0)3k_B T r^2} \tag{4.19}$$

where $k_B T$ is the thermal energy. Similarly, the interaction between two separate electric dipoles is:

$$E_i'' = -\frac{p_1 q_2 \Lambda}{(4\pi\varepsilon_0) r^3} \tag{4.20}$$

where Λ is constant. Ionic bonds between molecules typically have strength of the order of $\sim 500 \, kJmol^{-1}$. Electrostatic forces become even more important at larger distances for biological molecules to function correctly and provide dominant long range interaction.

4.2.4 Screened electrostatic interaction

The charges at the surface and the counter ions in the solution form a so-called electric double layer. Hence, the electrostatic repulsion is called a double-layer repulsion. An electric double layer screens the Coulombic interaction, which is important for determining the resultant electrostatic forces. These forces are easily experienced when hands are washed with soap. Adsorbing soap molecules makes the skin negatively charged and the slippery feeling is caused by the strongly repulsive double layer forces. The screening process allows a many-body problem involving two strongly charged objects immersed in an electrolyte containing large number of ions to be reduced to a simple two-body problem. The range of interaction of the double-layer repulsion is characterized by the Debye length $\mathcal{K}^{-1}$ defined as follows:

$$\mathcal{K}^{-1} = \sqrt{\left(\frac{\varepsilon_r\varepsilon_0 k_B T}{\sum_i \rho_i(\infty) e^2 z_i^2}\right)} \tag{4.21}$$

where ε_0 and ε_r are, respectively, the permittivity of free space and the relative permittivity of the dielectric in which ions are embedded, where Z_i is the valence of the charged groups on the surface, e is the electronic charge, and $\rho_i(\infty)$ is the density of counterions at infinity. As is seen from relation (4.20), the Debye length is inversely proportional to the concentration of ions in solution and a larger concentration of ions in solution reflects a small $\mathcal{K}^{-1}$ as a larger amount of ions effectively "screen" the interaction. The Debye length can be interpreted as the characteristic length over which the electrostatic potential decays with distance from the surface, as seen in Fig. 4.4. The significance of the Stern layer, shown in Fig. 4.4 is that ions in solution have a finite particle size, the decay in the potential begins where the ions are freely mobile, not perfectly at the surface of a charged material, but at a finite distance away from the surface.

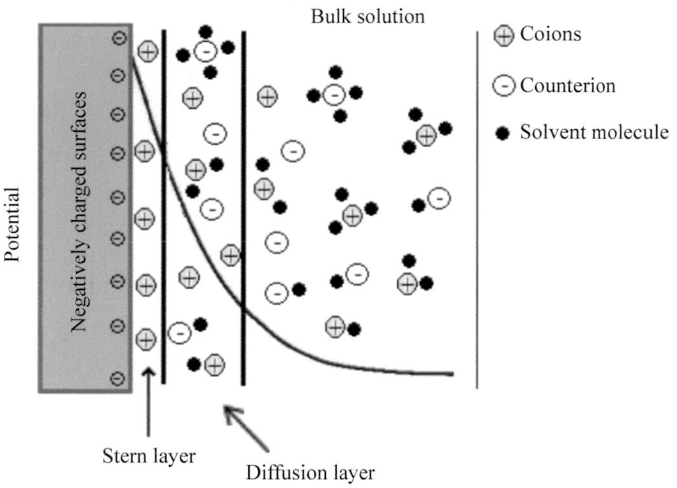

Figure 4.4. An electric double layer indicating the distribution of co-ions and counterions diffusing into bulk solution.

The charging of a surface in a liquid occurs in two ways: (i) by the dissociation of surface groups and (ii) by adsorption of ions onto the surface. The adsorption of an ion from bulk solution onto an oppositely charged surface could charge the surface positively. The chemical potential ψ_c, i.e., total free energy per molecule for the electric double layer is given as:

$$\psi_c = z_i e\, \psi_e + k_B T \log \rho_i \tag{4.22}$$

where, ψ_e is the electric potential. The first term is due to the electrostatic energy and the second is the contribution of the entropy of the counterions. Equation (4.22) expresses Poisson's equation for electrostatics, which relates ψ_e to the density of free ion concentration ρ_{fi} immersed in a dielectric at a distance x from a charged surface.

$$\varepsilon_r \varepsilon_0 \frac{d^2 \psi_e}{dx^2} = -\rho_{fi} \tag{4.23}$$

Poisson's equation for electrostatics can be combined with the Boltzmann distribution for the thermal distribution of ion energies and gives the *Poisson-Boltzmann (PB) equation*, which describes the behaviour of ψ_e in an electrolyte solution.

$$\frac{d^2 \psi_e}{dx^2} = -\frac{z_i e \rho_i}{\varepsilon_r \varepsilon_0} e^{-z_i e \psi_e / k_B T} \tag{4.24}$$

The PB equation can be solved to give the potential (ψ_e), the electric field ($E = \partial \psi / \partial x$) and the ρ_i at any point in the space between two planar surfaces. However, there are some limitations on the PB at a short separation distance, for example, in ion correlation effects, the ions are no longer point-like and the sharp boundaries between dielectrics affect the solutions of the electromagnetism equations. The pressure (P) between two charged surfaces in water can be calculated using the contact value theorem, which relates the force between two surfaces to the density of contacts at the midpoint,

$$P(r) = k_B T [\rho_i(r) - \rho_i(\infty)] \tag{4.25}$$

where $\rho_i(r)$ is the ion concentration at distance r. One biological example, where the screened electrostatic interactions play a major role and the interface pressure is determined by the ion concentration enhancement at the surfaces as they approach each other is the example of a charged membrane. Let us suppose that. two surfaces with a charge density of $0.4\ Cm^{-2}$ are placed at a distance of 2 nm and the inverse Debye screening length κ, is $1.34 \times 10^9\ m^{-1}$. Substituting the Eq. (4.21) in Eq. (4.24) for ρ_i to calculate pressure we get:

$$P(r) = k_B T \rho_{is} = 2\varepsilon_r \varepsilon_0 \left(\frac{k_B T}{z_i e}\right)^2 \kappa^2 = 1.68 \times 10^6\ Nm^{-2}, \text{ where } \rho_{is} \text{ is the charge density on the surfaces.}$$

4.2.5 The forces between charged spheres in solution: DLVO theory

A successful theory that explains the forces between colloidal particles and the aggregation of aqueous dispersions quantitatively is known as the Derjaguin, Landau, Verwey and Overbeek (DLVO) theory. The theory explains the aggregation of aqueous dispersions quantitatively and describes the force between charged surfaces interacting through a liquid medium. The potential is used to explain a situation when two particles approach one another and their ionic atmospheres begin to overlap and a repulsion force is developed. It combines the effects of the van der Waals attraction and the electrostatic repulsion or Coulombic (Entropic) forces due to the so-called double layer of counterions discussed in the preceding section. At the maximum energy barrier, repulsion is greater than attraction and the particles rebound after interparticle contact, hence, remain dispersed throughout the medium. The maximum energy needs to be greater than the thermal energy, otherwise the particles will aggregate due to the attraction potential. The height of the barrier indicates the stability of the system. If the barrier is cleared, then the net interaction is all attractive, and as a result the particles aggregate. The electrostatic part of the DLVO interaction is computed when the potential energy of an elementary charge on the surface is much smaller than the thermal energy scale, $k_B T$. However, it must be emphasized that the concept and hence, the effects of agglomeration or clustering under optical interaction irradiation, are different from the situation where high numbers of single particle dispersions exist within the medium. This can further be understood and clarified by noting that basically, the agglomeration process for colloidal particles results from the coupling between two main interactions: (1) particle-fluid interactions, which play a role in the motion of particles within a flow and govern the number of particle–particle encounters, and (2) particle–particle interactions, which control whether colliding particles will adhere (adhesion or attractive interaction) or simply bounce (repulsive interaction). The second process, as in this case, is described by the DLVO theory which defines inter-particle forces as the sum of van der Waals and double layer electrostatic contributions.

For a number of colloidal materials it has been found that the critical coagulation concentration, $\rho_i(\infty)$ varies as the inverse sixth power of the valency of the electrolyte counterions, i.e., $\rho_i(\infty) \propto z_i^{-6}$. Total DLVO interaction potential ψ_{DLVO} (r), between two spherical partic les that interact at a constant surface potential is defined as:

$$\psi_{DLVO}(r) = [(64\pi k_B T R \rho_i \psi_s^2)1/\mathcal{K}^2]\,e^{-\mathcal{K}r} - \frac{AR}{6\,r} \tag{4.26}$$

where r is the interparticle distance, A is the Hamrker constant, ψ_s is the surface potential and R is the radius of the colloid.

4.2.6 Depletion forces

A depletion force often is regarded as an entropic force and is an effective attractive force that arises between large colloidal particles that are suspended in a dilute solution of *depletants*, which are smaller solutes that are preferentially excluded from the volume between the approaching colloidal spheres (Fig. 4.5). When colloidal spheres and polymers are mixed in a solution (e.g., water), the colloides can experience an effective attractive interaction force in the absence of polymers in the space between colloidal spheres, i.e., the excluded volume. The depletion force is defined as:

$$F_d = -\Pi V_d = -\Pi\ 4/3\ \pi\ R_g^3 \tag{4.27}$$

where $\Pi = \dfrac{N}{V} kT$ is the osmotic pressure, N/V is the number density of polymer chain, kT is the thermal energy, V_d is the depleted volume, R_g is the radius of gyration of large molecules.

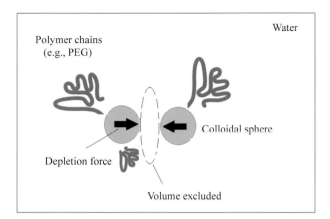

Figure 4.5. Depletion forces between two colloids in a solution of water soluble polymer chains, for example, polyethelyene glycol (PEG).

4.2.7 Steric forces

As discussed, atoms occupy a certain amount of space within a molecule and in doing so, they are brought close together and by decreasing the space between them, their wavefunctions overlap. However, overlapping due to the Pauli and Born exclusion principle will affect the molecules' conformation and reactivity. For example, interacting membranes experience a repulsive steric force due to the fluctuations of membranes structures which are called membrane forces (Fig. 4.6).

The entropic force per area (the pressure P(r)) between two surfaces is given by contact value theorem:

$$P(r) = kT[\rho(r) - \rho(\infty)] \tag{4.28}$$

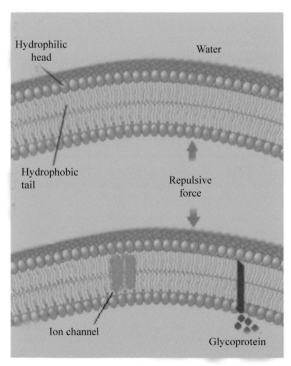

Figure 4.6. Repulsive forces occur between flexible membranes due to the thermally induced collisions.

where $\rho(r)$ and $\rho(\infty)$ are the volume densities of molecular contacts at a certain height (r) above a single membrane and infinity, respectively. The bending energy of membrane can be found using,

$$kT = \frac{2\pi x^2 B_r}{R^2} = \pi x^2 \cdot B_E \tag{4.29}$$

where $B_E = \frac{2B_r}{R^2}$ is the energy of the bending mode, R is the radius of curvature, and x is the radius of contact. Since, $x^2 \approx 2Rr$.

Then,

$$kT = \frac{4\pi r B_r}{R} \tag{4.30}$$

Now, the entropic force per unit area between two membranes can be determined using,

$$P(r) = \frac{kT}{\pi x^2 r} \approx \frac{kT}{2\pi R r^2} = \frac{(kT)^2}{B_r r^3} \tag{4.31}$$

i.e., $P(r) \propto r^3$

Other steric effects are:

a) *Shielding*: This occurs when a charged group on a molecule is apparently weakened or spatially shielded by less charged (or oppositely charged) atoms.

b) *Attraction*: This occurs when molecules have conformation or geometries that are optimized for interaction with one another.

c) *Repulsions*: These occur between different parts of a molecular system and show importance in governing the direction of transition-metal-mediated transformations and catalysis. Steric repulsion is also largely responsible for the stabilizing of colloids by coating the surface with a polymer, and can also cause bond length shortening, and compressional frequency enhancement in the IR spectrum.

4.3 Free electrons in solids

4.3.1 Introduction

If an electron is bound to an atomic orbit by electrostatic attraction, its energy tends to be limited to discrete permitted levels or bands. These energies are determined by the *state* of the electron and are normally designated by a wave function ψ. The various ψ_s correspond to the different probability distributions of the electron cloud which can occur around the nucleus. A particular energy may correspond to more than one independent ψ, which called *degeneracy*. If all the states in a set are occupied by electrons, then the completed set is known as a *closed shell* and it is very tightly bound to the nucleus. Thus, the electron bound to the nucleus of an atom can exist only in a series of states having sharply defined energies. To change this energy, the electron must make a transition from one state to another. During this process, it can emit or absorb a photon of electromagnetic radiation with a frequency proportional to the energy difference between the states defined by Eq. (1.12). The outer electrons, however, are not so strongly bound perhaps because the positive charge which attracts them to the nucleus will be reduced by the screening effect of the inner closed shells. The energy level model where it is assumed that the electrons are tightly bound to atomic nuclei can be used to explain many of the properties of materials which are electrical insulators and the outer electrons are responsible for the electrical properties of materials.

4.3.2 The energy and distribution of free electrons

In solid-state physics, the free electron model is a simple model for the behaviour of valence electrons in a crystal structure of a metallic solid. It was developed by Sommerfeld, who combined the classical Drude model with quantum mechanical Fermi–Dirac statistics and hence, it is also known as the Drude–Sommerfeld model. The free electron is successful in explaining a number of experimental phenomena, namely:

- the Wiedemann–Franz law which relates electrical conductivity and thermal conductivity
- thermal electron emission and field electron emission
- the temperature dependence of the heat capacity
- the shape of the electronic density of states
- the range of binding energy values
- electrical conductivities

We can assume that an outer atomic electron can move freely within the material. To calculate the possible states or wave function ψ and the energy E of an electron in a crystal (i.e., the box), the Schrodinger equation is suitable. The wave function of free electrons is in general described as the solution of the time independent Schrödinger equation for free electrons. A particle moving under the influence of potential energy V(x) is a free particle since the force acting on it is F = –dV(x)/dx = 0. We know from classical mechanics, that a free particle can either be at rest or be moving with constant momentum. In either case, its total energy E is constant. The 1–D time-independent Schrodinger equation is:

$$E\psi(x) = -\frac{\hbar^2}{2m}\frac{d^2\psi}{dx^2} + V(x)\,\psi(x) \tag{4.32}$$

Regardless of the value of the constant and setting V(x) = 0, the Eq. (4.32) does not lose its generality and is re-written as:

$$E\psi(x,t) = -\frac{\hbar^2}{2m}\frac{d^2\psi}{dx^2} \tag{4.33}.$$

The solutions are:

$$\psi(x,t) = \psi_0\, e^{-iEt/\hbar} \tag{4.34a}$$

and

$$\psi(x,t) = e^{i\,(kx - \omega t)}$$

$$\psi(x,t) = e^{i(kx - \omega t)} = e^{ikx}\, e^{-i\omega t} = e^{ikx}\, e^{-iEt/\hbar} \tag{4.34b}.$$

Comparing (4.29a) with (4.29b) we get:

$$\psi_0 = e^{\pm ikx} \text{ where } k = 2\pi/\lambda \text{ is wave number or } k = \frac{P}{\hbar} = \frac{\sqrt{2mE}}{\hbar} \tag{4.35}.$$

Hence, the maximum electron energy is:

$$E_{max} = \frac{\hbar^2 k^2}{2m} \tag{4.36}$$

That is, the complex exponential of (4.34b) gives the form of a free particle eigenfunction corresponding to the eigenvalue E. Since E is entirely kinetic energy ½ mv² we may write:

$$1/2\ mv^2 = \frac{\hbar^2 k^2}{2m} \tag{4.37}$$

So, the momentum is mv = ℏk.

Note that, the nodes of the real part of the oscillatory wave function are located at positions where kx – ωt = (n+1/2) π, with n = 0, + 1, + 2. The reason is that the real part of Ψ(x,t) which is cos(kx – ωt), has the value zero wherever kx – ωt = (n+1/2)π. Therefore, the nodes occur wherever x = (n+1/2)

$\pi/k + \omega t/k$ and, since these values of x increase with the increasing t, the nodes travel in the direction of the increasing x. According to the Pauli principle, the electrons in the ground state occupy all the lowest-energy states, up to some Fermi energy E_F. Since the energy is given by,

$$E(k) = \frac{\hbar^2 k^2}{2\,m} \qquad (4.38)$$

this corresponds to occupying all the states with wave vectors $|k| < k_f$, where k_f is the so-called Fermi wave vector, given by,

$$k_f = \left(\frac{3\pi^2 N_e}{V}\right)^{1/3} \qquad (4.39)$$

where N_e is the total number of electrons in the system, and V is the total volume. The Fermi energy is then:

$$E_F = \frac{\hbar^2}{2m}\left(\frac{3\pi^2 N_e}{V}\right)^{2/3} \qquad (4.40).$$

At 0 K, the first free electron will be in the lowest energy state, and the subsequent electrons will occupy the next higher states, thus if there are N electrons altogether, the N lowest energy states will be filled up to an energy E_{max}.

$$N = \frac{V(2m_e\,E_{max})^{3/2}}{3\pi^2 \hbar^3} \qquad (4.41)$$

where V is the volume of the sample and m_e is the mass of the electron. However, first we need to have some kind of idea about the average energy of these electrons. For a monovalent metal such as copper or gold, the electrons in the atom are arranged in closed shells with one extra electron on the outside. It is this one electron per atom which is the "free" electron. In one mole of material containing 6×10^{23} atoms, this will also correspond to the N free electrons. One mole of material contains 6×10^{23} atoms, which will also be N free electrons for monovalent metals. If the molar volume is about 10 mL then by substituting this in Eq. (4.41), $E_{max} \approx 10^{-18}$ J is calculated, where all N free electrons may occupy allowed states.

4.3.3 Physical significance of the amplitude $\psi(x)$

In the field of wave, the square of amplitude represents the intensity of the wave. At a position of high amplitude, the wave is more intense, i.e., more energy is localized there. The amplitude of the wave function varies from point to point within the small region in which the particle is to be found. This concept was first successfully explained by Max Born. Briefly, the square of the absolute value of the wave function is defined as:

$$|\psi(x,t)|^2 = \psi^*(x)\,\psi(x) \qquad (4.42)$$

where $\psi^*(x)$ denotes the complex conjugate that has a physical connection between the properties of the wave function $\psi(x,t)$ and the behaviour of the associated particles in terms of *probability density,* i.e., the quantity specifies the probability, per unit length of the axis, of the finding the particle near the coordinate x at time t. In short, the probability of finding the particle described by the wave function $\psi(x,t)$ in the interval dx around the point x is $|\psi(x,t)|^2$ dx. In 3-D, a wave function would be of the form $\psi(x,y,z)$ and the probability of finding the particle in the unit volume element surrounding the point xyz is:

$$P(xyz) = |\psi(xyz)|^2 \qquad (4.43).$$

The probability of finding the particle within a finite volume V is:

$$P_V = \int_V |\psi(xyz)|^2 dx\ dy\ dz \qquad (4.44).$$

The particle must always be somewhere in space, thus, the probability becomes:

$$\int_{\text{all space}} |\psi(xyz)|^2 dx \, dy \, dz = 1 \tag{4.45}.$$

The process of integrating over all possible locations to give unity is known as normalization. In the potential well with width a, i.e., x = a, the normalized wave function is found as:

$$\psi(x,t) = \sqrt{\frac{2}{a}} \sin \frac{\pi n x}{a} \tag{4.46}$$

where a is width of the potential well.

Keywords: Mesoscopic forces, van der Waal forces, Hydrogen bonding, Electrostatic, Screened electrostatic interaction, DLVO theory, Depletion forces, Steric forces, Simple harmonic motion, Zero-point energy.

References

Barrat, J. and J. Hansen. 2003. Basic Concepts for Simple and Complex Fluids. Cambridge University Press.
Israelachvili, J. 1992. Intermollecular and Surface Forces. Academic Press.
Rose, R., L. Sherard and J. Wuff. 1966. The Structure and Properties of Materials. Vol. VI. John Wiley & Sons Inc., NY.
Rosenberg, H.M. 1984. The Solid State. Second Edition. Oxford Physics Series, Clarenton Press.
Rudden, M. and J. Wilson. 1992. Elements of Solid State Physics. John Wiley & Sons Inc., NY.

Part II
Nanobiophotonics: Biophotonics and Nanotechnology

5

Fundamentals of Biology and Thermodynamics

5.1 Introductory biological concepts

Biology is a natural science concerned with the study of life and living organisms, including their structure, function, growth, evolution, and distribution. Biological surface science is broadly defined as an interdisciplinary area where properties and processes at interfaces between synthetic material and biological environments are investigated and bifunctional surfaces are fabricated. Surfaces play a vital role in biology and medicine, with most reactions occurring at surfaces and interfaces. The advancement in surface science instrumentation that has occurred in the past quarter of a century has significantly increased our ability to characterize the surface composition and molecular structure of biomaterials. Similar advancement has been shown in material science and molecular biology. The combinations of these subjects have allowed us to obtain a detailed understanding of how the surface properties of a material can control the biological reactivity of a cell interacting with that surface. Main examples include: medical implants in human body, biosensors and biochips for diagnosis, tissue engineering, bioelectronics and biomagnetics materials, and artificial photo synthesis.

Light–matter interaction, which is the basis for optically probing structure and function at cellular and tissue levels, as well for the light-activated photodynamic therapy of cancer and other diseases; benefits from a molecular understanding of cellular and tissue structures and functions. This section starts with the description of a cell, which is the basic unit of the body. It describes the various structural components of the cell and their functions. An important part of a living organism is the diversity of cells that are present in various organs to produce different functions. A microscopical structure of an animal cell is shown in Fig. 5.1.

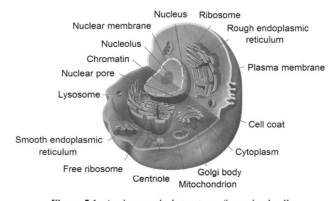

Figure 5.1. A microscopical structure of an animal cell.

Biological systems are essentially an assembly of molecules where water, amino acids, carbohydrates (sugar), fatty acids, and ions account for 75–80% of the matter in cells. The remainder of the cell mass is accounted for by macromolecules, also called polymers (or biopolymers in the present case), which include peptides/proteins (formed from sugars), DNA (deoxyribonucleic acid, formed from nucleotide bases and dioxyribose sugar), RNA (ribonucleic acid, formed from nucleotide bases and ribose sugar), and phospholipids (formed from fatty acids). These macromolecular polymers organize to form cells. The main structural components of a cell are:

5.1.1 Cell structure

Plasma membrane

This forms a semipermeable outer boundary of both prokaryotic and eukaryotic cells. This outer membrane, about 4–5 nm thick, is a continuous sheet of a doubly layer (bilayer) of long-chain molecules called phospholipids. A phospholipid molecule has a long tail of alkyl chain, which carries a charge (and is thus ionic). Phospholipid molecules spontaneously orient (or self-organize) to form a bilayer in which the hydrophobic tails are pointed inwards and embedded within the nonpolar interior of the lipid bilayer, and the hydrophilic heads, i.e., the ionic groups are pointed outwards in the exterior, and are thus in contact with the surrounding aqueous environment.

Many functions of membranes are most intimately connected to the membrane structure and its composition of (i) lipids and (ii) proteins. The former constituents are essential as a barrier function between two aqueous phases, while the latter are involved in the specific functions of the membranes, such as energy transductions, immune response, electrical insulation, protein secretion, pinocytosis, propagation of electrical impulses, controlling the transport of food, water, nutrients, and ions such as Na^+, K^+, and Ca^{2+} (through so-called ion channels) to and from the cell, as well as signals (cell signaling) necessary for proper cell function. The proteins associated with membranes may be classified into two categories of (i) peripheral and (ii) integral. Peripheral proteins are those that appear to be only weakly bound to their respective membrane and do not appear to interact with the membrane lipids, whereas the integral proteins are more strongly bound to the membrane and exhibit functionally important interactions with the membrane lipids.

Cytoplasm

Cytoplasm represents everything enclosed by the plasma membrane, with the exclusion of the nucleus. It is present in all cells where metabolic reactions occur. It consists mainly of viscous fluid medium that includes salts, lipids, vitamins, nucleotides, amino acids, RNA, and proteins which contain the protein filaments, actin microfilaments, microtubules, and intermediate filaments. These filaments function in animal and plant cells to provide structural stability and contribute to cell movement. Many of the functions for cell growth, metabolism, and replication are carried out within the cytoplasm. The cytoplasm performs the functions of energy production through metabolic reactions, biosynthetic processes, and photosynthesis in plants.

Cytoskeleton

The cytoskeleton structure, located just under the membrane, is a network of fibers composed of proteins, called protein filaments. This structure is connected to other organelles. In animal cells, it is often organized from an area near the nucleus. These arrays of protein filament perform a variety of functions:

- Establish the cell shape
- Provide mechanical strength to the cell
- Perform muscle contraction
- Control changes in cell shape and thus produce locomotion
- Facilitate intracellular transport of organelles

Nucleus

The nucleus is often called the control of the cell. It is the largest organelle in the cell, usually spherical with a diameter of 4–10 μm, and is separated from the cytoplasm by an envelope consisting of an inner and an outer membrane. All eukaryotic cells have a nucleus. The nucleus contains DNA distributed among structures called chromosomes, which determine the genetic makeup of the organism. The chromosomal DNA is packaged into chromatin fibers by association with an equal mass of histone proteins. The nucleus contains openings (100 nm) in its envelope called nuclear pores, which allow the nuclear contents to communicate with the cytosol. The inside of nucleus also contains another organelle called a nucleolus, which is a crescent-shaped structure that produces ribosomes by forming RNA and packaging it with ribosomal protein. The nucleus is the site of replication of DNA and transcription into RNA. In a eukaryotic cell, the nucleus and the ribosomes work together to synthesize proteins.

Mitochondria

Mitochondria are large organelles, globular in shape (almost like fat sausages), which are 0.5–10.5 μm wide and 3–10 μm long. They occupy about 20% of the cytoplasmic volume. They contain an outer and an inner membrane, which differ in lipid composition and in enzymatic activity. The inner membrane, which surrounds the matrix base, has many infoldings, called cristae, which provide a large surface area for attachment of enzymes involved in respiration. The matri space enclosed by the inner membrane is rich in enzymes and contains the mitochondrial DNA. Mitochondria serve as the engine of a cell. They are self-replicating energy factories that harness energy found in chemical bonds through a process known as respiration, where oxygen is consumed in the production of this energy. This energy is then stored in phosphate bonds. In plants, the counterpart of mitochondria is the chloroplast, which utilizes a different mechanism of photosynthesis to harness energy for the synthesis of high-energy phosphate bonds.

Endoplasmic reticulum

The endoplasmic reticulum consists of flattened sheets, sacs, and tubes of membranes that extend throughout the cytoplasm of eukaryotic cells and enclose a large intracellular space called lumen. It is close to the nucleus, and is the site of attachment of ribosomes. Ribosomes are small and dense structures 20 nm in diameter, and are present in great numbers in the cell.

Golgi apparatus

It consists of stacked, flattened membrane sacs or vesicles, which are like shipping and receiving departments, because they are involved in modifying, sorting, and packaging protein for secretion of delivery to other organelles, or for secretion outside of the cell. There are numerous membrane-bound vesicles (< 50 nm) around the Golgi apparatus, which are thought to carry materials between the Golgi apparatus and different compartments of the cell.

Lysosomes

There are vesicles of hydrolytic enzymes that are 0.2–0.5 μm in diameter and are single-membrane bound. They have an acidic interior and contain about 40 hydrolytic enzymes involved in intracellular digestions.

Chromatin

The material of a cell nucleus that stains with basic dyes and consists of DNA and proteins.

5.1.2 Types of cells

Cells come in many shapes and compositions. The human body is made up of over 200 different types of cells, some of which are living cells. The human body also consists of non-living matter such as hair, fingernails, and hard parts of bone and teeth, which are also made of cells. These cell variations are produced by cell differentiation. Also, different types of cells assemble together to form multicultural tissues or organisms.

Epithelial cells

Epithelial cells form sheets, called epithelia, which line the inner and outer surfaces of the body. Some of the specialized types of cells are: (i) absorptive cells, which have numerous hair-like microvilli projecting form their surface to increase the absorption area, (ii) ciliated cells, which move substances such as mucus over the epithelial sheet, (iii) secretory cells, which form exocrine glands that secrete tears, mucus, and gastric juices, (iv) endocrine glands, which secrete hormones into the blood, and (v) mucosal cells, which protect tissues from invasive microorganisms, dirt, and debris.

Blood cells

These cells are contained in blood, which in fact, is a heterogeneous fluid consisting of a number of different types of cells. These cells comprise about 45% of the blood's volume and are suspended in a blood plasma, a pale yellowish colour fluid which makes up about 55% of total blood volume. The three different types of blood cells are (i) erythrocytes (commonly known as red blood cells; often abbreviated ad RBC), (ii) leucocytes (commonly known as white blood cells), and (iii) thrombocytes (also known as platelets). Erythrocytes or red blood cells are very small cells, 7–9 μm in diameter, with a biconcave, discotic shape. They usually have no nucleus. One cubic centimeter of blood contains about 5 billion erythrocytes, with the actual number depending on a number of factors such as age, gender, and health. They contain an oxygen-binding protein called hemoglobin, and thus perform the important function of transporting O_2 and CO_2.

Muscle cells

These specialized cells form muscle tissues, such as skeletal muscles to move joints, cardiac muscles to produce heartbeat, and smooth muscle tissues found around the internal organs and large blood vessels. Muscle cells produce mechanical force by their contraction and relaxation.

Nerve cells or neurons

Neurons are cells specializing in communication. The brain and spinal cord, for example, are composed of a network of neurons that extend out from the spinal cord into the body.

Germ cells

Germ cells are haploids (cells containing one member or a copy of each pair of chromosome). The two types of germ cells specialized for sexual fusion, also called gametes, are (i) a larger, non-motile (non-moving) cell called the egg (or ovum) from a female, and (ii) a small, motile cell referred to as sperm (or spermatozoon) from a male. A sperm fuses with an egg to form a new diploid organism (containing both chromosomes). Bacteria are another example of haploid cells.

Stem cells

Another type of cell that has received considerable attention during recent years is the stem cell. Stem cells can be thought of as blank cells that have yet to become specialized (differentiated), giving them the characteristics of a particular type of cell, such as the ones described above. Stem cells thus have the ability to become any type of cell to form any type of tissue (bone, muscle, nerve, etc.). The three different types of stem cells are (i) embryonic stem cells, which come from embryos, (ii) embryonic germ cells, which come from testes, and (iii) adult stem cells, which come from bone marrow. Embryonic stem cells are classified as pluripotent because they can become any type of cell. Adult stem cells, on the other hand, are multipotent in that they are already somewhat specialized.

Molecules and energy

All living creatures are made up of cells. They exist in a wide variety of forms, from single cell in free-living organisms to those in complex biological organisms. Despite the great diversity exhibited by living systems, all biological systems, amazingly, are composed of the same types of chemical molecules and utilize similar principles in replication, metabolism, and, in higher organisms, the ability to organize at the cell levels. Even at the most elemental cellular level, microorganisms exhibit a large range of length scale, from viruses measuring 20–200 nm, to a eukaryotic cell measuring 10–100 μm. An important feature of the eukaryotic cell is its ability to differentiate and produce a variety of cells, each carrying out a specialized function. Schematic 5.1 shows the evolution of a living organism.

Without energy every molecule would be absolutely still, nothing would ever occur, and life as we know it would be impossible. Cells are packed with energy: chemical energy, potential energy, and kinetic energy. Every chemical reaction, every little movement of a molecule involves a transfer of energy. This is because organisms need a constant supply of energy to stay alive. Organisms contain a lot of energy, and by using a simple calorimeter one can get some idea how much energy is actually stored in an organism. The energy is stored in molecules making up the organism. These molecules are synthesized when energy is freely available and broken down to release energy when required. Energy is stored within an organism in two main forms: chemical energy and potential energy. In the former case, the amount of energy stored within a molecule is because of the particular bonds between the atoms of that molecule. For example, glucose contains five C-C bonds, seven C-O bonds, seven C-H bonds, and five O-H bonds, each of which contributes towards the energy content of the molecule. Most molecules in organisms are built to fulfill a particular function, for example, hemoglobin is synthesized in red blood cells to carry oxygen, or lysozyme is synthesized to act as an antibacterial agent in tears. Different molecules are used to store energy in different conditions. Macromolecules such as triglycerides and starch act as long term energy stores, while sugars such as sucrose and glucose act as short term energy storage molecules.

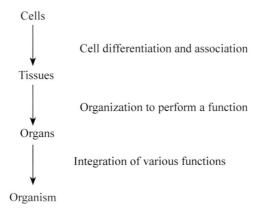

Schematic 5.1. Evolution of a living organism.

5.1.3 Chemical constituents of cells

Nucleic acids

These are biopolymers, or large biomolecules, which exist in two forms—as DNA (deoxyribonucleic acid) and RNA (ribonucleic acid), and are made from monomers known as nucleotides. Each nucleotide has three components: a 5-carbon sugar, a phosphate group (tetrahedral PO_4), and a nitrogen-containing ring, which could be either purine or pyrimidine. The four bases composing DNA are adenine (A), guanine (G), thymine (T), and cytosine (C). In the case of RNA, (T) is replaced by uracil (U). If the sugar is deoxyribose, the polymer is DNA. If the sugar is ribose, the polymer is RNA. When all three components are combined, they form a nucleic acid. Nucleotides are also known as phosphate nucleotides.

Proteins

Proteins are polymer chains made of amino acids linked together by peptide bonds.

Amino acids are biologically important organic compounds containing amine ($-NH_2$) and carboxylic acid ($-COOH$) functional groups, usually along with a side-chain known as R group specific to each amino acid. The key elements of an amino acid are carbon, hydrogen, oxygen, and nitrogen, though other elements are found in the side-chains of certain amino acids. During human digestion, proteins are broken down in the stomach to smaller polypeptide chains via hydrochloric acid and protease actions. This is crucial for the synthesis of the essential amino acids that cannot be biosynthesized by the body. Twenty different amino acids make a vast array of proteins capable of performing diverse tasks.

Properties of proteins

The native conformation of protein has a 3-D structure. *Primary structure* is the linear sequence of amino acids along the polypeptide backbone. *Secondary structure* is the folding of certain regions of the protein into helical arrays. *Tertiary structure* is the single polypeptide chain. *Quarternary structure* is the relative arrangement of polypeptide chains in higher order aggregates. *Denaturation* is a process in which proteins or nucleic acids lose the quaternary structure, tertiary structure, and secondary structure which is present in their native state, by application of some external stress or compound such as a strong acid or base, a concentrated inorganic salt, an organic solvent (e.g., alcohol or chloroform), radiation, or heat. If proteins in a living cell are denatured, this results in disruption of cell activity, and possibly cell death. Denatured proteins can exhibit a wide range of characteristics, from conformational change and loss of solubility to aggregation due to the exposure of hydrophobic groups. It should be noted that when proteins are coagulated they tend to clump into a semi-soft, solid-like substance. A chemical change has taken place because a new substance is produced.

Another important property of protein is that it does not pass through the cell membrane opening due to its large size, which normally forms colloids rather than solutions in water.

Types of proteins

Proteins are very diverse in their structure and function, and thus can be classified into various groups. Based on structure and shape, proteins can be divided into the following classes:

a) Fibrous Proteins, which are the main components of supporting and connective tissues such as skin, bone, and teeth. An example is a collagen, which is the most abundant protein in the body; it is a triple helix formed by three extended chains arranged in parallel.

b) Globular Proteins, which consist of polypeptides tightly folded into the shape of a ball. Most globular proteins are soluble in water. Examples are albumin and gamma globulins of the blood. Hemoglobin is another important proteins belonging to this class. However, it is also an example of a proteins group, often classified separately as conjugated proteins, which carry conjugated group for their function. In the case of hemoglobin, this conjugated group is a heterocyclic ring called heme, which binds and releases molecular oxygen.

Protein function

Proteins provide a wide variety of functions. Many functions involve binding with specific molecules called ligands or substrates that produce catalytic chemical reactions, as well as work as switches and machines. Some of these functions are described here.

- Enzymes, which act as catalysts for a specific biological reaction.
- Structural proteins such as collagen, which form major connective tissue and bone.
- Contractile proteins such as action and myosin, which are found in muscles and allow for stretching or contraction.
- Transport proteins like hemoglobin, which carry small molecules like oxygen through the bloodstream. Other proteins transport lipids and iron.
- Hormones, which consist of proteins and peptide molecules. These are secreted from the endocrine glands to regulate chemical processes. An example is insulin, which controls the use of glucose.
- Storage proteins, which act as reservoirs for essential chemical substances. An example is ferritin, which stores iron for making hemoglobin.
- Protective proteins, which provide protection to various cells and tissues. Antibodies are globular proteins that provide protection against a foreign protein called antigens. Others are fibrinogen and thrombin, which are involved in blood clotting. Interferons are small proteins that provide protection against viral infection.

Sugars

These are the main source of food molecules for a cell. They provide the required energy for various cellular functions. Polysaccharide is formed by the linkage of many monosaccharide units called *residues*. Polysaccharide complex forms important extracellular structures, which are covalently bound to proteins in the form of glycoproteins and to lipids in the form of glycolipids.

Lipids

Although the term *lipid* is sometimes used as a synonym for fats, fats are a subgroup of lipid called triglycerides. Lipids also encompass molecules such as fatty acids and their derivatives (e.g., phospholipids), as well as other sterol-containing metabolites, such as cholesterol. The main biological functions of lipids include storing energy, signaling, and acting as structural components of cell membranes. Lipids may be broadly defined as hydrophobic or amphiphilic small molecules; the amphiphilic nature of some lipids allows them to form structures such as vesicles, ultilamellar/unilamellar liposomes, or membranes in an aqueous environment, as discussed in §5.1.

5.1.4 Cellular processes

The functions of a highly dynamic living cell mainly include: replication,operation and communication between other cells. The processes involve both physical and chemical changes. Furthermore, the chemical changes can be permanent (such as protein synthesis, DNA replication), or cyclic (such as conversion of ATP into ADP and back). The chemical changes occurring are highly complex, often catalyzed by enzymes (reaction–specific proteins) and coenzymes (small molecules such NADH). The different dynamic processes occurring in a cell are illustrated in Schematic 5.2 (Khosroshahi and Mahmmodi 2009).

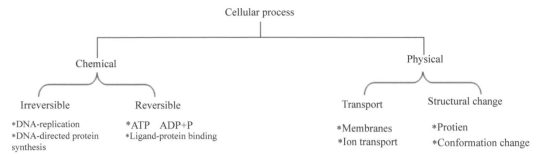

Schematic 5.2. The various dynamic processes occurring in a living cell.

Different types of cellular processes in biological system are as follows:

Cell replication

Process of producing new cells in two different ways: (a) *Mitosis* (nucleus is divided into two genetically equivalent daughter cells), and (b) *Meiosis* (a type of cell division that results in four daughter cells, each with half the number of chromosomes of the parent cell, as in the production of gametes, that reduces the number of chromosomes from diploid to haploid).

Cell biosynthesis

Process of producing cellular macromolecules: (a) *Transcription* (replication of single strand of DNA to complementary RNA), (b) *Translation* (Ribosome-mediated production of proteins from messenger RNA).

Cell energy production

This corresponds to conversion of one type of energy to another. (a) *Glycolysis* is conversion of chemical energy of carbohydrates to Adenosine triphosphate (ATP), which transports chemical energy within cells for metabolism. (b) *ATP synthesis* is the process of generating ATP from Adenosine diphosphate (ADT), either by (i) chemical bond energy (Mitochondria), or (ii) light energy (photosynthesis).

Cell signalling

This is part of a complex system of cellular communication that governs basic activities and coordinates cell actions. The ability of cells to perceive and correctly respond to their microenvironment is the basis of development, tissue repair, and immunity, as well as normal tissue haemeostasis. There are three types of signalings: (a) *Endocrine* corresponds to hormonal signaling of distant cells, (b) *Paracrine* is signaling from one cell to an adjacent cell, and (c) *Autocrine*, which is the same cell simulation signal.

Cell death

(a) *Necrosis* (i.e., the stage of dying, the act of killing) is a form of cell injury which results in the premature death of cells in living tissue by autolysis. Necrosis can be caused by factors external to the cell or tissue, such as temperature, infection, toxins, or trauma, and (b) *Apoptosis* is a programmed cell death through well-defined steps of morphological changes. There are two mechanisms by which apoptosis can occur. First, it is triggered by internal signals from within the cell, such as an internal damage to a protein in the outer membranes of the mitochondria, and the second is by external signals, sometimes known as death activators, which bind to receptors at the cell surface.

Cell transformation

This is a genetic conversion of a normal cell into a cell having cancer-like properties (i.e., oncogensis).

5.1.5 Tissue constituents

In biology, tissue is a cellular organizational level intermediate between cells and a complete organ, as seen in Schematic 5.1. A tissue is an ensemble of similar cells from the same origin that together carry out a specific function. Organs are then formed by the functional grouping together of multiple tissues. The study of tissue is known as *histology,* and in connection with disease is called *histopathology*. The functions of many types of cells within tissues are coordinated, which collectively allows an organism to perform a very diverse set of functions, such as its ability to move, metabolize, reproduce, and conduct other essential functions. The various constituents forming tissue are (Khosroshahi 2011):

Cells

They are normally organized in a defined form.

Cell-adhesion molecules (CAM)

Different membrane proteins act as glue on the cell surfaces to bind cells to each other. Adhesion between cells of the same type are known as "homophilic", and between different types as "hetrophilic". Most CAMs are uniformly distributed within plasma membranes that contact other cells. The five principal classes of CAMs are: cadherins, immunoglobulins (Ig), selection, mucins, and integrins.

Extracellular matrix (ECM)

This is a network of proteins and carbohydrate polymers in the spaces between cells. The matrix helps bind the cells and acts as a reservoir for hormones controlling cell growth and differentiation. It also provides a lattice through which cells can move. Connective tissues, which largely consist of the extracellular matrix, form the architectural framework of an organism. A diversity of tissues forms (skin, bone, spinal cord, etc.) is derived from a variation in the relative amount of the different types of matrix macromolecules, and the manner in which they organize in the extracellular matrix. Connective tissues consist of cells sparsely distributed in the extracellular matrix, which is rich in fibrous polymers such as collagen. The cells are attached to the components of the extracellular matrix. In contrast, epithelial tissues consist of cells that are tightly bound together into sheets called epithelial. The extracellular matrix consists of three major proteins: (i) highly viscous proteoglycans providing cushions for cells, (ii) insoluble collagen fibers, which provide strength and resilience, and (iii) multiadhesive matrix proteins, which are soluble and bind to receptors on the cell surface. Collagen is the single most abundant protein in all living species.

Cell junctions

Cell junctions occur at many points of cell-cell and cell-matrix contact in all tissues. There are four major classes of junctions:

- Tight junctions, which connect epithelial cells that line the intestine and prevent the passage of fluids, through the cell layers
- Gap junctions, which are distributed along the lateral surfaces of adjacent cells, and allow the cells to exchange small molecules for metabolic coupling among adjacent cells
- Cell-cell junctions which perform the primary function of holding cells into a tissue
- Cell-matrix junctions, which also perform the primary function of holding cells into a tissue.

5.1.6 Types of tissues

Epithelial tissues: Epithelial tissues form the surface of the skin and line all the cavities, tubes, and free surfaces of the body. They function as the boundaries between cells and a cavity or space. Their function is to protect the underlying tissues, as in the case of skin.

Muscle tissues

The three kinds of muscle tissues are

- Skeletal muscles, which are made of long fibers that contract to provide the locomotion force
- Smooth muscle lines of the intestines, blood vessels, etc.
- The cardiac muscle of the heart

Connective tissues

The cells of connective tissues are embedded in the extracellular materials. Examples of supporting connective tissues are cartilage and bone. Examples of binding connective tissues are tendons and ligaments. Another type are fibrous connective tissues, which are distributed throughout the body, and serve as a packing and binding material for most of the organs.

Nerve tissues

These tissues are composed primarily of nerve cells (neurons). They specialize in the conduction of nerve impulses.

Tissues provide coordinated functions of the constituent cells. The functions of the tissues, however, are not just those provided by the constituent cells, but are also derived from intercellular communications and from the extracellular matrix (ECM) components. ECM acts as a reservoir for many hormones that control cell growth and differentiation. In addition, cells can move through ECM during the early stages of differentiation. ECM also communicates with the extracellular pathways, directing a cell to carry out specific functions.

5.2 Thermodynamics basics

5.2.1 The laws of thermodynamics and controversy of disorder

All living things depend on energy for survival. Energy exists in many forms, from the energy locked up in the atoms of matter itself to the intense radiant that are emitted by the sun, and between these limits energy sources are available, such as the chemical energy of fuels and the potential energy of large water masses evaporated by the sun. Applied thermodynamics is the science of the relationship between heat, work, and the properties of systems. It is concerned with means necessary to convert heat energy from available sources, such as chemical fuels or nuclear piles into mechanical work. The laws of thermodynamics are natural hypotheses based on the observations of the world in which we live. The classical form was developed in the nineteenth century by Gibbs (1876). In his monograph on 'The Equilibrium of Heterogeneous Substances', thermodynamics was operated on with a black box and phenomenological approach, in which exchanges of matter, heat, and other forms of energy were related to macroscopic properties such as pressure, temperature, volume, etc. of the system in question. The state of a system (microstate) is determined by its properties just in so far as these properties can be investigated directly or indirectly by experiment. As Gibbs put it:

> *"So when gases of different kinds are mixed, if we ask what changes in external bodies are necessary to bring the system to its original state, we do not mean a state in which each particle shall occupy more or less exactly the same position as at some previous epoch, but only a state*

which shall be undistinguishable from the previous one in its sensible properties. It is to states of systems thus incompletely defined that the problems of thermodynamics relate".

A system, in general definition, is that portion of universe that is involved directly in a particular process. The rest of the universe is called the environment, as seen in Fig. 5.2. The system interacts with the environment across its boundary. These interactions are directly responsible for changes that occur to the state of the system. The knowledge of these interactions can be used to predict resulting changes that will occur to the system.

There are two different approaches to refer to the boundary of a system. In one case, the system is determined by a fixed mass, i.e., it is constant and includes nothing else. When this mass moves or changes its shape, so does the boundary. This is called a *closed system*, such as those studied in physics (Fig. 5.3a). A closed system is said to be isolated if no energy of any form passes across its boundaries, otherwise it is unisolated. In the other case, which is called an *open system*, as shown in Fig. 5.3b, mass and energy may enter or leave the system, i.e., there is an exchange across the boundary with the environment such as plants and animals, since they exchange materials with the environment (e.g., food, oxygen, waste products).

The state of system (macroscopic state) is determined by its *properties* just in so far as these properties can be studied directly or indirectly by experiment. The properties of a substance describe its present state without a record about the past. Therefore, when a system is considered in two different states, the difference in volume or in any other property between the two states depends merely on the states themselves, and not on the manner in which the system may pass from one state to another. There are two types of properties (i) *extensive* (extrinsic) where the properties depend on the amount of matter in the system, e.g., volume, heat , momentum, and electrical charge, (ii) *intensive* (intrinsic) where the properties are independent of the size of system, e.g., temperature, pressure, density, composition. In addition, transport properties such as viscosity, diffusivity, and thermal conductivity are intensive properties. The parameters that denote these properties are characteristics of the system in a given state. If the system changes from state A to the state B, each of these properties changes by a definite amount. Let us say the volume changes from V_A to V_B then $V_A - V_B = \Delta V$, where Δ is positive increase in the value of that parameter. In principle, the properties of the state of a system can be related mathematically and their variation is expressed by the differential and integral calculus. According to *Zeroth law*, if two systems are in thermal equilibrium with the third

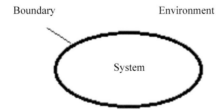

Figure 5.2. An illustration of a system with its boundary in thermal equilibrium with the surroundings.

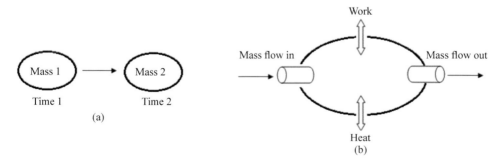

Figure 5.3. (a) A closed system where no mass or energy is exchanged through the boundary and (b) an open system where both mass and energy may enter or leave the system, i.e., there is an exchange across the boundary with the environment.

system, then they are in equilibrium with each other. All systems in such mutual thermal equilibrium are said to have the same temperature and those systems not in equilibrium have different temperatures.

The ***First law*** of thermodynamics is simply the formulization of law of conservation of energy which simply asserts that an entity 'energy' has many forms (thermal, electrical, mechanical, etc.) which are interchangeable with the conservation of its total amount. The first law of thermodynamics can be applied to processes at constant temperature, i.e., *isothermal*, at constant pressure, i.e., *isobaric* and at constant volume, i.e., *isochoric*. The first law states that:

When a system undergoes a thermodynamics cycle then the net heat supplied to the system from its surroundings is equal to the net work done by the system on the surroundings. Therefore, Gain in intrinsic energy = net heat supplied – net work done. For a non-flow process, we have

$$\Delta U = Q - W \tag{5.1}$$

where ΔU is the internal energy, Q is the amount of heat added to the system, and W is the work done by the system. Note that if work is done on the system, W will be negative and ΔU will increase. If heat leaves the system, Q is negative. Since Q and W represent energy transferred into or out of the system, ΔU changes accordingly. Also, note that the Eq. (5.1) applies to a closed system, but if we take into account the change in internal energy due to the increase or decrease in the amount of matter, then it can also be applied to an open system. For an isolated system, we have $W = Q = 0$, so $\Delta U = 0$ and when no heat is allowed to flow in or out of the system, it is said to be *adiabatic process* (i.e., $Q = 0$). Since internal energy is property then gain in internal energy in changing from state 1 to state 2 can be written as

$$U_2 - U_1 = \sum_1^2 dQ - \sum_1^2 dW \tag{5.2}$$

$$U_2 - U_1 = dQ - \int_1^2 PdV \tag{5.3}$$

$$dU = dQ - dW \tag{5.4}$$

When the system is moved from a state 1 to state 2, the Q and W depend on the particular process (or path) used. Q and W are different for different processes, even though the initial and final states of the system are the same for each process. The quantity Q-W is the same for all processes that take the system between the same two states. U is a function of the state of the system only, and does not depend on the past history. Therefore, the first law of thermodynamics is a statement by which we can define a function U, which is a property of the state of the system. For an isothermal process, we have

$$W = \int_1^2 PdV = nRT \int_{V_1}^{V_2} \frac{dV}{V} = nRT \ln \frac{V_2}{V_1} \tag{5.5}$$

and for an isobaric system, we have

$$W = P_2(V_2 - V_1) = nRT_2 \left(1 - \frac{V_1}{V_2}\right) \tag{5.6}$$

The ***second law***, which is also a natural law, deals with the question of the direction in which any chemical or physical process involving energy takes place. It is concerned with the uni-directional nature of our experiences: dropped eggs do not re-assemble, coffee cups and glasses can break simultaneously once dropped, but never go back together simultaneously, and we cannot re-fill the petrol tanks of our cars by pushing them backwards, etc. All these processes are uni-directional, and no real process is ever reversible in its entirety. To explain this lack of irreversibility, scientists in the latter half of the nineteenth century proposed a new principle known as second law of thermodynamics. This law is a statement about which processes occur in nature and which do not. One statement by Clausius (1867) is that heat flows naturally from a hot object to a cold object; heat will not flow spontaneously from a cold object to a hot object. Notice the special role of heat (thermal energy) as that form of energy available for conversion into directed mechanical work. A device which does the job is called *heat engine*. The thermal efficiency of heat engine is defined as

$$\eta_Q = \frac{W}{Q_1} \tag{5.7}$$

where Q_1 is heat supplied by the source, but

$$Q_1 - Q_2 = W \tag{5.8}$$

where Q_2 is the heat rejected, $Q_1 > W$ and rewriting Eq. (5.7)

$$\eta_Q = 1 - \frac{Q_2}{Q_1} \tag{5.9}$$

Entropy and controversy of disorder

Order is to do with everything in its proper place and behaving in its proper manner. Disorder is the opposite. Order is a well-tuned machine with all its parts moving in perfect coordination with all other parts. Thus, a machine with parts not behaving as they should implies the machine is out of order. Order does not necessarily involve movement, for instance books in library shelves do not move but they are in order by resting in their proper place. So what is entropy? Probably the most common answer you hear is that entropy is a kind of measure of disorder. Equating entropy with disorder is misleading and creates unnecessary confusion in evaluating the entropy of different systems. Historically, the concept of entropy originated around the mid-19th century, from the study of heat, temperature, work, and energy, known as thermodynamics. This was the era of the steam locomotive. The term entropy was coined in 1865 by Clausius, who thought of it as representing a kind of "internal work of transformation". It simply stated that *entropy is the relationship between the temperature of a body and its heat content*. A quantity, S known as *entropy* was postulated to measure the degree of irreversibility and was assigned to zero value for ideal processes (dS or $\Delta S = 0$). Entropy is the heat content divided by the body's temperature.

$$S = Q/T \tag{5.10}$$

In other words, the heat stored in an object at a given temperature is its entropy multiplied by its temperature. It is important to note that the definition of entropy, as originally conceived in classical thermodynamics, had nothing to do with order or disorder. It had everything to do with how much heat energy was stored in a body at a given temperature. The entropy of system is the average heat capacity of the system averaged over its absolute temperature. Based on the molecular description of heat content and temperature, Boltzmann showed that entropy must represent the total number of '*different ways the molecules*' could move. It therefore appears that a more descriptive word for the essence of entropy is '*diversity*', rather than an aimless disorganization or disorderliness. As we will see, a living system is complex and has a high degree of order as well as a high degree of entropy. More on this is discussed in §5.7. Energy measures the capability of an object or system to do work, and if entropy is used to show the measure of the disorder of a system, it really means the number of different microscopic states a system can be in, given that the system has a particular fixed composition, volume, energy, pressure, and temperature. By *microscopic states*, we mean the exact states of all the molecules making up the system. Just knowing the composition, volume, energy, pressure, and temperature does not tell us much about the exact state of each molecule making up the system as there can be billions of different microscopic states, all of which correspond to the sample having the same composition, volume, energy, pressure, and temperature. The analysis of the relationship between heat, work, and temperature for a reversibly-operating heat engine showed that S could be a property of the state of the system if it was equated, for reversible processes, to the heat absorbed reversibly divided by the temperature, i.e.,

$$dS = \frac{dQ}{T} \tag{5.11}$$

The Eq. (5.11) describes the infinitesimal increase in entropy of a system at constant temperature when infinitesimal energy is added as heat. This is NOT the same as change in entropy of a system by increasing the temperature, $\partial T/\partial S$. We can integrate Eq. (5.11) to get entropy increase due to temperature increase, i.e., $\Delta S = Q \ln (T_2 - T_1)$. This is an important result. It tells us that the difference in entropy, $S_b - S_a$, between equilibrium states of a system does not depend on how we get from one state to the other. Though dQ is not a perfect differential, the change in the entropy dS, which is given by the Eq. (5.11) is a perfect differential. The quantity $1/T$ is integrating factor for dQ. The entropy is a state variable; its value depends only on the state of the system and not on the process or the history of how it got there. This is a clear distinction to Q and W which are not state variables; their values depend on the processes undertaken. The second law then could be stated in the form of: '*In any real process, there is always an increase in entropy*'. The greater the value of the increase in entropy in a natural process occurring in a particular system, the greater the extent of its irreversibility. In other words, the system is less available for performing mechanical work and becomes more chaotic. Thus, changes in entropy measured something to do with 'character' and not simply the quantity of energy in a system. Boltzmann clearly explained the relationship between this character and the availability of directed mechanical work in terms of statistical thermodynamics—that the energy states of any system are all discrete and not continuous even for translational (i.e., linear) energy. The *character* of the energy states relates to entropy, which represents the so-called 'spread' or distribution of matter over the possible available energy states-the degree of randomness or disorderliness of the matter-energy distribution. Therefore, when entropy is loosely related to measure of disorder or randomness, it is this kind of orderliness that is being referred to: The greater the entropy, greater the number of available complexions or the number of possible microstates corresponding to a given macrostate. This is not same as the classical geometrical orderliness that normally is spoken, e.g., books in the library shelves or atoms in their crystal lattice position, etc. Entropy represents the *diversity* of internal movement of a system. The greater the diversity of movement on the molecular level, the greater the entropy of the system.

5.2.2 Entropy and direction

The importance of entropy is that it can be used to specify the direction in which a physical process will go. Consider two subsystems A and B in thermal contact with corresponding temperatures of $T_1 = 350$ K and $T_2 = 300$ K, respectively. According to Clausius's statement of the second law of thermodynamics, heat will only flow from A to B, never the other way round. This flow of heat is *irreversible*. Using Eq. (5.10), the change in the entropy of A is $\Delta S_A = -1/350$ JK^{-1} and similarly for B is $\Delta S_B = +1/300$ JK^{-1}, thus, the total change in ΔS is

$$\Delta S_A + \Delta S_B = - (1/350) + (1/300) = (1/2100) \text{ JK}^{-1}$$

The total entropy of A + B increases. If, however, 1 J of heat flowed the other way round (i.e., from B to A), the total entropy would decrease by $(1/2100)$ JK^{-1}. The latter process in never observed in the real world. Hence, the direction of heat flow is given by

$$(\Delta S_A + \Delta S_B) > 0.$$

In the limit of $T_1 = T_2$, the change would be reversible and $(\Delta S_A + \Delta S_B) = 0$ and hence, $S_A + S_B$ is maximum. As an example of an irreversible process, consider the above subsystems, A and B with an equal volume, V as shown in Fig. 5.4.

The subsystem A consists of a mole of molecules, whereas B is a vacuum. If the partition is removed, the molecules will diffuse to fill the vacuum and occupy the whole volume, as seen in Fig. 5.4c. This is an irreversible process, because once the partition is removed and distribution is done, the molecules will never return to their initial state, i.e., to fill the left hand side of the system again. In this example,

$$\Delta S = R \ln 2 \tag{5.12}$$

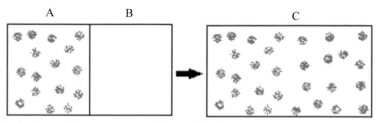

Figure 5.4. Example of an irreversible process, where if the partition is removed between the subsystems A and B, the gas expands and will fill whole space, (c). The gas molecules will never go back to subsystem A, as before, again.

The direction of the irreversible process is given by the condition that the total entropy of an isolated system increases in an irreversible process. For a system interacting with its surroundings,

$$(\Delta S_{sys} + \Delta S_{sur}) \geq 0$$

The equality sign holds for a reversible change (Adkins 1975). We can, therefore, make a general statement of second law of thermodynamics as follows:

The entropy of an isolated thermodynamic system never decreases. It either stays constant (reversible process) or increases (irreversible process).

But, since all real processes are irreversible, then we can state that:

The total entropy of any system plus of its environment increases as a result of any natural processes.

All irreversible processes arise and persist to produce entropy and will continue to do so whenever the global entropy production of the universe increases, and as long as all natural laws and constants are respected (Prigogine et al. 1972). This is true for the burning flame of a candle and of course, life itself. Entropy production is thus not incidental to the processes of life, but gives life its vitality and reason for being through the existence of entropy production. It is therefore, highly crucial to emphasize that the change of the entropy is the arrow of direction indicating the spontaneous processes in complex systems. In a biological thermodynamically *open* system, the rate of entropy production and its net flow of direction is determined by the resultant fluxes of entropy of individual constituting components of the system. The direction of entropy flow between normal (system A) and cancerous tissues (system B) is determined by thermodynamic differences between solid tumors and surrounding normal environment, i.e., normal tissue. Since cancer development is an exergonic process, it implies that heat (Q) flows from tumor (B) at higher temperature to its surrounding (A) at lower temperature, hence forcing healthy tissue to gain heat. Since always $S_B > S_A$, normal cells develop towards the entropy minimum, whereas for cancerous cells, towards entropy maximum. The rate of entropy production of cancerous cells is always greater the normal cells. As mentioned earlier, an irreversible process, as in this case and all other natural phenomena, takes place via different dissipation mechanisms driven by differences in heat production, chemical potential gradients, Gibbs energy, pH, conductance, membrane potential gradients, membrane response to the exposure of external force fields. The applied field force is very important as it can reverse the direction of the entropy-flow information between A and B.

5.3 Statistical mechanics and microstates

Statistical mechanics is a branch of physics in which statistical methods are applied to the microscopic constituents of a system in order to predict the microscopic properties. In classical statistical mechanics, each particle is regarded as occupying a point in phase space, i.e., it has a position and momentum at any particular instant. The probability that this point will occupy any small volume is given by *Maxwell-Boltzmann law*, which gives the most probable distribution of the particles in phase space.

However, in quantum statistics, the space is divided into cells each having a volume hf, where h is Planck constant, and f is the number of degree of freedom of the particles. Maxwell-Boltzmann statistics gives the average number of particles found in a given single-particle microstate, under certain assumptions

$$\frac{N_i}{N} = \frac{\exp\left(-E_i/k_B T\right)}{\sum_j \exp\left(-E_j/k_B T\right)}$$

(5.13)

where:

- i and j are indices of the single-particle microstates
- N_i is the average number of particles in the single-particle microstate *i*
- N is the total number of particles in the system
- E_i is the energy of microstate *i*
- T is the equilibrium temperature of the system
- k_B is the Boltzmann constant

The assumptions of this equation are that the particles do not interact, and they are in thermal equilibrium. The denominator in Eq. (5.13) is simply a normalizing factor so that the N_i/N add up to 1 and can be used to derive relationships between temperature and the velocity of gas particles. All that is needed is the density of microstates in energy, which is determined by dividing up momentum space into equal sized regions. The energy distribution is given

$$f_E(E)\, dE = f_p(p)\, d^3p$$

(5.14)

where d^3p is the infinitesimal phase-space volume of momenta corresponding to the energy interval dE. Making use of the spherical symmetry of the energy-momentum dispersion relation $E = |p|^2/2m$, this can be expressed in terms of dE as

$$d^3p = 4\pi|p|^2\, d|p| = 4\pi m\, \sqrt{2mE}\, dE$$

(5.15)

Substituting (5.15) in (5.14), and expressing in terms of the energy E, we get

$$f_E(E) = 2\sqrt{\frac{E}{\pi}} \left(\frac{1}{kT}\right)^{3/2} \exp\left(\frac{-E}{kT}\right)$$

(5.16)

By the equipartition theorem, this energy is evenly distributed among all three degrees of freedom, so that the energy per degree of freedom, ε is

$$f_\varepsilon(\varepsilon)\, d\varepsilon = \sqrt{\frac{1}{\pi\varepsilon kT}}\, \exp\left[\frac{-\varepsilon}{kT}\right] d\varepsilon$$

(5.17)

Statistical mechanics deals with the molecular levels and the physical laws use variables and effects such as temperature, pressure, energy, entropy, concentration, molecular motions, electrochemistry, reaction rates, and phase change that are applied at macroscopic level and related to thermodynamics. All these variables are crucial to the structure, function, operation, and integrity of cells. Needless to remind that biological systems are more complex to understand and describe than an ideal gas using macroscopic variables only. One simple example is the role of chemical potential, where both the macroscopic and molecular phenomena are strongly related. Before we continue, let us review some of the concepts that are related to thermodynamics and are useful in biology.

Equilibrium is a state obtained by a system where the variables no longer change with time, and neither energy nor matter enters or leaves the system. Usually, cells and their surroundings are almost at thermal equilibrium. So, if there are any temperature differences over a small distance between them, heat would flow from hotter to colder cells. Similarly, water can leave or enter cells quite rapidly due to the permeability of the membrane to water. We address conceptual issues related to the applicability of equilibrium concepts by using arguments about separation of time scales to determine when equilibrium ideas can be suitably used in a living biological context. In *steady state* on the other hand, despite constant condition of variables, energy or matter can enter or leave the system. Consider our own skin as an example. It loses heat via radiation and evaporation but gains it via conduction from structures such as subcutaneous tissue and blood flow. The point is that the maintenance of a steady state requires a continuous input of energy. Removing the source or sink of energy brings the living system to an equilibrium state, and it eventually dies.

5.3.1 Thermodynamics and biochemistry

To elaborate further, it would be convenient and informative to remind ourselves of the concept of energy quantization (hc/λ) discussed in chapter one. In biochemistry, the different amount of energy delivered by different wavelengths are either used for photosynthesis (useful energy), or photodissociation of molecules (dangerous energy). The living organism at surrounding temperature (i.e., room temperature) of ~ 300 K emits an IR wavelength of ~ 10 µm, corresponding to 2×10^{-20} J/photon (0.125 eV) that is ~ 10 kJ/mole of photons. The radiating temperature of the sun is ~ 6000 K, assuming most of the light is visible ~ 550 nm corresponding to 3.6×10^{-19} (2.27 eV), that is ~ 250 kJ/mole of photons. Therefore, we can see that one biological significance of energy quantization is that the quantum energy of visible or ultraviolet light is very close to quantized energy levels of electrons in atoms and molecules. The practical implication of this is its application for the activation of many chemical reactions directly similar to those in the process of photosynthesis. As for low IR energy level, it is comparable with kinetic energies of molecules due to their thermal motion, usually used for an indirect reaction activation.

A cell is normally considered a macroscopic object which contains roughly 10^{14} molecules, and we can define and measure different parameters such as temperature, the pressure inside cells, the stress in the membrane, etc. Indeed, it is the power of thermodynamics which enables us to investigate the behaviour of biological systems at a macroscopic scale without indelving in molecular details. Statistical mechanics, on the other hand, can help us by applying the laws of mechanics to understand the behaviour of a large number of atoms, molecules, and light at the macroscopic level. Hence, it links thermodynamics to quantum mechanical laws at the molecular level. The laws of thermodynamics apply to macroscopic systems, whereas the concepts of entropy and temperature have clear definitions. However, at microscopic level it may be applied to a large number of molecules in a statistical fashion but not to individual molecules or atoms. Considering the kinetic energy of a molecule to be heat, we may say that a collective organized motion of molecules can do work, whereas a random molecule can supply heat.

In chemical and biochemical processes, we need an energy that covers the reaction involved during work done on the surrounding and receiving heat from it. This is done by combining two thermodynamics quantities of *enthalpy* defined as H = U + PV, and *Gibbs free energy* defined by G = H – TS = U + PV – TS. The former is required, because in any biochemical process under normal conditions of constant pressure, the molecular volumes may change. The latter is also needed because biochemical processes occur at a constant temperature, thus the heat produced is transferred elsewhere, and the heat absorbed in a process is provided by surrounding areas. TΔS is the amount of heat gained at a constant temperature, so Gibbs free energy adds to the internal energy, the work done in volume changes, as does the heat that the process loses to its environment. As far as biology is concerned, the term TS in the Gibbs free energy allows for entropic forces, which involve the internal or potential energy of a system. In biological systems, displacements, say in x-direction, change the Gibbs free energy, and so the force is $-\partial G/\partial x$. Thus, the forces depend on the changes in both energy and entropy.

5.3.2 Statistical entropy and microstates

The idea was originally suggested and formulated by Ludwig Boltzmann between 1872 to 1875, but later modified by Max Planck in about 1900. To quote Planck, "*the logarithmic connection between entropy and probability was first stated by L. Boltzmann in his kinetic theory of gases*". A macrostate has to involve an amount of matter sufficiently large so that we can measure its volume, pressure and temperature. However, in thermodynamics, this is not strictly true. A *macrostate* is the thermodynamic state of any system that is exactly characterized by measurement of the system's properties such as P, V, T, H, and number of moles of each constituent, and a *microstate* deals with the energy that molecules or other particles have. A microstate deals with the possibility of different accessible arrangements of the molecules' dynamical energy for a particular macrostate. A macrostate does not change over time if its observable and measurable properties do not change, while a microstate of a system is specifically concerned with time and the energy of molecules in that system. Therefore, a microstate is one of the many distinct ways that the microscopic objects making up our macroscopic system can be arranged. For example, let us suppose we are interested in disposition of a fluorescently labeled molecule on a surface. There are various ways of doing this, as each conformation is a specific microstate, but they all have one feature in common, i.e., the molecule is to be adsorbed on the surface.

Statistical mechanics can help us compute the relative probabilities of all the microstates consistent with the constraints imposed on the system such as temperature, mean distance between the ends of molecule, and the concentration of ligand in solution. From biological interest point of view, the challenge is to determine the number of biologically equivalent microstates, and then compute their probabilities. In other words, the task of statistical mechanics would be determining the probabilities of the microstates in the system by providing us with a thorough formula containing the Boltzmann factor. According to the principle of *a priori* probabilities, the probability P_i that a thermal equilibrium in small systems is its *ith* microstate is equal to the ratio of the number of microstates accessible to the composite system in which subsystem B, as denoted before, is in its *ith* microstate to the total number Ω_e of microstates accessible to the composite system.

$$P_i = A \exp(-\beta E_i) = A \exp(-E_i/k_B T) \tag{5.18}$$

where E_i is the energy of microstate, T is the temperature, k_B is Boltzmann constant (1.38×10^{-23} JK^{-1}), $\beta = 1/k_B T$, $k_B T$ (or RT where is molar gas constant = 8.314 J K^{-1} Mol^{-1}) is thermal energy and its value is $\sim 4 \times 10^{-21}$ J per molecule for ordinary temperatures. The probability that the small system is in its *ith* microstate with energy ε_i is proportional to $\exp(-\beta E_i)$. The quantity $\exp(-\beta E_i)$ is called the *Boltzmann factor* and the Eq. (5.18) is called *Boltzmann distribution or Canonical distribution*. Since the small system must be in one of its possible microstates, $\sum P_i$ must be equal to unity. Using Eq. (5.18) we have

$$\sum P_i = \sum A\exp(-\beta E_i) = A \sum \exp(-\beta E_i) = 1 \tag{5.19}$$

where,

$$A = \frac{1}{\sum_{(states)} \exp(-\beta E_i)}$$

In the Eq. (5.19), the summation is over all the possible microstates of the small system. Equation (5.18) can be rewritten in the form

$$P_i = \frac{\exp(-\beta E_i)}{Z} \frac{\exp(-E_i/k_B T)}{Z} \tag{5.20}$$

where

$$Z = \sum_{(states)} \exp(-\beta E_i) = \sum_{(states)} \exp(-E_i/k_B T) \tag{5.21}$$

is the *partition function*. The assumption in Eq. (5.21) is over microstates of the small system. For many biological experiments, it is easier to determine the probability of a state (e.g., concentration of ligand-bound receptors) than directly measure its energy.

Note that Boltzmann's formula applies to microstates of the universe as a whole, each possible microstate of which is presumed to be equally probable. However, in thermodynamics it is important to be able to make the approximation of dividing the universe into a system of interest, plus its surroundings; and then to be able to identify the entropy of the system with the system entropy in classical thermodynamics. The microstates of such a thermodynamic system are *not* equally probable—for example, high energy microstates are less probable than low energy microstates for a thermodynamic system kept at a fixed temperature by allowing contact with a heat bath. The statistical entropy reduces to Boltzmann's entropy when all the accessible microstates of the system are equally likely. Boltzmann›s entropy is the expression of entropy at thermodynamic equilibrium in the canonical ensemble. This postulate, which is known as Boltzmann›s principle, may be regarded as the foundation of statistical mechanics, which describes thermodynamic systems using the statistical behaviour of its constituents. In statistical mechanics, Boltzmann's equation is a probability equation relating the entropy S of an ideal gas to the quantity Ω_e, which is the number of complexions of the system, i.e., the number of possible disposition of matter over the available energy states, or more precisely, the number of *microstates* corresponding to a given *macrostates* identified through its macroscopic properties. In other words, it measures the number of ways in which the molecules can be assigned to the various energy states for the distribution in question. For now, the system volume is considered constant.

$$\ln \Omega_e = N \ln N - \sum N_1 \ln N_1 \tag{5.22}$$

$\ln \Omega_e$ defines the degree of probability of the system, and gives quantitative measure of the state of chaos which prevails. The properties of $\ln \Omega_e$ are closely related to thermal magnitudes, and it is one of the most highly regarded functions in physical chemistry. Rewriting Eq. (5.13)

$$N_1 = \frac{N \exp(-E_1/k_B T)}{\sum \exp(-E_1/k_B T)} \tag{5.23}$$

where, N_1 is number of molecules or particles in state 1 and denoting $G_e = \sum \exp(-E_1/k_B T)$. For convenience we multiply $\ln \Omega_e$ by k and denote

Entropy = (Boltzmann's constant k_B) x (logarithm of number of possible states Ω_e)

$$S_e = k_B \ln \Omega_e \tag{5.24}$$

Since the logarithm of a number always increases as the number increases, we see that the more possible states that the system can be in (given that it has a particular volume, energy, pressure, and temperature), the greater the entropy, hence greater the extent of its irreversibility. It turns out that S_e is itself a thermodynamic property, just like E or V. Therefore, it acts as a link between the microscopic world and the macroscopic. One important property of S_e follows readily from the definition: since Ω_e is a natural number (1,2,3,...), S_e is either zero or positive. Note that $\Omega = 1$ represents the maximum order in this respect, i.e., minimum entropy, since $\ln \Omega_e = 1$.

Importance of Ω_e

Before we proceed, it would be useful to consider an example in order to have an idea about the number of accessible microstates Ω_e for a macroscopic system. Consider a system of N spatially separated particles such as molecules. According to $\Omega_e = 2^N$ where $N = 6.02 \times 10^{23}$ so we obtain

$$\Omega_e = 2^{6.02 \times 10^{23}} = 10^{1.8 \times 10^{23}} \tag{5.25}$$

To illustrate how big the number $10^{1.8 \times 10^{23}}$ actually is, first we need to know how long the number would be if we wanted to type it. To type 10^4 in full implies writing one followed by four zeros, similarly, typing 1.8×10^{23} means writing one followed by 1.8×10^{23} zeros. Now, assuming a typical font size, there will be 5 digits/cm, i.e., 500 digits/m. Therefore, 2^N would be 1.8×10^{23} divided by $500 = 3.6 \times 10^{20}$ m long. Also, remembering that one light year is 3×10^8 m/s $\times$ 365 (d/yr) $\times$ 24 (h/d) $\times$ 3600 (s/h) = 9.5×10^{15} m. Thus, the number in Eq. (5.25) would be 3.8×10^4 light years long, which, with a simple calculation, is about the radius of our galaxy. This is the distance required in order to write down the number of microstates that is the statistical weight of a typical macrostate of a macroscopic system. Thus,

$\ln \Omega_e = \ln 2^N = N \ln 2 = 4.17 \times 10^{23}$ and using Eq. (5.24),

$S_e = k_B \ln \Omega_e = 1.38 \times 10^{23} \times 4.17 \times 10^{23} = 5.76 \text{ JK}^{-1}$

Therefore, the number Ω_e, which requires astronomical distances to write in full is now reduced to less than 10 digits, so we need to work with Boltzmann's idea after all. Let us continue with the discussion.

$$S_e = k_B N \ln N - \sum k_B N_1 \ln N_1 \tag{5.26}$$

Substituting N_1 for S_e in (5.24)

$$S_e = k_B N \ln G_e + k_B NT \, d\ln G_e/dT \tag{5.27}$$

$$S_e = R \ln G_e + RT \, d\ln G_e/dT \tag{5.28}$$

$$\frac{dG_e}{dT} = \frac{\sum (E_1 \exp E_1/k_B T)}{k_B T^2} \tag{5.29}$$

Hence,

$$\sum (E_1 \exp E_1/k_B T) = k_B T^2 \, dG_e/dT \tag{5.30}$$

After some substitution we get

$$S_e = R \ln G_e + \frac{E}{T} \tag{5.31}$$

Equation (5.31) indicated the relation of the entropy to the total energy, which is very important. We now take the differential coefficient of the entropy, S_e, with respect to the temperature, i.e., the function tells us how the degree of disorder changes with temperature increase, and molecules are transferred into higher energy states. Assuming the volume of the system is kept constant, and after some simplification, Eq. (5.31) is rewritten

$$\left(\frac{\partial S_e}{\partial T}\right)_v = \frac{1}{T}\left(\frac{\partial E}{\partial T}\right)_v \tag{5.32}$$

Now, the change of entropy due to an increase of temperature dT at constant volume is given

$$dS_e = \left(\frac{\partial Se}{\partial T}\right)_v dT = \left(\frac{C_v dT}{T}\right) \tag{5.33}$$

Clearly, as the temperature rises, S_e increases according to the relation

$$S_e = C_v \ln T + S_{e'} \tag{5.34}$$

where $S_{e'}$ is a function of volume. Again, it is important to have an intuitive understanding of increase of S_e with the temperature, as explained for Eq. (5.11). As the total energy of the system becomes greater, the higher energy states become accessible to more molecules. Consequently, as the distribution widens, so do the number of ways molecules can move. Therefore, it is correct to state that when a substance becomes hotter, its state becomes more probable. Similarly, as the volume increases, the state becomes more probable, and thus by analogy we may write

$$\left(\frac{\partial S}{\partial V}\right)_T = R\left(\frac{\partial V}{\partial V}\right)_v \tag{5.35}$$

$$S_V = R \ln V \tag{5.36}$$

Now, if we consider systems in which the temperature and the volume are both variables, then the above results are combined. There are number of ways in which the energy distribution can be realized as

$$S = S_e + S_V$$

$$k_B \ln \Omega = k_B \ln \Omega_e + k_B \ln \Omega_v$$
$$S = C_v \ln T + R \ln V \tag{5.37}$$

where S takes into account both the spatial positions of the molecules and their motions is called *statistical entropy of the system*. In its differential form it is

$$dS = C_v \, dT/T + R \, dV/V \tag{5.38}$$

Equation (5.38) indicates the increase in entropy and probability which accompanies increase in temperature or expansion of volume. As was mentioned in §5.2.1, entropy refers to the number of available microstates and NOT just to the geometrical aspect of *order*. This type of order is scarcely adequate as a measure of the complexity and *organization* of biological systems. A living system is complex and has a high degree of order and high degree of entropy, i.e., a live mouse has more entropy than its corpse and a stone because of the diversity of internal movement of the system on the molecular level and hence, more available microstates to offer. In short, entropy is a measure of our lack of knowledge and information. One may say that a state of low entropy is a necessary condition, but not a sufficient one for biological complexity and organization to occur.

5.4 Biological complexity, fractal and chaos

Life is an out-of-equilibrium thermodynamics process; its origin and evolution is strictly dependent on the entropy production (i.e., dissipation of an external thermodynamic potential) and the evolution of this potential in time. The evolution in physical science is normally referred to as the approach of a system to the thermodynamic equilibrium characterized by the increase of entropy of the second law of thermodynamics. The process of physical evolution always tends towards the continuous disorganization, meaning the destruction of structures introduced by the initial conditions (Prigogine and Nikolis 1971). On the contrary, the arrow of biological evolution is pointing to the opposite direction. Here, the idea of evolution is associated with an irreversible increase of organization, leading to the creation of more complex structures. Now, living organisms are open systems exchanging energy and matter with their surroundings, and the change in entropy in both the organism and the surroundings have to be assessed. Thus, it is perfectly possible for entropy to decrease due to say, metabolism, etc., occurring in a living system, while at the same time there is an increase in entropy of the surroundings due to the heat transfer from the system (note, S = Q/T). Therefore, the concept of physical and biological evolution can be reconciled by the *open-system* model of living organisms, and the second law of thermodynamics can be applied to it. Prior to any mathematical treatment or modeling of such system, the concepts of *complexity, stochastic, chaos* must be carefully considered, as they are all interrelated to each other.

Complexity: Figure 5.5 illustrates that subatomic particles can be organized into atoms, which are the components of molecules, and molecules can be organized into macromolecules, such as DNA and proteins, which can be built into cells. Cells can then be organized into tissues, which form organs, and organs can be grouped into organ systems, which are built into entire organisms—including humans like ourselves. Organisms are units that can form populations, and then biospheres, which go on to make up even greater levels of *complexity*.

Units of matter organized and integrated into levels of increasing complexity is a concept referred to as *integrative levels* of *organization*. Integrative levels of organization allow researchers to describe the evolution from the inanimate to the animate and social worlds (Novikoff 1945). Remember that the dynamics in both complexity and chaos is nonlinear. In this context, linearity means that the equations of motion do not contain any power of variables higher than 1.

Emergent properties

When units of biological material are put together, the properties of the new material are not always additive, or equal to the sum of the properties of the components. Instead, at each level, new properties and rules emerge that cannot be predicted by observations and full knowledge of the lower levels. Such

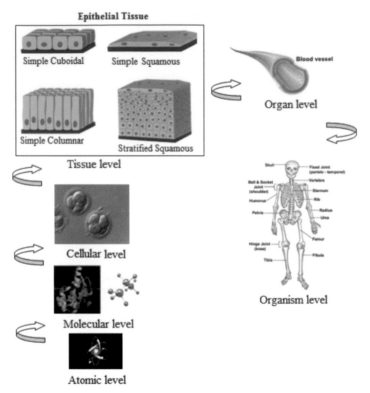

Figure 5.5. Hierarchy of complexity starting from the subatomic level, up to the formation of an organism structure.

properties are called *emergent properties* (Novikoff 1945). Thus, our understanding of physical and chemical properties in lower levels of organization helps us understand only some of the properties of living organisms, which prevents use of a reductionist approach. Adding to this, the fact is that chaos also destroys the reductionist approach that we can have a complete control or absolute power over the matter if we know enough about the details. The details whose sensitivity strongly depends on the initial conditions and prevents us from such absolute predictability. No matter how well we understand the physics and chemistry of living systems, we must recognize that living systems, and other high integrative levels, have new and unique properties that emerge through the combination of the lower-level units of matter. Likewise, our understanding of the new emergent properties at a higher level does not help us understand the properties of the lower levels, because each integrative level of organization has its own particular structure and emergent properties. Even if we do understand the cell's function, that does not mean we fully understand the organism's physiology. After all, the activity of each cell is affected by the activity of other cells in the tissues, organs, and organ systems within the organism. The combination of structure and emergence leads to self-organization, which is the effect of emerging behaviour on the structure or creating a new structure. To summarize the importance of complexity, Baranger (2000) in his enlightening paper, has enlisted the most prominent properties of complexities, as follows:

- Complex systems contain many constituents interacting nonlinearly.
- The constituents of a complex system are interdependent.
- A complex system posses a structure spanning several scales.
- A complex system is capable of emerging behaviour.
- Complexity involves an interplay between chaos and non-chaos.
- Complexity involves an interplay between cooperation and competition.

Chaos: is traditionally thought of as being confusion and turmoil, but in the sense of chaos theory, it is the idea that the state of final outcome of something is strongly sensitive upon initial conditions, as explained in Chapter 2. Actually one can find brief organized patterns within chaotic systems. Chaotic systems have three main properties of *sensitivity*, *topological mixing*, and *periodicity*. For example, a feature of many cancer cells is that the DNA in their chromosomes is all shuffled. A fraction of DNA containing one or more genes have escaped from their chromosome due to some mechanism of damage and positioned in a different place. Other lengths of DNA have been transferred to a different chromosome altogether. It has been shown that the proliferative activity of long-term cultured Fao rat hepatoma cells exhibit signs of complex dynamics system, with successive rises and falls in proliferation (Wolform et al. 2000). They used a geometric representation on a 2-D map to analyse the proliferation data in the three Fao cultures. The graphical construction suggested that the persistent oscillations of proliferation are partly due to chaotic dynamics.

Fractal: However, recently a much more encouraging aspect of research has been the discovery of *fractal pattern* of the cancerous cells (Dokukin et al. 2011). It has been shown using atomic force microscopy how the surface of human cervical epithelial cells demonstrate substantially different fractal behaviour when the cell becomes cancerous. Fractal patterns, as shown in Fig. 5.6, are self-similar, irregular curves, or shapes that repeat their patterns when zoomed in and out (Mandelbrot 1998).

We can say that they are "infinitely complex", the very signature of chaos itself. These patterns are usually formed in a far-from equilibrium condition (Meakin 1998), or emerge from chaos (MacCauley 1993). There is a wide spectrum of examples including the universe, trees, minerals, clouds, and biological tissues. It is generally believed that an imbalance of various biochemical reactions, which is typically associated with cancer, could lead to chaos and fractal behaviour of cancers (Sedivy and Mader 1997). A crucial difference between healthy cells and cancerous cells may be the presence of fractal patterns. Previous studies had already found traces of fractal patterns in the biochemistry and mechanics of cancerous tissue, but never before on the surfaces of single, isolated cancer cells. The work could provide us a better understanding of how the surface of cells affects the progression of some cancers, which could in turn lead to new strategies for fighting the disease. Although the origin of many cancers is still a mystery, some scientists believe that these diseases are linked to complex processes in living cells becoming unbalanced, which could lead to chaotic behaviour. Indeed, signs of chaos have already been seen in biochemical and physical studies of cancerous tissue—with the structure of some cancerous tissues, for example, having fractal properties associated with chaotic systems. Fractal patterns had, however, never been seen before on the surfaces of single cancer cells. The new observation could be significant because scientists already know that the surface of a cancer cell plays an important role in "metastasis". This is the process whereby cancer cells manage to leave a primary tumor—often forcing their way through healthy tissue—and travel to other parts of the body to create secondary tumors.

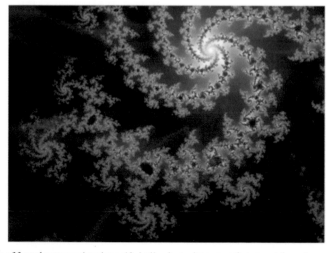

Figure 5.6. An example of fractal patterns showing self-similar, irregular curves that repeat the patterns when zoomed in and out.

5.4.1 Statistical dynamical complexity

Introducing the concept of entropy and complexity above and remembering that a system which consists of a large number of interacting elements or interrelated components is referred to as a *complex system*, now we attempt to describe how one can actually measure it. The key role is played by statistical mechanics, particularly that entropy is related to information theory. Boltzmann-entropy production rate leads to the well-known Pesin-type identity, which provides a simple measure of dynamical complexity in terms of Lyapunov exponents (Hilborn 2009). The relationships of dynamical complexity have been found very useful for studying the increase of complexity. Clearly, a statistical model is essential considering the large number of accessible microstates acting as points along different trajectories between the initial and present states. Also, since these variables are moving along a path in phase space, thus statistical mechanics is used to deal with such chaotic systems, which is characterized by exponential separation of close trajectories expressed by Lyapunov exponents. Let us suppose a biological system consisting of n interacting elements of concentration p^i, (i = 1,2,....n). The current state as a dynamical model consists of a set of nonlinear rate equations in state space defined by

$$\dot{p} = f(p, q) \tag{5.39}$$

where $p = (p_1, p_2,.....p_n)$ is a point in the n-dimensional state space, and $q = (q_1, q_2,...q_n)$ is the control parameter. Assuming that for a given value of q, the system has a stationary solution, i.e., a fixed point for example, $p^* = (p_1^*, p_2^*,.....p_n^*)$. Now, the next point to p^* is

$$p(t) = p^* + \delta p \tag{5.40}$$

where δp represents the deviation of p(t) from initial fixed point p^*. The time-evolution of $\delta p(t)$ is

$$\delta\dot{p}(t) = A(p^*)\,\delta p(t) \tag{5.41}$$

where $A(p^*) = \left[\left(\dfrac{\partial q_i}{\partial q_j}\right)_{p^*}\right]$ is the Jacobian matrix of the function q at the stationary state p^*. The time-derivative in the left hand side represents the local derivative $\delta/\delta t$ instead of the total time-derivative d/dt. The solution in Eq. (5.41) is given by

$$\delta p(t) = e^{At}\delta p(0) \tag{5.42}$$

$\delta p(0)$ is deviation of the initial state from the initial point p^*. For orthonormal representation of the Jacobian matrix $A(p^*)$ we have

$$A(p^*) = Diag(\lambda_1, \lambda_2,..... \lambda_n) \tag{5.43}$$

where $(\lambda_1, \lambda_2,..... \lambda_n)$ are the eigenvalues of the matrix $A(p^*)$. So, the solution in Eq. (5.42) becomes

$$\delta p_i(t) = \delta p_i(0)\, e^{\lambda_i t}, (i = 1,2,....n) \tag{5.44}$$

The asymptotic stability of stationary state described by Eq. (5.44) shows that the real parts of the eigenvalues must have negative values, i.e., $Re(\lambda_j < 0)$, meaning that all the deviations $\delta p_i(t)$ approaches to zero with time. If any of one of the eigenvalues posses a positive real part, the stationary state is unstable. This result can be applied to chaotic systems.

Aside background

Various types of *stability* may be discussed for the solutions of differential equation describing dynamical systems. The most important type is that concerning the stability of solutions near a point of equilibrium. This may be discussed by the theory of Lyapunov. In simple terms, if the solutions that start out near an equilibrium point P_e stay near P_e forever, then P_e is *Lyapunov stable*. In other words, if P_e is Lyapunov stable and all solutions that start out near P_e converge to P_e, then P_e is *asymptotically stable.*

(Lyapunov stability gives a definition of asymptotic stability for more general dynamical systems, and all exponentially stable systems are also asymptotically stable). The notion of *exponential stability* guarantees a minimal rate of decay, i.e., an estimate of how quickly the solutions converge. Remembering that the definition of asymptotic is that it is a line that approaches a curve but never touches it. Consider a simple scalar equation $y'(t) = ay(t)$. The solution is, of course, $y(t) = y_0 e^{at}$, where $y_0 = y(0)$. In particular, $y(t) \equiv 0$ is a solution. What happens if we start at some point other that 0? If $a < 0$, then every solution approaches 0 as $t \rightarrow \infty$. We say that the zero solution is (*globally*) *asymptotically stable*. Figure 5.7 shows the graphs of a few solutions and the direction field of the equation, i.e., the arrows have the same slope as the solution that passes through the tail point.

Now let us suppose two trajectories for the dynamical model system defined by Eq. (5.39), one point due to the reference point p_r, and another from the neighbouring point $\delta p(t)$, thus, $p(t) = p_r + \delta p(t)$. The distance between two trajectories at time t is given by

$$\delta p(t) = \left[\delta p_1^2(t) + \delta p_2^2(t) + ...\delta p_n^2(t) \right]^{\frac{1}{2}} \tag{5.45}$$

Recalling Eq. (5.44),

$$\lambda_i = \lim_{t \to \infty} \frac{1}{t} \log \left[\frac{\delta p_i(t)}{\delta p_i(0)} \right], \quad (i = 1,2,...n) \tag{5.46}$$

It should be noted that the Lyapunov exponent is the value of the real part of the eigenvalue averaged over the trajectory under study. Now to measure the complexity of a system, we need to measure the entropy characterizing the evolution of the system from the initial state $p(0)$ to the current state $p(t)$. Rewriting the Eq. (5.44)

$$\Delta p(t) = e^{\lambda_i t} \delta p(0) = B(t) \delta p(0) \tag{5.47}$$

where $B(t) = e^{\lambda_i t}$ is the matrix of evolution and plays a vital role in evolution of the system. The diagonal elements $e^{\lambda_i t} = \text{diag}(e^{\lambda_1 t}, e^{\lambda_2 t},... e^{\lambda_n t})$ characterize the different trajectories concerning the initial state to the final state. The accessible microstates (i.e., the statistical entropy) along the trajectories $e^{\lambda_i t}$ are characterized

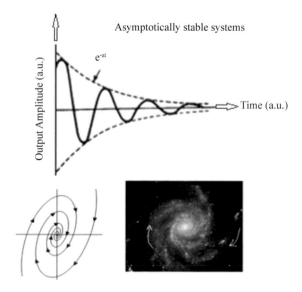

Figure 5.7. Asymptotically stable system defined by Lyapunov stable. The exponential stability guarantees a minimal rate of decay.

by $e^{\lambda_i t}$. The measure of all accessible microstates lying on the trajectory $e^{\lambda_i t}$ are therefore considered to be proportional to the quantity $e^{\lambda_i t}$, so the quantity

$$\Omega(t) = \Pi_{i=1}^{n} \, e^{\lambda_i t} \tag{5.48}$$

is proportional to the measure, i.e., the volume of the totality of all accessible microstates lying on the different trajectories for evolution, in other words $\delta p(0) \rightarrow \delta p(t)$. Now by considering the quantity $\Omega(t)$, one can define a Boltzmann-like entropy of the macrostates consisting of all accessible microstates in the evolution process of $\delta p(0) \rightarrow \delta p(t)$,

$$G_B(t) = \ln \Omega(t) = \ln\Pi_{i=1}^{n} \, e^{\lambda_i t} = \sum_{i=1}^{n} e^{\lambda_i t} \tag{5.49}$$

The relation (5.49) is the measure of entropy associated with the evolution, $\delta p(0) \rightarrow \delta p(t)$. Now, the complexity of an evolving system is connected to entropy of the evolving matrix $B(t) = e^{At}$. Thus, the Eq. (5.49) can be rewritten as

$$G_B = \ln|B(t)| = \Pi_{i=1}^{n} \, e^{\lambda_i t} \tag{5.50}$$

where $\ln|B(t)|$ is determinant of e^{At}. Since the exponential in Eq. (5.50) with negative Lyapunov exponents λ_i must be replaced by 1, there is only one microstate with negative Lyapunov exponent being occupied $\delta p_i = 0$. Hence, the entropy in Eq. (5.49) becomes

$$G_B(t) = \sum_{i=1}^{n^*} \lambda_i t \tag{5.51}$$

where the summation in the right-hand side extends over the positive Lyapunov exponents only. Clearly, the entropy $G_B(t) = 0$ at initial time $t = 0$, and it increases with the time of evolution. The dynamical complexity, which is a property of the evolution of a state, and not of the state itself, is defined as the rate of change of entropy, Eq. (5.51), i.e., the Boltzmann-entropy production rate

$$Z_D = \dot{G}_B(t) = \sum_{i=1}^{n^*} \lambda_i t \tag{5.52}$$

The right-hand side represents the sum of all positive Lyapunav exponents. Pesin-like identity plays a significant role in the characterization of complexity of various type of dynamical systems. Equation (5.52) indicates that complexity measure is dependent on the positive Lyapunov exponents of the system.

5.5 Thermodynamics of cancer cells

Cancer is a generic name given to a collection of related diseases and a group of malignant cells which have lost their control over normal growth. Malignant cancerous tumors mean they can spread into, or invade, the nearby tissues. In addition, as these tumors grow, some cancer cells can break off and travel to distant places in the body through the blood or the lymph system in a process known as metastasis and form new tumors far from the original tumor. Unlike malignant tumors, benign tumors do not spread into, or invade, nearby tissues. Thermodynamics is essential for an understanding of the processes maintaining the living state and conditions resulting in weak links in biological processes, leading to various diseases. The mechanism of cancer development may involve a thermodynamic explanation, where a series of effects induce disorder in healthy tissues. But let us first look at the relationship between nutrients, thermodynamics, and cancer.

The human organism continuously takes up nutrients to build up macromolecules and functionally active structures. The nutrients are converted to high entropy and low Gibbs energy-containing waste products that are excreted by the host. On the basis of the first law of thermodynamics ($\delta Q = \delta U + \delta W$), the energy of nutrients is transformed, proceeding towards minimum entropy production and the release of heat and "waste products" in our biological open system. Part of the heat produced during exothermic processes supports the optimal efficiency of the endothermic biological reactions in the organism, and the rest is dissipated in the environment on the basis of the second law of thermodynamics. During the growth, there are some differences between the healthy tissues and the growing tumor, including metabolic, structural, and thermodynamic differences for heat production. Both structural and thermodynamic differences can be used to follow the entropy differences between cancerous and normal tissues. Entropy production results from the transport of heat and matter between the two phases of the system, and also from the chemical reactions taking place. Thus, the rate of increase of entropy production, i.e., dS/dT is the result of bidirectional currents, the sum of individual fluxes flowing in opposite directions between cancerous and normal tissues. It is well known that normal tissues develop towards minimum entropy production, while a cancer moves towards the maximum entropy. The informational entropy production rate is concerned with a solid tumor embedded in healthy tissues, where the entropy flow is equivalent to the amount of entropy flowing in and out of the boundary defined at a thermodynamic distance. The irreversible processes communicated via various dissipation mechanisms are by differences in heat production, chemical potential gradients, Gibbs energy, intercellular acidity (pH), conductance, membrane potential gradients, membrane potential of cells, and the response to external force fields.

Organisms and their compartments are thermodynamically open systems; they have been analyzed by means of structural entropy. Such morphological studies give information about the entropy changes from a directed exchange with the environment. In the host, the relationship between healthy tissues and malignant tissues can be described by the second law of thermodynamics. This defines the direction of physical and biological processes resulting in tumor growth. Entropy always increases for any non-equilibrium system due to the more disordered sub-cellular structures of the cancerous cells with their different sub-cellular structures. The information inherent in a cancerous cell is different from that in a normal cell. In living healthy cells, the free energy is high (increases) and their entropy is low (decreases) due to the altered metabolism at the expense of the environment. The entropy production of healthy cells is lower than that of cancerous cells if no external energy input is applied to the tissues. However, when appropriate external energy is applied, the rate of entropy production of normal tissues may exceed that of cancerous tissues. Cancerous tissues develop towards the maximum entropy, but maximum entropy involves the total amount of energy not available for work in the cells (Molnar 2009).

The life of cancer is ordered at the expense of disordering its surroundings, when cancer becomes a parasite of the living state. The mitochondrial activity decreases continuously in cancer. Damage to the mitochondria results in a compensatory increase in glycolytic ATP production in the malignant cells, together with a decreased level of oxidation of NADH linked substrates. The mitochondrial defects contribute to tumor progression in several ways, such as by modified energy production, free radical generation, and programmed cell death (Van Ness 1969, Carew and Huang 2002). Cell population systems operate at thermodynamic non-equilibrium, which continuously acquires free energy, heat, and work from the surrounding. The life of cancer is ordered at the expense of disordering its surroundings, when cancer becomes a parasite of the living state. The mitochondrial activity decreases continuously in cancer. The disorder of tumors and the long-range correlations in ordered tissues are in competition with each other. Tumor cells break the ordering of processes in the host and resulting propagation in existing structures. Their difference in entropy development increases with time. It is assumed that the entropy for the two different living systems increases monotonously with time from zero to infinity, but the differences are constant in time. The process of informational entropy flow thus introduces the arrow of time into cancer dynamics.

The malignant cells are non-linear dynamic systems which self-organize in time and space far from thermodynamic equilibrium and exhibit high complexity, robustness, and adaptability. The robustness is thought to be due to functionality in the face of various external and internal perturbations (Kitano 2003, 2004). Adaptability is the response to cellular stress induced by an energetic overload which eventually results in cellular entropy. The entropy production rate of cancer cells, which is a Lyapunov function, is always higher than that of healthy cells. One important aspect of thermodynamics, as we will see, is that the entropy production rate of avascular tumor is the *"Hallmark of cancer"*.

5.5.1 Cancer hallmarks

According to Hanahan and Weinberg (2000), virtually all cancers can be characterized by the following hallmarks: (1) Self-sufficiency in growth signals, (2) Insensitivity to anti-growth signals, (3) Anti-growth signals, (4) Tissue invasion and metastases, (5) Limitless replicative potential, (6) Sustained angiogenesis, and (7) Evasion of apoptosis. From a physical point of view, additional characteristics can be considered as both common and important for cancer initiation and progression: (a) Mechanical and structural: (i) Change in viscoelasticity of cells, i.e., a higher level of rigidity of the extracellular matrix (ECM) and a lower level of rigidity of the cancer cells compared to the normal cells, (ii) Change in membrane composition, i.e., over-expression of signaling proteins or p-glycoproteins, (iii) Epithelial-to-mesenchymal transition in cell morphology and associated reduction in the cells function synchronization and higher level of motility, (iv) Elimination of various signaling pathways, particularly apoptotic, allowing cancer cells to survive, spread in foreign organs, (v) Manufacturing and secretion of specialized proteins to dissolve basement and other membranes to facilitate cell motility, (b) Metabolic: (i) Warburg effect, which results in an increased production of metabolic energy using the glycolytic rather than oxidative phosphorylation pathways, (ii) Hypoxia, which is correlated with the glycolytic switch, (iii) A decrease of the trans-membrane potential, and (iv) A reduction in the cellular pH value which is likely also related to the Warburg effect.

5.5.2 Biophysics and phase transitions

A vast amount of information is available in literature about biochemistry, genomics, and cell biology of cancer. However, not so much has been discussed about the biophysics of the cancer state. Physics has introduced an essential and necessary theoretical and experimental approach to understand dynamic non-equilibrium systems such as living cells, which can be integrated with knowledge of biochemical and biophysical achievements furnished by cell biology and biochemistry. One interesting and key playing issue in this field is phase transitions, for example solid-liquid or liquid–gas, which may occur at critical value of external parameter, such as temperature. Take a soft tissue as an example, which mainly contains water. Under direct effect of an irradiating heat source, the tissue gradually warms up until at a critical value of energy, the temperature of water is increased from 37°C reaches to 100°C; which corresponds to a transition from liquid to gas, and hence a transition in the tissue constituent molecules. Cells in living matter can exist in two distinct ways: (a) normal cells, which are differentiated, proliferated, and undergo apoptosis when damaged, and can also adhere to each other to form regular tissues or organs, (b) cancer cells, which are not differentiated as well as normal cells, and reproduce themselves quite irregularly and without limit, evade apoptosis, and colonize organs where they do not belong.

Two types of organizational changes can occur at cell level if a normal cell undergoes a transition so that it evades apoptosis due to accumulating genetic mutations or somatic damage, say because of ionizing radiation (Nunney 1999): (a) cancer initiation at cell level, and (b) cancer progression at population level. The former case is divided into three types of changes: (i) Physiological, where there are some changes in cell metabolism, such as from oxidative phosphorylation to glycolysis which is known as *Warburg effect,* (ii) Morphological, the epithelial to mesenchymal transition characterized by changes in morphology and motility, and (iii) Molecular, where activation of a host of signalling and protein expression alterations can occur. These three changes are related and derived from epigenetic transformations. The structural organization and metabolic functioning of the above changes are driven by genetic instability, physical, and chemical forces. In the latter case, however, the changes involve the replacement of one group of cells, which adhere to each other to form a differentiated tissue, by another group of cells and thus, form a highly heterogeneous and more motile aggregate, i.e., tumor or neoplasm. Similarly, the changes here are driven by forces of natural selection.

It is possible to apply the extensive knowledge of phase transitions obtained from physics and chemistry to both aforementioned groups of (a) and (b) in order to achieve a quantitative physico-chemical description of the initiation and progression of cancer with potential applications to more effective cancer diagnosis and therapy. Therefore, from the diagnostic point of view, a transition stage of cancer can be the critical stage of this dynamical system and similarly, from a therapeutic point of view, it can be argued that if the stability condition of cancer is reversed in favour of the normal state, the cancer is being cured. Early advances in concept of phase transitions in physical systems was made by Ma (1976). The *control parameters* (e.g., temperature and pressure) derive the systems to instability when approaching their critical values and the corresponding changes in *order parameters* (e.g., density difference between liquid and gas) describe the major physical changes occurring in the system under investigation. It is, therefore, the second law of thermodynamics that acts as an underlying principle to determine the equilibrium state of a macroscopic system. However, phase transitions usually occur in systems that are not isolated from their surroundings, but are in continuous contact with a heat source. At a fixed temperature T, the minimizing of the free energy function G (Gibbs free energy) is required. Gibbs energy describes the thermodynamic state of the system in terms of its entropy and its internal energy, the latter taking account of molecular interactions within the system

$$G = H - TS \tag{5.53}$$

where H, the total energy or enthalpy is the sum of free energy and a function TS of the entropy.

The most striking difference between living systems and non-living systems from thermodynamics point of view is that the former exist in states far from thermodynamic equilibrium (Haken 1978). Living systems survive only because there is a flow of energy and matter between them and their surroundings. Entropy is lost into surroundings as heat to compensate for the generation and maintenance of structural order (entropy reduction) and functional organization (Prigogine 1980). However, there exist phase transitions in far-from equilibrium physical systems, too. Prior to applying thermodynamics to cancer, we need to determine the relevant control and order parameters mentioned above. In the case of a transition from normal to cancer cells, the nature of change is one of molecular or cellular rearrangement leading to elimination of different cell cycle check points. Although cancer triggering can occur at molecular level, thermodynamic treatments are normally expressed in terms of macroscopic variables. Cells function as metabolic networks defined by a large ensemble of interacting enzymes within a substance mediated by processes typically described using chemical kinetics transforming one metabolic into another (Klevecz et al. 2008). Such networks support the concept of describing cells in terms of aggregate variables-macroscopic parameters that are functions of structure of the network and the biochemical interactions between the elements. During the normal-cancer phase transition, many macroscopic changes occur that are in fact used as cancer diagnosis factors. For example, cancer cells exhibit significant changes in viscoelastic properties, morphology, nuclear structure, and chromatin structure, and heterogeneity (Navin et al. 2010), as well as changes in metabolism, pH values, and trans-membrane potentials. In the case of control parameter, the first important parameter would be temperature. But because most biological systems are mostly isothermal, thus it is likely that temperature change can be used as control parameter in a limited number of heat-sensitive conditions, such as testicular cancer. Knowing that the biological systems are complex and a large variety of cancer cell types exist, for example there are 200 distinct pathological conditions, thus there are a variety of control and order parameter options for different types of cancer. Although most of the research in the past has been focused on biochemical and chemical carcinogens, it is increasingly being noticed that living cells are also profoundly affected by physical forces including shear stress, surface adhesive forces (Fuhrman et al. 2011), and pressure (Basan et al. 2009). How the cancer cells respond to different macroscopic chemical and physical variables is one of the current interesting subjects in this field, which undoubtedly leads to a better understanding of the origin of cancer. Based on this, other possible control parameters can be: chemical gradients, mechanical stresses and pressure, thermodynamic fluxes, electromagnetic radiation, ionizing radiation, electric fields, and concentration gradients of toxic carcinogens. It is expected that classification of cancer cells in terms of discussed variables should provide a deeper insight of the processes leading from healthy or normal to malignant cells. An ideal theory is believed to predict the following: (i) The physico-chemical conditions at which carcinogenesis will occur, (ii) The transition point to metastasis, and (iii) optimized course therapy in a given situation.

5.5.3 Phase transitions and cancer

The hallmarks of cancer described in §5.5.1 are physiological attributes factors representing differences in cell-cell signaling, the apoptotic and metabolic dysregulation. These differences are associated with underlying physical changes. One hypothesis is that the transition from a healthy to malignant cell may be analyzed by a dynamical phase transition both in physical and informational space owing to well-known changes in the genetic material due to accumulated mutations, chromatin distributions. The progression of cancer must involve a population-level shift because of better adaptation of the cancer cells to the prevailing conditions and competition between the two co-existing phenotype: normal and cancerous. The population shift in the direction of greater malignancy can be viewed as a tendency towards greater stability, and hence a maximum entropy or a minimum Gibbs free energy. Static physical systems achieve thermodynamic equilibrium by reaching a free energy minimum within the given physical constrains, such as constant temperature, volume or pressure, while living systems achieve dynamic stability as a competitive advantage over species within the external environmental conditions such as a nutrient supply, a lower oxygen concentration, or increased pH.

The thermodynamic state of matter can be characterized by macroscopic physical parameters which can be grouped into three classes: (a) Intensive variables, which are bulk variables and independent of the system's size, temperature, pressure, electric and magnetic fields, (b) Extensive variables, such as entropy, volume, electric polarization, and (c) Stare functions such as entropy, enthalpy, free energy, and internal energy. Phase transitions are characterized by extreme sensitivity to small perturbations and by infinite correlations across the system. There is a difference between first and second order phase transitions. In the first order phase transition, a discontinuity occurs in the order parameter. Thus, in the transition from a liquid to a gas the density changes sharply as the temperature is raised through the boiling point. In the second order transition, the gradual changes in the control parameter may move the system in and out of the equilibrium state, for example, in the case of the ferromagnetic to paramagnetic transitions of iron oxides heated above the Curie temperature (Lowrie 1997). There are a large number of phase transitions that may occur in thermodynamically open systems, for example in open physical systems transitions tend to occur when the system is far from thermodynamic equilibrium and the resulting stable states exchange material and energy with the environment. Prigogine (1980) used the term "dissipative structure" to describe a system which may exhibit structural stability, but nevertheless continuously produce entropy by energy dissipation and hence remains stable by exporting this entropy to its surrounding. In this sense, a living matter is a dissipative structure, i.e., being far from the equilibrium, dissipative, and thermodynamically open. The transition from normal to cancer is a first order far from thermodynamic equilibrium phase transition. Under normal conditions, healthy cells represent a more stable state, whereas cancer is a metastable. Once the cells suffer from an increased damage due to, for example, internal dysregulation, metabolic impairment, or genetic changes, then the relative stability between the two types of states (i.e., healthy and cancerous) shifts. When the system is moved into one of the two stable states, it becomes much harder to separate them due to a potential energy barrier between them. Therefore, it is by reversing the condition globally, such as shifting control parameter values that can lead to total eradication of cancer from the body. As mentioned before, there are a number of control parameters that may encourage the shifting from normal to cancerous state: oxygen reduction, higher concentration of carcinogens, pH reduction, i.e., higher acidity, increase damage due to ionizing radiation. On the other hand, the order parameter of the system defines the response to external perturbation. In the case of a living system, a typical example is the mitotic index. Although there is much to be discussed about this new aspect and vision of cancer diagnosis and therapy, we can at this stage accept that advance mathematical models point towards the fact that cancer can be viewed and analyzed as a dynamical first order phase transition. By that it is meant that the phase transitions suggests a truly successful therapy would require a change of conditions disfavoring the cancer phenotype, and not just simply carrying out a local excision or destruction of cancer cells in their micro-environment. A better understanding of cancer thermodynamics also suggests a more effective therapeutic strategy away from radiation and chemotherapy alone towards novel types of interventions based on both control and order parameters which will hopefully open a new era of early effective cancer treatment.

5.5.4 Entropy and tumor

As mentioned in §5.5, the entropy production rate for tumor growth can be considered as hallmark of cancer. According to the second law of thermodynamics, the net entropy of a system together with the environment increases as a result of any natural process. Because entropy can be transferred from the system to the environment, the actual system can then have a decrease in entropy. However, an isothermal system at constant pressure must suffer a decrease in free energy. In an equilibrium state, free energy has a minimum value and the difference ΔG in free energy between the system's actual state and its equilibrium state is, in effect, a measure of the system's tendency to change. At any given temperature T, the difference in entropy ΔS and, the change in ΔG and ΔH are related from Eq. 5.53 as $\Delta H/T = \Delta G/T + \Delta S$. The second law requires an overall production of entropy of energy from the environment and system, i.e.,

$$\Delta S(e) + \Delta S > 0 \tag{5.54}$$

where $\Delta S(e)$ is the increase in entropy of the environment. Now, we know from classical thermodynamics that if the constraints of a system are the temperature T and the pressure P, the entropy production can be evaluated using Gibbs's free energy as

$$\delta S_i = -\frac{1}{T} dG \tag{5.55}$$

Taking time derivative,

$$\frac{\delta S_i}{dt} = -\frac{1}{T} \frac{dG}{dt} \tag{5.56}$$

where $\delta S_i/dt$ represents the entropy production rate, $\dot{S}_i$. The term dG/dt can be developed by means of the chain rule as a function of the degree of advance of reaction as

$$\frac{dG}{dt} = \left(\frac{\partial G}{\partial \xi}\right) \frac{d\xi}{dt} \tag{5.57}$$

where $\left(\dfrac{\partial G}{\partial \xi}\right)$ represents affinity A with opposed sign (Donder and Van Rysselberghe 1936). Affinity is often addressed in works that attempt to find a thermodynamic basis or thermodynamic causes of chemical reactions rates. Two principle relations are used

$$\sum_{j=1}^{R} A_j\, r_j \geq 0 \tag{5.58a}$$

$$A = RT \ln (\vec{r}/\overleftarrow{r}) \tag{5.58b}$$

The above relations 5.58a and b are called de Donder inequality. Here $\vec{r}$ and $\overleftarrow{r}$ are the forward and reverse reactions respectively, and $r = \vec{r} - \overleftarrow{r}$ is the overall rate. Negative reaction rate means that reaction is running in the opposite direction. A reaction with negative affinity, called non-spontaneous, may be coupled to another reaction of positive affinity and may run with a positive overall reaction rate. So, for example, reaction 1 with negative affinity, $A_1 r_1 < 0$ is coupled with reaction 2 giving

$$A_1 r_1 + A_2 r_2 > 0 \tag{5.59}$$

Thus, a reaction can be forced in their ono-spontaneous direction by other one. A general chemical reaction j is supposed in a reacting mixture with the total number of components equal to n symbolized by [i], so

$$\sum_{i=1}^{n} v_{ij}[i] = 0 \tag{5.60}$$

v_{ij} is the stoichiometric coefficient, negative for reactions and positive for products. The affinity of this reaction is defined as

$$-\sum_{i=1}^{n} v_{ij}\, \mu_i = A_j \tag{5.61}$$

where μ_i is the chemical potential component i. The thermodynamic equilibrium constant (K_j) can be identified with the kinetic equilibrium constant, which is given by the ratio of the forward $\vec{K}_j$ and reverse $\overleftarrow{K}_j$ rate constants.

$$K_j = \vec{K}_j / \bar{K}_i \tag{5.62}$$

which is known as Guldberg-Waage constant and the term $\dot{\xi} = \dfrac{d\xi}{dt}$ is the reaction rate. Taking Eqs. (5.56) and (5.57) we get

$$\dot{S}_i = \frac{\delta S_i}{dt} = \frac{1}{T} A \dot{\xi} \tag{5.63}$$

And the relation 5.58 can be rewritten for affinity as

$$A = RT \ln \left(\frac{K_j}{\Pi(C_i)^{V_{ij}}} \right) \tag{5.64}$$

Here, C_i is the concentration of species i whose stoichiometric coefficients v (i) are negative for reactants and positive for products. Rewriting the Eq. (5.64)

$$A = RT \ln \left(\frac{\vec{k} \Pi C_{\vec{i}}^{V_i}}{\bar{k} \Pi C_{\bar{i}}^{V_i}} \right) \tag{5.65}$$

The reaction rate $\dot{\xi}$ can be evaluated according to the difference between forward and backward reaction rates as

$$\dot{\xi} = (\dot{\xi}_f - \dot{\xi}_b) = \vec{k} \Pi C_{\vec{i}}^{V_i} - \bar{k} \Pi C_{\bar{i}}^{V_i} \tag{5.66}$$

Substituting (5.66) and (5.65) in (5.63) gives

$$\dot{S}_i = R (\dot{\xi}_f - \dot{\xi}_b) \ln \frac{\dot{\xi}_f}{\dot{\xi}_b} \geq 0 \tag{5.67}$$

According to the second law of thermodynamics, the Eq. (5.67) is always positive and is also a Lyapunov function, and thus provides a directional criterion and stability for the dynamical system. In other words, it characterizes a complexity of the system. In fact, one can postulate the entropy production introduced by Eq. (5.67) as a "*hallmark of cancer*", which can be used for prognosis of tumor proliferation.

5.5.5 Fractal, entropy and tumor

While it is not intended here to fully describe the details of fractal mesoscopic model, a brief introduction, however, is presented to show the importance of the relation between fractal and tumor in thermodynamical understanding of diagnosis and treatment. It is known that there exists a close relationship between entropy production rate and fractal structure of cancer cells. Fractals are "self-similar" irregular temporal and spatial shapes that repeat their pattern when zoomed in and out (Dokukin et al. 2011). Both cancer and normal cells exhibit fractal behaviour but with different fractal dimensionality. It was shown by Dokukin et al. that the cell surface can indeed develop fractal behaviour when cells become cancerous. This occurs at nanoscale, when analyzing the distribution of adhesive properties over the two-dimensional surface of biological cells using, for example, atomic force microscopy (AFM). Fractals can be measured by their dimension, whereas the human entropy product may be determined by oxygen and glucose metabolism. These complex disordered patterns are typically formed under far-from equilibrium conditions. There has been a long-standing hypothesis that an imbalance of various biochemical reaction, which are typically associated with cancer, could result in chaos and the associated fractal behaviour of cancer (Sedivy and Mader 1997). Diagnosis of tumor proliferation capacity and invasion capacity is very complex because these terms include many fractals, such as tumor aggressiveness, which is related with the tumor growth rate $\dot{\xi}$ with fractal dimension Φ_f among other fractals. A detailed account on cancer aggressiveness is reported by Waliszewski (2016). Let us suppose the tumor growth rate ($\dot{\xi} = \dot{\mu} - \dot{o}$), where $\dot{\mu}$ and $\dot{o}$ are macroscopic parameters representing moitosis and apoptosis rates respectively. Re-writing the Eq. (5.67)

$$\dot{S}_t \approx R(\dot{\mu}-\dot{o}) \ln \frac{\dot{\mu}}{\dot{o}} \tag{5.68}$$

The repression (5.68) represents the entropy production rate and in terms of moitosis and apoptosis rates.

The fractal dimension as a function of Mitosis and apoptosis rates, which quantitatively describes the tumor capacity to invade healthy tissue is defined by Norton (2005),

$$\Phi_f = \left(\frac{5-\dfrac{\dot{\mu}}{\dot{o}}}{1+\dfrac{\dot{\mu}}{\dot{o}}} \right) \tag{5.69}$$

Substituting the Eq. (5.69) in Eq. (5.68) it gives

$$\dot{S}_t = R(\dot{\mu}-\dot{o}) \ln \left(\frac{5-\dfrac{\dot{\mu}}{\dot{o}}}{1+\dfrac{\dot{\mu}}{\dot{o}}} \right) \tag{5.70}$$

In the relation (5.70), two properties are observed: (a) the growth rate, which is associated with its invasive capacity ($\dot{\xi} = \dot{\mu}-\dot{o}$), and (b) the complexity, a morphology characteristic, such as the fractal dimension of the tumor interface. According to Norton (2005), this quantifies the tumor capacity to invade and penetrate the healthy tissue.

5.6 A note on the philosophy of biological system

Biological systems are considered irreversibly organized (Prigogine 1971, Rubin 2014). They do not explode or decay under ordinary conditions, but seem to grow and evolve towards a singularity or limit cycle if energy and matter is available. The rules of their network composition, their underlying network hierarchy, and their order in time and space remain to be understood. The relationships between biology and the physicochemical sciences, and between organisms and inorganic matter, are of significant interest to the philosophy of science both from theoretical as well as practical points of views. It is for this reason that perhaps it would be useful at this stage to remind ourselves that part of the main theme and direction of the book is to launch an effort to integrate the individual components of subject including nanoparticles, laser light, tissue, cells (healthy and malignant), imaging, and therapy in a neat and comprehensible package. To begin with, let us remember that a biological system is a complex network of biologically relevant entities. A biological organization spans several scales from micro to the nanoscopic scale, for example cells, organelles, macromolecular complexes, and regulatory pathways. During the so-called packing process and hence representing it in a straight forward technical approach for many biomedical issues, we may encounter a number of technical questions whose answers, to my belief, greatly exist in non-technical or philosophical aspect of the problem. That is to say, quite often to gain a better understanding of our results, we have to employ a cognitive approach to recognize and acknowledge the necessity of outlining some of the principal features of the biology and of the controversies that surround some parts of it. These considerations are divided between those scientific research methodologies that are holistic, examining entities in their wholeness using '*top-down*' approach and those that are reductionistic, examining the part that make up wholes, i.e., '*bottom-up*' approach. It is interesting to note that, as will be discussed in Chapter 7, these approaches are similarly used in nanotechnology and nanobiotechnology.

The panorama of the sciences in the first half of the twentieth century was undoubtedly dominated by the revolutions of quantum and relativity theory. The similar reverberations then continued to echo in other branches of science, such as particle physics and cosmology. After the advent of "new physics", it was time for "new biology" to play a part in the development of science, which in fact exhibited itself as interaction of the "modern synthesis" of biology with physics and chemistry. The combination of physicists and biologists (Watson and Crick 1953) led to the determination of the 3-D chemical structure of DNA, that carries hereditary biological information, which resulted in a new research known as "*molecular biology*". Molecular processes and structures that are involved in the dynamics of a living organism offered powerful quantitative techniques for probing these structures at the subcellular and molecular levels. Historically speaking, molecular biology is well rooted in (a) informational school: dealing with genetic information, and (b) structural school: dealing with the three dimensional structures of biological molecules throughout the evolved hierarchy of living organisms. Let us consider an example of DNA. As we know, in the nuclei of any particular cell of an organism, within its DNA double helices there are specific sequences which perform a unique set of functions, say, enzymes. This particular base sequence in this DNA has a meaning, i.e., a defined readout via the code, only when the DNA has been assembled in that organism and can have its biochemical function as a genetic blueprint for the production of, for instance, protein. Remembering that chemical processes are indeed the means by which bases are incorporated into chains of DNA, but the sequence in which the bases are assembled in DNA is a function and property of the whole organism. Therefore, the concept of *information transfer*, which is required to understand what is actually going on biologically when DNA functions in an actual cell cannot be simply articulated in terms of the concepts of physics and chemistry, despite the fact that they explain the fundamental laws and how the molecular machinery operates to convey information. To this end, the concept of *information* is meaningless except with reference to the functioning of the whole cell. Therefore, a biological scientist is certainly eagerly conscious not only that biological organization is hierarchy of parts making wholes at different levels, but also that dynamic processes are themselves interlocked dynamically in space and time in more complex networks. Hence, it would be very naive to imagine the hierarchy of systems to simply be a static assembly of building blocks constituting different levels, which certainly do not correspond to the dynamic complexity observed by biologists in living organisms. Adding to this is the fact that stochastic processes (i.e., a random process of collection of random variables representing the evolution of some system of random values over time), which is the probabilistic counterpart to a deterministic process, has also been implicated by other biological systems (Frehland 1982). Stochastic and chaotic elements are essential parts of many biochemical processes and as it was mentioned earlier, the biochemical reactions, which is typically associate with cancer, could result in chaos and the associated fractal behaviour of cancer. Therefore, the very early question, and hence the subsequent questions, which ought to be considered and answered during any one given related investigation is that is biology nothing but physics and chemistry?

Classification of domains

Issues about the relationship between biology and the physical sciences, or between organisms and their physical components, arise in three main domains:

Ontological reductionism (OR)

This is the structural and constitutive domain where the issue is whether or not physicochemical entities and processes underlie all living phenomena (Ayala and Dobzhansky 1974). Are organisms made up and composed of the same components as those making up inorganic matter? Is it the case that organisms consist of other entities besides molecules and atoms? In other words, are they nothing but an aggregation of atoms and molecules? Do organisms exhibit properties other than those of their constituent atoms and molecules? In other words, do organisms exhibit '*emergent*' properties? In this constitutive approach, the mechanistic position is that organisms are ultimately made up of the same atoms that make up inorganic objects, and of nothing else. This view date backs to the seventeenth century, when Rene Decartes (1596–1650) proposed that animals are nothing but complex machines. OR claims that organisms are eventually composed of nonliving parts, so no substance or other residue remains after all atoms making up an organism are taken into account. Also, OR implies that the laws of physics and chemistry fully apply to all biological processes at the level of atoms and molecules. Early founders of molecular biology (Francies 1966) claimed that the ultimate aim of the modern movement in biology is to explain *all* biology in terms of physics and chemistry. In making such a claim, he was asserting a philosophical position that biological concepts and theories and laws can be *reduced* to those of physics and chemistry, that living organisms are '*nothing but*' atoms and molecules. It is this '*nothing but*' fallacy, which is relevant to our main theme, whether or not biology can in fact be reduced to physics and chemistry? After all it is not very hard to imagine that a computer is not *nothing but* just pile of wires, semiconductors, plastic, and other materials, as much as an engine is not *nothing but* iron and other materials.

It is very true that organisms are made up of atoms and molecules, but these organisms and the living processes are certainly highly complex patterns, special and highly improbable patterns of physical and chemical processes. Therefore, the formulation of the question that whether properties of an organism are those of physical component parts or those of the '*emergent*', is very crucial in our analysis of the problem. For example, are the properties of common salt, sodium chloride, simply the properties of sodium (Na^+) and chlorine (Cl^-) when they are associated according to the formula NaCl? The answer is 'yes' only when we take into account their association into table salt and the combined (emergent) properties.

Methodological

It is concerned with the strategy of research and the acquisition of knowledge.

The general question is whether a particular biological problem should be addressed by studying the underlying processes or should also be referred at higher levels of organization, such as cell, the organism population, and other factors. One such example amongst others, as discussed in the preceding sections, is application of thermodynamics; particularly the second law; in understanding and therapy of tumors in terms of entropy.

Methodological reductionism (MR)

This claims that the best strategy of research is to study living phenomena at increasingly lower level of complexity, and eventually at the level of atoms and molecules. For example, genetic scientists seek to understand heredity ultimately in terms of the behaviour and structure of DNA, RNA, enzymes, and other macromolecules rather than only in terms of whole organisms, which is indeed the level at which Mendelian laws of inheritance are formulated and expressed. In its extreme end, MR claim that biological research should be conducted only at the level of the physicochemical component parts and processes. Pursuing the question at other levels is not fruitful, since the biological phenomena must ultimately be understood at an atomic and molecular scale.

Methodological compositionist (MC)

This 'holistic' approach is counterpart to MR and claims that in order to understand organisms, one should be able explain their organization, i.e., how organisms and groups are organized and what functions they serve. According to MC, organisms must be investigated as wholes and not only in their component parts. Similarly, at its extreme end, MC makes the opposite claim—only biological research at the level of whole organism, populations, and communities worth following. For this group, research at lower level of organization may be good in physics and chemistry, but it has no biological significance. It is unlikely that any modern scientist would sincerely sponsor any of the above extreme line of thought, because this would imply the support of unreasonable claim of MR that genetics research should have not have been undertaken in the first place until the discovery of DNA as hereditary material. Similarly, MC, which implies that understanding the structure of DNA or the enzyme processes involved in replication is of no significance to the study of heredity or the investigation of physicochemical reactions in the transmission of nerve impulses is of no use or interest to the understanding of animal behaviour. Therefore, it seems reasonable to adopt a moderate position—that the best strategy to study a biological phenomena is at increasingly lower level of organization and ultimately at the level of atoms and molecules. As Dobzhansky (1969) argued, the biologist does not really have to choose between MR and MC approach, as both are equally necessary; they are complementary to each other; incomplete without the other, and indeed at the present state of knowledge, each is incomplete by itself.

Epistemological reductionism (ER)

The fundamental issue here is whether or not the theories and laws of biology can be derived from the laws and theories of physics and chemistry. ER deals with the organization of knowledge and the logical connection between the strategies of research and the acquisition of knowledge as it was the prime concern of MR. Therefore, for ER, the *derivability* and the *connectability* are two important conditions. The former states that in order to reduce a branch of science to another it is essential to show that the laws and theories of the secondary science can be derived as logical consequences from the laws and theories of the primary science. Generally, the experimental laws and theories of a branch of science contain distinctive terms that do not appear in other branches of science. To establish an epistemological reduction, it is necessary that suitable connections be held between the terms of the secondary science and those used in the primary science. This is the condition of connectability. The reduction of thermodynamics to statistical mechanics required the definition of terms such as 'temperature' by means of terms such as 'kinetic energy'. Similarly, the reduction of theories and experimental laws of genetics to physicochemistry requires the terms such as 'gene' and 'chromomosome' to be defined by means of terms such as 'hydrogen bond', 'nucleotide', 'DNA', and other terms. The integration of diverse scientific theories and the laws into more comprehensive ones simplifies science and extends the explanatory power of scientific principles, and hence conforms to the goals of science. Epistemological reductions are of great importance to science, as it greatly contributes to the advances of scientific knowledge. One clear and established example is the reduction of thermodynamics to statistical mechanics made possible by the discovery that the temperature of a gas reflects the mean kinetic energy of its molecules. Similarly, the number of branches of physics and astronomy have been extensively unified by their reduction to the new theories of great generality, including quantum mechanics and relativity.

Epistemological antireductionism (EAR)

As it was mentioned above, biological organization is certainly a hierarchy of parts making wholes at different scales, but also that dynamic processes are themselves interlocked dynamically in space and time in a very complex network. Thus, processes at molecular scale, such as enzymatic reactions, are part of a complex network of interlocked reactions of this metabolic web, which itself is distributed spatially over a structurally hierarchical framework of organelles. The organelles are themselves interconnected by structures and by chemical messengers in a larger whole, i.e., cell, which itself is incorporated into organs. It is for this reason that biologists are inclined to emphasize the concepts that have to be employed in order to describe and understand such complexities, which clearly indicate new kinds of interlocking at each new level of biological organization and hence, the emergence of new kinds of interlocking relationships. These new relationships themselves require new concepts to order them and render them coherent, as well as special experimental techniques to verify and validate them.

Such a biologist who strongly supports the '*autonomy*' of biological concepts is referred to as EAR. In short, an EAR claims that the biological research should be pursued at all levels of integron of the living systems, including the atomic and molecular levels. For example, Jacob (1974) believed that such distinctive ideas in biology cannot solely be envisaged or translated into conceptual terms of physics and chemistry:

"*From particles to man, there is a whole series of integration, of levels, of discontinuities. But there is no breach that takes place in them; no change in 'essence'... . At each level of organization, novelties appear in both properties and logic. To reproduce is not within the power of any single molecule by itself. This faculty appears only with the simplest integron deserving to be called a living organism, that is the cell... . Biology can neither be reduced to physics, nor can do without it.*"

Question 1

So when did the association between entropy and disorder originate? The information about the role of molecules in determining the classical thermodynamic variables such as pressure, temperature, and heat was gradually completed. Pressure was defined as the total force exerted by individual molecules, colliding with themselves and the walls of the container, averaged over the surface area of the container. Temperature was determined to be the average kinetic energy of all the different ways the molecules could move, and it was Ludwig Boltzmann who first formulated the mathematical relationship between entropy and molecular movement. Based on the molecular description of heat content and temperature, Boltzmann showed that entropy must represent the total number of *'different ways the molecules'* could move. Heat flowed from a hot body to a cold body as kinetic energy was transferred through molecular collisions occurring at the boundary between the two bodies and further distributed throughout the body as molecules collided with each other within the body. At each collision, kinetic energy was exchanged. On average, molecules with more kinetic energy lost kinetic energy as they collided, and molecules with less kinetic gained kinetic energy as they collided, until, on average, the kinetic energy was optimally distributed among all the molecules and their various modes of movement.

The net result was that the more ways a system could move internally, the more molecular kinetic energy the system could hold for a given temperature. This was because temperature was just the average kinetic energy per mode of movement. In Boltzmann's mind, the more ways a system could move internally, the more disorderly the system was. From his point of view, a system in *perfect order* was one in which all the molecules were organized in perfect array without any freedom of movement.

Question 2

Is disorder really the best word to describe entropy? It seems there are a number of issues with using disorder to define entropy. The first problem is that the systems having multiple levels of organization might be more or less 'orderly' on one level and not so much on another. For example, an ice cube as a system is disorderly, but on the molecular level, the ice molecules are neatly arranged in place in an orderly way. Thus, it appears that the application of the term (disorder) be limited to only one clearly specified level at a time. The second problem with disorder as a definition for entropy, even on the molecular level, is its misinterpretation (in my opinion) that: disorder implies things are not where they are supposed to be. This cannot be the case as movement on the molecular level is still governed by Newtonian mechanics otherwise, the equations correlating molecular movement with the observable variables of classical thermodynamics, such as temperature and pressure, could not have been derived as they were. Indeed, the molecules are exactly where they should be. Where else could they be? They are not free to make any random turn or jump between collisions. They continue straight between collisions and then strictly obey the laws of conservation of energy and conservation of momentum during the collisions. If we could observe the individual sequence of moves of each molecule in a system and if a particular sequence had particular significance, for instance because it led to a kind of replication or evolution, then we might perceive that combination of moves as having more order than some other combination. Entropy is independent of our perception of order in the system, i.e., the amount of heat a system holds for a given temperature does not change based on our perception of order. Entropy, like pressure and temperature is an independent thermodynamic property of the system that does not depend on our observation.

Keywords: Complexity, Chaos, Cancer hallmarks, Emergent properties, Entropy, Epistemological reductionism, Fractal, Laws of thermodynamics, Methodological reductionism, Ontological reductionism, Phase transition, Statistical mechanics.

References

Ayala, F. and Th. Dobzhansky. 1974. Studies in the philosophy of biology. Macmilian, London and University of California Press.

Baranger, M. 2000. Chaos, Complexity and Entropy. New England Complex Systems Institutes, Cambridge 1–17.

Basan, M., T. Risler and J. Joanny. 2009. Homostatic competition drives tumor growth and metastasis nucleation. HFSP J. 3: 265–272.

Carew, J. and P. Huang. 2002. Mitochondrial defects in cancer. Molecular Cancer Biomed. Central I: 9: 1–12.

Crick, F. 1966. Molecules and man. University of Washington Press, Seattle p. 10.

Clausius, R. 1867. The Mechanical Theory of Heat. Taylor and Francis, London.

De Donder, Th. and P. Van Rysselberghe. 1936. Thermodynamic theory of affinity: A book of principles. Oxford University Press.

Dobzhansky, Th. 1969. On Cartesian and darwinian aspects of biology. pp. 165–178. *In*: Philosophy, Science and Method. Macmillan. New York, 1974.

Dokukin, M., N. Guz and R. Gaikwad. 2011. Cell surface as a fractal: normal and cancerous cervical cells demonstrate different fractal behavior of surface adhesion maps at the nanoscale. Physical Rev. Lett. 107: 028101-1-4.

Francis, H and C. Crick. 1966. Of molecular and man. Univ. of Washington Press. seattle, P. 10.

Frehland, E. 1982. Lecture notes on biomathematics: stochastic transport processes in discrete biological systems. Springer-Verlag.

Fuhrman, A., J. Staunton and V. Nadakumar. 2011. AFM stiffness nanotomography of normal, metaplastic and dysplastic human esophageal cells. Phys. Biol. 8: 015007.

Gibbs, W. 1876. The Equilibrium of Heterogeneous Substances. Transactions of the Connecticut Academy of Arts and Sciences 3: 108–408.

Haken, H. 1978. Synergetics: An Introduction: Non-equilibrium Phase Transitions and Self-Organization in Physics, Chemistry and Biology. 2nd edition, Springer-Verlag, Berlin.

Hanahan, D. and R. Weinberg. 2000. The hallmarks of cancer. Cell 100: 57–70.

Hilborn, R. 2009. Chaos and Non-Linear Dynamics. Oxford University Press, Oxford.

Jacob, F. 1974. The logic of living systems: a history of heredity. Nature 326: 555–55a.

Khosroshahi, M.E. 2011. Characterization and evaluation of surface modified titanium alloy by long Nd: YAG laser for orthopaedic applications: An *in-vivo* study, (Chapter 8) in Biomedical Engineering Trends in Material Science., Intech Publisher, Croatia.

Khosroshahi, M.E. and M. Mahmoodi. 2009. Fundamentals of biomedical applications of lasers Induced surface modification of titanium alloys. (Chapter 1) in Titanium Alloys Preparation, Properties and Applications. NOVA Publisher, USA.

Kitano, H. 2003. Cancer robustness: tumor tactics. Nature 426: 125–131.

Kitano, H. 2004. Cancer as robust system: Implications for anticancer therapy. Nature Review Cancer 4: 227–235.

Klevecz, R., C. Li, I. Marcus and P. Frankel. 2008. Collective behavior in gene regulation: the cell is an oscillator, the cell cycle a development process. FEBS J 275: 2372–2384.

Lowrie, W. 1997. Fundamentals of Geophysics. Cambridge University Press.

Ma, S. 1976. Modern Theory of Critical Phenomena reading, Mass: W.A. Benjamin. Advanced Book Program.

MacCauley, J. 1993. Chaos, Dynamics and Fractals: An Algorithmic Approach to Deterministic Chaos. Cambridge University Press, p. xxi.

Mandelbrot, B. 1998. Letters: Is nature fractal. Science 279: 785–786.

Meakin, P. 1998. Fractals, Scaling and Growth far from Equilibrium. Cambridge University Press, p. xiv.

Molnár, J. and B. Thornton. 2009. Thermodynamics and electrobiologic prospects for therapies to intervene in cancer progression. Current Cancer Therapy Rev. 5: 158–169.

Navin, N., A. Kranitz and L. Rodgers. 2010. Inferring tumor progression from genomic heterogeneity. Genome Res. 20: 68–80.

Norton, L. 2005. Conceptual and practical implications of breast tissue geometry: toward a more effective, less toxic therapy. Oncologist 10: 370–381.

Novikoff, A. 1945. The concept of integrative levels and biology. Science 101: 209–15.

Nunney, L. 1999. Lineage selection and the evolution of multistage carcinogenesis. Proc. Biol. Sci. 266: 493–498.

Prigogine, I. and Nikolis, G. 1971. Biological order, structure and instability. Quarterly Review of Biophysics 4: 107–148.

Prigogine, I., G. Nikolis and A. Babloyantz. 1972. Thermodynamics of evolution (I). Physics Today 25: 23–28.

Prigogine, I. 1980. From being to becoming: time and complexity in the physical sciences. San Francisco: W.H. Freeman.

Rubin, A. 2014. Thermodynamics of irreversible processes in biological systems near equilibrium. Fundamentals of Biophysics. Wiley Online Library.

Sedivy, R. and R. Mader. 1997. Fractals, chaos, and cancer: Do they coincide? Cancer Investigation 15: 601–607.

Van Ness, H. 1969. Understanding thermodynamics. McGraw-Hill Book Company, New York.

Watson, J. and F. Crick. 1953. Molecular structure of nucleic acids: A structure for DNA. Nature 171: 737–738.

Wolform, C., N. Chau, J. Maigne and J. Lambert. 2000. Evidence for deterministic chaos in aperiodic oscillations of proliferative activity in long-term cultured Fao hepatoma cells. J. Cell Sci. 113: 1069–1074.

Waliszewski, P. 2016. The quantitative criteria based on the fractal dimensions, entropy and lacunarity for the spatial distribution of cancer cell nuclei enable identification of low or high aggressive prostate carcinomas. Frontiers in Physiology 1–6.

6

Biophotonics

6.1 Some definitions

The term *biophotonics* represents a combination of *biology* and *photonics,* where photonics in turn is the combination of *photons* and *electronics*, which deals with the science and technology of generation, manipulation, and detection of photons. Photons play a central role in information technologies, such as fiber optics, the way electrons do in electronics. Photonics includes optical and non-optical technologies that deal with electromagnetic radiation. Therefore, biophotonics can be described as the development and application of optical techniques, such as imaging, to the study of biological molecules, cells, and tissue. One of the main benefits of using optical techniques is that they preserve the integrity of the biological cells being examined. Biophotonics has become the established general term for all techniques that deal with the interaction of photons with biological systems. This refers to absorption, emission, detection, and creation of radiation from biomolecular cells, tissues, organisms, and biomaterials. Areas of application are life science, medicine, agriculture, and environmental science. There are other terms with some differences and similarities between them, which ought to be defined more carefully: *biomedical photonics* and *biomedical optics*. The field of optics, in general, involves 'optical' light or 'visible' light (400 nm–750 nm), which covers only about 10 percent of the whole electromagnetic spectrum. *Biomedical photonics*, which is the application of photonics as defined above in biomedical science and technology, employs the use of entire range of electromagnetic spectrum. Figure 6.1 schematically describes the inter-relation between these areas.

6.2 Fundamentals of tissue optical properties and light transport

6.2.1 Tissue structure

It is well known that in medical applications, a laser can be used to produce a variety of effects such as photochemical, coagulation, vaporization, and ablation, which is discussed in detail in §6.3. Therefore, the optical properties of tissue are of prime importance to be taken into account when analyzing the laser-tissue interaction, mainly because the properties are closely related to optical parameters, such as wavelength, pulse duration, power density, etc. Optical properties not only depend on tissue composition, but are also related to the microscopic structure of the tissue as well. Thus, any change in the tissue composition or structure could alter the optical properties (Duck 1990).

Human skin is a uniquely engineered organ that allows life cycle by regulating heat and water loss from the body whilst preventing it from noxious chemicals or microorganisms. Skin membranes can be examined at various levels of complexity, and more information about the degree of complexity itself can be obtained by examining the structures and functions of the membrane. With regard to transdermal drug delivery, the membrane can be considered a simple physical barrier, while for bioimaging applications, the skin components play a major limitation. Figure 6.2 demonstrates the skin tissue structure.

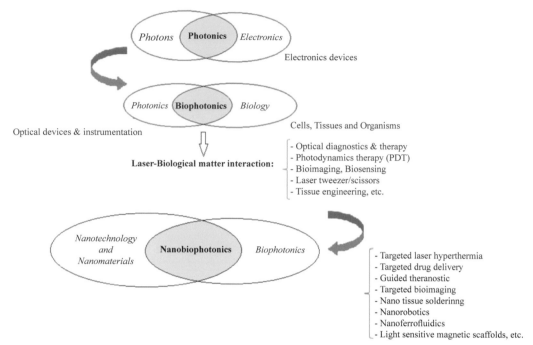

Figure 6.1. Basic illustration of photonics and biophotonics with examples of devices and biomedical applications.

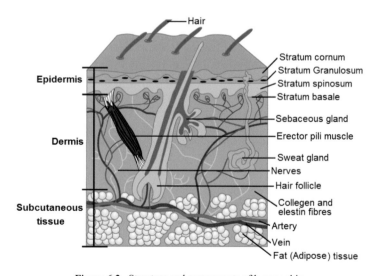

Figure 6.2. Structure and components of human skin.

Epidermis (i.e., the outermost layer): This layer forms the waterproof, protective wrap over the body's surface, which also serves as a barrier to infection. Epidermis is a complex multiply layered membrane with thickness varying between 0.06 mm on the eyelids to 0.8 mm on the palm and soles of the feet. This layer does not contain blood vessels, and hence nutrients and waste products must diffuse across dermo-epidermal layer in order to maintain tissue integrity. The cells in the deepest layers are nourished almost exclusively by diffused oxygen from the surrounding air, and to a far lesser degree by blood capillaries extending to the upper layers of the dermis. The main type of constituting cells are Merkel cells, keratinocytes, with melanocytes, and Langerhans cells.

Stratum corneum: This layer comprises of dead cells providing the main barrier to transdermal drug delivery of drugs. This layer typically comprises only 10 to 15 cell layers and is around 10 μm thick when dry, but may swell to several times thicker when wet. This layer regulates water loss from the body whilst preventing the entry of harmful materals, including microorganisms. The barrier nature of the stratum corneum depends critically on its unique constituents; 75–80% is protein, 5–15% lipid with 5–10% unidentified on a dry weight basis. The protein is located primarily within the keratinocytes: 70% alpha-keratin; 10% beta-keratin; 5% proteinaceous cell envelope; and 15% enzyme and other proteins. In addition to the keratinocytes and lipid lamellae, water plays a major role in maintaining stratum corneum barrier integrity. Water is also a plasticizer, and thus prevents the layer from cracking due to mechanical damage.

Stratum granulosum: This layer is only one to three cell layers thick, containing enzymes that begin degradation of the viable cell components, such as the nuclei and organells.

Stratum spinosum: This layer consists of two to six rows of keratinocytes that change morphology from columnar to polygonal cells. Within this layer the keratinocytes begin to differentiate and synthesize keratins that aggregate to form tonofilaments. The cell membranes of adjacent keratinocytes are connected by desmosomes, which is also responsible for maintaining a distance of about 20 nm between the cells.

Stratum basale: The cells which are metabolically active are similar to other tissues within the body containing organells such as mitochondria and ribosomes. In addition to keratinocytes, the stratum basale contains other cell types. Melanocytes synthesize the pigment melanin from tyrosine. There are two forms of melanin: eumelanin, which is more black/brown form, and phaeomelanin, which is red or yellow. Melanins provide an energy pathway within the skin where they absorb ultraviolet (UV) radiation, and are free radical scavengers. Despite equal number of melanocytes in a given body, darker-skinned people have more active and efficient melanocytes. Other cells found within the basale layers are Langerhans and Merkel cells, where the former are recognized as the antigen-presenting cells of the skin which readily bind to the cell surfaces, and the latter associated with nerve ending, found on the dermal side of the basement membrane, and it seems they have a role in cutaneous sensation.

Dermis is typically 3–5 mm thick, and is the major component of human skin. It is composed of a network of connective tissue, predominantly collagen fibrils, providing support and elastic tissue providing flexibility, embedded in a mucopolysaccharide gel. This layer causes a minimum physical barrier when considering transdermal drug delivery, as it essentially contains gelled water, however, it can be a serious problem if delivering highly lipophilic molecules. The extensive vasculture of the skin is essential for regulation of body temperature, as well as delivering oxygen and nutrients to the tissue. The vasculture is also important in wound healing and repair, as will be discussed in Chapter 14. The blood flow around 0.05 mL/min per mg of skin is very efficient for the removal of molecules that have traversed the outer skin layers and are influenced by shunt route transport.

6.2.2 Tissue optical properties

Figure 6.3 illustrates a typical light-matter interaction situation where in principle, five main optical effects can occur: Reflection, refraction, absorption, scattering, and transmission.

Normally during the interaction process, one may use the wave theory to study the energy propagation in a medium or the particle theory for interaction of photons with material. The amount of reflection and refraction depends on the refractive index of the medium and the absorption coefficient, $\alpha(cm^{-1})$ depends on the medium, the wavelength, and intensity of beam. The type of reflection also depends on the quality of the tissue surface, where a smoother surface will show more *specular* reflection (i.e., the angle of reflection is close to angle of incident), and a more irregular surface will suffer from *diffuse* reflection (i.e., the angle of reflection deviates from the angle of incident).

Refractive index (n): This describes how light propagates in the medium, and is defined as $n = c/V_m$ where V_m is the phase velocity of light in the medium and c is the speed of light. Any changes in n, either continuous or abrupt, produces reflection, refraction, and scattering. Since tissues are heterogeneous in composition, so one may be interested to know about the refractive indices of constituents or an averaged

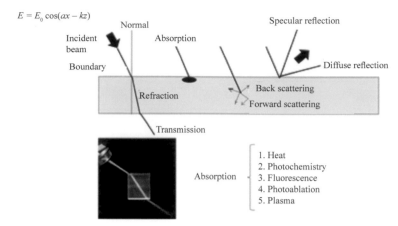

Figure 6.3. Geometrical representation of light-tissue interaction effects.

value for the tissue as a whole. Water makes up a significant portion of most tissues, with (n = 1.33), which represents the minimum value for soft-tissue constituents. Other soft-tissue components are melanin particles mainly found in the epidermal layer of the skin with n = 1.6. Whole tissues such as brain, lung, kidney, bladder, etc. cover a range of 1.36–1.40. Extracellular fluids and intercellular cytoplasm have a value between 1.35–1.38, and for fatty tissues it is about 1.45. The membranes that enclose cells and subcellular organells is the origin of scattering in cellular tissues.

When light passes through a medium, some part of it will always be attenuated. This can be conveniently taken into account by defining a complex refractive index,

$$\underline{n} = n + ik \tag{6.1}$$

Here, n is the real part of the refractive index and indicates the phase velocity, while k is the imaginary part called the extinction coefficient, which indicates the amount of attenuation when the electromagnetic wave propagates through the material. The complex wave number $\underline{k}$ is related to the complex refractive index $\underline{n}$ through $\underline{k} = 2\pi\underline{n}/\lambda_0$ where λ_0 is the vacuum wavelength. This can be inserted into the plane wave expression as

$$E(z,t) = \mathrm{Re}\,[E_0 e^{i\,(kz-\omega t)}] \tag{6.2a}$$

$$E(z,t) = \mathrm{Re}[E_0 e^{i\,2\pi\,(n+ik)z/(\lambda_0-\omega t)}] \tag{6.2b}$$

$$E(z,t) = e^{-i\,2\pi kz/\lambda_0}\,\mathrm{Re}\,[E_0 e^{i(kz-\omega t)}] \tag{6.2c}$$

We see that k gives an exponential decay as expected from the Beer–Lambert law. Since intensity is proportional to the square of the electric field, $|E|^2$, it will depend on the depth into the material as $\exp(-4\pi kz/\lambda_0)$ and the attenuation coefficient becomes $\alpha = 4\pi k/\lambda_0$. This also relates it to the penetration depth or *absorption mean free path*, δ_a, the distance after which the intensity is reduced by 1/e ($\approx$ 37%), $\delta_a = 1/\alpha = \lambda_0/(4\pi k)$. Both n and k are dependent on the frequency. In most circumstances k > 0 (light is absorbed) or k = 0 (light travels without loss).

Reflection/refraction: When a light wave propagates in a medium with a given refractive index, it can possibly encounter other components with different refractive indices, which causes the light to deviate from its path. If the width of the light beam is small compared to the dimension of boundary or its curvature, reflection and refractive transmission may occur. The amount of light reflected by the transmission through a boundary depends on the refractive indices of the two materials, the angle of incidence, and the polarization of the incoming wave.

$$\sin \theta_2 = \frac{n_1}{n_2}\sin \theta_1 \tag{6.3}$$

For normal incidence onto a planner boundary, the refraction of the incident energy that is transmitted across its interface is given by

$$T = \frac{4n_1 n_2}{(n_1 + n_2)^2} \tag{6.4}$$

This reflection from the interface is known as Fresnel reflection and is distinct from the diffuse.

Absorption: The ability of light to penetrate tissue depends on how strongly it is absorbed by the tissue, which in turn depends on number of factors, mainly the electronic constitution of its atoms and molecules, and the wavelength of light. The inverse of absorption coefficient gives the value of optical penetration depth or absorption depth. As the laser beam passes through the medium, it will be absorbed according to Beer-Lambert's law, $I = I_0 e^{-\alpha z}$ which is due to various intercellular as well as extracellular constituents of the tissue. After the absorption, the light can appear within tissue as heat, photochemistry, fluorescence, photoablation, or ionization (plasma), as can be seen in Fig. 6.3. Now let us start with considering the effects of tissue properties on the light behaviour within tissue. The manner in which the radiation is absorbed is explained as follows. When the beam passes over a small elastically bound charged particle, the particle will be set into motion by the electric force of the electric field. Provided that the frequency of the radiation does not correspond to a natural resonance frequency of the particle, then fluorescence or absorption will not occur, but a forced vibration would be initiated. The force induced by the electric field is very small and is incapable of vibrating an atomic nucleus. We are therefore discussing photons interacting with electrons which are either free or bound. This process of photon being absorbed by electrons is known as the "inverse bremsstrahlung effect". (The bremsstrahlung effect is the emission of photons from excited electrons.) As the electron vibrates, it will either re-radiate in all directions, or be restrained by the lattice phonons (the bonding energy within a sold or liquid structure). In the latter case, the phonons will cause the structure to vibrate, and this vibration will be transmitted through the structure by the normal diffusion type processes due to the linking of the molecules of the structure; the vibrations in the structure we detect as heat. The biomedical applications of absorption are: *Diagnostic*, where transitions between two energy levels of molecule can provide some spectral information about the molecules such as fluorescence spectroscopy about diseased tissue, and *therapeutic*, where absorption of energy is the primary mechanism that permits light from a laser to produce physical effects on tissue for treatment purposes. 'Therapeutic window' is the term given to the spectral range (600–1300 nm), where most tissue are sufficiently weak absorbers to permit significant penetration of light, as we can see from Fig. 6.4.

At the short-wavelength end, the window is bound by the absorption of hemoglobin in both its oxygenated and deoxygenated forms. At shorter wavelengths, many absorbing biomolecules become important, including DNA and the amino acids tryptophan and tyrosine. At the IR end of the window, penetration is limited by the absorption of water. The volume fraction of blood in typical tissues is in the range of 1–5%, so the average absorption due to hemoglobin in a tissue is about 20–100 fold lower than that of the whole blood. Within the therapeutic window, scattering is dominant over absorption, and so the propagating light becomes diffused. Consider, for example, the oxygenated molecule. The size of the molecule is about 6.8 nm in diameter, so the cross-sectional area $= 3.6 \times 10^{-13}$ cm^{-2}, but the porphyrin ring, the active site of the absorption, is about 1 nm in diameter giving an area of 0.8910^{-15} cm^{-2}. The extinction coefficient for 805 nm is 0.8910^3 cm^{-1} M^{-1} (Wray 1988). Therefore, the effective cross sectional area σ_a of absorber is

$$\sigma_a = \frac{0.89 \times 13^3 \,\text{cm}^{-1}}{\text{mols/lit}} \frac{1000 \,\text{cm}^3}{\text{lit}} \frac{1 \,\text{mole}}{6.0 \times 10^{23} \,\text{molecules}} = 1.5 \times 10^{-18} \,\text{cm}^{-2}/\text{molecule}$$

Therefore, the effective cross area is much smaller than the actual geometrical cross sectional area, i.e., $\sigma_a \ll A_a$. Now, the efficiency factor $Q_a = \sigma_a / A_a = 1.9 \times 10^{-4}$. At 415 nm, the extinction coefficient, k, is about 4.4×10^{-5} cm^{-1} M^{-1}, which yields a value of $\sigma_a = 7.3 \times 10^{-16}$ cm^{-2} and $Q_a = 0.092$.

For a localized absorber, the absorption cross section σ_a can be defined as

$$\sigma_a = \frac{P_a}{I_0} \tag{6.5}$$

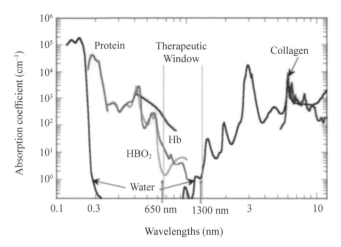

Figure 6.4. Absorption spectra of major constituents of skin and blood with therapeutic window between 650–1300 nm.

where P_a is the amount of laser power absorbed. σ_a makes an approximation that the cross section is independent of the reactive orientation of the impinging light and the absorber. A medium with a uniform distribution of identical absorbing particles can be characterized by the absorption coefficient, α

$$\alpha = \rho_a \sigma_a \tag{6.6}$$

where ρ_a is the number density of absorbers. As stated above, the reciprocal of absorption coefficient provides the optical penetration depth. Figure 6.5 shows a diagram of the various medical laser wavelengths penetration depths inside skin.

Scattering: This occurs when there is a spatial variation in the refractive index. The scatterers are the subcellular organells with dimensions approximately between 100 nm and 6 μm. Most of these scatterers fall in the Mie region, exhibiting anisotropic forward-directed scattering patterns. The mitochondria with sizes of 0.5–2 μm are the dominant scatterers among the organells. The lipid folds inside mitochondria structure gives them a high optical contrast to the surrounding cytoplasm, hence producing a strong scattering effects. The largest of the cellular organells is the cell nucleus with a diameter of about 4–6 μm. The cell varies in shape and size among different tissue types with dimensions of a few microns and larger. An isolated cell can be a strong scatterer, but within the tissue the scattering is largely of a subcellular origin. Normal whole blood consists of about 55 vol% plasma (90% water, 10% proteins: albumin, globulin, fibrinogen, waste substances, minerals (Na, Ca, K, Cl)), 45 vol% cells (99% red blood cells-RBCs or erythrocytes), and 1% white blood cells (WBCs; leukocytes and thrombocytes). A normal RBC is mainly characterized by a flat bioconcave shape with volume, surface area, and diameter ranging from 80–108 μm^3, 119–151 μm^2 and 7–8 μm, respectively. The RBC membrane contains proteins and glycoproteins embedded in, or attached to, a fluid lipid bilayer that gives it a viscoelastic behaviour. The RBC protein is almost entirely hemoglobin, while roughly 60% of the total plasma protein is albumin. The normal range of RBCs is about 4.32–5.66$10^{12}$ cells/L in men and 3.88–4.99$10^{12}$ cells/L in women. Total hemoglobin concentration in whole blood ranges from 13.3–16.7 g/dL for men, and 11.8–14.8 g/dL for women. The hematocrit is the volume fraction of cells within the whole blood volume and ranges between ≈ 37%–49% under physiological conditions. Therefore, the scattering properties of blood are dependent on the haematocrit (i.e., volume fraction of RBC).

Tissue cells and extracellular proteins such as elastin, collagen, and elastin provide mechanical strength and durability. The scattering properties of these tissues are subject to small-scale inhomogeneities and large-scale variations in the structures they form. Similar to absorption, scattering also has some important biomedical applications in both diagnostic and therapeutic: *Diagnostic*: Scattering depends on the size, morphology, and structure of the components in tissue (e.g., lipid membrane, nuclei, collagen fibres). Variations in these components due to disease would affect scattering properties, hence providing

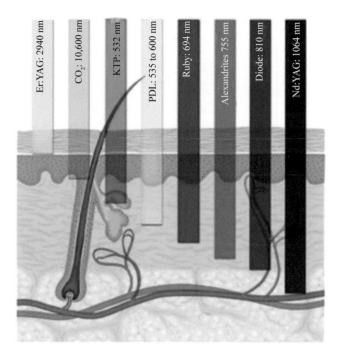

Figure 6.5. Penetration depth of different laser wavelengths in human skin, starting from Er:YAG laser as minimum depth to Nd:YAG laser as highest.

a means for diagnostic purposes, particularly in imaging applications. *Therapeutic*: Scattering signals can be used to determine optimal light dosimetry and provide useful feedback during therapy. In principle, given the refractive indices of the two materials and the size and shape of the scatterer, the radiation can be calculated. When a monochromatic plane wave that has an intensity interacts with the scattering object, some of the beam power will be redirected, i.e., scattered. The ratio of scattered power to the incident intensity is called *scattering cross section*.

$$\sigma_s(\hat{s}) = \frac{P_s}{I_0} \tag{6.7}$$

where $\hat{s}$ is the propagation direction of the plane wave relative to the scatterer. The scattering cross section has units of area. Note that scattering depends on the polarization of the incoming wave, but we can assume the Eq. (6.7) as an average over the orthogonal polarization states. The angular distribution of the scattered radiation is given by the differential cross section

$$\frac{d\sigma_s}{d\Omega}(\hat{s},\hat{s}') \tag{6.8}$$

where $\hat{s}'$ represents the axis of a cone solid angle $d\Omega$ originating at the scatterer. Assuming the scattering cross section is independent of the relative orientation of the incident light and the scatterer, i.e., it is a spherically symmetric object, then the scattering cross section at a given wavelength is

$$\sigma_s(\hat{s}) = \sigma_s \tag{6.9}$$

   A medium containing uniform distribution of identical scatterers is characterized by scattering coefficient $\beta(cm^{-1})$

$$\beta = \rho_s \sigma_s \tag{6.10}$$

where ρ_s is the number density of scatterers. The *scattering mean free*, δ_s, path represents the average distance a photon travels between consecutive scattering events

$$\delta_s = \frac{1}{\beta} \tag{6.11}$$

In biological tissues, scattering interactions are often dominant mechanisms affecting the light propagation. The scattering is divided into three categories defined by the size of the scattering object relative to the wavelength of light (Saidi et al. 1995):

1) The *Rayleigh* limit, where the size of the scatterer, ϕ_s, is smaller than light wavelength (i.e., $\phi_s < \lambda$) and the scattering varies with fourth power of the wavelength of the illuminating light. Those structures include cellular components, such as membrane and cell subcomponents, and extracellular components, such as the ultrastructure of collagen fibrils. In the classical description (i.e., e.m.w.), this condition produces a dipole moment in the scatterer, a spatially redistribution of the charges in the scatterer. This dipole moment oscillates in time with the frequency of the incident light field and consequently generates dipole radiation. However, in the quantum picture, Rayleigh scattering is called 'elastic', because the charged particles in a medium are set into oscillatory motion by the electric field of the incident light and re-emit light of the same frequency as the incident, i.e., the energy of the scattered photon is same as the incident photon. In contrast, in an 'inelastic' scattering, the energy is changed. For example, in Raman scattering, the frequencies of scattered photons are shifted from the incident frequency by amounts that are characteristic of molecular transitions, normally between vibrational energy states. The term inelastic refers to the case where the scattered photons either lose energy to Stokes, or gain energy from (anti-Stokes) the molecules. Raman scattering is very small compared to Rayleigh scattering (roughly 1 Raman-shifted photon for every 10^6 Rayleigh photons).

2) The *Mie regime*, where the size of the scatterer is comparable or larger than the light wavelength ($\phi_s \approx \lambda$). Various cellular structures, such as mitochondria and nuclei, and extracellular components like collagen fibers, have sizes on the order of hundreds of nanometers to a few micrometers, comparable to laser wavelengths between 500–1000 nm.

3) The *geometric limit*, where the size of scatterer is much larger than the wavelength ($\phi_s \gg \lambda$).

   Single scattering: In the case of single scattering, a new exponential relationship can be defined for the collimated beam intensity I, relative to the incident intensity I_0, and a transmitted distance z through an absorbing medium as

   $$I(r,z) = I_0(r,z)e^{\gamma} \tag{6.12}$$

   where $\gamma = \alpha + \beta$ is total attenuation coefficient (cm^{-1}) and γ^{-1} which is known as mean free path gives the distance travelled by a photon between interaction. There are two cases:

   a) *Homogeneous medium* ($\beta = 0$)

   $$I(r, z) = I_0(r, z) \cdot e^{-\alpha z} \tag{6.13}$$

   and the amount of heat deposited per unit volume after photons absorption is

   $$Q(r, t) = I \alpha(r, z) \ (Wcm^{-3}) \tag{6.14}$$

   b) *Inhomogeneous medium* ($\beta \neq 0$)

   $$I(r, z) = I_0(r, z) \cdot e^{-(\alpha + \beta)z} \tag{6.15}$$

   $$Q(r, t) = I \alpha(r, z) + I \beta(r, z) \tag{6.16}$$

   For a beam width with Gaussian profile,

   $$I(r, z) = I_0(r, z) \cdot e^{-2r^2/w^2} \tag{6.17}$$

   $$I(r, z) = I_0(r, z) \cdot e^{-2r^2/w^2} \cdot e^{-(\alpha + \beta)z} \tag{6.18}$$

where, r is the radial distance from the interaction point and w is the beam width. Figure 6.6 represents the distribution of beam intensity within tissue after interaction, (a) and the corresponding beam profile (b). As the laser intensity propagates through the tissue, its amplitude is exponentially reduced and similarly, during this process heat is lost to the surrounding and the temperature is gradually decreased.

As mentioned before, on encountering a scattering particle within a homogeneous medium, photons travelling in a direction $\hat{s}$ are scattered into a new direction $\hat{s}'$. The new directions generally do not occur with equal probability, and can be decreased by the differential scattering coefficient, $d\beta$ $(\hat{s},\hat{s}')$. Integrating over all angles gives β, the total scattering coefficient

$$\beta = \int_{4\pi} d\beta(\hat{s},\hat{s}')\, d\hat{s}' \qquad (6.19)$$

Here it is assumed that the scattering coefficient is independent of the original direction $\hat{s}$ of the photons, and that it depends only on the scattering angle between the incident and scattered photons. This may hold true for randomly structured media, but many media have orientation-dependent structure and the scattered intensity distribution will therefore, depend on the incident direction. The scattered phase function p is the normalized version of the differential scattering coefficient

$$p(\hat{s},\hat{s}') = \frac{1}{\beta} d\beta\, (\hat{s},\hat{s}') \qquad (6.20)$$

such that $\int_{4\pi} p(\hat{s},\hat{s}')\, d\hat{s}' = 1$. The mean cosine g of the scattering angle θ, the angle between the incident $\hat{s}$, and new scattered $\hat{s}'$ directions is known as anisotropy factor

$$g = \int_{4\pi} p(\theta) \cos(\theta)\, d\hat{s}' \qquad (6.21)$$

If the scattering is completely isotropic, then p is equal for all angles and g = 0. For tissues, g ranges from 0.4 to 0.99, which indicates that scattering is strongly forward directed. The g parameter is in fact a measure of scattered retained in forward direction following a scattering event. For a Rayleigh scatterer, the scattering phase function varies as $1+\cos^2\theta = 1+(\hat{s}\cdot\hat{s}')^2$, where $p(\hat{s}\cdot\hat{s}')$ describes the fraction of light energy incident on the scatterer from the $\hat{s}'$ direction that gets scattered in the $\hat{s}'$ direction. As the particle size increases, however, the intensity distributions increases in the forward direction, and p for small angles is much higher than for all other angles. Therefore, the mean cosine tends towards a value of unity, the higher the g value, the more forward-peaked the scattering. *Reduced scattering* is defined as combining the scattering coefficient and anisotropy factors, which takes in to account that the anisotropy of the scattering has an impact on the effective attenuation of light due to scattering.

$$\beta' = (1-g)\beta \qquad (6.22)$$

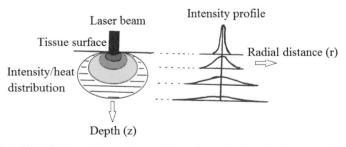

Figure 6.6. Distribution of laser intensity or temperature at the surface and within the tissue sample. The curve widens and the peak intensity/temperature decreases with time and distance.

It follows for the transport attenuation coefficient $\gamma' = \alpha + \beta'$ and $1/\gamma'$ represents the transport mean free path. Most of the scattering processes of interest in tissue optics are in Mie limit and the phase function can be difficult to calculate without detailed knowledge of the system. Normally, an approximation known as Henyey-Greenstein function is used for this purpose defined as

$$P_{HG} = (\cos\theta) = \frac{4\pi\sigma_s}{\sigma_a + \sigma_s} \frac{1 - g^2}{(1 + g^2 - 2g\cos\theta)^{3/2}} \tag{6.23}$$

Henyey-Greenstein function describes the angular dependence of light scattering by small particles.

Multiple scattering: Now let us consider a medium with a uniform distribution of scatterer, each with σ_s and ρ_s as defined before. The medium can be imagined as a number of layers with thickness Δz, and the field incident onto the first layer is a plane wave with intensity I_0. Figure 6.7 illustrates such a medium, where after a multiple scattering, photons are deviated from their main path and continuous with their *random walk* within the tissue.

The power incident on a local region of the layer with cross-sectional area A is $I_0 A$. The power scattered out of the wave as it crosses it is

$$I_0\rho_s\sigma_s A\Delta z = I_0\beta \, A\Delta z = I_0\sigma_s N_{layer} \tag{6.24}$$

where N_{layer} is the number of scatter encountered in the layer. After passing through the layer, the power remaining in the wave is

$$P_r = I_0 A - I_0\rho_s\sigma_s A\Delta z = I_0 A(1 - \sigma_s\Delta z) \tag{6.25}$$

When $\sigma_s A\Delta z = 1$ for a layer, the effect saturates, i.e., there is no further physical effect by increasing this quantity. The light intensity is decreased by an amount $(1 - \sigma_s A\Delta z)$ as it passes through each layer, and if the total number of layers is N_L then the total distance (depth) traveled Z is $Z = N_L \Delta z$, then

$$P_r(N_L) = I_0 A (1 - \rho_s\sigma_s\Delta z)^{N_L} = I_0 A(1 - \sigma_s\rho_s\frac{Z}{N_L}) \tag{6.26}$$

As N_L increases, Eq. (6.26) converges to an exponential and because there is no absorption $(\alpha = 0)$, the total power in the scattered field is defined by

$$P_{total} = I_0 A (1 - e^{\rho_s\sigma_s Z}) = I_0 A(1 - e^{[\frac{\sigma_s}{A}N_s]}) \tag{6.27}$$

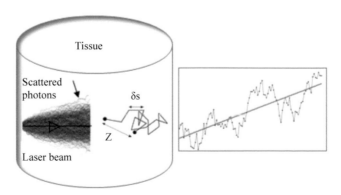

Figure 6.7. Illustration of photons random walk (i.e., mean free path) as a result of multiple scattering within tissue. Thus, photons deviate from the main optical path covering a wider angular distribution.

where N_s is the total number of scatterers encountered in the medium. The quantity $\rho_s \sigma_s Z$ is proportional to the number of scatterers encountered along the entire path from 0 to Z. Since $\rho_s \sigma_s Z = \frac{\sigma_s}{A} N_s$ when $\rho_s \sigma_s Z \ll 1$ then the scattered power can be approximately

$$P_{total} \approx I_0 \sigma_s N_s \tag{6.28}$$

Therefore, the power is proportional to the number of scatterers. Physically, it is like saying that the scattered power is completely due to waves that have scattered. However, an extra care should be taken into account when the approximation

$$1 - e^{\rho_s \sigma_s Z} \approx \rho_s \sigma_s Z \tag{6.29}$$

breaksdown, since it may become nonlinear relationship with N_s and thus, the power contained in number of scattered waves becomes significant. Therefore, the criterion for defining a system as a single scattering medium is

$$\rho_s \sigma_s Z \ll 1 \quad \text{or} \quad \beta Z \ll 1 \tag{6.30}$$

The importance of multi-scattering effect is in providing the mechanism for *'decohering'* the scattered field and eventually justify the use of radiation theory (RT) in which coherence processes are not rally playing the main role during an interaction.

6.2.3 Light transport in tissue

Optical propagation or diffusion in strongly scattering media is of prime importance in several fields including biomedical and has been extensively studied (Welch et al. 1987), (Jacques and Prahl 1987), (Arnfield et al. 1988), (Patterson et al. 1989), (Tromberg et al. 1993), and (Chan et al. 2005). Most human tissues are considered turbid, which are heterogeneous structures and correspondingly have spatial variations in their optical properties. The spatial variation and density of these fluctuations make these tissues strong scatterers of light. As seen in Fig. 6.7, a significant fraction of the photons' encounters with these tissues are scattered multiple times, causing a diffused and largely incoherent field of penetrating beam. The transport of radiant energy in a medium containing uniformly distributed scattering and absorbing particles is governed by an integro-differential known as the equation of transfer. The relationship between light scattering and cellular structure can also be studied by the spatial variation in the refractive index on a microscopic level. The phase shift $\Delta\varphi$ of an incident wave on passing through a tissue is related to the difference in refractive index Δn between the tissue and the surrounding medium.

$$\Delta\varphi = \frac{2\pi Z \Delta n}{\lambda} \tag{6.31}$$

where Z is the thickness of tissue and λ is the laser wavelength. Light propagating through tissue can be classified into types: coherent and incoherent. Coherency refers to the ability of a light field to maintain a definite, i.e., nonrandom phase relationship in space and time and exhibit stable interference effects. Speckle patterns are such examples which occur when laser light is reflected from a rough surface or when coherent light passes through a scattering medium. On the other hand, an incoherent source such as flash lamp, LEDs exhibit random patterns both temporally and spatially and thus, is not capable of producing stable or observable interference effects. In tissues, light that is scattered many times can exhibit coherent and incoherent properties, as discussed in Chapter 2. A more suitable description is one in which the wave like behaviour of light is ignored and the transport of individual photons, which can be absorbed or scattered, is considered. The fundamental equation describing in the RT model is the radiation transport equation (known as Boltzmann equation), which describes the basic dynamics of the intensity. Light is specifically treated as a collection of localized incoherent photons. Let us suppose a photon energy defined by its position $\mathbf{r}(t)$ and the direction of propagation $\hat{s}$. As the photon propagates in space over the time interval dt, it loses energy due to absorption and scattering out of $\hat{s}$, but also gains energy from light scattered into ŝ-directed photon from other directions and from local source of the light at **r** (t). The general RT equation is (Chantrasekhar 1960)

$$\frac{1}{c_m}\frac{\partial I(r,\hat{s},t)}{\partial t} + \hat{s}.\nabla L(r,\hat{s},t) = -\gamma I(r,\hat{s},t) + \frac{\gamma}{4\pi}\int_{4\pi} p(\hat{s},\hat{s}')\, I(r,\hat{s},t)d\Omega' + Q(r,\hat{s},t) \tag{6.32}$$

where c_m (ms^{-1}) is the velocity of light in the medium, I (Wm^{-2}) is intensity, sometimes also called fluence rate or irradiance, L (Wcm^{-2} sr^{-1}) is the energy radiance, $\gamma = \alpha + \beta$ is total attenuation, $\Omega = A/r^2$ is the solid angle (steradian, sr), A and r are the area and radius of sphere respectively, Q is the source term. The dynamics of intensity is interpreted through the change in I(r,ŝ,t) with time, i.e., the intensity will increase with time if the spatial derivative in the direction is decreasing, so it will flow from high intensity region to low intensity. The decrease of $-\gamma I(r,\hat{s},t)$ in Eq. (6.29) will always cause a decrease of I(r,ŝ,t) to account for the scattering and absorption losses. The intensity is related to energy radiance as follows (Tromberg et al. 1993)

$$I(r,t) = \int_{4\pi} L(r,\hat{s},t)\, d\Omega \tag{6.33}$$

The steady-state RT equation in a source-free region is written as

$$\hat{s}.\nabla L(r,\hat{s},t) = -\gamma I(r,\hat{s}) + \frac{\gamma}{4\pi}\int_{4\pi} p(\hat{s},\hat{s}')\, I(r,\hat{s})d\Omega' \tag{6.34}$$

In the diffuse model, I(r,ŝ,t) can be divided into coherent, I_c and incoherent (diffuse), I_d terms

$$I(r,\hat{s},t) = I_c(r,\hat{s},t) + I_d(r,\hat{s},t) \tag{6.35}$$

But in tissue optics with regard to light transport, it is the diffused field which is the penetrating component of light, thus the determination of the intensity of the diffused field is the main objective. The diffusely reflected light within tissue after multiple scattering is different to a typical surface reflection in that it contains some information about the bulk of the mediums such as tissue, because it has collectively sampled an extended volume of the tissue. Thus, we can rewrite the Eq. (6.32)

$$\frac{1}{c_m}\frac{\partial I_d(r,\hat{s},t)}{\partial t} + \hat{s}.\nabla L(r,\hat{s},t) = -\gamma I_d(r,\hat{s},t) + \frac{\gamma}{4\pi}\int_{4\pi} p(\hat{s},\hat{s}')\, I_d(r,\hat{s},t)d\Omega'$$
$$+ \frac{\gamma}{4\pi}\int_{4\pi} p(\hat{s},\hat{s}')\, I_c(r,\hat{s},t)d\Omega' \tag{6.36}$$

where

$$Q(r,\hat{s},t) = \frac{\gamma}{4\pi}\int_{4\pi} p(\hat{s},\hat{s}')\, I_c(r,\hat{s},t)\, d\Omega' \tag{6.37}$$

or

$$\frac{1}{c_m}\frac{\partial I_d(r,\hat{s},t)}{\partial t} + \hat{s}.\nabla L(r,\hat{s},t) = -\gamma I_d(r,\hat{s},t) + \frac{\gamma}{4\pi}\int_{4\pi} p(\hat{s},\hat{s}')\, I_d(r,\hat{s},t)d\Omega' + Q(r,\hat{s},t) \tag{6.38}$$

Diffusion Approximation (Scattering dominant): When the absorption is sufficiently low to allow significant penetration of light into tissue, scattering becomes dominant transport process. This scattering-dominant limit is known as diffusion limit because photons are able to move through the tissue although scattering disperses the light randomly. The assumption made in the derivation of the diffusion equation are that the source and scattering within tissue are both isotropic. The time-dependent diffusion equation is

$$\frac{1}{c_m}\frac{\partial I(r,t)}{\partial t} - D\nabla^2 I(r,t) + \alpha I(r,t) = Q(r,t) \tag{6.39}$$

where D is the diffusion coefficient defined as

$$D = \frac{1}{3[\alpha + \beta(1-g)]} = \frac{1}{3[\alpha + \beta']} \tag{6.40}$$

$$\delta_0 = \sqrt{\frac{D}{\alpha}} \tag{6.41}$$

where $\beta' = \beta(1-g)$ is the transport scattering coefficient or 'reduced scattering', which explains the anisotropy of the scattering in an essentially isotropic model, and δ_0 is the optical penetration depth. The principle of similarity states that two media illuminated by a diffuse source will have similar photon distribution if the following conditions are met

$$\alpha_1 = \alpha_2 \text{ and } \beta_1(1-g_1) = \beta_2(1-g_2) \tag{6.42}$$

Therefore, the transport scattering coefficient effectively represents the isotropic medium, with $g = 0$, that gives an equivalent light distribution to an anisotropic medium of scattering coefficient β, and anisotropy factor g. Hence, by using g in this way, the diffusion approximation can model a 'linear anisotropy' that is applicable to biological media. Provided $\beta' > \alpha$, therefore, light can be considered to be propagating diffusely through a scattering medium beyond a depth from the surface, Z_θ, from the source. Consequently, $\Phi(r,t)$ exponentially decays with increasing depth into medium. The decay constant is known as the effective attenuation coefficient, γ_{eff}, and is predicted by diffusion theory to be

$$\gamma_{eff} = \sqrt{3\alpha\,(\alpha+\beta')} \tag{6.43}$$

The time-resolved solution to Eq. (6.35) is

$$I(r,t) = \frac{E_p c_m N}{(4\pi Dt)^{3/2}} e^{-\alpha c_m t} \cdot e^{-r^2/4Dt} \tag{6.44}$$

where E_p is the photon energy (hv) and N exp $(-\alpha c_m t)$, contains the total number of photons that exist at time t, which is decreasing in time due to absorption and $|r = \mathbf{r} - \mathbf{r_0}|$. The spatial distribution of the light is Gaussian with time-varying 1/e radius of $r_{1/e} = \sqrt{4Dt}$. The steady-state equation is (Jacques 1995)

$$-D\nabla^2 I(r) + \alpha I(r) = Q(r) \tag{6.45}$$

The solution to Eq. (6.45)

$$I(r) = P.\frac{e^{-r/\delta_0}}{4\pi Dr} = P.\frac{e^{-r\,\gamma_{eff}}}{4\pi Dr} \tag{6.46}$$

where P is an isotropic point source power (W). Substituting relation (6.43) in (6.46), we obtain

$$I(r) = P.\frac{e^{-r.\sqrt{3\alpha[\gamma(1-g)]}}}{4\pi Dr} \tag{6.47}$$

6.3 Laser-tissue interaction mechanisms

The interaction of laser radiation with matter, in general, can be studied and discussed in terms of mechanism(s) that may play a major role during the process. However, it must be noted that despite similar mechanisms in action, the laser interaction with a biological system is not same as interaction with an inorganic matter, and that the acute or chronic effects must be seriously taken in to consideration in the former case. For all intents and purposes, one should be able to predict the type and expected outcome of an interaction beforehand in order to prevent from unexpected results or even possible undesirable accidents. Undoubtedly, the paramount importance of this statement can readily be confirmed by studying not so remote history of lasers in medicine. For any type of interaction, we have to consider in advance the key optical parameters of given laser mainly the wavelength, pulse duration, energy per pulse, as these parameters determine other factors governing the interaction quality such as: fluence (Jm^{-2}), irradiance or power density (Wm^{-2}), and temperature change. Therefore, it is possible to implement various types of interaction, which may be linear, non-linear, single or multi-photon, etc., and thereby induce different effects in tissue, as shown in Fig. 6.8. Equally important, one should be also aware of the optical and thermal properties of the target matter and their importance so that can match the aforementioned expectations with the given laser optical parameters.

When considering such interaction one should take into account the inhomogeneous character of their various properties namely: biological, chemical, and physical (such as mechanical, optical, acoustical, electrical, or others). A simple and naive example would be like using a highly absorbing laser wavelength for hair removal applications, which gives us nothing but a disastrous scene. This is because we do not expect photons with, say about 1 μ penetration depth as with Er:YAG lasers, to be able to penetrate the dermis layer to reach the hair follicle, and what makes it even worse is the false notion of using a prolonged exposure of skin in the hope of getting there. Other unfortunate experienced example, optimistically speaking in the early days, is that an ophthalmologist used such prolonged exposure of argon laser at 488 nm for retinal photocoagulation, and just because the desirable results were not achieved, he then increased the laser output power hoping for better results, but not surprisingly, the patient's agony was the only sensible observation. Keeping this in mind, we can look at the mechanisms in terms of power density and the exposure time, as illustrated in Fig. 6.8. depicted and modified from (Boulnois and Marshall 1986). The interaction of laser with biological systems occur at various levels in the order of hierarchy, as shown in Fig. 6.5: molecules, cells, tissue, organs, and whole organism. The applications are divided into: (1) Laser diagnostics, (2) Laser therapy, and (3) Laser surgery.

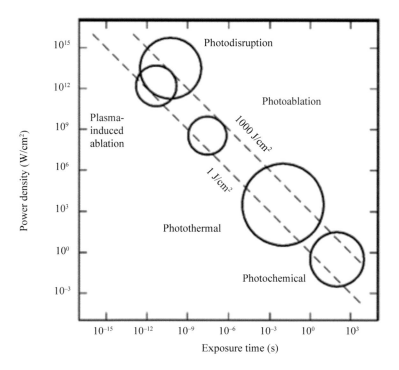

Figure 6.8. Laser-tissue interaction mechanisms shown as a variation of power density with irradiation time (Modified version of Boulnois (1960)).

6.3.1 Photochemical

Photodynamic therapy (PDT) is an elegant light based oncologic intervention where it uses a light sensitive drug (a photosensitizer), in combination with light of a visible wavelength, to destroy target cells (e.g., cancerous or pre-cancerous cells). PDT is generally used either as a primary treatment (usually in skin conditions) or as an adjunctive treatment alongside surgery, radiotherapy, or chemotherapy. Studies during the 1950s to 1960 revealed not only tumor ablation, but the inter-related ability of photosensitizing agents to fluoresce and demarcate tumors (Lipson and Baldes 1960). However, it was not until the 1970s when Dougherty (1975), working with porphyrin compounds (Hematoporphyrin derivative-HPD), accidentally rediscovered PDT. In contrast to previous iterations, Dougherty created a commercially suitable photosensitizing drug, reliable light sources, and appropriate clinical trials proving the value of PDT to the oncologic community. Some of commercial photosensitizers are: M-tetrahydroxophenyl chlorine (mTHPC) (Foscan), Mono-L-aspartyl chlorine e6 (NPe6), Aminolevulinic acid (ALA), Fotosens. HPD, AL A, MACE, and Foscan can activate at multiple light wavelength from blue to green to red, again allowing for more selective illumination depth based on the individual tumor's depth and location of surrounding critical structures.

Mechanism: As is shown in Fig. 6.8, PDT operated at low power densities and long exposure times. A two-step modality in which the delivery of a light–activated and lesion-localizing photosensitizer is followed by a low, non-thermal dose of light irradiation. The cytotoxic effect occurs because of the absorption of a photon of appropriate wavelength in a photosensitizer molecules, followed by intersystem cross-over and transfer of energy to an oxygen molecule and oxidation of critical cell structures by the reactive singlet oxygen. Almost all photochemical reactions are dependent on reactive oxygen species (ROS). Among the ROS, the singlet oxygen $^1O_2$ is the most important one. As is seen in Fig. 6.9, when the photosensitizer is exposed to specific wavelengths of light, it becomes activated from a ground to an excited state. As it returns to the ground state, it releases energy, which is transferred to oxygen to generate oxygen ROS, such as oxygen and free radicals to mediate cellular toxicity.

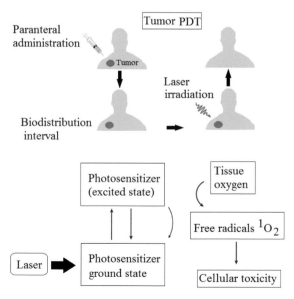

Figure 6.9. Photodynamic therapy cycle.

Normally, after a sensitizer is being injected into the body, it remains inactive until it is excited by a suitable laser wavelength, such as 632 nm, after 48–72 hours during which it is almost cleared from whole body except from the tumor where it is concentrated. The effective absorbed dose D* (J/kg) may be defined as

$$D^* = (A_s/\rho_t)CI\eta't \tag{6.48}$$

where A_s (m⁻¹/µg/g) is specific absorbance of photosensitizer, ρ_t(kg/m⁻³) is tissue density, C is concentration of photosensitizer (µg/mL), I (Wcm⁻²) is intensity, η' is relative photodynamic effectiveness, and t(s) is exposure time. If dose rate turns out to be significant in some conditions, then an effective absorbed dose rate can be defined by deleting the exposure time, and the biological response correlated to the dose rate time. The rate of drug clearance from healthy tissue is much faster than tumoric tissue. Generally, some of the typical technical issues with PDT are: mode of light delivery, light scattering, and distribution within tumor and light detection. Usual lasers used for PDT includes He-Ne, Dye, Diodes, and Gold vapour.

6.3.2 Photothermal

Photothermal effects cover a wide range of temperature dependent phenomena including:

i) *Photothermolysis*: Thermal dynamics effects, microscale overheating
ii) *Photohyperthermia* (37–43°C): No irreversible damage of tissue
                         (45–60°C): Loosening membrane (edema), tissue welding, denaturation of enzymes
iii) *Photocoagulation* (60–100°C): Coagulation, necrosis (cell death)
iv) *Photovaporization* (≥ 100°C): Water vaporization, drying out
v) *Photocarbonization* (≈ 300°C): Carbonization, pyrolysis

Therefore, in addition to tissue heating and thermal injury, laser irradiation can result in tissue vaporization, melting, ejection, and pyrolysis, all of which can lead to removal of biological material. These effects are collectively referred to as 'tissue ablation'. Briefly, the photothermal ablation takes place through a number of stages, which are explained as follows and shown in Fig. 6.10.

1. Light absorption: After light interaction with tissue, it is absorbed (i.e., α >>β) and heat is generated.
2. Temperature rise: As the tissue is heated via direct energy deposition and conduction, the temperature increases. The instantaneous and delayed heating will be discussed shortly in this section.
3. Tissue response: Primarily, dehydration and protein denaturation occurs, which can affect the optical and thermal properties of tissue.
4. Subsurface temperature: This is followed after tissue response.
5. Subsurface pressures: After temperature increase, the internal pressure builds up, whose magnitude and location are determined by other parameters: heat source distribution, rate of energy deposition, heat of ablation, number of nucleation sites which affect the time of ablation onset.
6. Tissue explosion: This depends on the temperature and the amount of built up pressure. When explosion happens, it is accompanied by surface tissue rupture and hence the cellular materials are ejected and leave the surface as kinetic energy. This causes the surface temperature of the tissue to decrease.

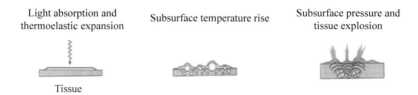

Figure 6.10. Schematic representation of photothermal steps for laser-induced tissue removal.

7. Continued heating: If heating is continued after the removal of the material, soon all water content is completely vaporized, and depending on the rate of heat transfer, ignition threshold is soon reached.
8. Pyrolysis: Carbonization (charring) and burning occur until a high degree of unwanted perforation is observed.

Figure 6.11 demonstrates the photothermal scheme where tissue optical properties defines the amount of light absorption, the thermal properties governs the heat transfer within the tissue, and the thermal effects are determined by corresponding rate coefficients. The laser thermal effects on tissue can take different forms.

As is seen in Fig. 6.12a, where if the beam is focused, the result will be a sharp incision with a relatively deep cut. However, when the beam is slightly widened or defocused so to speak, it will not

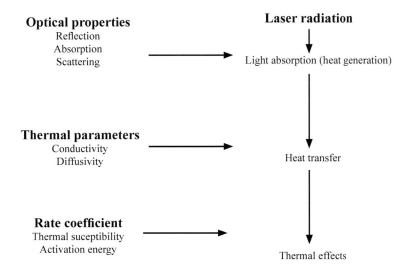

Figure 6.11. Diagrammatic representation of photothermal mechanism showing the inter-ration of optical properties, thermal parameters and rate coefficients of tissue with laser radiation.

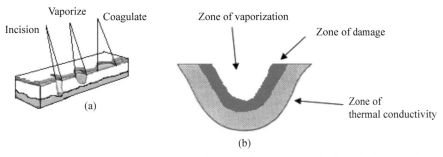

Figure 6.12. Schematic representation of focused and defocused effects of laser radiation on tissue. Note that the thermal damage due to conductivity can be reduced under adiabatic condition.

cut as much as before, but mainly vaporizes the intermediate layers. Coagulation, which is a superficial effect, is achieved when the beam is quite defocused and the intensity is dramatically reduced. Suppose, the tissue is now sliced for histological studies, as seen in Fig. 6.12b. The central portion represents the vaporized section, but because of heat transfer to the surrounding area, some degree of thermal damage can occur that strongly depends on the heat confinement condition (i.e., adiabatic or diffusion condition). This will be discussed shortly. The furthest region indicated possible effects of thermal conductivity on the healthy part of tissue. This is not necessarily interpreted as damage.

Heat transfer

Heat generation for homogeneous and inhomogeneous media is described by Eqs. (6.13) and (6.15), respectively. The heat losses in a laser-material interaction including tissue or biomaterials are:

(i) Heat conduction, (ii) Heat convection, (iii) Heat radiation

The heat flow, jQ is proportional to the temperature gradient according to the general diffusion equation;

$$jQ = -K\nabla T \tag{6.49}$$

where $K = D_t/\rho c$ (Wm^{-1} K^{-1}) is the thermal conductivity, D_t is the thermal diffusivity (m^{2}s^{-1}), ρ is the density of material (Kg m^{-3}), and c is the heat capacity of material (Jg$^{-1\circ}$C^{-1}). The equation of continuity, which describes the temporal change in heat per unit volume, is defined by the divergence of the heat flow,

$$\nabla. jQ = \nabla. K\nabla T = K\nabla^2 T \tag{6.50}$$

where ∇ is the *Laplace operator*. Using

$$dQ = mc\, dT \tag{6.51}$$

and after some simplification we get

$$\frac{\partial T}{\partial t} = -1/\rho c\, (\nabla. jQ) = -1/\rho c\, (K\nabla^2 T) \tag{6.52}$$

If we combine Eq. (6.49) with Eq. (6.52) we get

$$\frac{\partial T}{\partial t} = K\nabla T \tag{6.53}$$

Equation (6.53) is called *homogeneous*, equation, which describes the decrease of temperature after laser exposure due to heat diffusion. The general solution is

$$T(r,z,t) = T_0 + \frac{\xi}{(4\pi Kt)^{-3/2}} e^{(-\frac{r^2+z^2}{4Kt})} \tag{6.54}$$

Here ξ is the integration constant. Now, by adding a heat source, Q such as laser, one obtains

$$\rho c\frac{\partial T}{\partial t} = K\nabla^2 T + Q(r) \tag{6.55}$$

This is an *Inhomogeneous equation or Fourier parabolic* heat equation, which describes the temperature distribution in laser irradiated tissue. In this case, it is assumed that after laser-tissue interaction, the heat generated is *instantaneously* transferred to the surrounding region. The solution strongly depends on temporal and spatial dependences of Q(r,z,t), but for simplicity an isotropic heat conduction is assumed

$$Q(r,z,t) = Q_0\delta(z-z_0)\, \delta(t-t_0) \tag{6.56}$$

The general solution can be expressed by 1-D Green's function as

$$G(z-z_0, t-t_0) = \frac{1}{\sqrt{4\pi K(t-t_0)}} e^{\left[-\frac{(z-z_0)^2}{4K(t-t_0)}\right]} \tag{6.57}$$

But, the Fourier's law, which is simple in mathematics, has been widely used in various research areas, even though it is only an empirical relationship. In principle, however, the Fourier's law leads to an unphysical infinite heat propagation speed within a continuum field for transient heat conduction processes because of its parabolic characteristics, which is in contradiction with the theory of relativity

(Joseph and Preziosi 1989, Cahill et al. 2003). To overcome this spatio-temporal challenge, especially in ultra-small scales, a model is proposed by Cattaneo and Vernotte, which is known as CV model (Cattaneo 1958, Vernotte 1961).

$$\rho c \tau_r \left(\frac{\partial^2 T}{\partial t^2} \right) + \rho c \left(\frac{\partial T}{\partial t} \right) = K \nabla^2 T + Q \tag{6.58}$$

where τ_r denotes the relaxation time that tissue responds to the heat perturbation. The CV model (Eq. 6.58) gives rise to a wave-type of heat conduction equation and is called *hyperbolic* or *non-Fourier* heat conduction equation. The introduced time-derivative term in the CV model describes a wave nature of heat propagation at a finite speed, which has been proved in both theory and experiments (Vernotte 1961). The propagation speed is defined as:

$$V_t = \sqrt{\frac{K}{\rho c \tau_r}} \tag{6.59}$$

Equation (6.56) is also called "thermal wave speed". For $\tau_r = 0$, V_t is infinitely high in accordance with the instantaneous heat propagation predicted by the Fourier model. However, the most commonly used heat transfer equation for either a biological fluid or tissue is Pennes' (1948) bioheat equation because of its conciseness and validity.

$$\rho c \frac{\partial T}{\partial t} = \nabla.(K \nabla T) + C_b \dot{V}(T_a - T) + \dot{Q}_s + \dot{Q}_m \tag{6.60}$$

where ρ, C, $\dot{V}$, $\dot{Q}_s$, $\dot{Q}_m$, C_b and T_a are density of tissue, specific heat of tissue, blood perfusion rate (Kg/m³s), heat generation due to external heat source (W/m³), tissue metabolic heat generation (W/m³), specific heat of blood, and artery temperature, respectively.

In an experiment (Khosroshahi et al. 2014) investigated theoretically and experimentally, the effects of Fourier and non-Fourier heat conduction due to magnetic-gold nanoshells (MNS) were observed on lung cancer cells using a diode laser. It was observed that experimentally measured temperature distribution is in good agreement with that predicted by simulation of non-Fourier hyperbolic heat conduction model. Temperature contours of irradiated cancer cells incubated with 0.01 mg/mL of MNS based on Fourier and non-Fourier conduction model are shown in Fig. 6.13.

Temperature changes of irradiated cancer cells at 184 W/cm² using 0.01 mg/mL of MNS for experimental, 2-D and 3-D simulation are shown in Fig. 6.14. The boundary and slice representation of 3-D temperature gradients are presented in Fig. 6.15, where the spatio-temporal temperature distribution of irradiated MNSs-laden cancer cells is clearly distinguished with its maximum at the center shown by red.

Thermal process

After the interaction, laser radiation locally heats the material resulting in some phase change, e.g., melting, vaporization. In general, a fraction of radiation is reflected, R and partly is transmitted. We have

$$I(z) = (1-R)I_0 \, e^{-\alpha z} \tag{6.61}$$

Where

$$R = \frac{[n_m - n_a]^2}{[n_m + n_a]^2} \tag{6.62}$$

with n_m and n_a being refractive indices of medium and air, respectively. From Eq. (6.62), the local intensity is

$$-\frac{dI(z)}{dt} = (1-R)I_0 \alpha \, e^{-\alpha z} \tag{6.63}$$

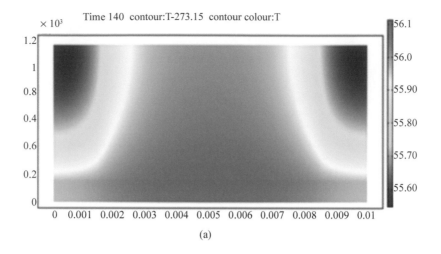

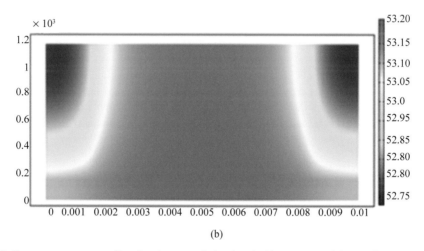

Figure 6.13. Temperature contours of irradiated cancer cells incubated with MNPs-containing medium (MNPs concentration = 0.01 mg/ml) at power density of 184 W/cm². (a) Numerically-obtained heat gradient based on Fourier and (b) non-Fourier conduction model.

Assuming now this creates heating, so the change in energy is

$$\Delta E = \rho c \Delta T \tag{6.64}$$

or in terms of laser power we write

$$\frac{dE}{dt} = \rho c \frac{dT(z)}{dt} \tag{6.65}$$

Equating Eqs. (6.63) and (6.65)

$$\rho c \frac{dT(z)}{dt} = (1\text{-}R)I_0 \alpha\, e^{-\alpha z} \tag{6.66}$$

The Eq. (6.65) reflects rate of temperature rise to absorption coefficient and thermal properties of material. It neglects, however, heat loss from heated zone by thermal conduction. The heat flow depth (i.e., thermal diffusion depth) in time t is

$$X_t = \sqrt{4D_t \tau_p} \tag{6.67}$$

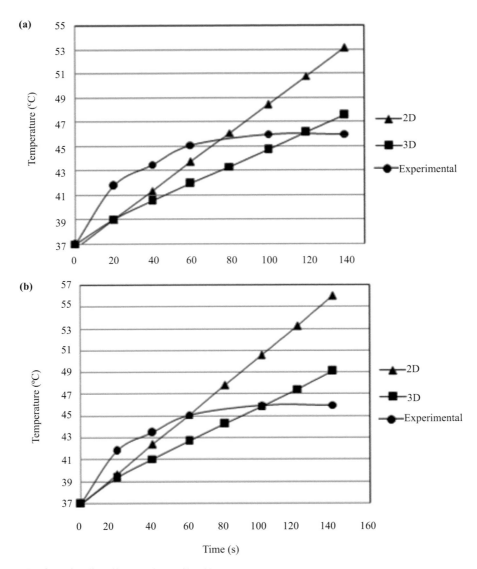

Figure 6.14. Dimensionality effects on the profile of irradiated QU-DB lung cancer cells incubated with MNPs-containing culture medium (MNPs concentration = 0.01 mg/ml) over a period of 150 seconds at the power density of 184 W/cm². Simulation trials conducted based on both (a) non-Fourier and (b) Fourier conduction model.

where τ_p is laser pulse duration. There are two possible distinct situations:

1. ***Adiabatic limit***: This refers to 'thermal confinement' condition where laser-induced heat is confined to the interaction point and its transfer to the surrounding region is neglected. This is normally considered for nanosecond and shorter laser pulses. The following conditions are considered for an adiabatic case:

   a) Absorption dominates the scattering (i.e., $\alpha \gg \beta$)
   b) Optical penetration depth is smaller than thermal diffusion depth (i.e., $\delta_0 \gg X_t$)
   c) Laser pulse duration is smaller than thermal relaxation time (i.e., $\tau_p \ll \tau_r$, i.e., $\tau_p/\tau_r \leq 1$)
   d) Energy density (fluence) is below the ablation threshold (i.e., $F \ll F_t$)
   e) Reflection from the material surface has a non-zero value (i.e., $R \neq 0$)

(a)

(b)

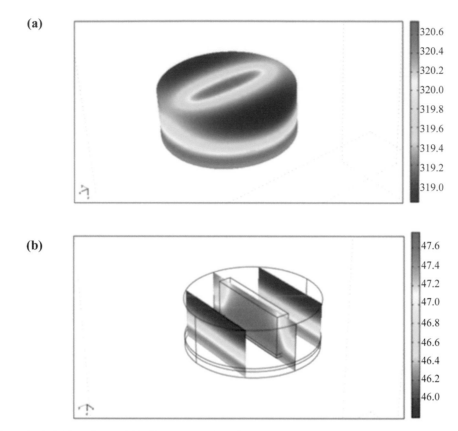

Figure 6.15. (a) Boundary and (b) slice representation of 3-D temperature contours of irradiated cancer cells incubated with MNPs-containing medium (MNPs concentration = 0.01 mg/ml) at power density of 184 W/cm^2. Black edges in (b) indicates the computational domain.

For example, if we assume that a pulse of an Er:YAG laser (2.94 μm) interacts with a soft tissue, say skin, with absorption coefficient of about 13000 cm^{-1}, i.e., a photon penetration depth of ≈ 0.8 μm, then the thermal relaxation time would be equivalent to 1.2 μs. This means it takes about this much time for heat to diffuse from the interaction zone to the surrounding area. Thus, any pulse duration less than this value would be suitable to prevent the heat transfer.

So,

$$\delta_0 = \frac{1}{\alpha} >> \sqrt{4D_t\tau_p} \tag{6.68}$$

$$\tau_r = \frac{\delta_0^2}{4D_t} = \frac{\left(\alpha^{-1}\right)^2}{4D_t} \tag{6.69}$$

From Eq. (6.65), temperature rise at the end of pulse is

$$\Delta T(z) = \frac{(1-R)}{\rho c} I_0 \alpha \tau_p . e^{-\alpha z} \tag{6.70}$$

At the surface (z = 0)

$$\Delta T_0 = \frac{(1-R)}{\rho c} I_0 \alpha \tau_p = \frac{(1-R)}{\rho c} F\alpha \tag{6.71}$$

For z > 0 (at a depth within the material), and α >> β the Gaussian beam profile may be written as

$$T(r,z) = \frac{\alpha I \tau_p}{\rho c} e^{-\alpha z} \cdot e^{-2r^2/w_0^2}$$ (6.72)

where w_0 is radius of the Gaussian beam. This solution is valid up to the onset of ablation. At the onset of ablation and in the ablation regime, an ablation front energy balance equation is coupled with equation (6.52). Temperatures are then obtained by simultaneous solution of the two equations. Thermal confinement is important in microsurgery to limit the thermal injury of structures outside the focal volume as well as to minimize the energy dose necessary to produce the desired cellular effect.

Thermoelastic stress generation

In the absence of vaporization, the temperature increase due to transient heating produced by the energy deposition in the focal volume leads to thermal expansion of the tissue, as a result of which a momentum is set up within tissue. Consequently, a rarefaction inside the heated volume is responsible for the compressive and tensile stresses. The thermal expansion directed into the tissue generates positive stress (compressive wave), and the outgoing wave or outward expansion directed towards the free surface generates negative stress (rarefaction wave). At nanosecond subablation regime, some useful information can be deduced from the thermoelastic response about the thermal relaxation of excited states and optical properties of the materials (Dyer 1989). However, in contrast to short pulses, it has been demonstrated that more depth information can be achieved by using longer laser pulses as chirps (i.e., modulated) in frequency-domain mode (Fan et al. 2004). Generally, there are two possible limiting cases during stress wave generation by thermal expansion accompanying the rapid laser heating of surfaces:

a) *Short-pulse limit*: (acoustic penetration depth $\delta_a \ll \delta_o$), we have $c_a \tau_p \ll 1/\alpha$. Here, the volume that absorbs laser energy cannot expand during the laser-pulse heating and the tissue is in the compression stage. If A is the spot size, then the total laser energy absorbing volume, $V = A/\alpha$, then the thermal expansion of the volume is

$$\Delta V = \frac{E\beta}{\rho C_p}$$ (6.73)

where C_p is specific heat capacity at constant volume and β is volumetric thermal expansion coefficient defined as

$$\beta = \frac{\Delta P C_p}{c_a^2 \alpha F}$$ (6.74)

The pressure increase due to the volume expansion is given by

$$\Delta P = \rho c_a^2 \frac{\Delta V}{V}$$ (6.75)

By substituting the above equations for ΔP, we obtain

$$\Delta P = \frac{\beta c_a^2}{C_p} \frac{E}{V} = \Gamma \alpha F$$ (6.76)

where $\Gamma = \beta c_a^2/C_p$ is called Grüneisen coefficient, which is an intrinsic thermophysical property of material and is defined as the change of internal stress within a material per unit increase of energy density under constant volume (isochoric) conditions.

b) *Long-pulse limit,* corresponds to $\tau_p \gg \tau_a$ (the acoustic transient time), thus $c_a \tau_p \gg 1/\alpha$. In this case, the acoustic pulse traverse in the absorption region with finite speed during the laser pulse heating. Hence,

$$\Delta P = \rho c_a \frac{\Delta V}{A \tau_p} = \frac{\beta c_a}{C_p} \frac{E}{A \tau_p}$$ (6.77)

$$\Delta P = \frac{\beta c_a}{C_p} \frac{F}{\tau_p} \tag{6.78}$$

Moreover, because the absorption of photons imparts no significant momentum to the sample, the transient stresses will contain both compressive and tensile components that can produce mechanical damage (Paltauf and Dyer 2003). To reduce the magnitude of the thermoelastic stresses, one must deposit energy on a time scale longer than that required for an acoustic wave to propagate out of the heated volume.

2. **Non-adiabatic or Diffusion limit**: In this case, heat is not confined at the interaction zone and it is conducted to the surrounding medium.

The conditions are: $\beta \gg \alpha$, $\tau_p > \tau_r$ and $\delta_0 \ll X_t$. Therefore, If $\delta_0 = \frac{1}{\alpha} \ll \sqrt{4D_t\tau_p}$ then heat flows out of interaction zone and the average power per unit volume is

$$\langle P \rangle = \frac{I_0(1\text{-}R)}{\sqrt{4D_t\tau_p}} \tag{6.79}$$

Using Eq. (6.62)

$$\frac{dT}{dt} = \frac{I_0(1\text{-}R)}{\rho c \sqrt{4D_t\tau_p}} \tag{6.80}$$

And at the end of pulse temperature rise is

$$\Delta T = \frac{I_0(1\text{-}R)\tau_p}{\rho c \sqrt{4D_t\tau_p}} = \frac{F(1\text{-}R)}{\rho c \sqrt{4D_t\tau_p}} \tag{6.81}$$

Now both the fluence and pulse duration are related and influential, whereas in adiabatic case, only fluence remains. This situation readily arises when the adiabatic conditions are not satisfied. For example, (Khosroshahi et al. 2007, 2008) 200 μs Nd:YAG laser has been used for surface modification of Ti6Al4V alloy for orthopaedic applications. Equation (6.52) was used to evaluate the variation of the surface temperature of Ti6Al4V during the heating and cooling cycles. During heating $t < \tau_p$, the solution is

$$T(x,t) = T_h (x,t) = \left[\frac{I_0\alpha}{K} \left(\frac{4D_t t}{\pi} \right)^{1/2} \exp\left(\frac{x^2}{4D_t t} \right) - x \text{ erfc} \frac{x}{\sqrt{4D_t t}} \right] + T_0 \tag{6.82}$$

During cooling the temperature drops for all $t > \tau_p$ and

$$T(x,t) = T_c (x,t) = \frac{I_0\alpha}{K} \left(4D_t \right)^{1/2} \left[\sqrt{t} \times i \text{ erfc} \frac{x}{\left(4D_t\right)^{1/2}} - \sqrt{t\text{-}\tau_p} \times i \text{ erfc} \frac{x}{\sqrt{4D_t (t\text{-}\tau_p)}} \right] + T_0 \tag{6.83}$$

where $i \text{ erf} (x)$ is the integral of the complementary error function defined as

$$i \text{ erfc} = \int_x^{\infty} \text{erfc} (y) \, dy = \frac{1}{\sqrt{\pi}} e^{-x^2} \, x \text{ erf} (x) \tag{6.84}$$

where T_h and T_c are heating and cooling temperatures, respectively. Figure 6.16 shows the calculated surface temperature variation with the time for the Ti6Al4V irradiated by the pulsed Nd:YAG laser.

Figure 6.17 indicates an example of sharply defined irradiated area after ten laser pulses. The depression observed at the center of ablated spot is thought to be due to laser Gaussian profile, where most of the pulse energy is concentrated at its peak.

It is also important to note that in some respects, physicists have extended the concept of wave to a large number of phenomena corresponding to physical situations described by a varying field that propagates in both space and time. Such situations can be due to the interaction of intensity modulated or frequency modulated continuous laser with biological systems, including tissue and fluids. The importance of this point is in appreciating the fact that such waves have direct effects on the material due to their behaviour. For example, does perturbation in the temperature field lead to propagation as thermal waves within the medium? And if so, what are the physical consequences? There are many similar questions. The goal of this discussion is not to go into a detailed analysis of the question, but to address some of the issues that are crucial to know and how it may be different to single pulse mode.

It is well established that the temperature oscillations produced by a periodic heat source have the same mathematical expression as a highly damped wave similar to electromagnetic waves propagating through other media, e.g., metals (Almond and Patal 1996). However, heat conduction is a diffusive process governed by a parabolic differential equation which lacks second-order derivative with respect to time. As mentioned above, its main limitation is it does not take propagation speed into account. To overcome this limitation, a relaxation time is introduced between temperature gradient and heat flux, which takes the form of hyperbolic equation. Let us suppose a tissue surface is uniformly irradiated by a laser beam of periodically modulated intensity,

$$I_0 = \left(\frac{1 + \cos \omega t}{2} \right) = \mathrm{Re}\left(\frac{I_0(1 + e^{i\omega t})}{2} \right) \tag{6.85}$$

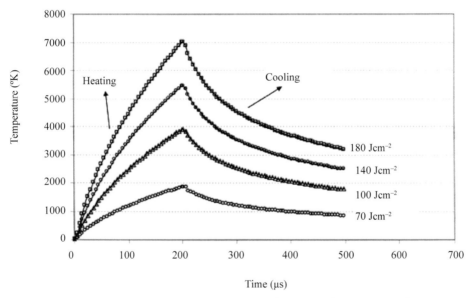

Figure 6.16. Numerical evaluation of surface temperature variation of Ti6Al4V with time using MATHCAD computer program.

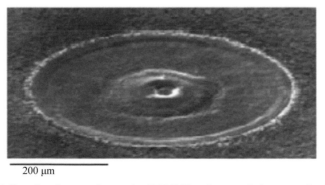

200 μm

Figure 6.17. Scanning electron micrograph of Ti6Al4V surface morphology treated at 210 Jcm^{-2}.

where I_0 is the intensity of the beam and $\omega = 2\pi f$, with f being the modulation frequency. The temperature at any point of the tissue is given by

$$T(x,t) = T_{amb} + T_{dc}(x) + T_{ac}(x,t) \qquad (6.86)$$

where T_{amb} is the ambient temperature, T_{dc} is time-dependent temperature rise above the ambient, and T_{ac} is a periodic temperature oscillation of the same frequency as the incident radiation expressed as $T_{ac}(x,t) = \text{Re}\left[\theta(x)e^{i\omega t}\right]$. Thus, Helmholtz's equation

$$\frac{d^2\theta(x)}{dx^2} - q^2\theta(x) = 0 \qquad (6.87)$$

Where

$$q = \sqrt{\frac{i\omega}{D_t}} \qquad (6.88)$$

By solving the Eq. (6.87) and using as boundary condition the heat flux continuity on the sample surface

$$-K\frac{d\theta(x)}{dx}\bigg|_{x=0} = \frac{I_0}{2} \qquad (6.89)$$

The time-dependent component of the temperature is obtained as

$$T_{ac}(x,t) = \text{Re}\left[\frac{i_0}{2Kq}e^{-qx}e^{i\omega t}\right] = \frac{I_0}{2e_t\sqrt{\omega}}e^{-x/D_e}\cos\left(\frac{x}{D_e}-\omega t+\frac{\pi}{4}\right) \qquad (6.90)$$

where $e_t = \frac{K}{D}$ and $X_t = \sqrt{\frac{2D_t}{\omega}}$ are thermal effusivity and thermal diffusion depth, respectively. One of the important results of this discussion is that only the temperature oscillations (i.e., T_{ac} as thermal waves) with respect to the ambient temperature appears and does not carry energy. The energy is transported through the tissue by T_{dc} component (Salazar 2006). In other words, there are two possibilities that one should consider under such condition: (a) The tissue components (e.g., molecules, cells) behaviour or oscillations subject to thermal wave oscillations and (b) The effect of temperature rise due to T_{dc} component on tissue.

Tissue mass removal and damage prediction

Basically, two models can be considered for tissue ablation: (a) Beer's Law and (b) Linear mass removal. The former model predicts a linear relationship between the depth of ablation and the logarithm of the fluence. This model is sometimes referred as 'blow off' model, It is implicitly assumed that no material is removed from beam path during the laser pulse and that it gives the penetration of the light into the tissue during the pulse. Beer's Law states:

$$F(z) = F_0 e^{-\alpha z} \qquad (6.91)$$

where F_0 is the fluence at the surface and $F(z)$ is the fluence at depth z. If the ablation process has a threshold fluence F_{th}, then ablation will occur to a depth D_e, called etch depth (Srinivasan 1986).

$$D_e = \frac{1}{\alpha}\ln\left(\frac{F_0}{F_{th}}\right) \qquad (6.92)$$

Ablation occurs by explosive vaporization or 'blow off' of the material above the depth D_e. The mass of tissue removed is given by integration of the depth of the crater across the entire irradiated area A,

$$M_r = \int (\rho_t D_e)\,dA \qquad (6.93)$$

where ρ_t is tissue density. For a beam with a uniform intensity profile, the depth of the crater will be constant across the entire crater and the mass removed will be

$$M_r = \rho_t A\, D_e \tag{6.94}$$

By substituting in Eq. (6.92) it yields

$$M_r = \frac{\rho_t A}{\alpha} \ln\left(\frac{F_0}{F_{th}}\right) \tag{6.95}$$

Thus, there is a linear relationship between the mass of tissue removed and the logarithm of the fluence.

In the second model, there is a linear relationship between the incident fluence and the etch depth. This model is more appropriate for the situation where the material at the surface of tissue leaves the beam path during the ablation pulse and does not attenuate the beam once ablated.

$$D_e = \frac{(F_0 - F_{th})}{H_a} \tag{6.96}$$

where H_a is the heat of ablation, and so by combining with Eqs. (6.93) and (6.96) we get

$$M_r = \frac{\rho_t A(F_0 - F_{th})}{H_a} \tag{6.97}$$

Thus, there is a linear relationship between the mass removed and the fluence. Figure 6.18 illustrates the mass removal at different values of fluence for both models.

It worth noting that some important phenomena such as superheating of subsurface tissue, explosive removal of tissue, and scattering of the incident radiation are not included in the model, although one of the assumptions is $\alpha \gg \beta$. It is also assumed that the absorption of laser beam does not decrease during the laser pulse (i.e., by laser-induced removal of material out of beam). Surface dehydration plays a major role in the rate of ablation and affects the thermal damage region. This is due to change of absorption coefficient during laser irradiation. The effect of dehydration on ablation was experimentally observed when a hard tissue such as enamel was irradiated by a mid-IR multi-wavelength hydrogen fluoride (HF) laser operating between 2.6–3 μm (Khosroshahi and Ghasemi 2004). The experimental set up is shown in Fig. 6.19, where the energy uniformly and suitably is imaged on the tissue. More information was achieved regarding the interaction mechanism using PTD and spectroscopic techniques.

A fit to the data using Eq. (6.79) yields $F_{th} \approx 47$ Jcm^{-2} and $\alpha \approx 1780$ cm^{-1} for the threshold and effective absorption coefficient, respectively. By assuming a Gaussian profile for the probe beam, one can write the dependence of the photodiode response ΔV on the beam deflection as follows (Diaci and Mozina 1992),

$$\Delta V = V_0 \; \text{erf} = \frac{2}{\sqrt{2}} \frac{\varphi}{\theta} \tag{6.98}$$

With φ and θ being the beam angular deflection due to change in index of refraction and angular divergence, respectively, V_0 is the photodiode output voltage at $\varphi = 0$, therefore only for $\varphi \ll \theta$, ΔV is linear. Figure 6.20 shows the output voltage (hence deflection) as a function of laser pulse number at 23 Jcm^{-2}. The origin of the signal is due to heat emitted from the surface of the tissue, hence causing the deflection of the probe beam. It can be seen that the voltage amplitude decreases with pulse number due to water vaporization from the enamel surface. The signal amplitude then remained constant after four pulses and reached a minimum value indicating the onset of absorption by hydroxyapatite.

In order to inhibit the enamel surface from dehydration and changing of its optical properties, it was sprayed with water after a defined number of pulses. One possible reason for having a rather smooth wall is the fact that thermal relaxation time, τ_r of enamel is much greater than the pulse width (i.e., $\tau_p \ll \tau_r$). In this case, the optical penetration depth $\delta_0 \approx 5.6$ μm and thermal diffusivity of enamel $D_t \approx 4.7 \times 10^3$ (cm^{2}s^{-1}), using Eq. (6.69) the value of, τ_r is found to be 16 μs. Since, it is assumed that thermal conduction loss is

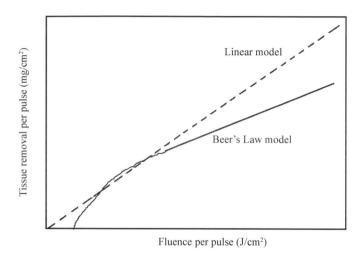

Figure 6.18. Theoretical models of linear and Beer-lambert's law for tissue removal as a function of laser fluence.

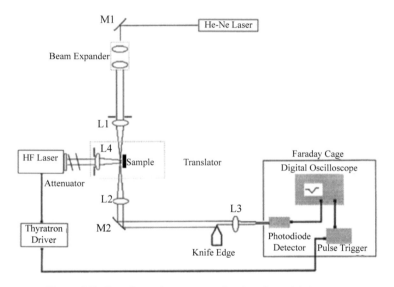

Figure 6.19. Experimental arrangement for photothermal deflection.

negligible during the ablation phase, which is valid, provided the spot size and characteristic absorption depth are large compared with the thermal diffusion depth X_t, then using the Eq. (6.64), (i.e., $\delta_0 >> X_t \approx 0.86\,\mu m$). Consequently, it satisfies the condition defined by adiabatic case.

A simple relation can be used to estimate the depth of damage, D_d that denatures the tissue at a particular critical temperature, T_c (Walsh et al. 1988)

$$D_d = \left(\frac{1}{\alpha}\right) \ln\left[\frac{F_{th}\alpha}{(T_c - T_0)\rho c}\right] \tag{6.99}$$

T_0 is the initial tissue temperature. Also, the thermal damage, which is due to thermal denaturation, $\Omega(t)$ or inactivation of enzymes is a temperature-dependent rate process derived from the Arrhenius equation

$$\Omega(t) = A \int_0^t \dot{R}\, dt \tag{6.100}$$

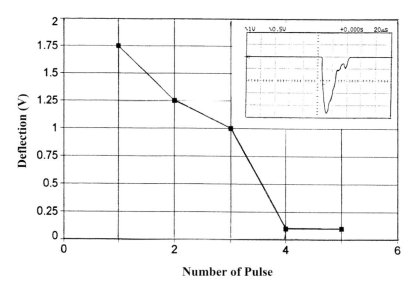

Figure 6.20. Variation of photodiode output voltage amplitude as a function of laser pulse number at 23 Jcm^{-2} and 2 mm separation of probe beam from the surface of tooth.

$$\Omega(r,z) = A \int_{t_i}^{t_f} \exp\left[\frac{\Delta E}{RT(r,z,t)}\right] dt \qquad (6.101)$$

where A is the pre-exponential or frequency factor (S^{-1}), $\dot{R}$ is the reaction rate and $\Delta E = T\Delta S + \Delta H$ is the activation energy of the reaction (J mol^{-1}), and $\Delta H = U + P\Delta V$ is the enthalpy, R is the universal gas constant (8.31 J mol^{-1} K^{-1}) and t_f and t_i are time after and before laser exposure respectively. Equation (6.101) can be rewritten in terms of cells population

$$\Omega(r,z) = \ln\left[\frac{C_d}{C_0}(t)\right] \qquad (6.102)$$

That is, damage index is equivalent to ratio of damaged cells to initial healthy cells. Thus, the damage coefficient varying between 0 and 1.

$$C_\Omega = \frac{\Omega}{(\ln 2 + \Omega)} \qquad (6.103)$$

Therefore, if $\Omega = 0$ no molecules or cells are said to be damaged (i.e., Cd/C0 = 0), if $\Omega = 1$, it implies about 63% damage, and if $\Omega > 1$ means that most of the molecules or cells are damaged. However, normally for damage threshold Ln $\Omega = 2$ (i.e., 0.693) or 50% is considered.

Generally, molecules such as enzymes, whose entropy ΔS and enthalpy ΔH is relatively low are more sensitive to whole process of thermal damage, whereas other molecules such as collagen molecules with higher ΔS and ΔH are more sensitive and show reaction to peak temperature.

Cavitation, photoacoustic and tissue ablation

The concept and interest in understanding the behaviour of cavitation bubbles in liquids has been extensively investigated since the late 1800s, when propeller-driven ships were first developed. Indeed, one of the earliest theoretical models of the collapse of a spherical void in an incompressible liquid was solved by Rayleigh in 1917. This was followed by many other good work in this field including Lauterborn and Bolle (1975), Tomita and Shima (1986), Vogel and Lauterborn (1988), and Ward and Emmony (1991). Basically, cavitation is formation and activity of bubbles in a liquid. The bubbles may contain gas, vapour, or a mixture of both gas and vapour. If bubbles contain gas, then the expansion may be by diffusion of dissolved gases from the liquid into the bubble, or by pressure reduction, or by temperature increase. If, however, the bubbles contain mainly vapour, reducing the ambient pressure low enough at constant temperature causes an explosive vaporization into the cavities, which is called 'cavitation'. There are four different types of cavitation (Young 1989).

a) Hydrodynamic cavitation: This is produced by pressure change in a flowing liquid.
b) Acoustic cavitation: This is produced by acoustic/sound waves in a liquid due to pressure changes.
c) Optical cavitation: This is produced by photons of high intensity such as laser causing liquid rupturing.
d) Particle cavitation: This is produced by elementary particles such as proton.

In a non-flowing system, the ambient pressure can be changed if it is subject to sound waves travelling through it. Now, if the pressure amplitude is high enough to reduce the local pressure down to or even below the vapour pressure in the second, i.e., negative cycle of the sound, any small amount of cavities or bubbles will grow. If the pressure amplitude is increased to give zero and a negative pressures (tensions) locally in the liquid, then the bubble growth will increase. Once this small bubble is set to motion, it expands and contracts in the sound field. There are two distinct types of motions: *stable* and *unstable*. In the former, the bubbles oscillate for many periods whereas in the latter are transient cavities that exist for less than one cycle (Young 1989). It should be noted that the first type is generally a non-linear process in that the change of bubble radius is not proportional to the sound pressure. The second type, however, due to high compressibility of gas bubbles high potential energy is obtained from the sound wave when the bubbles expands and the kinetic energy is concentrated when the bubbles collapse. In the transient cavitation, this transformation of a low energy density sound wave into a high energy density collapsing bubble occurs because the motion is non-linear. Since it concentrates the energy into very small volumes, it can generate very high pressures and temperatures resulting in possible material erosion, initiate chemical reactions, and produce luminescence called sonoluminescence. Interest in mid-IR lasers for clinical applications is mainly due to their high absorption by tissue water content. However, their applications may vary depending on the quality of controllable parameters and priority of the goal, such as tissue cutting, welding, coagulating or possibly transmitting through a suitable optical fiber for remote application. On the other hand, some surgical treatments including angioplasty, ophthalomolgy, orthopaedic and urology are performed in a liquid environment (e.g., saline, blood, plasma) which implies a high fraction of light energy is being absorbed by the surrounding medium and less is reaching the target. An earlier work of Lin (Lin et al. 1990) on the dynamics studies of fiber coupled laser-induced cavitation for tissue ablation showed that laser spikes produced by Er:YAG laser at free running mode can propagate through the bubble and damage tissue on the distal side of the bubble. This was followed by the work performed by Dyer et al. (1993) using a short pulse HF laser where the creation the role of a hot, high pressure, vapour cavity at the fibre tip was demonstrated by shadowgraphy, as we can see in Fig. 6.21.

A multiline HF laser (2.67–2.96 µm) with 400 ns pulse duration at full-width at half maximum (FWHM) was coupled into IR fluoride glass fibre with 480 µm core diameter. The fibre output was photographed using a 4 ns duration N_2 pump dye laser operating at ~ 573 nm (rhodamine 6G). Pressure transients produced in tissue samples were recorded using a 9 µm thick poly vinylidene fluoride (PVDF) film piezoelectric transducer. Figure 6.22 indicates the plot of the transverse radius of the bubble, r, as a function of time for fiber output at various fluences. In each case, the bubble reaches a maximum size and the time scale for growth and collapse decreases as the fluence decreases. The bubbles in each example appeared to become unstable in the final stage of collapse, dissipating through the generation of minute bubbles.

A sequence of shadowgraph is shown for the fibre tip located 2.5 mm away from a cornea tissue with its maximum diameter, as seen in Fig. 6.23a. Notable is the collapsing cavity in frame 6.24 (b), where the bubble front surface is deformed due to high pressure opposing in the opposite direction, and finally the 'jetting' occurs at the final stage near the tissue the boundary, seen in Fig. 6.23c.

For SEM evaluation, the tissues were fixed in glutaraldehyde-formaldehyde and dried using a critical point drying apparatus to minimize structural deformation or collapse. Figure 6.24 a shows an SEM of the corneal surface damage that resulted following 20 pulses at an output fluence of 5 Jcm^{-2} with fiber tip located about 200 µm from the surface. There is an extensive damage in the form of disruption and distortion of stromal collagen fibrils over a zone exceeding 1 mm in diameter. An example of SEM

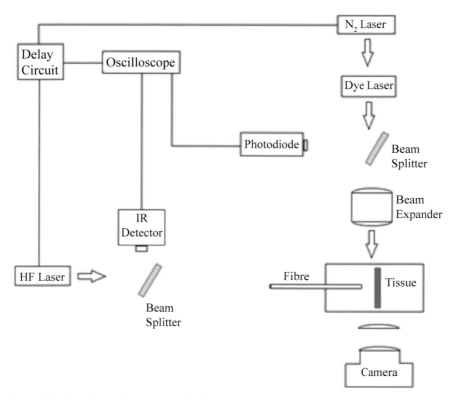

Figure 6.21. Experimental arrangement for dynamic study of cavitation using shadowgraph technique.

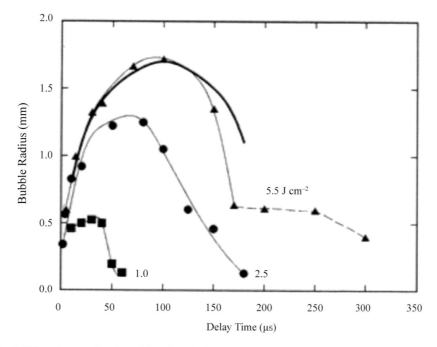

Figure 6.22. Bubble radius as a function of time for exit fluences from the fibre of 1, 2.5 and 5.5 J cm⁻². The broken lines are fits to the data to guide the eye. The solid line is the calculated bubble radius suitably scaled to have the same maximum radius as the experimental value at 5.5 Jcm⁻².

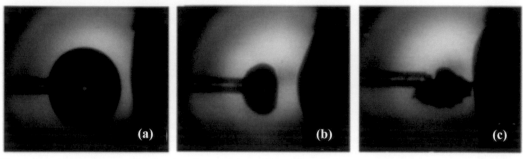

Figure 6.23. Bubble sequence for fibre in saline with tip positioned 2.5 mm from a cornea sample. (a) 100 μs, (b) 300 μs, (c) 480 μs at 5 J cm⁻².

photograph of the ablation site for the contacted fibre is shown in Fig. 6.24b for exposure at 5 J cm⁻² for 100 pulses. The interaction region is significantly smaller in diameter than the fibre core, possibly because of some fluence nonuniformity at the exit surface. It is evident that the ablated surface is essentially free of debris, and that a sharply defined incision is produced that clearly penetrates the epithelium and superficial stroma. This behaviour is closely similar to that for an air-based contacted fibre (Dyer et al. 1992), but is in contrast to Fig. 6.24.

Measurements of the transient pressure pulse accompanying ablation for the contacted fibre ($d = 0$) were made for a ~ 300 μm thick section of cornea mounted on the PVDF piezoelectric transducer. The transducer output shown in Fig. 6.25 for an exit fluence of 2.5 Jcm⁻² exhibited a fast rise time (~ 80 ns), a duration of ~200 ns (FWHM) and some ringing following the main pulse.

The oscilloscope trace was triggered by the laser pulse using an IR photodiode, and it was observed that the delay between pulses decreased as the fluence was raised. This delay has a fixed component set by the acoustic transit time in the sample (neglecting shock effects), and a component that depends on when ablation commences during the laser pulse. It can thus be deduced that ablation occurs at earlier times as the fluence is increased. The peak output voltage from the PVDF transducer can be converted to a corresponding normal force (Cross et al. 1988), and hence, to a pressure if the area of infuence of the acoustic pulse can be defined. For this purpose, we assume that a plane acoustic wave propagates between the tissue surface and transducer and takes the area as that of the fibre core. It should be noted, however, that this is a relatively poor assumption in the present case, because the transducer lies beyond the nearfield range, Z_R. This is given by (Cross et al. 1988)

$$Z_R = \frac{a^2}{\lambda} \qquad (6.104)$$

where a is the fibre core radius and λ, is the characteristic acoustic wavelength generated in the interaction. Taking $a = 240$ μm, $\lambda \cong 2c_a \Delta t$, where Δt is the width of the pressure pulse (Fig. 6.26) and c_a the sound speed for bulk longitudinal waves in the tissue ($c_a \sim 1.5 \times 103$ ms⁻¹), $Z_R \sim 100$ μm. This is considerably smaller than the tissue sample thickness (~ 300 μm) so that significant "edge" effects will occur, i.e., three-dimensional expansion effects cannot strictly be neglected. This transition to nonplanar propagation may explain why a rarefaction component develops on the pressure pulse. Figure 6.26 shows the pressure amplitude as a function of fluence. It is clear that large stresses are generated for the contacted fibre geometry, values exceeding 10⁸ Pa being recorded for output fluences above ≈ 7 Jcm⁻².

The dynamics of laser-induced cavitation bubbles have been extensively studied and analysed for cases where a focused laser produces spherical bubbles either in free liquid or liquid in the vicinity of a plane solid or air boundary (Lauterborn 1980). For cavitation initiated by a fibre-delivered laser, the situation is more complicated, because aspherical growth is promoted by the planar geometry of the initial vapour cavity formed at the fibre tip and by the perturbing influence of the fibre during "bubble" growth. This is evident from Fig. 6.24, where the vapour bubble is observed to be somewhat flattened in the direction parallel to the fibre axis. Given the lack of a readily applicable theory for aspherical growth (Lauterborn 1980), an analysis based on a spherical-cavity model is retained hereby assuming that it is justifiable to

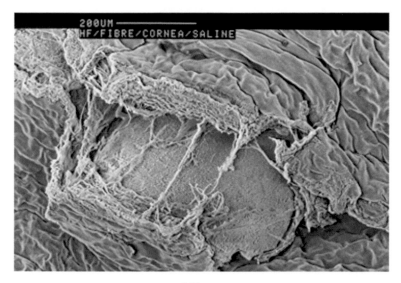

200 μm

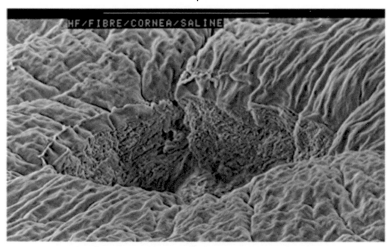

Figure 6.24. Surface of cornea following exposure to 20 pulses from HF laser with fibre tip located ~ 200 μm from the sample in saline at 5 Jcm^{-2} (a) and contacted fibre in saline at 5 Jcm^{-2} after 100 pulses (b).

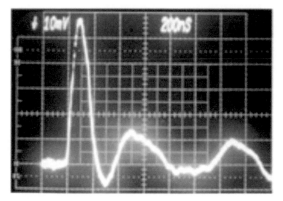

Figure 6.25. Transient pressure pulse produced by ablation of cornea with contacted fibre in saline at 2.5 Jcm^{-2}. The start of the trace is triggered by the HF-laser pulse.

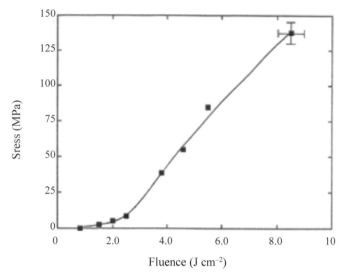

Figure 6.26. Peak stress deduced from the photoacoustic transducer as a function of fluence for HF-laser ablation of cornea. Contacted fibre in saline.

define an equivalent spherical radius for the bubble. In Fig. 6.22 the bubble radius (transverse to the fibre axis)—time plot is seen to be approximately symmetrical and is similar to the behaviour observed for the growth and collapse of spherical bubbles (Lauterborn 1980, Young 1989). The characteristic collapse (and growth) time for gas filled spherial bubbles is given by (Young 1989):

$$\tau_c = 0.91 R_m (\rho/P_0)^{1/2} (1 + P_f/P_0) \tag{6.105}$$

where R_m is the maximum bubble radius, ρ is the liquid density, P_0 is the liquid pressure (atmospheric pressure as the hydrostatic contribution from the liquid is negligible), and P_f is the pressure in the fully expanded bubble. Estimates discussed below show $P_f/P_0 < 2.7 \times 10^{-2}$ so that τ is very close to that for collapse of an empty cavity, i.e., with $P_f = 0$. At an exit fluence of 5.5 J cm^{-2} we obtain from Fig. 6.23 $\tau \approx 100$ µs so that with $P_0 = 10^5$ Pa, R_m is calculated from Eq. 6.102 to be 1.1 mm compared with $r_m = 1.7$ mm for the measured maximum transverse radius of the bubble. On this basis, the effective radius is substantially lower than r_m, which is not unreasonable given that the bubble is a flattened sphere into which the fibre protrudes. In addition, volume may be lost due to liquid that penetrates into the axial regions of the bubble, but is not detected in the shadowgraph, which only delineates the cavity boundary.

The growth of a spherical vapour cavity can be described by the following equation which can be derived from energy considerations (Young 1989):

$$\rho \dot{R}^2 = \frac{2P_i}{3(\gamma-1)} \left[(R_i/R)^3 - (R_i/R)^{3\gamma} \right] - \frac{2P_0}{3} \left[1 - (R_i/R)^3 \right] \tag{6.106}$$

Here R is the radius of the cavity and $\dot{R}$ the corresponding wall velocity. At t = 0, the cavity velocity satisfies $\dot{R} = 0$, R = R_i and the vapour pressure is P_i. It is assumed that in the subsequent expansion the vapour obeys an ideal adiabatic gas law of the form PV^γ = constant, where $\gamma \approx 4/3$ is the ratio of specific heats. In deriving Eq. 6.106, it is assumed that surface tension and viscous effects are negligible, and that the liquid incompressible. The assumption of incompressibility leads to the cavity wall velocity being zero at t = 0 and only increasing slowly with time at early stages of the expansion. This follows because the corresponding acoustic velocity in the liquid is infinite in this approximation, and the gas cavity cannot accelerate a finite mass of liquid instantaneously. Whilst this treatment is adequate for analyzing the long-term expansion and contraction phase of bubbles, it is necessary to take compressibility into account when estimating acoustic pressure levels produced in the initial stages of the laser interaction. To evaluate Eq. 6.106, we take $P_i = 8.5 \times 10^7$ Pa based on the peak stress estimated from the photoacoustic transducer at 5.5 Jcm^{-2} (Fig. 6.27) and $P_0 = 10^5$ Pa. The resulting variation in velocity with radius is shown in Fig.

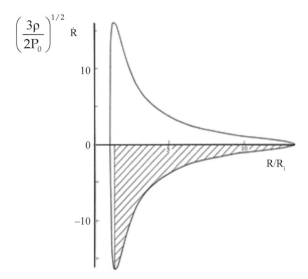

Figure 6.27. Normalised velocity of bubble $(3\rho/2P_0)^{1/2} \dot{R}$, as a function of R/R_i; for this calculation the initial radius $R_i = 8.2 \times 10^{-2}$ mm, the initial pressure $P_i = 8.5 \times 10^7$ Pa, $\gamma = 1.33$ and $P_0 = 10^5$ Pa. In the shaded region the liquid accelerates the wall of the vapour cavity.

6.27, where $(3\rho/2P_0)^{1/2} R$ is plotted as a function of R/R_i. In this case the maximum expansion ratio is $R_m/R = 13.3$ which with $R_m = 1.1$ mm gives $R_i = 8.2 \times 10^{-2}$ mm for the radius of the initial (equivalent) spherical cavity. Assuming no dissolved air enters from the liquid, the pressure P_f, in the fully expanded cavity can be estimated using $P_f = P_i (R_i/R_m)^{3\gamma}$ to be 2.7×10^3 Pa. This corresponds to $P_f/P_0 = 2.7 \times 10^{-2}$, indicating that the final pressure is substantially lower than the local hydrostatic pressure. A corresponding R-t plot derived by integrating Eq. 6.103 numerically is shown for comparison with the experimental data obtained at 5.5 J cm^{-2} in Fig. 6.22.

Laser-liquid interaction at the fibre tip

Water exhibits strong absorption at the wavelengths emitted at 2.94 µm and 10.6 µm, and in this case by the multiline HF laser and as a result energy is deposited in a very shallow region adjacent to the fibre tip. For low fluences the heated depth, neglecting thermal conduction, is $\alpha^{-1} \approx 1.6$ µm, where α is the average absorption coefficient ($\alpha \approx 6 \times 10^3$ cm^{-1}). Heating will lead to thermoelastic stress being generated due the water expanding, and if the fluence is high enough boiling can take place, i.e., if $T \geq 373$ K for $P_0 \sim 10^5$ Pa. Under conditions where the characteristic laser pulse duration, τ_p, is much longer than the timescale, $(\alpha c_a)^{-1}$, for an acoustic wave to travel across the heated zone, the peak thermoelastic stress can be shown to be (Cross et al. 1988):

$$\sigma_T \cong \frac{f \Gamma I_0}{C_a} \qquad (6.107)$$

Here I_0 is the peak laser irradiance, $F \sim 0.1$ is the Grüneisen constant for water (Cross et al. 1988) and $f < 0.5$ is a factor that depends on the precise laser pulse shape. For the present conditions, estimates give $f = 0.1$ so that for $I_0 < 10^6$ Wcm^{-2}, $\sigma_T \sim 7 \times 10^4$ Pa, i.e., the thermoelastic stress is relatively small. This is because stress relaxation by the propagation of an acoustic wave across the heated zone occurs on a timescale (~ 0.6 ns) that is much smaller than τ_p (< 400 ns). In principle, boiling of the heated water layer can take place once its temperature exceeds ~ 373 K under conditions where the local pressure in the liquid is $\sim 10^5$ Pa. However, because of the strongly non-equilibrium nature of the interaction we postulate that substantial superheating occurs, i.e., the temperature exceeds $T(P_v) = 373$ K, where $P_v \sim 10^5$ Pa is the vapour pressure that exists under equilibrium conditions. This can be justified by noting that heat extraction by bubble growth from microscopic vapour pockets can only take place if the temperature and vapour pressure is sufficiently high to overcome surface tension effects (Flowers and Mendoza 1970). In addition, even if bubble growth is initiated, the large difference in volume between the liquid and vapour below the critical point together with the finite bubble growth velocity will limit the maximum rate at which energy can be transferred to the vapour. If this falls below the rate at which energy is input from the laser, then the liquid temperature will continue to increase, i.e., superheating occurs. On this basis we argue that the liquid is heated at approximately constant pressure ($\sim 10^5$ Pa) to the critical temperature ($T_c = 647$ K), at which point distinction between liquid and vapour is lost. The pressure then increases sharply and growth of a vapour cavity can take place. An estimate of the threshold fluence, F_T, for attaining the critical temperature can be obtained from

$$F_T \, \alpha' = \Delta H_v \tag{6.108}$$

where α' is the mass absorption coefficient of water for the multiline HF laser and ΔH_v is the enthalpy difference between water at room temperature and the critical point (~ 2000 Jg^{-1}). If $\alpha' = \alpha/\rho$ is assumed to be constant with a value of approximately 6×10^3 cm^2 g^{-1} derived from available room temperature data (Hale and Querry 1973) suitably weighted for the laser spectrum, then $F_T = 0.33$ J cm^{-2}. A correction to account for heat loss by conduction to the fibre tip can be estimated from

$$F_f = S \, (T_c - T_R) \, (4D_t \, \tau_p)^{1/2} \tag{6.109}$$

where $S \approx 3.7$ J cm^{-3} K^{-1} is the mean volume heat capacity and $D \sim 1.8 \times 10^{-3}$ cm^2 s^{-1} is the mean thermal diffusivity of the fluoride glass fibre (Parker and France 1990). This gives $F_f \approx 0.07$ Jcm^{-2} and raises the threshold fluence to ~ 0.4 Jcm^{-2}. This is considerably lower than the fluence at which a detectable cavity is revealed by the shadowgraph technique, i.e., around 0.6 Jcm^{-2}. It is noted, however, that this calculated "threshold" corresponds to the attainment of the critical temperature at the water surface in contact with the fibre tip; substantially higher fluences are probably necessary to ablate a sufficiently large volume to promote bubble growth.

Photoacoustic response

Photoacoustic measurements made for the fibre contacted to the tissue surface show that detectable pressures occur for exit fluences from the fibre exceeding ~ 0.9 J cm^{-2} and that the peak pressure increases steadily above this value (Fig. 6.26). An estimate of the peak pressure generated under these conditions can be made as follows; we assume that ablation commences at that time, t_a, during the pulse when the net fluence delivered to the surface reaches the threshold value and that the ablation products expand by compressing the tissue surface. If as a result of ablation a layer of material of thickness Δx is converted to an ideal gas, the pressure P is found using

$$P = (\gamma - 1) \, \Delta F / \Delta x \tag{6.110}$$

where ΔF is the fluence delivered to the layer in a characteristic time $\Delta \tau_p$ for pressure release to occur by expansion. $\Delta \tau_p$ is estimated as

$$\Delta \tau = \Delta x / u = \Delta x \rho c_a / P \tag{6.111}$$

where u is the expansion rate of the gas cavity given by the local particle velocity produced in the confining tissue by the passage of a plane acoustic wave of pressure P (shock effects are neglected and it is assumed that the fibre is incompressible). Then using $\Delta F = I(t_a) \, \Delta \tau_p$, where $I(t_a)$ is the laser irradiance at t_a, we obtain from (6.110) and (6.111):

$$P = \left[\rho c_a I(t_a)(\gamma - 1) \right]^{1/2} \tag{6.112}$$

It is implicitly assumed in deriving (6.112) that the peak pressure occurs at the inception of ablation. This is reasonable if the laser irradiance satisfies $I < I(t_a)$ for $t > t_a$, making the expression applicable to fast rising but finite duration (and monotonically decreasing) laser pulses. A similar expression has been used by Zweig and Deutsch (1992) to describe pressures generated in the excimer-laser ablation of polyimide in a liquid environment. In that case, provided ablation commences at a fixed time near the peak of the laser pulse, the pressure scales as $(F/\tau_p)^{1/2}$, where F is the fluence. In the present experiments using a fast rise-time but relatively long duration laser pulse ($\approx$ 900 ns full duration) the pressure fluence dependence is anticipated to be more complicated than $F^{1/2}$. This is because for fluences near to but exceeding the threshold, ablation will commence near the end of the pulse producing low pressures because $I(t_a)$ is low. As the fluence is raised, ablation will progressively occur at earlier times in the pulse leading to an increase in pressure that depends not only on fluence but the detailed shape of the laser pulse. Ultimately at high fluence, ablation will occur at a fixed time near the peak of the laser pulse and the pressure will exhibit an $F^{1/2}$ dependence (Zweig and Deutsch 1992). This behaviour at least qualitatively can be used to explain the form of the variation observed in Fig. 6.26, where the pressure increases quite rapidly with fluence near threshold but starts to level out at high fluences. The fast rising form of the pressure transient (Fig. 6.25) and observation that the appearance of the pressure pulse moves to earlier times with increasing fluence also provides qualitative support for the model. The peak pressures predicted using (6.112) are in broad agreement with the experimental findings; for example, at 5.5 J cm^{-2}, assuming ablation occurs near the peak of the laser pulse, a calculated value of P = 1.8×10^8 Pa, is obtained using $\gamma = 1.16$ (Zweig and Deutsch 1992), compared with a measured value of $\sim 8.5 \times 10^7$ Pa. Given that there is likely to be amplitude loss due to acoustic attenuation and beam expansion over the $\approx$ 300 µm tissue path between the tissue surface and transducer, and that the model neglects fibre compression this agreement can be taken as satisfactory. The acoustic energy radiated into the tissue during the initial high-pressure phase of the cavity expansion can be estimated as

$$\Delta E_A \simeq P^2 A\, \Delta t\, /\rho c_a \qquad\qquad (6.113)$$

where A is the fibre core area, Δt the duration and P the peak pressure, respectively, of the pressure pulse. At 5.5 Jcm^{-2} where P $\sim 8.5 \times 10^7$ pa and $\Delta t = 200$ ns this corresponds to $\sim$170 µJ so that only a small fraction ($\sim$ 2%) of the input energy is converted to sound in the early phase of the expansion. Unfortunately, as noted earlier, it was not possible to measure any pressure transients associated with the long time expansion and contraction phase of the bubble because of the complicating effect of acoustic reflections. In later research, it was suggested (Pratisto et al. 1996) that because an IR laser pulse creates a water-vapour channel bridging the water-filled space between the fibre tip and the tissue surface, the use of a short (200 µs, 100 mJ) holmium (Ho:YAG) laser pulse at 2.1 µm as a prepulse to generate a vapour bubble through which the ablating Er:YAG laser pulse can be transmitted increases the cutting depth in meniscus from 450 to 1120 µm as compared with the depth following a single erbium pulse.

6.3.3 Photoablation

The term *'ablation'* refers to evaporation followed by expulsion of evaporated material. The absorption of strong laser pulses causes small explosions. The UV laser-induced ablation is called *'photoablation'*. In 1982, Srinivasan and Mayne-Benton discovered that many polymers can be etched with submicron resolution and without apparent thermal damage using an ArF (193 nm) excimer laser with intensity of 10^7–10^8 W/cm^{-2}. This was called ablative photodecomposition (APD), where it referred to a process whereby the absorption of 6.4 eV photons of 193 nm laser caused a direct bond breaking of biopolymers without apparent thermal damage or charring. Since then the ablation of organic polymers and biological tissues has been studied extensively by many investigators to understand the photochemistry of ablation. Organic polymers are made of carbon, hydrogen, nitrogen, and oxygen. The importance of APD is in its wide spectrum of medical and industrials applications including: micro-machining of biodegradable polymers in enhancing the efficacy of many drugs and constructing new therapeutic modalities (Toenshoff et al. 2000), pattern generation (Kyung-Bok et al. 2004, Aguilar et al. 2005), tissue engineering (Schmalenberg and Uhrich 2005), lithography (Jain and Wilson 1982). Further investigations showed that with ArF (193 nm) and KrF (248 nm), the dominant mechanism in ablative decomposition whereby fast ablation occurs is photochemical and that at longer excimer lasers, i.e., XeCl (308 nm) and XeF (351 nm), is

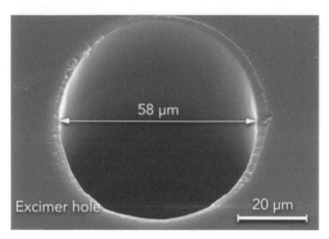

Figure 6.28. An example of photoablation of polymer (PET) with excimer KrF laser (Broude 2012).

primarily both photothermal and photochemical in nature (Dyer and Sidhu 1986). Figure 6.28 shows an example of photoablation of polyethylene terephthalate (PET) with KrF laser (Broude 2012).

The APD mechanism

The infrared photons with energies of < 1.5 eV per photon give rise to vibrational and rotational excitation of the absorber and by absorption of many repeated photons (multiphoton absorption), thermal decomposition of the material is achieved. In the UV range, the principle coupling of laser wavelength is to chromophores in the structural proteins. In the UV-laser-tissue interaction rapid bond breaking is believed to be a photochemical process that occurs from a high-lying electronic state. This will in turn, will cause a local increase in the pressure in the irradiated volume which will lead to ablation. The APD does not exist for the fluences below a certain threshold depending on material. Once the threshold is exceeded a single pulse can remove material. The thickness of the ablated tissue with one pulse increases with fluence. Generally, the physical process involves: absorption of the photon, bond breaking, and ablation of the products. To understand the chemistry of the decomposition of organic materials, it is essential to have some information about the rate of material transformation, the time scale in which the reaction occurs, and the composition of the products (Srinivasan 1982). The main reasons for considering this process as non-thermal are because the heat transfer to non-irradiated regions can be neglected and because of short pulse duration, the ablated tissue material takes most of the absorbed laser energy away from the remaining tissue as products leaves the surface. Thus, very thin layer of material is ablated in a controlled fashion.

Let us assume that two atoms A and B of a biopolymer, which are bound covalently by an electron is subject to laser exposure. Due to the structure of macromolecules, each electronic level is split into vibrational states. Upon absorption of energetic photons, the atoms may be promoted to an excited state, i.e., (AB)*. According to Franck-Condon's principle, the radial distance between the two nuclei of atoms A and B is not changed during the excitation process because of small electron mass. If a UV photon is absorbed, the energy gain is normally sufficiently high to reach an electronic state and exceeds the bond energy. Consequently, the two atoms may undergo dissociation at next vibrational level. So, one can express this as:

Excitation: $AB + h\upsilon \rightarrow (AB)^*$
Dissociation: $(AB)^* \rightarrow A + B + K.E.$ (kinetic energy)

The underlying steps are shown in the Fig. 6.29.

Useful information such as ablation onset (i.e., threshold) and absorption coefficient of the material can be derived from removal measurements by applying the Beer's-Lamberts law (Eq. 6.92) to describe the etch depth per pulse. The law in its simplest form states that no material is actually removed until the absorbed photon energy per unit volume has reached a critical value known as 'fluence threshold,

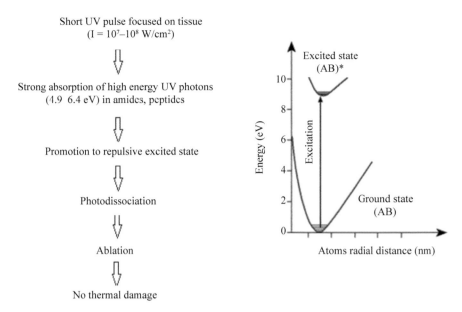

Figure 6.29. Schematic illustration of photoablation mechanism where the atoms are excited and their potential energy varies with the nuclei radial distance. Photodissociation occurs once the repulsive force at excited state becomes dominant.

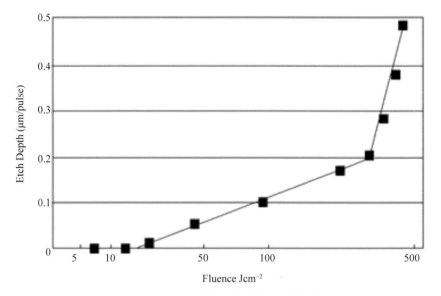

Figure 6.30. Ablation of 70 μm thick PET with KrF laser.

F_t'. Here, the plume (ablated particles) retains the same absorption coefficient as the condensed phase. An experiment (Khosroshahi 1993) used a fiber-delivered KrF laser to ablate PET. Figure 6.29 shows that the etching begins at fluence ≈ 25 mJcm^{-2} and then increased quite rapidly at higher values of fluenece. In the range of 25–300 mJcm^{-2}, a fit to data gives $\alpha \approx 12\,10^4$ cm^{-1} beyond which the etch rate increases more rapidly possibly due to increasing plume transparency. Under these conditions (i.e., transparent plume) the etch rate is described by an equation similar to 6.96, where the latent heat is replaced by energy per volume, αF_t. The increased transparency of plume is likely due to strong heating of the ablation products formed in the early stages of the laser pulse at high fluence, and hence resulting in their degradation to lower mass species which absorbs less strongly. In this experiment an assumed linear dependence beyond

≈ 300 mJcm^{-2} yields $\alpha F_t \approx 710^3$ Jcm^{-2} and considering the above F_t, and using (6.96), it gives a value of 2810^4 cm^{-1} for the effective absorption coefficient.

Safety issue

It is highly recommended to notice and take appropriate action when such materials are ablated either by IR or UV lasers, as they may produce hazardous plume and products. Dyer and Sidhu (1988) used spectroscopy and fast photography to study the luminous plume produced by ablative etching of PET and polyimide with XeCl laser. In air, the emission spectra of the plumes for PET and polyimide are characterized by strong CN and C2 emission bands and their observed emission greatly exceeded their radiative life-times. This latter observation suggests that these excited species to be produced during the expansion phase and are not solely produced in the initial ablation. The presence of CN in the plume of PET, a polymer containing no nitrogen, is indicative that this is formed by reaction with the environmental gas.

6.3.4 Photodisruption

The word '*rupus*' in latin denotes *burst* or *breaking*, so photodisruption in principle would imply a mechanical damage or tearing up the material caused by light absorption. This mode is sometimes referred to as photomechanical where typically nanosecond and shorter pulses are used. Photodisruption basically, has four known stage: plasma, shock wave, cavitation, and jetting. The first two occur in air (or a gaseous medium) but the third and the last one can also occur in a liquid medium following the formation of a plasma depending on the laser optical parameters. If the appropriate conditions are not satisfied, as for long pulse duration, then one may only observe the material photodisruption as a result of cavitation and jetting effects only, as discussed in §6.3.2. When a high peak power laser pulse is focused on the target, it creates high irradiances of about 10^{10} Wcm^{-2} for ns pulses and 10^{12} Wcm^{-2} for ps pulses, which generates a local high electric fields (10^6–10^7 V/cm) comparable to average atomic intramolecular Coulomb electric fields. Such laser fields are capable of inducing a dielectric breakdown of the target material, resulting in the formation of a microplasma, i.e., an ionized volume with significant number of free electrons or electron density. This is accompanied by a sudden adiabatic rise in plasma temperature due to kinetic energy of free electrons up to about 10,000K where a bright spark and noise can be observed. Following the plasma expansion, a shock wave is generated, which propagates spatially interacting with the surrounding medium causing the disruption of the material.

Figure 6.31a shows that a shock front is formed at very early stages of plasma formation and propagates with a velocity in the order of a few thousands of kms^{-1} and soon reaches its plateau, and after this point it decreases to acoustic velocity. Similarly, the plasma temperature, Fig. 6.31b, also gradually decreases exponentially and it eventually cools down.

At the microscopic level, the mechanism responsible for optical breakdown is the considerable production of free electrons. It is, however, possible to distinguish the initiation process, which corresponds to localized electron 'seeding' by ionization involving a few electrons only from the massive photodisruption. In the initial phase the ionization mechanisms, in which energies of about 7–10 eV must be applied in order to separate the individual electrons from the bound electrons, depending on pulse duration (Puliafito and Steinert 1984, Fradin et al. 1973).

i) Thermionic emission: Here, a Q-switched laser (≤ 10 ns) causes a local heating of the material, where temperatures exceeding several tens of thousands of degrees are reached. The presence of impurities accelerates the process.

ii) Multiphoton ionization: (MPI): This is a non-linear process where a very short mode-locked (ps) pulse trains causes molecular ionization called MPI. The threshold for optical breakdown is higher for mode-locked pulses than for Q-switched pulses. In air, the threshold for a single 25 ps pulse is about 10^{14} Wcm^{-2} whereas it is only 10^{11} Wcm^{-2} for a 10 ns pulse (Fradin et al. 1973). In biological solutions, these numbers are reduced by a factor of 100.

The key physical element of such photomechanical force interaction lies in a process known as '*electron avalanche*' or '*Inverse Bremsstralung*' effect. Bremsstralung is a process during which the electrons are

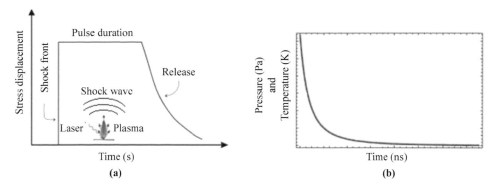

Figure 6.31. Variation of shock wave stress displacement with time (a) and exponential decay of shock wave pressure and plasma temperature with time (b).

accelerated and emit radiation. Thus, the inverse effect would be the absorption of photons by atoms and consequently emission of electrons. In the field of molecules or ions, free electrons already present or seeded so do speak absorb incoming photons and convert this energy into kinetic energy, thereby, increasing their velocity. During the collision of electrons with each other, further ionization is made, and this effectively continues as a chain reaction known as *avalanche*, as in snow avalanche. Thus we can write:

$$h\nu + e + A^+ \longrightarrow e + A^+$$

Therefore, the avalanche process grows exponentially and in within a few hundreds of ps a very large electron density, e.g., about 10^{21} cm^{-3} is achieved in focal volume of the laser pulse. This is called *laser-induced breakdown* of dielectric medium. The condition for plasma growth and sustainment is that losses due to inelastic collision or free electrons diffusion do not quench the Bremsstralung avalanche. The plasma oscillation frequency, ω_p is written as

$$\omega_p{}^2 = \frac{N_e{}^2}{\varepsilon_0 m_e} \tag{6.114}$$

where N_e is the total number of free electrons or electron density, $m_e = 9.1 \, 10^{-31}$ kg is mass of electron and $\varepsilon_0 = 8.85 \, 10^{-12}$ Fm^{-1} is the permittivity of free space. For the case, where the mean collision rate of electrons is much smaller than laser frequency, i.e., $\bar{\upsilon}_e \ll \omega_1$, then

$$\alpha_p = \frac{\bar{\upsilon}_e}{nc} \frac{\omega_p{}^2}{\omega_1{}^2} \tag{6.115}$$

where α_p is the plasma absorption, n is the refractive index, and c is the velocity of light. Thus, it can be seen that by increasing the light to longer wavelengths, e.g., IR, the plasma absorption is increases. It is deduced from (6.114) and (6.115) that $\alpha_p \simeq \sqrt{N_e}$ and that the electrons density soon reaches its critical value, N_c. At this stage, the incoming photons are no longer absorbed or converted, but instead are scattered. This condition is called '*plasma shielding effect*'.

$$N_c = \frac{\varepsilon_0 m_e}{e^2} \omega_1{}^2 \tag{6.116}$$

In terms of radiation wavelength,

$$N_c \leq \frac{\pi}{\lambda^2 r_e} \tag{6.117}$$

where $r_e = 2.8 \, 10^{-13}$ cm is the classical electron radius.

Recently, Khosroshahi et al. (2009) used a 200 ns CO_2 laser for surface modification of stainless steel for biomedical applications. Figure 6.32 illustrates the formation of plasma plume at about 800 mJ which grows in volume with the pulse energy, but as it can be seen, the size of plume remains constant for first few pulse number. Assuming that all pulse energy is used to ionize steel components particularly Fe with

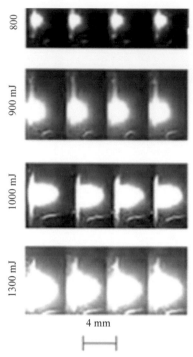

4 mm

Figure 6.32. Plasma profile as a function of pulse energy. The profile seems remain constant for first few laser pulses t a given energy.

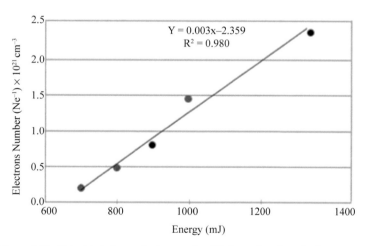

Figure 6.33. Calculated plasma electron number (Ne⁻) as a function of pulse energy.

63% constitution, which has a singlet ionization energy of $E_i \approx 16$ eV. Thus, the number of free electrons is approximately given by $N_e^- \approx (E_p/E_i)/eV$.

Figure 6.33 shows that number of free electrons, N_e^- linearly increases with pulse energy, which in this case gives a range of $(2.7–5) \times 10^{17}$. However, a rough estimate of the plasma plume volume can be obtained from magnification of pictures taken by CCD camera (Fig. 6.32). Hence, the free electron density per unit volume varies between $(0.2 \times 10^{21}$ and $2.3 \times 10^{21})$ cm⁻³ and between 800 mJ and 1300 mJ, respectively. The angular distribution of the material ejected by the target during ablation can be represented by the equation $I(\theta) - I_0\cos^n\theta$ where $I(\theta)$ is the flux intensity along a direction forming an angle θ with

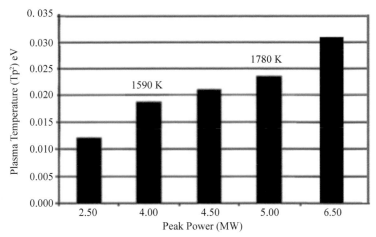

Figure 6.34. Calculated plasma temperature as a function of laser peak power.

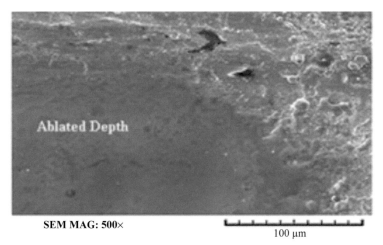

SEM MAG: 500×

100 μm

Figure 6.35. Ti6Al4V surface irradiated at 1350 J cm^{-2} with 4 pulses, where a clean crater wall and edge is obtained.

the normal to the target surface. I_0 is initial intensity corresponding to $\theta = 0$ and n is parameter related to the anisotropy of the distribution. In fact n = 1 corresponds to a perfectly spherical distribution, and n > 1 implies a more directional plume shape, as in our case in Fig. 6.32.

The electron temperature can reach a few to tens of electron volts (1 eV = 11,600 K) during the laser pulse duration, while the ions remain relatively cold. The corresponding plasma temperature can be calculated, to a close approximation using Eq. (6.118) (Dreyfus 1992).

$$T_p \approx \beta \left[P_\lambda \sqrt{\tau_p} \right]^{1/2} \qquad (6.118)$$

where β is a constant depending on material and P_λ is the laser peak power and τ_p is the laser pulse duration.

The variation of plasma plume temperature with laser peak power is shown in Fig. 6.34. As it is expected plume temperature steadily increases with increase in peak power.

Figure 6.35 demonstrates an example of the material surface smoothened due to plasma temperature at 1350 Jcm^{-2}. As it is evident from the Fig. 6.32, in this case, no plasma shielding effect was observed even at highest level of laser fluence since no decoupling effect had occurred.

6.4 Laser-induced fluorescence spectroscopy (LIFS)

6.4.1 Physical principles

There are two types of photoluminescence: (a) Fluorescence which has a life time in the range of 10^{-8} s, and (b) Phosphorescence with a life time of several seconds up to a few minutes. Several quantum mechanical considerations are important in the absorption and loss of interacting radiations: (1) The discrete steps that exist between one electronic, vibrational, and rotational levels, and (2) if the absorbed photon has more energy than required for a simple electronic transition, the excess energy is usually absorbed as rotational and vibrational energy. Figure 6.36 demonstrates the typical stages of a molecular excitation, where the transition to excited state is in the order of 10^{-15} s. Transitions to lowest singlet state are less rapid about 10^{-11} s and the probability of the transition to ground state is about 10^{-9} s. If light is absorbed by the absorption band of lowest energy (i.e., longest wavelength) then the molecule will likely undergo a transition from the ground state to the next highest electronic energy level (S1) and if, however, more energetic light is absorbed by molecules, it will make a transition to higher electronic level (S2) or (S3). In this case, the excess energy is quickly lost and the molecule returns from S2 vibrational energy levels to the lowest excited state (S1) via a process known as *'internal conversion'*.

When the incident photons are absorbed by an atom or molecule, it returns to the ground state via number of routes. (i) *Non-radiative* or radiationless relaxation process since no photons are emitted where the excited molecule converts all of the excitation energy into rotational and internal vibrational energy (internal conversion) in which case, the excited energy is dissipated as heat and the molecule returns to the ground state. The excited molecule can convert part of the excitation energy into vibrational and rotational energy, and can exist for some time in the lowest excited state (S1), (ii) *Radiative* relaxation process where the molecule is very efficient energy absorber and it can return directly from the excited state to ground state during which it emits photons. This emission of light is called *fluorescence*. The category of molecules capable of undergoing electronic transitions that result in fluorescence are known as *fluorophores* or fluorochromes. If, however, the molecule makes a transition from lowest vibrational state of singlet state (S1) to excited triplet state where it then is transferred to the ground state, is called *phosphorescence* which has a longer lifetime compared to fluorescence. Internal conversion and vibrational relaxation are

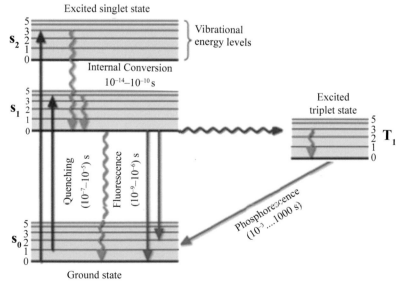

Figure 6.36. Electronic transition from ground state to excited state. Molecule can return directly to ground state to produce fluorescence or via triplet state producing phosphorescence.

responsible for the emitted photon with lower energy level than the incident photon. This shift to longer wavelength is known as '*Stokes shift*'. This is essential for sensitivity of fluorescence detection because it allows an effective separation of the fluorescence emission signal from Rayleigh-scattered excitation singlet. If, however, the emitted wavelength is shorter than the incident, i.e., a shift to shorter wavelength, it is called '*anti-stokes shift*'. Usually, LIFS uses a monochromatic laser light source, coupled to a small diameter fiber optic probe illuminating the target and the emitted fluorescence is then collected by another fiber which guided to a multichannel analyzer, computer or a UV-Vis spectrometer. In the clinical cases, it is often advanced through the instrument channel of an endoscope. Laser-induced fluorescence endoscopy (LIFE) is real time fluorescence imaging system incorporated in a standard endoscope enables the screening a large surface area of mucosa. By illuminating the entire endoscopic field of view, fluorescence images can be collected in parallel with the standard images. Such a system allows or improves dysplasia detection and directed biopsy sampling. The advantages of using LIFS, particularly for clinical applications such as diagnosis, are that the measurements are safe, noninvasive and can be performed quantitatively and quickly. The fluorescence technique can be automated and offers real-time detection and differentiation with a precision, selectivity and sensitivity. These can be further facilitated by using a tunable laser.

6.4.2 Fluorescence parameters

The main parameters that describe a fluorescence process are: Extinction coefficient (ε), fluorescence brightness (B) and quantum yield (q) or the efficiency of fluorescence emission relative to all other pathways of relaxation and is expressed as a dimensionless ratio of the number of photons emitted to the total number of photons absorbed by a fluorophore.

$$q = \frac{k_r}{k_r + k_{nr} + k_x} \tag{6.119}$$

$$q = \frac{\text{number of photons emitted}}{\text{number of photons absorbed}}$$

where $k_r = 1/\tau_0$, k_{nr} and k_x are the radiative, non-radiative, and intersystem crossing rate constants respectively, and τ_0 is the average lifetime of the excited state.

$$B = q. \varepsilon \tag{6.120}$$

High fluorescence molecules have high values of both ε and q, and thus high absorbance and efficient emission.

6.4.3 Measurement of fluorescence lifetime (FLT)

Fluorescent lifetime is an intrinsic property of fluorescence probes that is extensively used for studying biomolecules, microenvironment, and molecular associations. FLT has a high information content, which can also be used as a characteristic of a fluorophore and is concentration independent, unaffected by variation in excitation intensity and therefore, likely to be more reliable. Also, FLTs are very sensitive to variation of tissue pH and its oxygenation content. When a sample containing an initial population (n_0) of fluorophores is excited by a pulse of light, they are excited to a higher level with a population of $n(t)$. This population subsequently decays back to the ground state in a short scale of time due to fluorescence emission and non-radiative process,

$$dn(t)/dt = -(k_r + k_{nr}) n(t) \tag{6.121}$$

where n(t) is the number of molecules in the excited state at time t following the excitation. This results in an exponential decay of the excited state,

$$n(t) = n_0 e^{(-t/\tau)} \tag{6.122}$$

where τ is the fluorescence life time of the molecule and is defined as

$$\tau = (k_r + k_{nr})^{-1} \tag{6.123}$$

The fluorescence life time and quantum yield are related by,

$$\Phi = k_r/(k_r + k_{nr}) = \tau/\tau_0 \tag{6.124}$$

τ_0 is the natural or radiative lifetime of the fluorescence, $\tau_0 = k_r^{-1}$.

The decay of the fluorescence intensity as a function of time in a uniform population of molecules is,

$$I(t) = I_0(t) e^{(-t/\tau)} \tag{6.125}$$

Fluorescence lifetime can be measured in two distinct ways, see Fig. 6.37.

a) *Time-domain*: Here the sample is excited using a short pulsed source and the time dependent intensity of emission is measured following the excitation pulse.
b) *Frequency-domain:* Here, the sample is excited by an intensity modulated cw source at a very high frequency. The resulting fluorescence emission is thus also modulated at the same frequency. However, due to finite lifetime of fluorescence, the emission is delayed in time relative to the excitation. This delay is measured as a phase shift (φ) which can be used to calculate the decay time, called phase lifetime (τ_φ) and given by,

$$\tau_\varphi = \omega^{-1} \tan \varphi \tag{6.126}$$

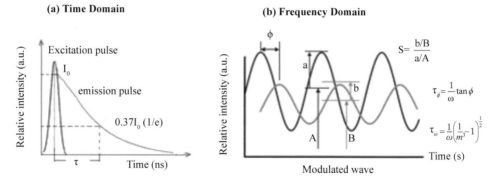

Figure 6.37. A time domain (a) and frequency domain (b) measurement of fluorescence lifetime.

6.4.4 Tissue autofluorescence

There are basically two methods for detection of fluorescence: One approach is to use tissue autofluorescence, i.e., the fluorescence originating from naturally occurring fluorophores called *endogenous* that are specific to normal or dysplastic tissue. The second approach is to use external agents or fluorophores called *exogenous* that tend to accumulate preferentially within malignant tissue. All tissue exhibit endogenous fluorescence, which is referred to as autofluorescence when is exposed to a particular exciting wavelength. Some of the significant biological fluorophores among others are: Nicotinamide adenine dinucleotide (NADH), Nicotinamide adenine dinucleotide phosphate (NADPH), Flavin adenine dinucleotide (FAD), Flavin mononucleotide (FMN), amino acids, vitamins, and lipids. Some of these are important indicators of tissue metabolic activity. As metabolism is activated, there is a shift to oxidized forms (NAD^+, FAD^+, etc.). The lack of these oxidized forms results in a reduction of fluorescence signal intensity. Equally important are the other tissue fluorophores, including the connective tissue proteins, collagen, elastin, and porphorines, i.e., the intermediates of haem synthesis (i.e., is a cofactor consisting of an Fe^{2+} (ferrous) ion contained at the center of a large heterocyclic organic ring called a porphyrin, made up of four pyrrolic groups joined together by methine bridges). Table 6.1 shows the peak excitation and corresponding peak emission wavelengths for some fluorophores in tissue (Bottiroli et al. 1995).

Note that a variety of pathological processes, such as inflammation, can cause metabolic changes, which in turn affect certain fluorophore concentration, thus producing a different and distinct autofluorescence compared to the original sample.

Table 6.1. Fluorescence excitation and emission wavelengths of various tissue fluorophores (Bottiroli et al. 1995).

Fluorophores	Peak excitation wavelength (nm)	Peak emitted wavelength (nm)
NADH	350	500
Flavin	455	495
Collagen	250	330
Elastin	285	350
Porphyrin	405	610

Wavelengths classification

1. UV range (100–400 nm)

UV-C (Far): 100–280 nm
UV-B (Mid): 280–315 nm
UV-A (Near): 315–400 nm

Main absorbers: Protien, Nucleic acids, Peptide bonds

2. Visible (400–750 nm)

Main absorbers: Melanin, Haemoglobin, Oxyhaemoglobin

3. IR (750–1 mm)

IR-C (Far): 1 mm–3 μm
IR-B (Mid): 3–1.4 μm
IR-C (Near): 1.4–750 nm

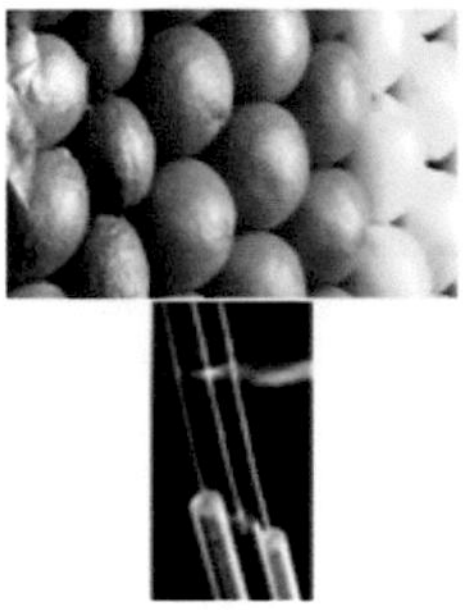

Main absorbers: Water (soft tissue, e.g., skin, eye)

Water absorption peaks: 1.45 μm, 1.90 μm and 2.94 μm

Schematic 6.1. Spectra classification of UV, Visible and IR wavelengths in terms of dominant absorbing components.

Short laser pulse focused at target:

$$I = \frac{\left(\dfrac{E_p}{\tau_p}\right)}{W^2}$$

⇩

High power density: $I \sim 10^{12}$ Wcm^{-2}

⇩

High electric field: $E = \left(\dfrac{2I}{c\varepsilon_0}\right)^{1/2} \approx 10^6$ V/cm

⇩

Dielectric breakdown (multiphoton process): $E_{laser} \sim E_{ionization}$

⇩

Plasma formation free electrons: $Ne \sim 10^{21}$ cm^{-3}, $T > 20{,}000°C$

⇩

Spherical shock wave propagation: $P \sim 13Ep/R^3$

⇩

Localized photodisruption

Schematic 6.2. Schematic illustration of photodisruption mechanism.

6.4.5 Detection and evaluation of normal and malignant cells using laser-induced fluorescence Spectroscopy (Khosroshahi and Rahmani 2011)

The aim of this research is to study the normalized fluorescence spectra (intensity variations and area under the fluorescence signal), relative quantum yield, extinction coefficient, and intracellular properties of normal and malignant human bone cells. Using Laser-Induced fluorescence spectroscopy (LIFS) upon excitation of 405 nm, the comparison of emission spectra of bone cells revealed that fluorescence intensity and the area under the spectra of malignant bone cells was less than that of normal. In addition, the area ratio and shape factor were changed. We obtained two emission bands in spectra of normal cells centered at about 486 and 575 nm, and for malignant cells about 482 and 586 nm, respectively, which are most likely attributed to NADH and riboflavins. Using fluorescein sodium emission spectrum, the relative quantum yield of bone cells is numerically determined.

Introduction

Osteosarcoma represents the most common sarcoma of bone, accounting for about one-quarter of all primary malignancies of bone and about one-third of all bone sarcomas. The incidence rates and 95% confidence intervals of osteosarcoma for all races and both sexes are 4.0 (3.5–4.6) for the range 0–14 years and 5.0 (4.6–5.6) for the range 0–19 years, per year per million persons. Among childhood cancers, osteosarcoma generally occurs in 2.4% of all malignant tumor cases. The incidence rates of childhood and adolescent osteosarcoma in Blacks and Hispanics is more than Caucasian, and it has always been considered to be higher in males than in females, occurring at a rate of 5.4 per million persons per year in males, vs. 4.0 per million in females. Osteosarcoma has a bimodal age distribution, having the first peak during adolescence (10–14-year-old age group) and the second peak in older adulthood (in adults older than 60 years old) (Ottaviani and Jaffe 2010, Mirabello et al. 2009). Bone marrow metastases are detected by imaging, such as skeletal scintigraphy (Even-Sapir 2005), radiography (Rybak and Rosenthal 2001), computed tomography (Fogelman et al. 2005), or magnetic resonance imaging (MRI) (Mentzel et al. 2004) and the other methods, such as positron emission tomography or single-photon emission computed tomography have a potential of evaluating it. When luciferase (Lus) or the green fluorescent protein (GFP) transfected cells are used, whole-body bioluminescent reporter imaging (BRI) (Yang et al. 2000) can detect microscopic bone marrow metastases, too. Polymerase chain reaction-based (PCR) methods with serious limitations (Zippelius et al. 1997) and immunocytochemical techniques (Pantel et al. 1993) are the other useful detection and quantification of cancerous bone marrow cells. In recent years, many optical methods are applied for biological and biomedical investigations. Light-induced fluorescence spectroscopy (LIFS) is one of the most widely spread spectroscopic methods which finds biomedical applications especially in diagnosis of cancer (Silveira et al. 2008, Benmansour et al. 2010). Fluorescence is the emission of light typically from aromatic molecules and depends on the nature of the excited state. In singlet excited states, the electron in excited orbital is paired (by opposite spin) to the second electron in the ground-state orbital. Consequently, return to the ground state is spin allowed and occurs rapidly by emission of a photon (Lakowicz 1999). This technique has been applied for the *in vitro* and *in vivo* analysis. In LIFS low-power laser light is directed toward biological component (such as biologic fluids, single cells, cell suspensions, frozen tissue sections, and bulk tissues), inducing fluorescence emission at wavelengths characteristic of the chemical composition of the biomaterials. The excitation light used for fluorescence measurements is usually in the near-UV and visible region. The advantages of using LIFS diagnosis are that the measurements are safe and noninvasive and can be performed quantitatively and quickly (Ramanujam et al. 1994).

The fluorescence technique can be automated and offers real-time detection and differentiation with a precision, selectivity, and sensitivity. In general, the predictive accuracy of spectroscopy is better than prediction based on biopsy solely. In contrast to conventional biopsy techniques, light and laser-induced fluorescence spectroscopy can be conducted to characterize tissues or to detect cancers without removing them (Chidananda et al. 2006, Vladimirov et al. 2007). If fluorescence could be used as a complementary method; then it could be of great interest in many clinical specialties. This would hopefully reduce the sampling error and help avoid unnecessary biopsies. Fluorescence spectroscopy also introduces other advantages, such as short pulse excitation, wavelength tunability, and narrow bandwidth excitation. By using different excitation wavelengths and spectral analysis techniques, fluorescence spectroscopy was subsequently used for distinguishing premalignant, malignant, and normal tissues in a variety of organ systems, such as lung and breast (Alfano et al. 1997), bronchus (Hung et al. 1991), colon (Romer et al. 1995), cervix (Ramanujam et al. 1994), esophagus (Vo-Dinh et al. 1998), and head and neck (Schantz et al. 1998). These alternations that occur as tissue progresses from a normal to a diseased state are reflected in the spectral characteristics of the measured fluorescence. The endogenous fluorophores such as the reduced form of nicotinamide adenine dinucleotide (phosphate) (NA(P)DH) and riboflavins (flavin mononucleotide (FMN) and flavin adenine dinucleotide (FAD)), collagen, elastin, amino acids, vitamins, lipids, and porphyrins have a significant variation in the concentration in different tissue types. These differences, together with alternations in the local environment within the tissue, are the basis for the discrimination between tumor and normal tissue by fluorescence spectroscopy. Characterizing biological samples, such as cells or tissues can be performed by steady-state fluorescence measurements in terms of overall intensity, peak wavelength, and spectral shape (Lakowicz 1999, Ramanujam 1994). The complicated analysis of tissues spectra due to strong light scattering because of structural heterogeneity and the need for improved sensitivity and specificity in cancer diagnosis has led to interest in native cellular fluorescence instead of frozen tissue section or bulk tissue fluorescence (Schantz et al. 1997). In diagnostic method for cancer detection, it is essential to separate malignant tumors from normal tissues. The goal of this study was to use LIFS to discriminate normal and malignant human bone cells and systematically characterize the differences in fluorescence properties, such as area ratio, shape factor, extinction coefficient, and quantum yield on emission spectra upon excitation at 405 nm.

Materials and method

Preparation of cell suspensions. Human osteosarcoma cell line (G 292, NCBI-C565), which was initiated from a primary bone tumor osteosarcoma, purchased from national cell bank of Pasteur institute of Iran. Normal osteoblast cell (HOB) were extracted by MACS (Magnetic activated cell sorting) method and measurements were made on cells having passage numbers of 30 or less. The G 292 cells were grown in Dulbecco modified Eagle medium (DMEM, GIBCO 116-12800) supplemented with 10% fetal bovine serum (FBS, GIBCO 106-10270). The HOB cells were grown in DMEM and HAM'S F12 (Sigma-Aldrich N6658) in ratio of 1:1, supplemented with 12% FBS. Both cells supplemented with 1% Antibiotic-Antimycotic Solution (PAA, P11-002), and then cells were incubated at 37°C with 5% CO_2. Upon reaching confluence for G 292 cells and pre-confluence for HOB cells (generally 3 days after passage), these cells were collected from culture flasks by trypsinization to yield a suspension and washed with phosphate-buffered saline (PBS) (GIBCO 18912-014). After washing, the cells were resuspended in a volume of 2 mL PBS. The cell suspensions pipetted into a cuvette with 1 cm path length for LIFS analysis. Cell concentration was determined by counting the number of cells per milliliter (cells/mL) manually in a standard manner with a hemocytometer from Neubauer and light microscope. The average cell viability determined with a manual viability count after addition of Trypan Blue 0.25% in PBS. The measurements were repeated independently three times for each sample.

Fluorescence spectroscopy of cell suspensions

A laser with 405 nm wavelength (CSI-405) with 100 mW maximum output power was used as an excitation source. An optical fibre with 600 μm core diameter and 0.22 NA (Ocean Optic LIBS-600-6-SR) was used to collect the fluorescence signal and guide it to the spectrometer (Ocean Optic, UV–VIS USB2000). The background spectrum was first recorded from cuvette filled with PBS solution and then the fluorescence measurements of cell suspensions were made at room temperature. After obtaining the spectra of samples, they were smoothened by Gaussian model using Find Graph software. In order to determine the relative quantum yield, 10^{-2} mM fluorescein sodium solution was used as a reference solution. The measurement was carried out after solving the fluorescein sodium powder (Merck, 518-47-8) in distilled water and filtration.

Results

The spectrum of the excitation light source is shown in Fig. 6.38. The average cell viability was $89.3 \pm 3.8\%$ and cell concentration for normal human osteoblast (HOB) and Human osteosarcoma cell line (G 292, NCBI-C565) were 9.4×105 and 8.6×10^5 cell/lit, respectively.

The 405 nm laser induced-fluorescence spectra of normal HOB and malignant G 292 cell, which is normalized to the HOB fluorescence peak at 486 nm (peak intensity of normal cell), are shown in Fig. 6.39. It can be seen that after samples excitation two peaks are observed at 486 and 575 nm corresponding to HOB cells, while that of malignant G 292 cells are slightly shifted to 482 and 586 nm, respectively. A considerable decrease in fluorescence amplitude of malignant G 292 cells compared to normal HOB cells can be seen and the main difference is observed in the region of 470–590 nm. This decrease can be explained in terms of biochemical and microstructural changes due to abnormalities. Main broad emission in the region of 470–490 nm were attributed to NADH (Colasanti et al. 2000, Kim et al. 2005) and secondary broad emission in the region of 570–590 nm is most likely attributed to riboflavins (Anidjar et al. 1998).

The comparison of laser induced-fluorescence spectra normalized to the main peak is presented in Fig. 6.40. When the peak intensities of the normal and malignant spectra are normalized, the differences in spectral line shape become more evident. The spectral line shapes of normal HOB and malignant G 292 cells are slightly different in the region of 530–610 nm. In order to develop an algorithm for disease classification based on the spectral differences, the ratio between two fluorescence peaks in each spectrum as shape factor, R_1 ratio, must be considered.

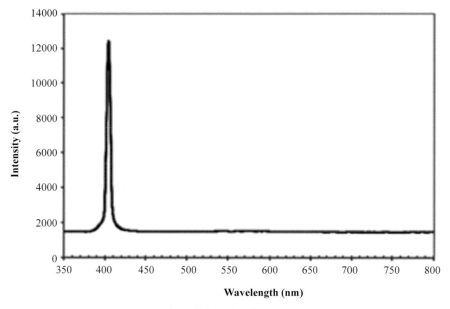

Figure 6.38. 405 nm laser beam spectrum.

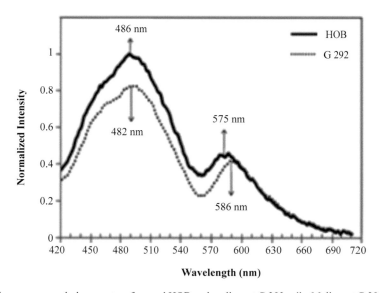

Figure 6.39. Fluorescence emission spectra of normal HOB and malignant G 292 cells. Malignant G 292 cell is normalized to the HOB fluorescence peak at 486 nm by Find Graph.

The peak fluorescence intensities and R_1 ratio is shown in Table 6.2. Also, R′ parameter, which is defined as intensity ratio of normal HOB over malignant G 292 cell, is shown in the Table 6.3. A decrease of fluorescence intensities of malignant G 292 comparing with normal HOB is noticeable, and is stronger at about 484 nm.

To intensify spectral structure differences of the fluorescence signal, each fluorescence spectrum was evaluated by area under the normalized fluorescence peak signal and area ratio (R_s). It became possible to notice slight differences among the spectra and identify parameters with the best distinction. It is visually obvious in Fig. 6.39 that the spectrum of G 292 malignant sample have smaller area than the HOB normal. Although these differences are not always visually obvious, the area under the fluorescence peak signals and Rs parameter is calculated by Find Graph software, as shown in Table 6.4. Based on normalized area

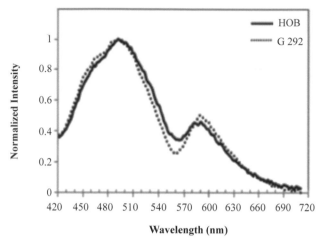

Figure 6.40. Fluorescence emission spectra of normal HOB and malignant G 292 cells normalized to main peak by Find Graph.

Table 6.2. Fluorescence intensities at ~484 and ~580 nm and intensity ratio (R_1) for malignant and normal cells.

	I_{max} (~ 484)	I_{max} (~ 580)	$R_1 = I_{484}/I_{580}$
G 292 0.80	0.44	1.82	
HOB 0.98	0.45	2.18	

Table 6.3. Intensity ratio (R') of normal HOB over malignant G 292 cell samples.

	λ = 484 nm	λ = 580 nm
$R' = I_{HOB}/I_{G292}$	1.23	1.02

Table 6.4. The area under the peak of normalized fluorescence signals and area ratio.

$S = x2 \int_{x1}^{x2} Ydx$ (x1 = 420, x2 = 680)
G 292   104.13
HOB   129.95

measurement, the decrease of area under the fluorescence peak of malignant G 292 cell compared to normal HOB cell is significant. Note that R_s is 1.25 ($R_s > 1$), thus, the discrimination is numerically meaningful. Using fluorescein sodium as a reference emission spectrum, the relative quantum yield of bone cells was numerically determined as 2.9% and 3.3% for G 292 and HOB, respectively.

Relative quantum yield

Since in our case some problems are associated with absolute quantum yield measurements, such as complicated calculations and instrumentation, several simple relative methods have been devised, which substitute a compound of "known" quantum yield in place of a standard scattered as a reference. This method consists simply of comparing the fluorescence intensity of sample under study to the intensity of a dye of known quantum yield. For the calculation of relative quantum yield, the Eq. 6.127 was used:

$$\frac{F_X}{F_s} = \frac{Q_X I_{EX} \% A_X G(\theta)_X}{Q_s I_{ES} \% A_s G(\theta)_s} \qquad (6.127)$$

where F_X is the measured fluorescence of unknown and F_s is that of the standard dye solution, Q_X and Q_s is the quantum yield of known and the standard dye solution, I_{EX} and I_{ES} is the intensity of exciting light of known and the standard dye solution, $\%A_s$ and $\%A_X$ is the percent absorption of solution (100-T%), $G(\theta)_s$ and $G(\theta)_X$ is geometry factor of standard dye solution and measured fluorescence of known (< 1 since not all of the fluorescent light observed), respectively. By exciting both samples at the same wavelength, having the solutions of equal absorbency at this wavelength and using the same set-up, the value of Eq. 6.128 will also be unity:

$$\frac{I_{EX}\%A_X G(\theta)_X}{I_{ES}\%A_s G(\theta)_s}=1 \tag{6.128}$$

Consequently, the ratio of the quantum yield of standard and unknown sample is:

$$\frac{F_X}{F_s}=\frac{Q_X}{Q_s} \tag{6.129}$$

To estimate the quantum yields for compounds emitting below 600 nm, Eq. 6.129 is suitable and practical. If a spectrometer system is used instead of monochromator-photomultiplier, one must integrate the total area under emission spectrum for both unknown and standard sample and use the area ratio $\left(\frac{S_X}{S_s}\right)$ in preference to intensity ratio in Eq. 6.129 (Demasa and Crosby 1971, Pesce et al. 1996). Among many possible dyes to choose from as a reference standard for quantum yield determination, we choose 10^{-2} mM fluorescein sodium solution with 0.79 ± 0.06 reported quantum yield (Pesce et al. 1996). Its emission spectrum in arbitrary unit is shown in Fig. 6.41. The area under the peak of reference solution in the region of 500–650 nm, which was calculated by Find Graph software, is 46487.6. By considering the main fluorescence peak of cell samples, the area under the fluorescence peak in arbitrary unit was calculated. Table 6.5 shows the quantum yield calculations of normal HOB and malignant G 292 cells using Eq. 6.129.

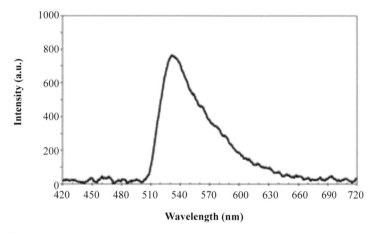

Figure 6.41. The spectrum of fluorescein sodium solution used as a standard reference and excited by 405 nm.

Table 6.5. The quantum yield calculation of normal HOB and malignant G 292 cells using Eq. 6.128. The area under the main peak of reference solution and cell samples is calculated by Find Graph.

Cell sample	$S_{(435–545\,nm)}$	$Q_x = \dfrac{S_x Q_s}{S_s}$		%Q
Malignant G292	1709.16	$Q_{G\,292} =$	$\dfrac{1709.16 \times 0.79}{46487.6} = 0.029$	2.9%
Normal HOB	1962.91	$Q_{HOB} =$	$\dfrac{1962.91 \times 0.79}{46487.6} = 0.033$	3.3%

Extinction Coefficient Calculation. A fundamental aspect of fluorescence spectroscopy is the evaluation of light absorption and extinction coefficient. The Lambert-Beer low is used to measure the absorption experimentally, and is expressed by Eq. (6.130):

$$\log \frac{I_0}{I} = \epsilon\, c d \tag{6.130}$$

where I_0 and I are the light intensities as the light enters and leaves the absorbing medium, ε is the molar extinction coefficient in $M^{-1}cm^{-1}$, c is the concentration in moles/liter (M), and d is the path length in cm. Assuming 10% light absorption by cell suspension ($I_A = 0.1 I_0$) occurred and $c \cong 9.0 \times 10^5$ cell/ml, ϵ is calculated by Beer-Lambert law:

$$\log \frac{I_0}{0.9\, I_0} = \epsilon \times 9.0 \times 10^5 \times 10^{-3} \times 1 \rightarrow \epsilon \cong 5 \times 10^{-5}\ (cm^2 \cdot cell^{-1})$$

Discussion

In this study, we observed a significant difference between the fluorescence spectra of normal and malignant cell samples. This is due to differences in intrinsic fluorescence properties of normal and malignant cells reflecting the amount of different present fluorophores and the properties of surrounding microenvironment. Previous studies on fluorescence-Excitation Emission Matrix (EEM) of different cells revealed the role of three principal endogenous fluorophores in cellular fluorescence. Depending on the excitation wavelength, it is provided by tryptophan, NAD(P)H, and riboflavins (FMN, FAD). NADH and riboflavins which correlate specifically with cellular activity can provide information about the metabolic changes within cells (Palmer et al. 2003, Drezek et al. 2001). In fact, we found the NADH and riboflavins fluorescence spectra decreased with malignancy, and it is due to deficiency of aerobic oxidation system. In other words, when malignant cells proliferate quickly, the ratio between the oxidized (NAD^+) and reduced form (NADH) of NAD alters and the accumulation of less fluorescent NAD^+ results in the decreased fluorescence in cancer (Yicong et al. 2007, Na et al. 2001). It seems that the observed blue and red shifts of NADH and riboflavins band from normal to malignant cells to be due to the physiological and biochemical transformation of normal cells into cancerous cells. Membrane potential abnormalities, mineral cell content, and membrane composition changes are due to changes in the dielectric properties of normal cells during its transformation to a cancer cell (Alfano et al. 1997, Bieling et al. 1996). However, the influence of multiple light elastic scattering of cells arising from Rayleigh scattering on the wavelengths shifts has to be considered (Grossman et al. 2001). Based on normalized intensity evaluation, the fluorescence peak decrease would allow clear discrimination between normal and malignant cells. To overcome the limitations of numerical intensity measurements, the use of a dimensionless ratio $R_1 = I_{484}/I_{580}$ as a shape factor is preferred. The fact that both intensities are equally influenced by experimental parameters indicates the very distinct shapes of normal and malignant spectra. A major advantage of this ratio is that the difference in intensity ratio at these two wavelengths can be attributed to the difference in the fluorescence yield of the native fluorophores (i.e., NAD(P)H, riboflavins) for various cell types. Ratio R1 was found to have a definite diagnostic potential in different kinds of cancer (Heintzelman et al. 2000, Mayinger et al. 2004). The shape distortion of the fluorescence spectra due to absorption of native fluorophores could lead to appearance of false maxima (Troyanova et al. 2007). In order to avoid this misunderstanding, normalized fluorescence spectra of both cells were evaluated. It's obvious that the spectral line shape of normal and malignant cell samples are slightly different. In addition to intensity changes, it can be seen that the spectral shape of normal and malignant bone cells alters by increasing ratio R_1. The R' value is found to be maximal at about 484 nm NADH emission with greatest spectral discrepancy. Thus, this wavelength should be convenient to maximize cancer discrimination. Hage et al. (2003), Chen et al. (1996) believe that one of the most accurate parameters that showed the best performance in the discrimination of different samples were the area under the peak of fluorescence signals. We expect that the area under the fluorescence peak of normal cell should be larger than the malignant one due to the intense metabolic activity of the malignant tumor cell and our experimental fluorescence spectra indicated a significant decrease with malignancy. Finally, in our case, RS = 1.25 (RS > 1), which is a suggestive ratio for indicating the discrimination between normal and malignant bone cells. The comparison of emission spectra of bone cells revealed that fluorescence intensity and the area under the spectra of malignant bone cells was less than that of normal. In addition, the area ratio and shape factor were changed. Two emission bands were observed in spectra of normal cells centered at about 486 and 575 nm and for the malignant cells at about 482 and 586 nm, respectively, which are most likely attributed to NADH and riboflavins.

6.4.6 *Comparison of blue wavelengths and scan velocity on the detection of enamel surface caries using steady-state laser-induced autofluorescence spectroscopy* (Khosroshahi and Taghizadeh 2014)

Fluorescence detection is a noninvasive technique which is well suited for both *in vitro* and *in vivo* measurements. The aim of this study is to report the results of sound and carious enamel fluorescence emission using (i) Different blue wavelengths, (ii) Different scan velocity, and (iii) Spectral ratio. The samples were irradiated using a tunable argon laser (459 nm, 488 nm), and a 405 nm laser at two different scan velocities of 0.23 and 0.5 mm/s. The results showed a spectral band of (443–492) nm for 405 nm, (493–522) nm for 459 nm and (526–625) nm for 488 nm lasers for sound teeth. It was found from the emission spectra that with increasing the excitation wavelength, the corresponding primary peaks of the carious samples showed a Stokes shifts of 4 nm, 6 nm, and 2 nm, respectively. No significant change was observed for the secondary peaks. Also, in all cases, the intensity of fluorescence signals of sound teeth were higher than those of carious. The highest shape factor of 1.82 and integrated intensity ratio of 1.20 were achieved with 405 nm which provides relatively a better tissue discrimination. Also, increasing the scan velocity reduced the signal amplitudes in both sound and carious samples.

Introduction

The crystalline enamel of a tooth is a biological composite consisting of 4% water, 95% mineral such as carbonated hydroxyapatite, and 1% organic matter. Dental caries, also known as 'tooth decay' or 'dental cavity', is a most prevalent chronic infectious disease that arises from an overgrowth of specific bacteria that can metabolize fermentable carbohydrates, hence producing acids as waste products of their metabolism. Caries can be described as a process resulting in structural changes to the dental hard tissue, and its onset is usually characterized by microscopically visible surface demineralization on dental tissue, but visual inspection is less sensitive and subjective. Thus, quantitative methods would provide early occlusal caries detection, which has always been a difficult task in dentistry due to the widespread use of fluorides, continuous surface mineralization and remineralization, and the complex anatomy of pits and fissures (Ketley and Holt 1993). Therefore, it is important that hidden caries be diagnosed at an early stage so that appropriate preventive and restorative treatment can be applied promptly. Traditional diagnostic methods, including visual inspection, tactile probe, and bitewing radiography have unavoidable drawbacks because of subjectivity and destructivity fissures (Ketley and Holt 1993). Since these techniques cannot detect carious lesions in its early stages, development of new diagnostic methods is of significance to detect the earliest signs of enamel demineralization with high specificity and sensitivity. Some of these techniques used for diagnosis of dental caries and minerals are as follows: plasma spectroscopy (PS) (Khosroshahi and Ghasemi 2004, Thareja et al. 2008), polarized Raman spectroscopy (PRS) (Ko et al. 2008), optical coherence tomography (OCT) (Popesca et al. 2008), fibre-delivered confocal microscopy (FCM) (Rousseau et al. 2007), quantitative light fluorescence (QLF) (Amaechi and Higham 2001), photothermal radiometry (PTR) (Hellen et al. 2011), photothermal imaging (PTI) (Gadalla et al. 2010), near IR imaging (NIRI) (Darling et al. 2010), and diagnodent laser fluorescence (DLF) (Boltzan et al. 2011).

While each method has its own potential and capability, none are without drawbacks and limitations, and at the moment there is no such system which is 'all in one'. Thus, choosing any of these methods is dictated by their particular application and goal. For example, QLF is based on measurement of relative loss of fluorescence, which is limited by its inability to distinguish a demineralized tooth area from initial enamel caries. Diagnodent fluorescence measures the level or quantity of fluorescence from carious lesion in the red region due to the presence of bacteria by-products such as porphyrins, using a 655 nm diode laser (Konig and Schneckenburger 1994). While diagnodent fluorescence can detect small caries at relatively larger depth compared with blue light, it suffers from drawbacks such as false signals when dealing with polishing pastes, plaque, calculus, and composite (Hibst et al. 2001). Also it is not suitable for detecting deeper root caries at its operating wavelength and may not provide the most accurate early detection, since it monitors the porphyrin fluorescence only, which is not related to the enamel crystal status (Abrams 2009). PTR is based on the analysis of thermal emission kinetics (i.e., non-radiative) from tissue irradiated by pulsed or modulated laser heating, providing a contrast-based image. While techniques such as PTR have shown its success as a depth profiling imaging system of soft and hard tissues defects (Jeon et al. 2007, Hellen et al. 2011), it however, lacks by definition, the capability of detecting radiation dependent properties of dental surface caries at shorter non-thermal radiation wavelengths. Laser-induced autofluorescence spectroscopy (LIAF) is another method where autofluorescence refers to the fluorescence of natural substances or endogenous fluorophores (Borisova et al. 2004a, 2006b). This technique is one of the most widely used spectroscopic methods in biomedical applications, especially of cancers (Gupta and Majumder 1997). The alternations occur as tissue progresses from a normal to a diseased state and are reflected in the spectral characteristics of the measured fluorescence. The endogenous fluorophores such as the reduced form of nicotinamide adenine dinucleotide (phosphate) (NADPH) and riboflavins (flavin mononucleotide (FMN) and flavin adenine dinucleotide (FAD)), collagen, elastin, amino acids, vitamins, lipids, and porphyrins have a significant variation in the concentration in different tissue types. These differences, together with alternations in the local environment within the tissue, are the basis for the discrimination between diseased and normal tissue by fluorescence spectroscopy. The limitations of QLF are avoided in LIAF spectroscopy, which obtains information on both the intensity changes and the changes in the shape of the spectra. This information can be useful in detecting the type of disorder. (Alfano and Yao 1981) first published the result of a systematic spectroscopic investigation comparing caries and non-caries teeth. The excitation light used for fluorescence measurements is usually in the UV-visible region, and the emitted light typically originates from aromatic molecules depending on the nature of the excited state. Characterizing biological samples such as cells or tissues can be performed in terms of overall intensity, peak wavelength, and spectral shape (Borisova et al. 2004). LIAF is a promising optical diagnostic tool due to the linkage of biochemical and morphological properties of tissues and, coupled with imaging, can provide information regarding biochemical, functional, and structural changes of biomolecular complexes in tissues that occur as a result of pathological transformation or therapeutic intervention (Fang et al. 2004).

Material and experimental techniques

Thirty male and female mandibular third molar (wisdom) teeth with the age ranging between (20–40), which were extracted for different reasons, such as periodontal problems, were provided and categorized by Tehran medical university school of dentistry for our investigation. The samples were classified during visual inspection as "sound" with clear enamel-intact tooth surfaces (lesion free) and those with visible superficial cavity as "carious", each group with fifteen specimen. Usually, the samples were collected in the same day of extraction or on the following day. Immediately after extraction, they were cleared of food particles, lesions or blood clot using a toothbrush under running tap water and then were stored at about 25°C in dark bottles filled with physiological saline solution containing 70% Ethanol. Before measurements, the samples were washed and dried with tissue paper so that they were free of influence of ethanol traces on fluorescence results. The LIAF measurements were carried out using the experimental set up shown in Fig. 6.42. The samples were irradiated in a dark room to avoid stray light interference using a suitably attenuated 1 mm beam of 150 mW tunable Argon laser (Melles Griot-35MAP431) at 488 nm and 459 nm wavelengths, and a 80 mW violet 405 nm (CSI). This was done to ensure that the samples are not photo-bleached and to avoid saturation effects. The fluorescence spectra of each tooth were recorded five times and then averaged for the final plotting. A simple programmable home-built XY scanner (Fig. 6.42) was used for displacement of samples at predetermined velocity which here were 0.23 and 0.5 mm/s. The output of scanner micro-controller was connected to computer for adjusting the required scan velocity. The fluorescence spectra were registered by a UV-VIS fibre optic spectrometer (Ocean Optics-USB 2000) consisting a 600-lines/mm grating with 10 nm spectral resolution. The LIF spectrum is recorded in the

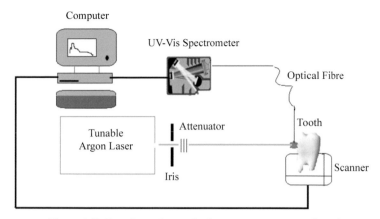

Figure 6.42. Experimental setup for fluorescence spectroscopic study.

430–730 nm spectral range. The output was then fed in to a computer to store and display the data. In the case of carious teeth, they were scanned in mesial-distal axis.

Experimental results

The fluorescence of dental tissue varies according to the chemical composition of pathological areas and the optical properties of tissue. In our case, the fluorescence intensity of all carious lesions was lower than sound teeth and varied with the extent of lesion. The lowest fluorescence amplitude was observed at the center of each lesion. Figure 6.43a illustrates the results for sound tooth at 405 nm where a broad band is observed between 430–530 nm at FWHM. As is seen, there are two peaks, one at 443 nm as the secondary (Is") and the other at 492 nm with a larger amplitude as the primary (Is'). This is very close to the results achieved by Ribeiro et al. (2005), who used a 405 nm laser and obtained a spectral range between 480–500 nm with a maximum peak around 490 nm. A similar result was obtained by Chen et al. 2010, using a 403 nm laser and a spectral range of 443–526 nm with a peak at 485 nm. When the laser beam gradually entered the carious zone during the scanning, the signal amplitudes of both peaks were decreased to 442 nm (Ic") and 488 nm (Ic'), due to the higher attenuation coefficient (mainly scattering) of photons by various fluorophore contents of the teeth (Fig. 6.43b). However, when the scan velocity was increased, the amplitudes of all peaks in all cases were decreased. Figure 6.43c demonstrates the averaged normalized fluorescence intensity when a tooth was scanned from gradually a healthy part 1 to the decayed region 2. The peak is reduced to its minimum value at the center, i.e., maximum attenuation 3 where the decay is worst, and at the exit it enters the healthy part again 4.

For the 459 nm, a broad band was recorded for sound tooth between 430–580 nm with Is" at 493 nm and Is' at 522 nm (see Fig. 6.44a). As is seen from Fig. 6.44b, a similar behaviour was observed for the carious sample at 516 and 493 nm, respectively, but with lower amplitudes. As is seen from Fig. 6.44c, there is a close overlap between regions 2 and 4, implying that not much of difference is made by 459 nm, i.e., it has a lower sensitivity.

Also, in the case of higher scan velocity, a distinctly similar pattern was observed, but at lower values. Figure 6.45 indicates that at a longer excitation wavelength of 488 nm, the sound and carious teeth show relatively four valleys located at about 526, 550, 580, and 625 nm. In order to evaluate the degree of tissue discrimination we need to define two parameters: the shape factor (Fs = I'/I") for both sound and carious teeth, and the fluorescence intensity ratio (R_i = Is'/Ic"). In fact, Fs is a dimensionless ratio that helps to overcome the limitation of numerical intensity measurements. A major advantage of this ratio is that the difference in R_i at these two wavelengths (primary and secondary) can be attributed to the difference in the fluorophore yield of the native fluorophores. The latter indicates the sensitivity of tissue differentiation, i.e., resolving power. In fact, this is similar to the signal-to-noise ratio; in other words, the higher the ratio the better the differentiation between the main signal and the background noise (i.e., the caries).

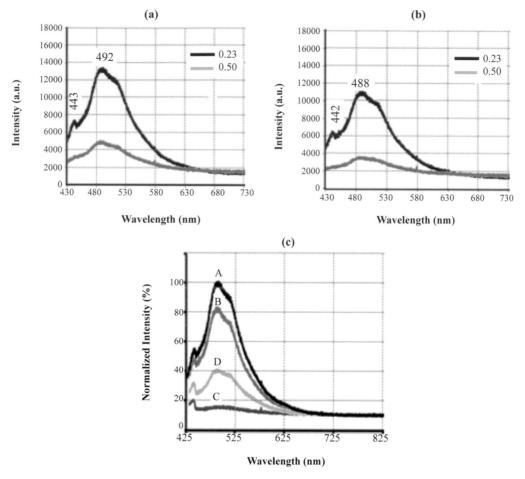

Figure 6.43. Autofluorescence spectra of sound (a) and carious (b) teeth excited at 405 nm at scan velocities of 0.23 and 0.50 mm/s; gradual changes (c) of spectra as laser scans from sound (A) to decay (B), center of decay (C), and sound area again (D).

But before calculation, each point had to be normalized such that the maximum fluorescence was a nominal one unit (100%) by dividing the fluorescence of each point by the maximum value.

In the case of some biological medium, such as dental tissue, $\pi–\pi^*$ transitions are more probable due to association of double bonds of, e.g., $C = C$ or $C = O$ with relatively high molar extinction coefficients. Another possible explanation for the changes in fluorescence lies with the variation in light scattering. This is readily demonstrated by the angular intensity function defined by Henyey–Greenstein intensity function (Eq. 6.23), which is relative to the structure of the mineral crystal in human dental enamel. Thus, crystals are responsible for the backward scattering, and the number of crystals and their scattering cross-section determine the scattering coefficient. Enamel demineralization results in an increase in the light scattering properties of enamel. Consequently, in dental caries, the light propagation directions are different as compared to sound tooth, so that more fluorescent photons are emitted in sound tooth than in carious lesion. Generally, it seems that the difference between the different results found in the literature can be attributed to a number of factors, such as lighting conditions, storage method of teeth, type and the specifications of teeth, and other factors. So far as the fluorescent signals are concerned in our study, there is clearly a Stokes shift in all cases. Therefore, by increasing the excitation wavelength, the emission primary peaks of the sound specimen (492, 522, and 526 nm) as well as the corresponding highest emission peaks from carious teeth (488, 516, and 524 nm) are shifted towards longer wavelength (Stokes). Also, two peaks at about 580 and 650 nm were observed in the red region when excited by 488 nm wavelength. Internal conversion and vibrational relaxation are responsible for the emitted photons that have lower

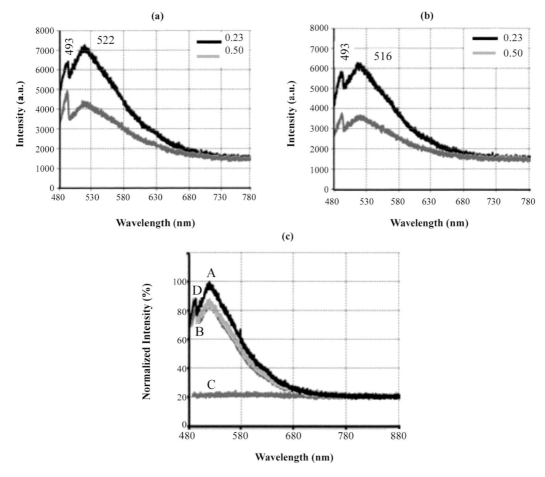

Figure 6.44 Autofluorescence spectra of sound (a) and carious (b) teeth excited at 459 nm can velocities of 0.23 and 0.50 mm/s; gradual changes (c) of spectra as laser scans from sound (A) to decay (B), center of decay (C), and sound area again (D).

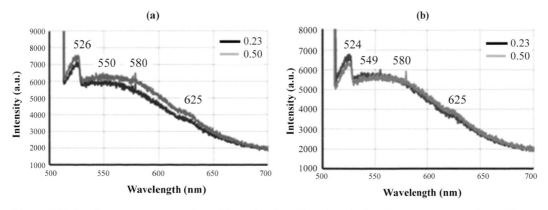

Figure 6.45. Autofluorescence spectra of sound (a) and carious (b) teeth excited at 488 nm at scan velocity of 0.23 and 0.50 mm/s.

energy than the incident photons. The amount of Stokes shift is a measure of relaxation process occurring in the excited state, populated by absorption. The difference in the energy of the absorbed photon and that of the emitted photon corresponds to the energy loss to the system due to non-radiative processes. The results showed a spectral band of 443–492 nm for 405 nm, 493–522 nm for 459 nm, and 526–625 nm for

488 nm lasers for sound teeth. It was found from the emission spectra that with increase in the excitation wavelength, the corresponding primary peaks of the carious samples showed Stokes shifts of 4, 6, and 2 nm, respectively. No significant change was observed for the secondary peaks. Also, in all cases, the intensity of fluorescence signals of sound teeth was higher than those of carious teeth. The highest shape factor of 1.82 and integrated intensity ratio of 1.20 were achieved at 405 nm, which provides relatively better tissue discrimination. Also, increasing the scan velocity reduced the signal amplitudes in both sound and carious samples.

6.5 Laser-induced plasma breakdown spectroscopy (LIBS)

6.5.1 Physical principles

Laser-induced plasma breakdown spectroscopy (LIBS) is a rapid chemical analysis technology, a type of atomic emission spectroscopy, which uses a short laser pulse to produce a micro-plasma on the sample surface. The main physical principle is the formation of high temperature plasma (ionized electrons) induced by a short laser pulse (ns and shorter). When such short pulse is focused onto the sample surface, a small volume of the sample is removed via photoablation mechanism, as seen in 6.3.3. The ablated material then further interacts with portion of pulse tail to form a highly energetic bright plasma that contains free electrons, excited atoms and ions. In typical research works, the plasma temperature can exceed 30,000 K.

At the high temperature during the early plasma, the ablated material dissociates (breaks down) into excited ionic and atomic species. During this time, the plasma emits a continuum of radiation which does not particularly contain any useful information about the species present. However, when it expands within a very short time frame, the plasma expands at supersonic velocities, and hence cools. During the plasma cooling process, the electrons of the atoms and ions at the excited electronics states returns into natural ground states, causing the plasma to emit light of different colors with discrete spectral peaks. Radiation in the visible spectral range originates from atomic and molecular electronics transitions. Thus, the heavy particles of low temperature plasmas, the neutrals and their ions basically characterize the color of a plasma. At this stage, the characteristic atomic emission lines of the elements can be observed and then identified by a suitable analyzer, such as optical spectrometer. For example, helium plasma is pink, neon plasmas are red, nitrogen plasmas are orange and hydrogen are purple. The intensities of plasma often are used to quantify the concentration of trace and major elements in the sample.

The central wavelength of line emission, λ_0 is given by the photon energy $E = E_p - E_k$ corresponding to the energy gap of the transition from level p with energy E_p to the energetically lower level k.

$$\lambda_0 = hc/(E_p - E_k) \tag{6.130}$$

Since the energy of a transition is a characteristic of the particle species, the central wavelength is identified for the radiating particle, unless the wavelength is shifted by the Doppler effect. The line intensity is quantified by the line emission coefficient,

$$\varepsilon_{pk} = n(p) \, A_{pk} \, \frac{hc}{4\pi \, \lambda_0} = \int_{line} \varepsilon_\lambda \, d\lambda \tag{6.131}$$

In units of W $(m^2 \, sr)^{-1}$, where 4π represents the solid angle $d\Omega$ (isotropic radiation), measured in steradian (sr). The line profile P_λ correlates the line emission coefficient with the spectral line emission coefficient ε_λ,

$$\varepsilon_\lambda = \varepsilon_{pk} P_\lambda \tag{6.132}$$

with

$$\int_{line} P_\lambda = 1 \tag{6.133}$$

A characteristic of the profile is the full width half maximum (FWHM) of the intensity. The line profile depends on the broadening mechanism. In the case of Doppler broadening, the profile is a Gaussian profile, and the line width correlates with the particle temperature.

The main advantages include:

- Entirely an optical technique
- On-line and real time analysis
- Broad elemental coverage
- Non-contact and possibility of remote operation
- No sample preparation is required as it can be used in field trial
- Extremely fast measurement time for a single spot analysis, normally within a few seconds
- Thin-sample analysis without a serious concern about the substrate interference.
- Versatile sampling protocols that include fast scanning of the sample surface and depth profiling by repeatedly discharging the laser. In the same position, effectively going deeper into the specimen with each shot

Limitations:

- Subject to variation of laser spark and resultant plasma which can limit reproducibility
- The measurements accuracy is typically better than 10% and precision is better than 5%
- Detection limits vary with type of elements and the experimental apparatus used
- Detection limit can range from > 100 ppm to < 1 ppm

6.5.2 *Interaction studies of multimode pulsed HF laser with enamel tissue using photothermal deflection and spectroscopy* (Khosroshahi and Ghasemi 2004)

In recent years much effort has been devoted to research on LIBS in diverse areas including archaeology (Giakoumaki and Melssanaki 2007), industry (Heilbrunner et al. 2012), biomedical engineering (Xian-Yun and Wei-Jun 2008), dentistry (Niemz 1994), cancer diagnosis (Corsi et al. 2003 and Imam et al. 2012), and nanoparticles (Ye et al. 2002, Brown and Rehse 2007). Similar to LIFS, LIBS also acts as an optical diagnosis technique, except that it is based on identification of target constituting chemical elements. In the field of dentistry, early detection of caries has always been a priority and though it deals with carious teeth, this study describes the results of healthy, or so called sound samples, for the purpose of comparison with carious teeth and as a reference. Twenty freshly extracted non-carious human third molars (wisdom) are used. Some of them were cut by an electric saw into facets of about 2 mm thick and of a 4.3 mm dimension and others were kept intact. Before the experiment the samples were stored in buffered saline containing 0.2% thymol solution to prevent bacterial growth. Immediately after the experiment the samples were placed in 0.9% sodium chloride solution. Prior to experiments the samples were air dried and mounted on a disk with paraffin wax. The experimental set up is shown in Fig. 6.46, where the plasma emission produced during interaction was photographed by a fast CCD camera (Panasonic Super Dynamic WV-GP450, Prior) and then conducted to a high resolution monochromator by an optical fibre for analysis of ablation plume. The time resolved signals were then detected by a photomultiplier tube (RCAS83010E) detector whose output was fed to the computer for data storage and further processing.

An example of laser-induced plasma is shown in Fig. 6.47, where the combustion of fast-ejected particles is clearly seen at the surface. The color of plasma gradually changed, as a function of pulse number, from blue when the enamel was dry, to orange-like when it was water sprayed, possibly indicating the different temperatures of hot ejecta. Figure 6.48 is the spectrum of enamel plasma spanning from (420–620 nm) with its strongest emission lines being those for neutral species of calcium at 526 nm and 559 nm, respectively.

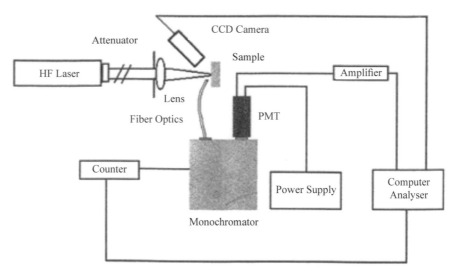

Figure 6.46. Experimental setup for plasma spectroscopic study.

Enamel Surface

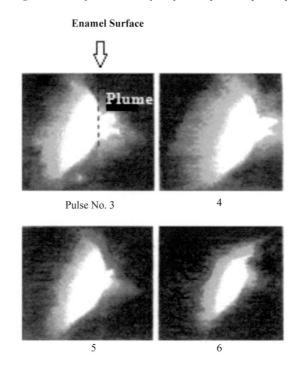

Figure 6.47. An example of HF laser-induced plasma and emission of hot ejected plume from enamel at 70 Jcm⁻² at various pulse numbers.

The evaluation of the plasma temperature is difficult due to its short lifetime. However, by comparing the intensities of two different calcium lines, one can estimate a mean plasma temperature. According to (Lochte-Holtgreven 1968), the following relation applies for two spectral lines of the same atomic species

$$\frac{I_1}{I_2} = \frac{A_1 g_1 \lambda_2}{A_2 g_2 \lambda_1} \mathrm{Exp}\left[-\left(\frac{E_1 - E_2}{KT}\right)\right] \tag{6.134}$$

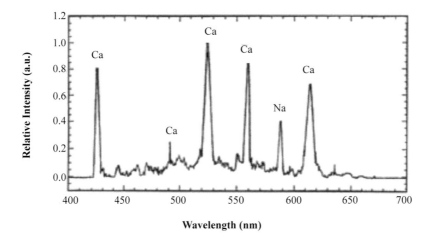

Figure 6.48. Spectrum analysis of plasma spark.

where I is the detected intensity, A is the transition probability, g is the statistical weight of the upper energy level, k is the detected wave length, E is the upper energy level, K is the Boltzmann's constant, and T is the plasma temperature with two calcium wavelengths of $\lambda_1 = 428.3$ nm and $\lambda_2 = 518.8$ nm. Using reference (Lide 1999), the corresponding parameters are:

$A_1 = 0.434 \times 10^8$ s^{-1}, $g_1 = 5$, $E_1 = 4.66 \times 10^{-19}$ J (2.9 eV)

$A_2 = 0.400 \times 10^8$ s^{-1} $g_2 = 5$, $E_2 = 3.84 \times 10^{-19}$ J (2.40 eV)

Also, the intensity ratio of the spectra shown in Fig. 6.48 is about $I_1/I_2 \approx 0.8$. Therefore, the corresponding mean plasma temperature of these spectra is about 53000 K (or 4.7 eV). This is slightly less than the value found by Niemz (i.e., 60000 K) using Nd:YLF laser (Niemz 1994). Assuming that all ≈ 500 mJ of energy is used for ionization of calcium which has an ionization energy of 10 eV. Therefore, the free electron density is approximately

$$N_e \leq \frac{500 \text{ mJ}}{10 \text{ eV}} \approx 3.3 \times 10^{17} \tag{6.135}$$

Also, a rough estimate of the plasma volume (=1000 μm)^3 was obtained from magnification of pictures taken by CCD camera, as seen in Fig. 6.46. Hence the free electron density becomes Ne < 3.13 × 10^{20} cm^{-3}. This shows that only 0.1% of the pulse energy is used for ionization. Also, the maximum power density is given by

$$I_m = \frac{E}{A\tau_p} \approx 0.6 \times 10^9 \text{ Wcm}^{-2} \tag{6.136}$$

which is less than the minimum value of 1×10^{10} Wcm^{-2} normally required for ionization process using nanosecond laser pulses. Therefore, it appears that spectroscopic studies can provide some useful opto-chemical information about biological tissues, which for example for a healthy dental enamel as in this case, calcium was the main chemical element observed in the plasma with emission spanning from 420 to 620 nm.

Keywords: Biophotonics, Rayleigh limit, Mie regime, Reduced scattering, anisotropy factor, Diffusion approximation, Adiabatic limit, Hyperbolic Fourier, Hyperbolic non-Fourier, Nanoshells, Thermoclastic stress, Cavitation, Jetting effect, Photoacoustic, Fluorescence spectroscopy, Osteobleast cells, Osteosarcoma, Plasma spectroscopy.

References

Abrams, S. 2009. Harnessing light and energy for the early detection of defected carries. Restor. Dent. 12: 10–16.

Aguilar, C., L. Yi and S. Mao. 2005. Direct micro-patterning of biodegradable polymers using UV and femtosecond lasers. Biomaterials 26: 7642–7649.

Alfano, R. and S. Yao. 1981. Human teeth with and without dental caries studied by visible luminescent spectroscopy. J. Dent. Res. 60: 120–122.

Alfano, R., G. Tang, A. Pradhan and W. Lam. 1997. Fluorescence spectra from cancerous and normal human breast and lung tissues. IEEE J. Quant. Electron. 23: 1806–1811.

Almond, D. and P. Patal. 1996. Photothermal Science and Techniques. Chapman and Hall, London.

Amaechi, B. and S. Higham. 2001. Diagnosis of dental caries using quantitative light-induced fluorescence. In: Papazoglou, T. and G.A. Wagnieres (eds.). Iiagnostic Optical Spectroscopy in Biomedicine. Proceedings of SPIE 4432: 110–117.

Anidjar, M., O. Cussenot, S. Vrillier and D. Ettori. 1998. The role of laser-induced autofluorescence spectroscopy in bladder tumor detection. Dependence on the excitation wavelength. Ann. N. Y. Acad. Sci. 838: 130–142.

Arnfield, M., J. Tulip and M. McPhee. 1988. Optical propagation in tissue with anisotropic scattering. IEEE Trans. Biomed. Eng. 35: 372–381.

Benson, R.C., R. Meyer, M. Zaruba and G. McKhann. 1979. Cellular autofluorescence: is it due to flavins? J. Histochem. Cytochem. 27: 44–48.

Benmansour, B., L. Stephan, J. Cabon and L. Deschamps. 2010. Spectroscopic properties and laser induced fluorescence of some endocrine disrupting compounds. J. Fluoresc. 20: 1–8.

Bieling, P., N. Rehan, P. Winkler and K. Helmke. 1996. Tumor size and prognosis in aggressively treated osteosarcoma. J. Clin. Oncol. 14: 848–858.

Boltzan de Paula, A., J. Campos, M. Dinizi and J. Hebling. 2011. In situ and *in vitro* comparison of laser fluorescence with visual inspection in detecting occlusal caries lesions. Laser Med. Sci. 26: 1–5.

Borisova, E., T. Uzunov and L. Avramov. 2004. Early differentiation between caries and tooth demineralization using laser-induced autofluorescence spectroscopy. Laser Surg. Med. 34: 249–253.

Borisova, E., T. Uzunov and L. Avramov. 2006. Laser-induced autofluorescence study of caries model *in vitro*. Laser Med. Sci. 21: 34–41.

Bottiroli, G., A. Croce and D. Locatelli. 1995. Natural fluorescence of normal and neoplastic human colon: a comprehensive *ex vivo* study. Laser Surg. Med. 16: 48–60.

Boulnois, M. and I. Marshall. 1986. He-Ne laser simulation of human fibroblast proliferation and attachment *in vitro*. Lasers Med. Sci. 2: 125–134.

Broude, S. 2012. Micro-hole drilling with lasers: comparing direct-write vs. mask projection for medical device manufacturing. Indust. Laser Solutions Magazine.

Brown, E. and S. Rehse. 2007. Laser-induced breakdown spectroscopy of Y-Fe$_2$O$_3$ nanoparticles in a biocompatible alginate matrix. Spectrochimica Acta Part B 62: 1475–148.

Cahill, D., W. Ford, K. Goodson and G. Mahan. 2003. Nanoscale thermal transport. J. Appl. Phys. 93: 793–818.

Cattaneo, C. 1958. Complex time-delay systems: theory and applications. Compt. Rend. 247: 431–433.

Chan, Y., J. Chou and J. Wu. 2005. Properties of a diffused photon-pair density wave in a multiple-scattering medium. Appl. Opt. 44: 1416–1425.

Chen, W., B. He, G. Wei, G. Gao and S. Li. 1996. Laser-induced fluorescence spectroscopy of human normal and cancerous tissues. Proc. SPIE 2887: 156.

Chen, Q., B. Lin, Z. Chen and H. Zhu. 2010. Pilot study on early detection of dental demineralization based on laser induced fluorescence. Laser Phys. 7: 752–756.

Chantrasekhar, S. 1960. Radiative Transfer. Dover Publisher, USA.

Chidananda, SM., K. Satyamoorthy, L. Rai, A. Manjunath and V. Kartha. 2006. Optical diagnosis of cervical cancer by fluorescence spectroscopy technique. Int. J. Cancer 119: 139–145.

Colasanti, A., A. Kisslinger, G. Fabbrocini and R. Liuzzi. 2000. MS-2 fibrosarcoma characterization by laser induced autofluorescence. Lasers Surg. Med. 26: 441–448.

Corsi, M., G. Cristoforetti, M. Hidalgo and S. Legnaioli. 2003. Application of laser-induced plasma spectroscopy technique to hair tissue mineral analysis. Appl. Opt. 42: 6133–6137.

Cross, F., R. Al-Dhair and P.E. Dyer. 1988. Ablative and acoustic response of pulsed UV laser-irradiated vascular tissue in a liquid environment J. Appl. Phys. 64: 2194–2199.

Darling, C., J. Jiao, C. Lee and H. Kang. 2010. Polarization resolved near-IR imaging of sound and carious dental enamel. Proc. SPIE. 7549: 75490.

Demasa, J.N. and G. Crosby. 1971. The measurement of photoluminescence quantum yields: a review. Phys. Chem. 75: 991–1024.

Diaci, J. and J. Mozina. 1992. A study of blast wave forms detected simultaneously by microphone and a laser probe during laser ablation. Appl. Phys. A 55: 84–93.

Dougherty, T.J. 1975. Photoradiation therapy. II. Cure of animal tumors with hematoporphyrin and light. J. Natl. Cancer Inst. 55: 115–21.

Dreyfus, R. 1992. Comparison of the ablation of dielectrics and metals at high and low laser powers. *In*: E. Fogarassy and S. Lazare (eds.). Laser Ablation of Electronic Materials, Basic Mechanism and Applications. p. 61. Elsevier Science Publishers B.V., North-Holland, Berlin.

Drezek, R., K. Sokolov, U. Utzinger, I. Boiko, A. Malpica and M. Follen. 2001. Understanding the contributions of NADH and collagen to cervical tissue fluorescence spectra: modeling measurements and implications. J. Biomed. Opt. 6: 385–396.

Duck, F.A. 1990. Physical properties of tissue. Academic Press, New York.

Dyer, P.E. and J. Sidhu. 1986. Direct-etching studies of polymer films using a 157-nm F_2 laser. J. Opt. Soc. Am. B3: 792–797.

Dyer, P.E. and J. Sidhu. 1988. Spectroscopic and fast photographic studies of excimer laser polymer ablation. J. Appl. Phys. 64: 4657–4663.

Dyer, P.E. and R. Srinivasan. 1989. Pyroelectric detection of ultraviolet laser ablation from polymers. J. Appl. Phys. 66: 2608–2612.

Dyer, P.E., M.E. Khosroshahi and S. Tuft. 1992. Optical fibre delivery and tissue ablation studies using a pulsed hydrogen fluoride laser. Laser Med. Sci. 7: 331: 1992.

Dyer, P.E., M.E. Khosroshahi and S. Tuft. 1993. Studies of laser-induced cavitation and tissue ablation in saline using a fiber-delivered pulsed HF laser. Appl. Phys. B. 56: 84–93.

Even-Sapir, E. 2005. Imaging of malignant bone involvement by morphologic, scintigraphic, and hybrid modalities. J. Nucl. Med. 46: 1356–1367.

Fan, Y., A. Mandelis, G. Spirou and I. Vitkin. 2004. Development of a laser photothermoacoustic frequency-swept system for subsurface imaging: theory and experiment. J. Acoust. Soc. Am. 116: 3523–3533.

Fang, Q., T. Papaioannou, A. Javier and J. Vaitha. 2004. Time-domain laser-induced fluorescence spectroscopy apparatus for clinical diagnostics. Rev. Sci. Instrum. 75: 151–162.

Flowers, B. and E. Mendoza. 1970. Properties of Matter. Wiley, London.

Fogelman, I., G. Cook, O. Israel and H. Van der Wall. 2005. Positron emission tomography and bone metastases. Semin. Nucl. Med. 35: 135–142.

Fradin, D., N. Blombergen and J. Letellier. 1973. Dependence of laser-induced breakdown field strength on plasma duration. Appl. Phys. Lett. 22: 635–638.

Gadalla, M. and M. El Sharkawi. 2010. Non-invasive technique for human caries detection and monitoring using time-resolved photothermal imaging. J. Med. Biol. Eng. 30: 113–118.

Giakoumaki, A. and K. Melssanaki. 2007. Laser-induced breakdown spectroscopy (LIBS) in archaeological science-applications and prospects. Anal. Bioanal. Chem. 387: 749–760.

Grossman, N., E. Ilovitz, O. Chaims and A. Salman. 2001. Fluorescence spectroscopy for detection of malignancy: H-ras overexpressing fibroblasts as a model. J. Biochem. Biophys. Methods 50: 53–63.

Gupta, P., S. Majumder and A. Uppel. 1997. Breast cancer diagnosis using N_2 laser excited autofluorescence spectroscopy. Laser Surg. Med. 21417–422.

Hage, R., P. Galhanone, R. Zângaro, K. Rodrigues and M. Pacheco. 2003. Using the laser-induced fluorescence spectroscopy in the differentiation between normal and neoplastic human breast tissue. Lasers Med. Sci. 18: 171–176.

Hale, G. and M. Querry. 1973. Optical constants of water in the 200-nm to 200-μm wavelength region. Appl. Opt. 12: 555–563.

Haringsma, J. and G. Tyget. 1999. Fluorescence and autofluorescence. Bailliere's Clinc. Gastroent. 13: 1–10.

Hellen, A., A. Mandelis, Y. Finer and B. Amaechi. 2011. Quantitative evaluation of the kinetics of human enamel simulated caries using photothermal radiometry and modulated luminescence. J. Biomed. Opt. 16: 1–13.

Hibst, R., R. Papulus and A. Lussi. 2001. Detection of occlusal caries by laser fluorescence: basic and clinical investigations. Med. Laser Appl. 16: 205–213.

Heilbrunner, H., N. Huber, H. Wolfmeir and E. Arenholz. 2012. Double-pulse laser-induced breakdown spectroscopy for trace element analysis in sintered iron oxide ceramics. Appl. Phys. A 106: 15–23.

Heintzelman, D.L., U. Utzinger, H. Fuchs and A. Zuluaga. 2000. Oral neoplasia using optimal excitation wavelengths for *in vivo* detection of oral neoplasia using fluorescence spectroscopy. Photochem. Photobiol. 72: 103–113.

Hung, J., S. Lam, J. LeRiche and B. Palcic. 1991. Autofluorescence of normal and malignant bronchial tissue. Lasers Surg. Med. 11: 99–105.

Imam, H., R. Mohamad and A. Eldakrouri. 2012. Primary study of the use of lser-induced plasma spectroscopy for the diagnosis of breast cancer. Opt. Photonics J. 2: 193–199.

Jacques, S. and S. Prahl. 1987. Modeling optical and thermal distributions in tissue during laser irradiation. Lasers Surg. Med. 6: 488–493.

Jacques, S. 1995. Modelling light optical properties. pp. 21–33. *In*: A.M. Verga Scheggi, S. Martellucci and A. Chester (eds.). Biomedical Optical Instrumentation and Laser-Assisted Biotechnology. NATO ASI Series. Vol. 325, Applied Sciences, Kluwer Academic Publishers, Dordrechet.

Jain, K., C. Willson and G. Lin. 1982. Ultrafast high resolution contact lithography using excimer lasers. SPIE: 334: 259–262.

Jeon, R., A. Hellen, A. Matveinko, A. Mandelis, S. Abram, B. Amaechi and G. Kulkarni. 2007. J. Biomed. Opt. 12: 034028.

Joseph, D. and L. Preziosi. 1989. Heat waves. Rev. Modern Phys. 61: 41–73.

Ketley, C. and R. Holt. 1993. Visual and radiographic diagnosis of occlusal caries in first permanent molars and in second primary molars. Br. Dent. J. 174: 364–370.

Khosroshahi, M.E. (R.R.A., unpublished data). 1993. Ablation of ophthalmic tissues using fiber-delivered UV and IR lasers. Phd Thesis. Hull University, England.

Khosroshahi, M.E. and A. Ghasemi. 2004. Interaction studies of multimode pulsed HF laser with enamel tissue using photothermal deflection and spectroscopy. Lasers Med. Sci. 18: 196–203.

Khosroshahi, M.E., M. Mahmoodi and J. Tavakoli. 2007. Characterization of Ti6Al4V implant surface treated by Nd:YAG laser and emery paper for orthopaedic applications. Appl. Surf. Sci. 253: 8772–8781.

Khosroshahi, M.E., M. Mahmoodi and J. Tavakoli. 2008. Effect of Nd:Yttrium-aluminum-garnet laser radiation on Ti6Al4V alloy properties for biomedical applications. J. Laser Appl. 20: 209–217.

Khosroshahi, M.E., F. Anoosheh pour, M. Hadavi and M. Mahmoodi. 2009. *In situ* monitoring the pulse CO_2 laser interaction with 316-L stainless steel using acoustical signals and plasma analysis. Appl. Surf. Sci. 256: 7421–7427.

Khosroshahi, M.E. and M. Rahmani. 2011. Detection and evaluation of normal and malignant cells using laser-induced fluorescence spectroscopy. J. Fluoresc. 22: 281–288.

Khosroshahi, M.E. and N. Taghizadeh Khoi. 2014. Comparison of blue wavelengths and velocity effects on the detection of enamel surface caries using steady-state laser-induced autofluorescence spectroscopy. J. Appl. Spect. 81: 347–353.

Khosroshahi, M.E., L. Ghazanfari and P. Khoshkenar. 2014. Experimental validation and simulation of fourier and non-fourier heat transfer equation during laser nano-phototherapy of lung cancer cells: An *in vitro* assay. J. Mod. Phys. 5: 2125–2141.

Kim, C., R. Kalluru, S. Willard and A. Musselwhite. 2005. Optimized optical fiber laser-induced fluorescence (LIF) sensor for human breast cancer cell lines diagnosis. Proc SPIE 5993: 60–65.

Ko, A., M. Hewko and M. Sowa. 2008. Early dental caries detection using a fibre-optic coupled polarization-resolved Raman spectroscopic system. Opt. Express. 16: 6274–6279.

Konig, K. and H. Schneckenburger. 1994. Laser-induced autofluorescence for medical diagnosis. J. Fluores. 4: 17–40.

Kyung-Bok, L., J. Dong and L. Zee. 2004. Pattern generation of biological ligands on a biodegradable poly(glycolic acid) film. Langmuir. 20: 2531–2535.

Lakowicz, J. 1999. Principles of Fluorescence Spectroscopy, 2nd edn. Kluwer/Plenum, New York.

Lauterborn, W. and H. Bolle. 1975. Experimental investigations of cavitation-bubble collapse in the neighborhood of a solid boundary. J. Fluid Mech. 72: 391–399.

Lauterborn, W. 1980. Cavitation and Inhomogeneities in Underwater Acoustic. Springer Series Electrophysics. Springer, Berlin.

Lide, D. 1999. Handbook of Chemistry and Physics, 80th edn. CRC, Boca Raton.

Lin, C., D. Stern and C. Puliafito. 1990. High speed photography of Er:YAG laser ablation in fluid. Invest. Ophthalmol. & Vis. Sci. 31: 2546–2550.

Lipson, R.L. and E. Baldes. 1960. The photodynamic properties of a particular hematoporphyrin derivative. Arch. Dermatol. 82: 508–516.

Liu, X. and W. Zhang. 2008. Recent developments in biomedicine fields for laser-induced breakdown spectroscopy. J. Biomed. Sci Eng. 1: 147–151.

Lochet-Holtgreven, W. 1968. Plasma Diagnostics. North Holland Press, Amsterdam.

Lord Rayleigh, J.W. 1917. On the pressure developed in a liquid during the collapse of a spherical cavity. Philos. Mag. 34: 94–98.

Mayinger, B., M. Jordan, T. Horbach and P. Horner. 2004. Evaluation of *in vivo* endoscopic autofluorescence spectroscopy in gastric cancer. Gastrointest. Endosc. 59: 191–198.

Mentzel, H., K. Kentouche, D. Sauner and C. Fleischmann. 2004. Comparison of whole body STIR-MRI and 99mTc-methylene-diphosphonate scintigraphy in children with suspected multifocal bone lesions. Eur. Radiol. 14: 2297–2302.

Mirabello, L., R. Troisi and S. Savage. 2009. Osteosarcoma incidence and survival rates from 1973 to 2004. Cancer. 15: 1531–1543.

Mondal, S., Sh. Gao, N. Zhu, R. Liang and V. Gruev. 2014. Real-time fluorescence image-guided oncologic surgery. Adv. Cancer Res. 124: 171–211.

Na, R., I. Stender and H. Wulf. 2001. Can autofluorescence demarcate basal cell carcinoma from normal skin? A comparison with protoporphyrin IX fluorescence. Acta Derm. Venereol. 81: 246–249.

Niemz, M. 1994. Diagnosis of caries by spectral analysis of laser-induced plasma sparks. Proced. SPIE 2327: 56–63.

Ottaviani, G. and N. Jaffe. 2010. The epidemiology of osteosarcoma. Cancer Treat Res. 152: 3–13.

Palmer, G., P. Keely, T. Breslin and N. Ramanujam. 2003. Autofluorescence spectroscopy of normal and malignant human breast cell lines. Photochem. Photobiol. 78: 462–469.

Paltauf, G. and P.E. Dyer. 2003. Photomechanical processes and effects in ablation. Chem. Rev. 103: 487–518.

Pantel, K., J. Izbicki, M. Angstwurm and S. Braun. 1993. Immunocytological detection of bone marrow micrometastasis in operable non-small cell lung cancer. Cancer Res. 53: 1027–1031.

Parker, J. and P. France. 1990. Fluoride glass optical fibers. Chapter 2. Blackie, Glasgow.

Patterson, M., B. Chance and B. Wilson. 1989. Time-resolved reflectance and transmittance for the non-invasive measurement of tissue optical properties. Appl. Opt. 28: 2331–2336.

Pesce, A., C. Rosen and T. Pasby. 1996. Fluorescence spectroscopy: an introduction for biology and medicine. Umi Books on Demand.

Pennes, H. 1948. Analysis of tissue and arterial blood temperatures in the resting human forearm. J. Appl. Physiol. 1: 93–122.

Popesca, D., M. Sowa and M. Hewko. 2008. Assessment of early demineralization in teeth using the signal attenuation in optical coherence tomography images. J. Biomed. Opt. 13: 054053.

Pratisto, H., M. Frenz, M. Ith, J. Hans, E. Altermatt, J. Duco and H. Weber. 1996. Combination of fiber-guided pulsed erbium and holmium laser radiation for tissue ablation under water. Appl. Opt. 19: 3328–3337.

Puliafito, C. and R. Steinert. 1984. Short-pulsed Nd:YAG laser microsurgery of the eye: biological considerations. IEEE. J. Quant. Elect. 12: 1442–1449.

Ramanujam, N., M. Mitchell, A. Mahadevan and S. Thomsen. 1994. Fluorescence spectroscopy: a diagnostic tool for cervical intraepithelial neoplasia (CIN). Gynecol. Oncol. 52: 31–38.

Romer, T., M. Fitzmaurice, R. Cothren, R. Richards-Kortum and R. Petras. 1995. Laser-induced fluorescence microscopy of normal colon and dysplasia in colonic adenomas: implication for spectroscopic diagnosis. Am. J. Gastroenterol. 90: 81–87.

Rousseau, C., S. Poland and J. Girkin. 2007. Development of fibre-optic confocal microscopy for detection and diagnosis of dental caries. Caries Res. 41: 245–251.

Riberio, A., C. Rousseau, J. Girkin and A. Hall. 2005. A preliminary investigation of a spectroscopic technique for the diagnosis of natural caries lesions. J. Dent. 33: 73–78.

Rybak, L. and D. Rosenthal. 2001. Radiological imaging for the diagnosis of bone metastases. Q. J. Nucl. Med. 45: 53–64.

Salazar, A. 2006. Energy propagation of thermal waves. Eur. J. Phys. 27: 1349–1355.

Saidi, I., S. Jacques and L. Zheng. 1995. Mie and Rayleigh modelling of visible light scattering in neonatal skin. App. Phys. 34: 7410–7418.

Schantz, S., H. Savage, P. Sacks and R. Alfano. 1997. Native cellular fluorescence and its application to cancer prevention. Env. Health Perspect. 4: 941–944.

Schantz, S., V. Kolli, H. Savage, G. Yu and J. Shah. 1998. *In vivo* native cellular fluorescence and histological characteristics of head and neck cancer. Clin. Cancer Res. 4: 1177–1182.

Schmalenberg, K. and K. Uhrich. 2005. Micropatterned polymer substrates control alignment of proliferating Schwann cells to direct netural regeneration. Biomaterials 26: 1423–1430.

Silveira, L., J. Betiol Filho, F. Silveira and R. Zângaro. 2008. Laser-induced fluorescence at 488 nm excitation for detecting benign and malignant lesions in stomach mucosa. J. Fluoresc. 18: 35–40.

Smith, S.R., K. Foster and G. Wolf. 1986. Dielectric properties of VX-2 carcinoma versus normal liver tissue. IEEE Trans. Biomed. Eng. 33: 522–524.

Srinivasan, R. 1986. Ablation of polymers and biologic tissues by ultraviolet lasers. Science 234: 559–565.

Srinivasan, R. and V. Mayne-Banton. 1982. Self-developing photoetching of poly(ethylene terephthalate) films by far-ultraviolet excimer laser radiation Appl. Phys. Lett. 41: 576–579.

Thareja, R., A. Sharma and S. Shukla. 2008. Spectroscopic investigations of carious tooth decay. Med. Eng. Phys. 30: 1143–1148.

Toenshoff, H., A. Ostendorf, F. Korte and T. Bauer. 2000. Micromachining using femtosecond lasers. SPIE 4088: 136–139.

Tomita, Y. and A. Shima. 1986. Mechanisms of impulsive pressure generation and damage pit formation by bubble collapse. J. Fluid Mech. 169: 535–564.

Tromberg, B., O. Svaasand and T. Tsay. 1993. Properties of photon density waves in multiple-scattering media. Appl. Opt. 32: 607–616.

Troyanova, P., E. Borisova and L. Avramov. 2007. Fluorescence and reflectance properties of hemoglobin-pigmented skin disorders. Proc. SPIE 6734: 673415.

Vernotte, P. 1961. Some possible complications in the phenomena of thermal conduction. Compte Rendus 252: 2190–2191.

Vladimirov, B., E. Borisova and L. Avramov. 2007. Delta-ALA mediated fluorescence spectroscopy of gastrointestinal tumors: comparison of *in vivo* and *in vitro* results. Proc SPIE 6727: 67271X.

Vo-Dinh, T., M. Panjehpour and B. Overholt. 1998. Laser-induced fluorescence for esophageal cancer and dysplasia diagnosis. Annals New York Acad. Sci. 838: 116–122.

Vogel, A. and W. Lauterborn. 1988. Time-resolved particle image velocimetry used in the investigation of cavitation bubble dynamics. Appl. Opt. 27: 1869–1876.

Walsh, J., T. Flotte, R. Anderson and T. Deutsch. 1988. Pulsed CO_2 laser ablation. Lasers Surg. Med. 8: 108–118.

Ward, B. and D. Emmony. 1991. Interferometric studies of the pressures developed in a liquid during infrared laser-induced cavitation bubble oscillation. Appl. Phys. Lett. 32: 489–515.

Welch, A., G. Yoon and J. Van Germet. 1987. Practical models for light distribution in laser-irradiated tissue. Lasers Surg. Med. 6: 488–493.

Wray, S., M. Cope and D. Deply. 1988. Characterization of the ear infrared absorption spectra of cytochrome aa3 and haemoglobin for the non-invasive monitoring of cerebral oxygenation. Biochemica et Biophysica Acta 933: 184–192.

Yang, M., E. Baranov, P. Jiang, F. Sun and X. Li. 2000. Whole-body optical imaging of green fluorescent protein-expressing tumors and metastases. Proc. Natl. Acad. Sci. 97: 1206–1211.

Ye, J., L. Balogh and T. Norris. 2002. Enhancement of laser-induced optical breakdown using metal/dendrimer nanocomposites. Appl. Phys. Lett. 80: 1713–1715.

Yicong, Wu, W. Zheng and J. Qu. 2007. Detection of cell metabolism via wavelength and time-resolved intracellular autofluorescence. Proc. SPIE 6430: 64300A.

Young, F.R. 1989. Cavitation. McGraw-Hill, Oxford.

Zippelius, A., P. Kufer, G. Honold, M. Köllermann and R. Oberneder. 1997. Limitations of reverse-transcriptase polymerase chain reaction analyses for detection of micrometastatic epithelial cancer cells in bone marrow. J. Clin. Oncol. 15: 2701–2708.

Zweig, A. and F. Deutsch. 1992. Shock waves generated by confined XeCl excimer laser ablation of polyimide. Appl. Phys. B. 54: 76–82.

7

Nanotechnology

7.1 Introduction

Let's start with the word '*nano*', which is derived from the Greek word: '*nanos*' meaning dwarf. When used as an unit, it represents one billionth of a meter (10^{-9} m). In other words, if we take one millionth of a meter and further divide it into thousand parts, one part would be one nanometer, which is equivalent to 10 hydrogen or 5 silicon atoms aligned in a line, or interestingly enough, is how fast a human nail grows per second. However, when it is used as a prefix for something, such as 'nanoscience', then nano implies the scale at which the science is seen. The study of fundamental relationships between physical properties, phenomena, and material dimensions in a nanometer scale is referred to as nanoscience. The first written concept about matter at nano scale was proposed by Feynman (1959), in his well-known 'Room at the bottom' lecture at Caltech:

> *"The principles of physics, as far as I can see, do not speak against the possibility of maneuvering things atom by atom. It is not an attempt to violate any laws; it is something, in principle that can be done; but in practice it has not been done because we are too big".*

Nanotechnology is the understanding and control of matter at dimensions approximately between 1 to 100 nm, where unique phenomena offers novel applications. It is thus, by definition, an engineering and manufacturing at a nanometer scale with atomic precision. Nanotechnology is not just a simple miniaturization from micro to nanoscale, since materials at micro level mostly exhibit similar properties as the bulk form. Appropriate laws of physics, such as quantum mechanics represented by Schrodinger's equation, can suitably predict the physical behaviour at nanoscale. At nanoscale, materials may exhibit very distinct physical and chemical properties compared to bulk, and scientists should be able to utilize these properties and continue with their quests at these ever smaller dimensions. It is for this reason that nanotechnology is truly and highly an interdisciplinary field of material science which involves physicists, chemists, biologists, engineers, and physicians to work together on: (i) understanding the physical properties of nanomaterials, (ii) synthesis and characterization of nanomaterials, (iii) design and fabrication of novel nanodevices, and (iv) design and construction of novel tools for characterization of nanomaterials and nanostructures. Quantum effects readily dominate properties of materials at such a small level; properties that are strongly size-dependent. In other words, when particle size is made at nanoscale. The properties including the melting point, electrical conductivity, magnetic permeability, chemical reactivity, and fluorescence vary as a function of the size of the particle. One such interesting quantum effect is the concept of 'tunability' of nanoparticle properties, i.e., by changing the size of the particle, its property of interest can be tuned. For example, size-dependent fluorescence color, which in turn can be used as markers for biomedical and industrial applications. An initial interest in the concept of nanotechnology stems from its connections with biology, where the smallest form of life, such as cells, contains nanometer-size active components. Nanobiotechnology is a subset of nanotechnology where, for example, molecular biologists are interested and inspired in 'Nano-biomimitics', i.e., atom-level engineering and manufacturing by employing biological precedence for guidance (Goodsell 2004). In molecular biology, the '*self-replicating*' machines at the atomic level are guided by DNA, replicated by RNA, some molecules are '*assembled*' by enzymes, and above all, the cells are nicely replete with molecular scale bioelectric motors, such as kinesin. On the other hand, the ion channels are beautifully doing their defined task, acting as biological security border where they allow or block specific ions (e.g., potassium or calcium) to enter a cell through its lipid wall membrane. It appears as though at this level, a delicate, subtle, and exquisitely engineered molecular scale device is relentlessly and reliably at work. Understanding the importance and the role quantum nanophysics plays in the molecular building blocks of our natural world can indeed inspire and guide us to a better design of man-made medical nanomachines or nanorobots in the future to come. For instance, machines that have the potential to serve as vehicles for the delivery of therapeutic agents, detectors, protection against early disease, or even repair of metabolic or genetic defects. Different nanosystems are shown in Schematic diagram 7.1.

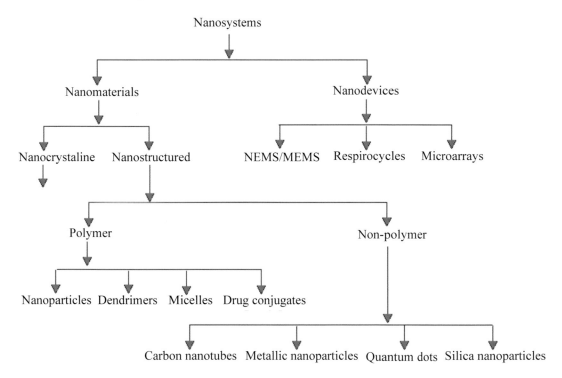

Schematic Diagram 7.1. Nanosystems with corresponding subdivisions.

7.2 Limitations and effects of small size

Clearly, by decreasing the size of the material, scientists and engineers are facing ever-increasing challenges in terms of design and application of system, partly imposed by technological maturity, which is expected to be resolved with time sooner or later, and partly by the very quantum nature of the sub-molecular particles. For example, power dissipation and overheating have become a serious problem in further reduction of metal-oxide semiconductor field effect transistor (MOSFET), since the off-currents in these devices increases exponentially with device scaling (Meindl et al. 2001). Widening the band gap of semiconductors occurs when the size of the materials reaches de Broglie's wavelength (Chapter 2). The limitation also occurs in other areas, such as nanomedicine, where in drug delivery and bioimaging, size plays a significant role in the efficacy and success of the treatment. It is true because we know that conventional micron-sized drug delivery methods in cancer therapy suffer from inefficacy of delivery and insufficient targeting.

7.2.1 Surface of nanoparticles

Undoubtedly, the first and most important consequence of a small particle size is its large surface area, i.e., the surface over volume ratio, or simply called the '*aspect ratio*'. Assuming spherical particles, each with the surface s and diameter ϕ, so that $s = \pi \phi^2$, and the corresponding volume is $v = (\pi/6) \phi^3$. Therefore, one obtains the aspect ratio

$$R = \frac{s}{v} = \frac{6}{\phi} \tag{7.1}$$

So the ratio is inversely proportional to the particle size and therefore, the surface ratio increases with decreasing particle size. If A is the surface per mol, which is a very important thermodynamic parameter, then we write

$$A = ns = \frac{M}{\rho \dfrac{\pi \phi^3}{6}} \pi \phi^2 \tag{7.2}$$

$$A = \frac{6M}{\rho \phi} \tag{7.3}$$

where n is the number of particles per mol, ρ is the density, and M the molecular weight of the material. Similar to aspect ratio, the area per mol increases inversely in proportion to the particle diameter. Therefore, for smaller particles, the area occupied by a volume of the nanoparticles is higher than that occupied by the same volume of micron sized particle. Thus, the number of particles available per square unit (i.e., area) in a nano system is much higher than a bigger sized system. The aspect ratio is very important since it determines the extent of activity of a nanoparticulate system. The limitation on how closely the nanoparticles can be physically placed next to each other is imposed by the simplest, yet most realistic model of quantum mechanics-the Bohr's model. By combining the energy of the classical electron orbit with the quantization of angular momentum, one obtains the Bohr's expression for the electron orbit radii and energies. The Bohr's radius can be derived by equating the centrifugal force of an electron following a circular trajectory around a proton and the electrostatic force experienced by the electron.

$$mv^2 = \frac{q^2}{4\pi\varepsilon_0 r^2} \tag{7.4}$$

Where, m is the mass of electron (Kg), v is the velocity of the electron (m/s), r is the radius of the orbit (m), q is the charge of electron (C), and ε_0 is the permittivity of free space (F/m). According to de Broglie's wavelength, $\lambda = \dfrac{h}{p}$ and according to the standing wave condition, the circumference of an orbit of an electron is equal to the whole number times the wavelength, i.e.,

$$2\pi r = n \lambda \tag{7.5}$$

For the first orbit $2\pi r = \lambda$. From $P = h/\lambda$ and $\lambda = 2 \pi r$

$$P = \frac{h}{2\pi r} \tag{7.6}$$

Therefore, substituting $v^2 = P^2/m^2$ for v in Eq. (7.4) and simplifying, we get

$$r = \frac{4\pi\varepsilon_0 h^2}{mq^2} \tag{7.7}$$

This radius is represented as Bohr's radius, $a_0 = 0.5 \times 10^{-10}$ m (or 12 pm). It defines the least distance from the nuclei at which a single electron revolves in an orbit which is at the lowest energy level. The model assumes that the energy of the particles in an atom is restricted or confined to certain discrete values, i.e., it is *quantized*. In simple words, it means only certain orbits are allowed, while the intermediate orbits are not allowed or, better say, do not exist.

7.2.2 Thermal effects

To have an idea of how much actually a nanoparticle surrounding temperature would affect its stability, we may consider a simple case of an isolated nanoparticle with a thermal energy of kT, where k is the Boltzmann constant. The nanoparticle has a property which depends on the volume v of the nanoparticle and the energy of this property may be w(v). If the volume is sufficiently small so that the condition

$$w(v) < kT \tag{7.8}$$

is satisfied, then one may expect some degree of thermal instability. This instability is usually seen in terms of nanoparticle displacement defined as

$$x.w(v) = \rho v x = kT \tag{7.9}$$

Let us assume a 100 nm gold nanoparticle with a density of 19300 kg m^{-3}. Using (7.9), we get x $\approx$ 42 μm or for 5 nm x $\approx$ 1 m !!. Although such displacements do not really occur physically, it definitely shows that under such conditions the nanoparticles are unstable and that they are on constant move.

Examples

a) If we take a closer look at nanoparticles on a carbon film using an electron microscope, this dynamic becomes more clear, where these nanoparticles are seen moving around on the carbon film. This may, on some occasions, cause major problems during electron microscopy investigations.

b) As it will be discussed in Chapter 8, in the case of superparamagnetism, the vector of magnetization fluctuates thermally to a zero coercivity between different so called '*easy*' directions of magnetization. These fluctuations are related to crystal magnetic anisotropy. Therefore, to distinguish between 'easy' (soft) and 'hard' magnetization, these directions are determining factors as to where the external field should be applied. Therefore, it seems, the stability condition of nanoparticles is important in some aspects of synthesis, characterization, and even biomedical applications where the stability and predictability of nanoparticles within the cells or during an *in vivo* targeting journey can be an issue.

7.3 Material properties at nanoscale

There are two broad categories of material properties: (a) *Intrinsic properties* such as resistivity, which is independent on the size and shape of the specimen. Many such properties at nanoscale are not predictable from those observed at macroscale. This is because totally new phenomena can emerge, e.g., quantum size confinement leading to changes in electronic structure, the presence of wave-like transport process and the interfacial effects, (b) *Extrinsic properties* such as resistance, which depends on the size of the material. Different types of properties are briefly outlined as follows:

1. *Structural*: The increase in surface area and surface free energy with decreasing particle size leads to changes in interatomic spacing.

2. *Thermal*: The melting temperature of a bulk material is not dependent on its size, but the above structural properties have significant effects on the properties. As the dimensions of a material decrease towards the atomic scale, the melting temperature scales with the material dimensions. The decrease in melting temperature can be on the order of tens to hundreds of degrees for metals with nanometer dimensions. For example, the melting point of gold nanoparticles has been observed to decrease rapidly for sizes less than 10 nm (Edelstein and Cammarata 1998). This phenomenon is very prominent in nanoscale materials, which melt at temperatures hundreds of degrees lower than bulk materials.

3. *Mechanical*: Many mechanical properties, such as toughness, are highly dependent on formation or presence of defects within a material. As the structural scale reduces to the nanometer range, the yield strength increases sharply. Many nanostructured metals and ceramics are observed to be superplastic, i.e., they are able to undergo an extensive deformation without necking or fracture.

4. *Magnetic*: (a) *Diamagnetism*—The magnetism is very weak and opposed to the applied magnetic field direction, (b) *Paramagnetism*—Magnetization develops parallel to the applied field as the field increases from zero, but the strength of the magnetization is weak, (c) *Ferromagnetism*—Materials which are intrinsically magnetically ordered and show spontaneous magnetization in the absence of applied field. These materials posses multiple magnetic domains, whereas nanoparticles often consist of one domain, which is known as *superparamagnetism*. This is discussed in more detail in Chapter 9.

5. *Optical*: The effect of reduced dimensionality on electronic structure has the most profound effect on the energies of the highest occupied molecular orbital—HOMO (the valance band) and the lowest unoccupied molecular orbit—LUMO (the conduction band). Semiconductors and metals show large changes in optical properties, such as color as a function of particle size. Colloidal solutions of gold nanoparticles have a deep red color which gradually becomes yellow as the particle size increases, as seen in Fig. 7.1.

In many applications, one may be interested to change the refractive index of, for example, a matrix such as polymer to a different value. This can be done by adding nanoparticles with an index of refraction which differs from that of the polymer. At low nanoparticle concentrations, we have

$$n_c = (1 - c)\, n_m + c\, n_p \tag{7.10}$$

where n_c, n_m, and n_p are index of refraction for composite, polymer matrix, and nanoparticle respectively, and c is the volume fraction nanoparticles. When a light interacts with the composite, it is partly scattered by nanoparticles, leading to loss of transparency of the composite. In other words, to maximize the composite transparency, the scattering should be kept at its minimum level. For spherical particles, i.e., particles with dimensions smaller than the light wavelength, the total power of the scattered light P_β in such medium, according to *Rayleigh*, is given

$$P_\beta = AP_0 c\, \frac{n_p - n_m}{n_m^{\,2}}\, \frac{\phi^6}{\lambda^4} \tag{7.11}$$

where A is constant factor, ϕ is the particle diameter, and $\lambda = \lambda_0/n_m$ where λ_0 is the vacuum wavelength of the incident light and P_0 is the initial power of the incident light. Clearly, it can be deduced from Eq. (7.11) that the particle size is crucial as it has the power of 6. To reduce the light scattering, the particle size must be kept as small as possible. Assuming, the particles are less than 10% of the light wavelength, then at the shortest visible wavelength (400 nm), the particles should be 40 nm if a material is to be transparent over entire visible spectrum. Since this is a maximum value and not an average, a very narrow particle size distribution is indispensable. It should be noted that as the particle size increases or clusters exist in the medium it will cause a dramatic increase in the light scattering. The effect of clustering is not seen in the Eq. (7.11), and we shall discuss about this effect in terms of bioimaging in Chapter 15. More on the effect of nanoparticle size on the light scattering is given in Chapter 9, where the changes of the optical properties of gold nanoshells during the shell growth based on self-assembly is discussed.

6. *Electronic*: The changes associated with electronic properties at small scale is mainly related to the increasing influence of the wave-like property of the electrons (quantum mechanical effects) and the

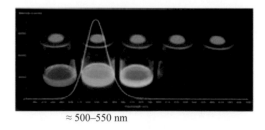

≈ 500–550 nm

Figure 7.1. Colloidal solutions of gold nanoparticles. Larger nanoparticles are observed at longer wavelength (Red-shift) and smaller particles at shorter wavelengths (Blue-shift).

scarcity of scattering centers. In a macroscopic system, the electronic transport is determined mainly by scattering with phonons and impurities but in a microscopic system, the system dimension is smaller than the electronic mean free path of inelastic scattering. Thus, electrons can travel through the system without random walk where the scattering centers are eliminated and the sample boundaries are smooth with specular reflections.

Keywords: Tunability, Nano-biomimitics, Nanorobot, Aspect ratio, Intrinsic properties, Extrinsic properties, Superparamagnetism.

References

Edelstein, A. and R. Cammarata. 1998. Nanotechnology: Synthesis, Properties and Applications. Institute of Physics, London.

Feynman, R. 1959. There is plenty of room at the bottom. The Vega Science Trust. The American Physical Society at CalTech California.

Goodsell, D. 2004. Bionanotechnology: Lessons from nature. Willey-Less. New Jersey. USA, pp. 1–8.

Meindl, J., Q. Chen and J. Davis. 2001. Limits on silicon nanoelectronics for terascale integration. Science 293: 2044–9.

Part III
Nanobiomaterials

8

Biomaterials and Surface Modification

8.1 Introduction

The main goal of this chapter is to discuss some applications of photonics in biomedical engineering, particularly with respect to biomaterials. At this stage '*nanomaterials*' are not involved and the biomaterials are treated in bulk form. Also, it is emphasized that it is not the intension of this chapter to cover the principles and technical discussion of biomaterials, as there are a number of concise and comprehensive text books available for those who are interested to obtain further information. The application of biomaterials whether for status, style, or medical purposes goes back to many centuries where for example, as it is generally agreed, that gold was first used in dentistry over 2500 years ago and it steadily increased, especially during the past 100 years (Crubezy et al. 1998). The first prototype for gold teeth as we know was introduced by dentist Giovanni d'Arcoli (1483), where teeth were cleaned, removing the decay and covered with gold leaf. The earliest successful implants were in the skeletal system (Bobbio 1972). Bone plates were introduced in the early 1900s to overcome the problems associated with fixation of fractures. During the World War II, the warplane pilots who were injured by plastic (polymethyl methacrylate-PMMA) air craft canopy did not suffer adverse chronic reactions from the fragments presence in the body. Since then, PMMA was widely used as intraocular lens (IOL) in ophthalmology.

The term '*Biomaterials*' is often applied to denote man-made materials used to construct prosthetic or other medical devices, e.g., pacemaker for implantation, e.g., stent in a human being. In other words, it is a synthetic material which can be used to replace part of a living system or to function in contact with living tissue (i.e., *in vivo*). '*Biological material*', however, is a material produced by biological systems, such as bone matrix and many others. It is noted that '*artificial*' materials, such as hearing aids or artificial limbs, which are in contact with the skin are not counted as biomaterials since they act as a barrier to external surrounding environment. It is important to note that in order for one to fully appreciate the problems inherent in an endeavour, to replace such organs with a prosthesis, it is essential not only to understand the properties of the original materials in various organs, but also to avoid the notion that even the best and modern technology has the ability to replace any part of our natural living organism with a biomaterial organ which will be superior to the original structure, partly due to the reasons discussed in Chapter 5. It is for this reason that one always finds that an organism as a whole will never operate better than when the original organ was in place. However, it does not imply that any such technological endeavour and quests should be limited, on the contrary, there is clearly an encouraging panorama of future on the horizon and perhaps with respect to prosthesis we should keep saying: '*It is as good as the first day*' more often. But that simply is not a science, though it may undoubtedly bear some positive psychological effects on the patient. The performance of biomaterials in the body can be considered from several different conceptual perspectives: (a) The problem area which has to be solved, (b) The body can be considered at the levels of tissue or organ, (c) Biomaterials may be considered as metals, polymers, ceramics, and composites. Biomaterial design is an important element of tissue engineering, incorporating physical, chemical, and biological cues to guide cells into functional tissues via cell migration, adhesion, and differentiation. Many biomaterials need to degrade at a rate commensurate with new tissue formation to allow cells to deposit new extracellular matrix (ECM) and regenerate functional tissue. In addition, biomaterials may need to include provisions for mechanical support appropriate to the level of functional tissue development.

The use of these materials in the body depends on a number of factors: (1) *Biocompatibility,* i.e., comparison of the tissue response produced through the close association of the implanted candidate material to its implant site within the host animal to that tissue response recognized and established as suitable with control materials (ASTM), or the capability of a prosthesis implanted in the body to exist in harmony with tissue without causing deleterious changes (Becker et al. 1986). A biocompatible material must not cause an irritation of surrounding structures, (2) *Nontoxicity,* i.e., the quality of not having toxic or injurious effects on biological systems, including an inflammation, or causing cancer. Thus, biocompatibility of a biomaterial involves the acceptance of an artificial implant by the surrounding tissues and by the body without the above indicators, (3) *Reliability*, this involves the health and condition of patient, the activities of patient and technique used by surgeon. The reliability can be expressed (Park and Lakes 1992)

$$r = 1-f \qquad (8.1)$$

where f represents the probability of implant failure. Normally, there are number of failure factors and the total rt is defined as

$$r_t = r_1 r_2 \ldots \ldots r_n \qquad (8.2)$$

For example (Park and Lakes 1992), if the failure of a knee replacement in the first five years are, 5% for infection, 3% for wear, 2% for loosening, 1% for surgical complication, and 4% for fracture, then reliability will be

$$r = (1-0.05)\,(1-0.03)\,(1-0.02)\,(1-0.01)\,(1-0.04) = 0.85\,(85\%)$$

Taking a further 10% for the pain, it gives, $(1-0.1) = 0.90$, thus, $0.85 \times 0.90 = 0.77$ (77%). It can be assumed that the failure processes are essentially independent.

Tissue engineering

Tissue engineering is evolved from the field of biomaterials development and refers to the use of combination of cells, biologically active molecules into functional tissues, and engineering and materials methods. The goal of tissue engineering is to assemble functional constructs that restore, maintain, or improve damaged tissues or whole organs, where it uses a scaffold for the formation of new viable tissue for a medical purpose. Artificial skin and cartilage are examples of engineered tissues that have been approved by the FDA, however, currently they have limited use in human patients. While most definitions of tissue engineering cover a wide range of applications, but most often it is closely associated with repairing or replacing portions of, or whole tissues (i.e., bone, cartilage, blood vessels, bladder, skin, muscle, etc.). The term *Regenerative medicine* is often used synonymously with tissue engineering, but it emphasises on the use of stem cells or progenitor cells to produce tissues. In other words, it incorporates research on self-healing where the body uses its own systems, sometimes with the help of foreign biological material to recreate cells and rebuild tissues and organs.

Significant developments in the multidisciplinary field of tissue engineering have produced a novel set of tissue replacement parts and implementation strategies. Scientific advances in biomaterials, stem cells, growth and differentiation factors, and biomimetic environments have created unique opportunities to fabricate tissues in the laboratory from combinations of engineered extracellular matrices, i.e., scaffolds, cells, and biologically active molecules. Among the major challenges now facing tissue engineering is the need for more complex functionality, as well as both functional and biomechanical stability in laboratory-grown tissues destined for transplantation. Finally, the success of tissue engineering, and the eventual development of true human replacement parts depends on the rate of harmonized convergence of engineering and basic research advances in tissue, matrix, growth factor, stem cell, and developmental biology, as well as materials science and bio informatics. For example, myocardial tissue engineering has become a prime goal of research in this field. Myocardial tissue engineering combines isolated functional cardiomyocytes and a biodegradable or nondegradable biomaterial to repair diseased heart muscle. The challenges in heart muscle engineering include cell issues, the design and fabrication of myocardial tissue engineering substrates, and the engineering of tissue constructs *in vitro* and *in vivo*.

Spiderman: A bio-mimic from nature

Spider webs are made of special spider silk, which is the strongest fibre known to man. It is five times stronger than steel. The strongest of all spider silk is produced by the Golden Orb Weaving spider. Spider's silk is mostly made up of the proteins fibroin and sericin (another natural fibre that is made up of protein). Because of its size, and the complex way spiders create the silk, it's very hard to copy, but much has been learned about the protein molecules in spider silk. A single strand that measures 3–5 microns across may be made up of thousands of individual sub-strands that are too small to be examined by any microscope. Silks from silkworms (e.g., Bombyx mori) and orb-weaving spiders (e.g., Nephila clavipes) have been explored to understand the processing mechanisms and to exploit the properties of these proteins for use as biomaterials. Spider silk from N. clavipes has been studied extensively and is characterized by its remarkable mechanical strength and thermal stability in fibre form (Wong Po Foo and Kaplan 2005). The different types of silks formed by spiders serve various functions. The mechanical properties of the different silks are due to structural differences derived from different amino acid compositions and sequences. Dragline silk for safety and web construction is one the strongest natural materials and is composed of two proteins: major ampullate spidroins protein 1 and 2 (MaSp1 and MaSp2). A molecular weight of 275 kDa is based on gel electrophoresis of MaSp1 (Kaplan et al. 1998) and 740 kDa based on the major ampullate gland silk by size exclusion chromatography (Jackson and O'Brien 1995). The amino acid composition of dragline silk, MaSp1 from N. clavipes, consists mainly of the amino acids glycine and alanine, like silkworm silk, while glutamic acid, proline, and arginine are also significant in content (Kaplan et al. 1998). This silk consists of repetitive blocks of peptides which give rise to the unique structural properties. Success in synthesizing spiderlike fibres could provide superstrong reinforcing fibres for advanced composites. The mechanical properties of silk fibres are based on the combination of high strength and high extensibility. Sider draglines and warm cocoon silk exhibits up to 35% elongation with tensile strengths in the naturally occurring fibre that are seen in some high-strength synthetic fibres. There are six silk types, including dragline and orb web proteins that act as support fibres for the orb frame and silk for wrapping prey. While silks from both silkworms and spiders have attractive properties, tests have demonstrated that the spider fibres have higher mechanical value (R&D 1993). The tensile strength values depend not only on the chemical structure, but also on processing parameters, particularly the rate of spinning.

Biometals

Biometals are metal ions used in biology, biochemistry, and medicine. The metals copper, zinc, iron, and manganese are examples of metals that are essential for the normal functioning of the human body. The biocompatibility of the metallic implants is of significant importance and concern from safety point of view. Metal compounds and ions can also produce harmful effects on the body due to the toxicity of several types of metals (Stephen 2014). For example, arsenic works as a potent poison due to its effects as an enzyme inhibitor, disrupting ATP production (Singh et al. 2011). Also, metals can corrode in the hostile body environment, which effectively weakens the implant in a defined period of time. Above all, the corrosion products escape into the tissue, leading to set of undesirable and adverse effects. The first stainless steel used for as implant material was type 302, which is stronger the vanadium steel and more resistant to corrosion. The former is no longer used due to its inadequate corrosion resistance. The next generation of stainless steel contained molybdenum in order to enhance its corrosion resistance in salt water, which is a close model to body physiological fluid. This type of steel was called 316 L and in the 1950s its carbon content was reduced from 0.08% to 0.03% (Park and Lakes 1992). Chromium as a reactive element is a major component of corrosion-resistant stainless steel. But the chromium and its alloys can be passivated to give a better corrosion resistance. However, for the purpose of biomedical applications such as implants, austenitic stainless steels including 316 and 316 L are widely used. These materials are nonmagnetic and have better corrosion resistance compared to other types. The inclusion of molybdenum improves the resistance to pitting corrosion. Finally, in order to stabilize the austenitic phase at room temperature, nickel is also added to enhance the corrosion resistance.

Currently, most artificial joints consist of a metallic component, either titanium alloy or Co-Cr tests against polymers, such as ultrahigh molecular weight polyethylene (UHMWPE). Cr-Co alloys have excellent wear resistance, and are stable due to the formation of a passive, tenacious, self-replenishing chromium oxide, a few atomic layers thick. Due to good wear resistance, Cr-Co alloys have a great potential application for metal-on-metal bearing surfaces for hip joints. Another widely used metal, such as in biomedical applications, is titanium and its alloys. Titanium alloys are metals that contain a mixture of titanium and other chemical elements. Such alloys have very high tensile strength and toughness. They are light in weight, have extraordinary corrosion resistance, and the ability to withstand extreme temperatures. Although commercially pure titanium has acceptable mechanical properties, and has been used for orthopaedic and dental implants, for most applications titanium is alloyed with small amounts of aluminium and vanadium, typically 6% and 4%, respectively, by weight. This mixture has a solid solubility which varies dramatically with temperature, allowing it to undergo precipitation strengthening. Grade five is also known as Ti6Al4V, which is the most commonly used alloy. It has a chemical composition of 6% aluminum, 4% vanadium, 0.25% (maximum) iron, 0.2% (maximum) oxygen, and the remainder titanium. It is significantly stronger than commercially pure titanium while having the same stiffness and thermal properties. This grade is an excellent combination of strength, corrosion resistance, weld, and fabricability (Murr et al. 2009).

Bioceramics

Bioceramics are usually polycrystalline inorganic silicates, oxides, and carbides. The ceramic materials used are not the same as porcelain type ceramic materials, but rather are closely related to either the body's own materials (e.g., calcium phosphate) or are extremely durable metal oxides. They are refractory in nature and possess high compressive strength. Bioceramics are classified into: inert, bioactive, and biodegradable materials (Park et al. 2004). Bioinert ceramics like alumina and zirconia maintain their physical and mechanical properties even in biological environments. Zirconia is highly wear resistant and tough; it undergoes stress-induced transformation toughening. A major application of zirconia ceramics is in total hip replacement (THR) ball heads. Ceramics such as phosphate and tricalcium phosphate (TCP) degrade when placed in a biological environment, and thus are considered biodegradable. Salts like hydroxylapatite (HA) can be crystallized from calcium phosphate. The main mineral of bone and teeth is HA, which explains its biocompatibility.

Bioceramics and bioglasses are ceramic materials that are biocompatible (Ducheyne and Hastings 1984), and are typically used as rigid materials in surgical implants, though some bioceramics are flexible. No bioinert ceramics exhibit bonding with the bone. However, bioactivity of bioinert ceramics can be achieved by forming composites with bioactive ceramics. Bioglass and glass ceramics are nontoxic and chemically bond to bone. Glass ceramics elicit osteoinductive properties, while calcium phosphate ceramics also exhibit non-toxicity to tissues and bioresorption. The ceramic particulate reinforcement has led to the choice of more materials for implant applications that include ceramic/ceramic, ceramic/polymer, and ceramic/metal composites. Among these composites, ceramic/polymer composites have been found to release toxic elements into the surrounding tissues. Metals face corrosion related problems, and ceramic coatings on metallic implants degrade over time during lengthy applications. Ceramic/ceramic composites enjoy superiority due to similarity to bone minerals, exhibiting biocompatibility and a readiness to be shaped. The biological activity of bioceramics has to be considered under various *in vitro* and *in vivo* studies. Performance needs must be considered in accordance with the particular site of implantation (Thamaraiselvi and Rajeswari 2004).

Bioceramics are meant to be used in extracorporeal circulation systems (e.g., dialysis) or engineered bioreactors. However, they are most commonly used as implants. Ceramics show numerous applications as biomaterials due to their physico-chemical properties. They have the advantage of being inert in the human body, and their hardness and resistance to abrasion makes them useful for bones and teeth replacement. Some ceramics also have excellent resistance to friction, making them useful as replacement materials for malfunctioning joints. Some bioceramics incorporate alumina (Al_2O_3), as their lifespan is longer than that of the patient's. The material can be used in inner ear ossicles, ocular prostheses, electrical insulation for pacemakers, catheter orifices, and in numerous prototypes of implantable systems, such as cardiac pumps (Thamaraiselvi and Rajeswari 2004). Alumino-silicates are commonly used in dental prostheses, pure or in ceramic-polymer composites. The ceramic-polymer composites are a potential way of filling cavities, replacing amalgams, suspected to have toxic effects. The alumina silicates also have a glassy structure. Zirconia doped with yttrium oxide has been proposed as a substitute for alumina for osteoarticular prostheses. The main advantages are a greater failure strength, and a good resistance to fatigue. Calcium phosphate-based ceramics constitute, at present, the preferred bone substitute in orthopaedic and maxillofacial surgery (Garrido et al. 2011). They are similar to the mineral phase of the bone in structure and/or chemical composition. The material is typically porous, which provide a good bone-implant interface due to the increase of surface area that encourages cell colonisation and revascularisation. Additionally, it has lower mechanical strength compared to bone, making highly porous implants very delicate. Since Young's modulus of ceramics is generally much higher than that of the bone tissue, the implant can cause mechanical stresses at the bone interface (Park et al. 1992). Calcium phosphates usually found in bioceramics include hydroxyapatite (HAP) $Ca_{10}(PO_4)_6(OH)_2$; tricalcium phosphate β (β TCP): $Ca_3 (PO_4)_2$; and mixtures of HAP and β TCP.

Biopolymers

Polymers (*poly*: many and *mer*: unit) are made by linking small molecules through primary covalent bonding in the main backbone with C, N, O, Si, etc. For example, polyethylene (PET), which is made from ethylene ($CH2 = CH2$), where the carbon atoms share electrons with two other hydrogen and carbon atoms.

On the other hand, biopolymers are polymers produced by living organisms, in other words, they are polymeric biomolecules. Since they are polymers, biopolymers contain monomeric units that are covalently bonded to form larger structures. A major defining difference between biopolymers and other polymers can be found in their structures. All polymers are made of repetitive units called monomers. Biopolymers often have a well-defined structure, the exact chemical composition and the sequence in which these units are arranged is called the *primary structure*, e.g., proteins. Many biopolymers spontaneously fold into characteristic compact shapes which determine their biological functions and depend in a complicated way on their primary structures. Structural biology is the study of the structural properties of the biopolymers. In contrast, most synthetic polymers have much simpler and more random (or stochastic) structures. In the structure of DNA is a pair of biopolymers, polynucleotides, forming the double helix. There are three main classes of biopolymers, classified according to the monomeric units used and the structure of the biopolymer formed: polynucleotides (RNA and DNA), which are long polymers composed of 13 or more nucleotide monomers; polypeptides, which are short polymers of amino acids; and polysaccharides, which are often linear bonded polymeric carbohydrate structures. Some biopolymers—such as polylactic acid (PLA) can be used as plastics, replacing the need for polystyrene or polyethylene based plastics. Some plastics are now referred to as being *'degradable'*, or *'UV-degradable'*. This means that they break down when exposed to light or air, but these plastics are still primarily oil-based and are not currently certified as *'biodegradable'* under the European Union directive on Packaging and Packaging Waste (94/62/EC). Polymers are considered for a wide range of biomedical applications because of their easy manufacturing, low cost, and sufficient mechanical and physical properties. Typically, they are used for orthopaedic, dental, cardiovascular, and soft tissue engineering. However, compared to metallic and ceramic systems, polymers tend to have low mechanical strength and poor wear resistance. Therefore, various surface modification techniques have been used to improve the functionality of these materials.

Composites

These materials are made from several different substances on microscopic or macroscopic level. The term composite usually is used to denote materials in which the distinct phases are separated on a scale larger than atomic and that the properties such as elastic modulus are very different to those of a homogeneous material. The properties of composites depend strongly on structure similar to homogeneous materials. The shape of inhomogeneities in a composite is divided into three broad categories: (i) particle, with no dimension, (ii) fibre with one long dimension, and (iii) platelet with two long dimensions.

8.2 Surface modification of biomaterials

Problems concerned with the physical (mechanical, thermal, optical, magnetic, and electrical) and chemical properties of different types of materials including strength, durability, flexibility, corrosion, and conductivity; which among the other properties are important determining factors; have caused some limitations with respect to their applications in various fields. Thus, a desire to overcome some of these drawbacks not only is a need, but certainly a challenging task whose complexity depends on the type of material and the scale at which the change is required. Needles to say that a further complication is added when a specific set of characterization must be done and approved before their applications. This latter requirement becomes more critical at nanoscale, as it will be discussed in the next chapter. As mentioned earlier, the surface of a biomaterial is in direct contact with living tissues in the body and the initial response of the living tissue to the biomaterial depends on its surface properties. However, it is rare that a biomaterial with good bulk properties also possesses the surface characteristics suitable for clinical applications. The main purpose of surface modification is to maintain the key bulk properties of the material, while modifying the surface to improve biocompatibility.

8.2.1 Modification techniques

1. Mechanical: polishing, sand blasting, carbide paper

Sandpaper or glass paper are generic names given to coated abrasive that consists of sheets of paper or cloth with abrasive material glued to one face. Sandpaper is produced in a range of grit sizes, and is used to remove material from surfaces, either to make them smoother to remove a layer of material (such as old paint layer), or sometimes to make the surface rougher (for example, making grooves on the surface). It is common to use the names: aluminium oxide paper, or silicon carbide paper. Abrasive blasting is the operation of forcibly propelling a stream of abrasive material against a surface under high pressure to smooth a rough surface, roughen a smooth surface, shape a surface, or remove surface contaminants. A pressurized fluid, typically compressed air, or a centrifugal wheel is used to propel the blasting material. Clearly, this mechanical methods cannot be suitable for a precise surface modification largely due to random size and direction of grooves and pits created by grits or sands on the surface, and also inclusion of impurities.

2. Electron beam

Free electrons in a vacuum can be manipulated by electric and magnetic fields to form a fine beam. Electron guns with powers of up to 150 kW are accessible, but normally about 60 kW is used. Where the beam collides with solid-state matter, electrons are converted into heat or kinetic energy. This concentration of energy in a small volume of matter can be precisely controlled electronically, which brings many advantages. The rapid increase of temperature at the location of impact can quickly melt a target material. In extreme working conditions, the rapid temperature increase can even lead to evaporation, making an electron beam an excellent tool in heating applications, such as welding. Electron beam technology is used in electron lithography of sub-micrometer and nano-dimensional images, in microelectronics for electron beam curing of color printing, and for the fabrication and modification of polymers, including liquid crystal films.

In polymers, an electron beam may be used on the material to induce effects such as chain scission (which makes the polymer chain shorter) and cross linking. The result is a change in the properties of the polymer which is intended to extend the range of applications for the material. The effects of irradiation may also include changes in crystallinity, as well as microstructure. Usually, the irradiation process degrades the polymer. The irradiated polymers may sometimes be characterized using DSC, XRD, FTIR, or SEM. In metals, melting is achieved by scanning the surface and it resolidifies again after the beam has passed over it. The major drawbacks are: (i) surface crack due to residual stress, which can be because of structural and chemical constituents of metal, (ii) Gaseous cavitation, possibly due to presence of, for example hydrogen, in the form of cavity or dissolved form in the base alloy, (iii) step-like layer after resolidification. This can be because of thermal gradient, which causes a stress gradient at the surface to push outward the molten material during the interaction with the electron beam.

3. Ion implantation

Ion implantation equipment typically consists of an ion source, where ions of the desired element are produced, an accelerator, where the ions are electrostatically accelerated to a high energy, and a target chamber, where the ions impinge on a target, which is the material to be implanted. Thus ion implantation is a special case of particle radiation. Each ion is typically a single atom or molecule, and thus the actual amount of material implanted in the target is the integral over time of the ion current. Typical ion energies are in the range of 10 to 500 keV. The lower energies in the range of 1 to 10 keV can be used, but result in a penetration of only a few nanometers or less. In some applications, for example prosthetic devices such as artificial joints, it is desired to have surfaces very resistant to both chemical corrosion and wear due to friction. Ion implantation is used in such cases to engineer the surfaces of such devices for more reliable performance. For example, the surface modification of steel by ion implantation includes both a surface compression which prevents crack propagation and an alloying of the surface to make it more chemically resistant to corrosion. The major limitations include: vacuum requirement ($\approx 10^{-5}$–10^{-7} mmHg), expensive, limited metals can be used for implantation.

4. Plasma spray

Plasma spray is a coating process. In these devices, the coating precursor is heated by electrical arc or plasma, which is formed between two electrodes in a plasma forming gas, usually consisting of either argon/hydrogen or argon/helium. As the plasma gas is heated by the arc, it expands and is accelerated through a shaped nozzle, creating velocities up to MACH 2. Temperatures in the arc zone can reach up to 20,000°K and the temperatures in the plasma jet can be 10,000°K several centimeters away from the exit of the nozzle. Nozzle designs and flexibility of powder injection schemes, along with the ability to generate very high process temperatures, enables plasma spraying to utilize a wide range of coatings, such as refractory materials including alloys, composites, tungsten, tantalum, ceramic oxides, and other refractory materials. They are fed in powder or wire form, heated to a molten or semi-molten state, and accelerated towards substrates in the form of micrometer-size particles. Combustion or electrical arc discharge is usually used as the source of energy for thermal spraying. Thermal spraying can provide thick coatings with thickness varying between a few microns to several mm, depending on the process. Coating quality is usually assessed by measuring its porosity, oxide content, macro and micro-hardness, bond strength, and surface roughness. Generally, the coating quality increases with increasing particle velocities.

Usual limitations of this technique are: weak interconnection between the particles microscopic structures, relatively weak adhesivity between the coating and substrate, probably because of non-uniform substrate heating, irregular surface (≈ 5–15 μm), non-uniform thickness of surface coating due to non-uniform distribution of particles from nozzle head, particle ventilation is required, a noise/sound isolating cabinet is needed (≈ 130 dB).

5. Radio frequency (RF) plasma

RF generator is used to ignite and produce the plasma by voltage or current sources inside a plasma reactor. The generator must be capable of reacting to the plasma's charging characteristics, ensuring that poer remains stable during operation. A typical device size is about 30 cm–1 m, and with the driving frequencies from DC to RF (13.56 MHz) to microwaves (2.45 GHz). The charged particle collisions with neutral particles are important and there are boundaries at which surface losses are important. Ionization of neutrals sustains the plasma in the steady state and the electrons are not in thermal equilibrium with the ions.

6. Chemical vapour deposition (CVD)

This is a chemically-induced process where some gas or vapour phase react chemically together inside a chemical furnace/reactor where the work piece is placed. In typical CVD, the substrate is exposed to one or more volatile precursors, which react and/or decompose on the substrate surface to produce the desired deposit. Frequently, volatile by-products are also produced, which are removed by gas flow through the reaction chamber, hence producing a thin solid layer deposited on the target. The layer could be monocrystalline. polycrystalline or even an amorphous material, depending on the chemical composition and metallurgical structure. In recent years, lasers have been used as heat source and chemical reactor, i.e., as an ignition (LCVD). In this case, a superior organometallic gas is used to provide 100% pure metal depending on the substrate, which is irradiated by a suitable laser. The absorption of photons by gas molecules above the substrate excite them to upper rotational level and after they return to the ground state, the whole process is repeated again. The laser-induced heat due to chemical reaction will consequently cause the gas to undergo a thermal dissociation, whereby the particles are deposited on the substrate.

For example: (i) Coating tungsten layer on Si, (ii) Growing thin diamond layer on Si.

7. Physical vapour deposition (PVD)

This is a physical process of material coating in vacuum where different technique such as vaporization, PLD, sputtering, and atomic bombardment are used. PVD is used in the manufacture of items which require thin films for mechanical, optical, chemical, or electronic functions. PVD can be performed as:

(a) Pulse laser deposition (PLD), (b) Matrix assisted pulse laser evaporation (MAPLE), and (c) Matrix assisted laser deposition ionization (MALDI).

(a) PLD

This is an example of PVD technique for coating development, where a high power pulsed laser beam is focused on the target surface inside a vacuum chamber, as seen in Fig. 8.1. The principle of operation is as follows:

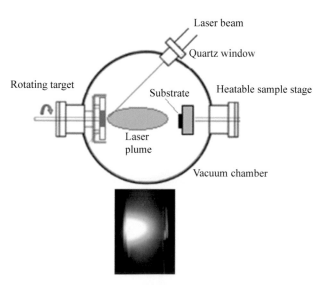

Figure 8.1. A typical setup for PLD experiment. Laser beam is focused on the target and the ablated particles are deposited on the substrate. Usually, the substrate disc is rotatable for preheating and uniform deposition.

(i) When the laser pulse is absorbed by the target, energy is first converted to electronic excitation and then into thermal, chemical, and mechanical energy resulting in evaporation, ablation, plasma formation, and even exfoliation, (ii) The ejected species expand into the surrounding vacuum in the form of a plume containing many energetic species including atoms, molecules, electrons, ions, clusters, particulates, and molten globules, before depositing on the typically hot substrate, (iii) The plume is then deposited as a thin film on a substrate (such as a silicon wafer facing the target). This process can occur in an ultrahigh vacuum or in the presence of a background gas, such as oxygen, which is commonly used when depositing oxides to fully oxygenate the deposited films.

One of the early PLD experiments with biomaterials was about deposition of HA on titanium alloy (Cotell 1993). It is known that calcium phosphate-based bioceramics have been used in non-bearing medical and dental implant devices. However, the use of these materials for orthopaedic applications where a substantial amount of applied load must be tolerated, as their lifetime is very limited due to the low tensile strength of these ceramics. On the other hand, possible corrosive products from metal surface in the long run can cause tissue irritation and inflammation. So, they coated the metal with one of the most stable calcium phosphate, i.e., HA ($Ca_{10}(PO_4)_6(OH)_2$). The results showed adhesion of crystalline HA film deposited at 600 C in Ar/H_2O was excellent, but films deposited at room temperature or in non-reactive environment did not adhere well to the substrate. Of course, since then many good and advanced research with different approaches have been suggested to improve different aspects of the work both on the technical side and the material selection.

(b) MAPLE

This technique has emerged for polymers and biomaterials deposition, since it provides a gentle mechanism to transfer small and large molecules weight species from condensed phase into the vapour phase. In this technique, organic or nanosized material is diluted in a volatile non-interacting solvent, with concentration of a few percent in weight, and frozen at the liquid nitrogen temperature. The frozen target is irradiated with a pulsed laser beam, whose energy is mainly absorbed by the solvent and converted to thermal energy, allowing the solvent to vaporize and be evacuated by the vacuum system. The solute materials have been deposited by this technique, like optical polymers, proteins, bacteria, and DNA (Chrisey et al. 2003). This technique has been used for number of biomedical applications, including drug delivery using KrF (248 nm) laser (Cristescu et al. 2007).

(c) MALDI

MALDI is a soft ionization technique used in mass spectrometry, allowing the analysis of biomolecules (biopolymers such as DNA, proteins, peptides, and sugars) and large organic molecules (such as polymers, dendrimers, and other macromolecules), which tend to be fragile and fragment when ionized by more conventional ionization methods. It is similar in character to electrospray ionization in that both techniques are relatively soft ways of obtaining ions of large molecules in the gas phase, though MALDI produces far fewer multiply charged ions. MALDI methodology is a three-step process: (i) the sample is mixed with a suitable matrix material and applied to a metal plate, (ii) a pulsed laser irradiates the sample, triggering ablation and desorption of the sample and matrix material, and (iii) the analyte molecules are ionized by being protonated or deprotonated in the hot plume of ablated gases, and can then be accelerated into whichever mass spectrometer is used to analyse them. An investigation was performed by Perera et al. (1995), which showed the formation of homo and hetro multimeric ions of large proteins in matrix assisted UV (337 nm) laser desorption/ionization of large proteins and their mixtures.

8. Micro/Nanopatterning

In order to improve the biocompatibility of materials used in medicine, a thorough understanding of cell-surface adhesion is essential. Cell membrane proteins are involved in the adhesion process, which include structural and metabolic changes of the cell. Predefined surface structure with nanometer dimension allow one to investigate the chemical and topological factors promoting cell adhesion. As for the improvement of the bicompatibility, it is essential for the tissue to maintain a specific architecture, which promotes appropriate morphogenesis in order to function properly. Ping et al. (2003) showed that laser patterned polymeric substrate have induced different degrees of directional growth of L929 cells, so that they grew in the direction aligned with the direction of microgrooves. However, the widths of the microgrooves showed a key role in morphology and growth orientation. Therefore, controlling the spatial orientation and the growth of cells have become an important investigation nowadays. In a research by Monsees et al. (2005), the effects of different titanium alloys and nanosize surface patterning on adhesion, differentiation, and orientation of osteoblast-like cells were studied. In the field of tissue engineering, for example, different approaches are used to produce scaffolds: gas foaming, fibre bonding, freeze-drying, and solvent casting. However, these methods are limited by their random micro-geometrics, low resolution features, random distribution of pores, residual particles, and solvents in the poly-matrix and limited oxygen/nutrient supply (Baran 2011). In this respect micro and nanofabrication technologies have emerged as versatile and powerful methods to produce such surface features by both direct and replication methods, where a 3-D scaffolds can be created by means of assembling techniques. Lima et al. (2014) used replication methods and produced a high resolution features as small as 5 nm on biodegradable polymers and assembling techniques to construct scaffolds.

9. *Selective laser sintering (SLS): See next section*

8.3 Some examples of laser surface modification

In this section, only the highlights of some of the published results of laser surface modification of materials for biomedical applications are briefly described, without going through the details.

8.3.1 *Evaluation of Mid-IR (HF) laser radiation effects on 316L stainless steel corrosion resistance in physiological saline* (Khosroshahi et al. 2004)

The effect of short pulsed ($\sim$ 400 ns) multiline hydrogen fluoride (HF) laser radiation operating on average at 2.8 µm has been studied on 316L stainless steel in terms of physical parameters. At low fluences ≤ 8 Jcm^{-2} (phase I), no morphological changes occurred at the surface, and melting began at about 8.8 Jcm^{-2} (phase II), which continued up to about 30 Jcm^{-2}. In this range melting zone was effectively produced by high temperature surface centres growth, which subsequently joined these centres together. Thermal ablation via surface vaporization began at about 33 Jcm^{-2} (phase III). The results of SEM evaluation and corrosion resistance experiment with cyclic potentiodynamic polarization method in a physiological (Hank's) solution indicated that pitting corrosion sensitivity was decreased, i.e., enhancement of corrosion resistance. Also, the XRD results showed a double increase of $\gamma(111)$ at microstructure, thus in effect a superaustenitic steel was obtained at optimized melting fluence with an increased corrosion resistance against physiological solution. Inclusions such as sulphides at the surface have been dissolved in the structure due to remelting or alternatively, they are covered by molten material. This is a highly important point to notice with regard to medical implantation inside a body.

Due to its favourable biocompatibility and mechanical properties, stainless steel and its alloys have become one of the promising implant materials for orthopaedic prosthesis applications. It is thus important to consider its corrosion resistance (CR) in a biological environment. Since it has been assumed that a satisfactory CR represents a necessary requirement for good biocompatibility, several studies have been performed on this subject. In particular some biocompatible metals like Ti base alloys rely on the presence of a passive film on its surface to develop an acceptable CR (Zitter and Plank 1987, Nakayamay et al. 1981). Although, adding chromium, molybdenum, and nickel could improve stainless steel CR, nevertheless these alloying elements can be scarce, expensive, and toxic. Therefore, laser surface modification (LSM) of biometals has become a considerable alternative for CR enhancement. LSM via heating effect involves a rapid melting of the surface layer, followed by subsequent rapid solidification of melted material to change its composition. It is important to note that the interaction of laser with metal surface (or other materials to that matter) affects the surface wettability characteristics, and hence the contact angle and the Gibbs free energy and its biocompatibility. Thus, the material can become either more hydrophobic or hydrophilic.

In this experiment a multiline hydrogen fluoride (HF) laser with a wavelength range between (2.67–2.96 μm) with an average wavelength of 2.80 μm, output energies of up to 600 mJ, and pulse duration of 400 ns at FWHM was used at 0.2 Hz. Throughout the experiment, an austenitic 316L stainless steel samples were used in the form of a cubic square with $10 \times 10 \times 5$ mm dimension. The specimens were first completely polished and finished with alumina powder using 300, 400, 600, 900 grit silicon carbide papers. Prior to tests, the samples were washed ultrasonically with alcohol, then degreased and rinsed with de-ionized water. The etching process was carried out for 30s using Marbel solution which consisted of distilled water (100 cc), HCl (100 cc), and CaSO4 (20 g). All the experiments were performed under ambient condition.

The standard potential dynamic polarization tests were carried out to study the metastable pitting corrosion behaviour. Specimens were first cathodically polarized from open circuit potential to −8-mV and then anodically polarized up to + 1600 mV with respect to standard calmol electrode until pitting occurred. This difference causes the libration of hydrogen and metallic ions, which in turn makes the current flow in the circuit. The metal corrosion behaviour can be studied by measuring this current and plotting the E-Log I diagram. All the experiments were conducted in Hank's solution at 37°C in order to simulate the body media. The effect of laser irradiation on sample is shown in Fig. 8.2, where the curve is divided into three zones. Zone I indicates that there is no morphological change below 8 Jcm⁻², but beyond that where zone II commences, the melting gradually occurs and continues up to about 33 Jcm⁻².

Since the melting threshold of grain boundaries is much lower than grain centres, thus the most probable melting points are considered to initiate at grain boundaries, which in turn is thought to be due to concentration of impurities. The comparison between two morphologically different areas, i.e., untreated and laser treated is shown in Fig. 8.3.

The grain boundaries and inclusions have disappeared and the scratches due to machining and polishing are sealed due to direct laser heating effect. Thus, a relatively smooth and reflective surface is achieved. Of course the plasma formation slowly took place above 40 Jcm⁻² and became stronger at higher levels. Whether this region has any biomedical application requires further research. Two other important findings are the effect of fluence and pulse number on the surface melting diameter. As it is indicated in Fig. 8.4, the melting diameter increases linearly up to about 40 Jcm⁻² where it reaches to about 450 μm, being consistent with the fact that the onset of ablation process is accompanied with ejection of material from the surface as gaseous and solid particles due to thermal vaporization, hence leaving the substrate with lower temperature. Beyond 40 Jcm⁻² the melting diameter decreases dramatically mainly because of intense interaction between laser pulse and laser-induced vapour plume.

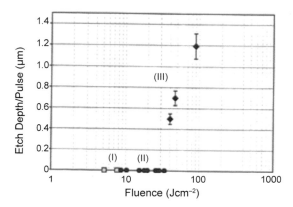

Figure 8.2. Etched depth per pulse of stainless steel with laser fluence: (I) no morphological change, (II) melting range and (III) vaporization and thermal ablation.

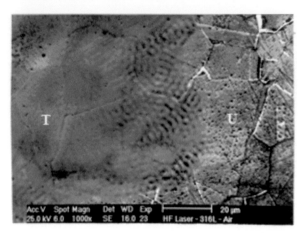

Figure 8.3. Morphology of untreated (U) and treated (T) surface at 15 Jcm⁻² after 10 pulses.

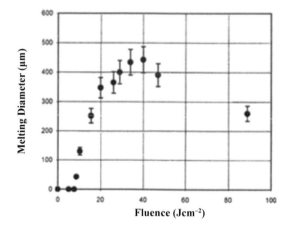

Figure 8.4. Variation of melting diameter as a function of fluence.

Also, it can be observed from Fig. 8.5 that the size of melting diameter increases with laser pulse, but saturates beyond a certain point.

The experimental results obtained from corrosion test is given in Table 8.1. Figure 8.6 illustrates typical cyclic potentiodynamic curves for untreated and treated 316 L stainless steel in Hank's salt balanced physiological solution.

It is noted that in the cathodic section of the curve, the laser treated sample is placed at a higher position, which means it releases hydrogen easier and acts as an electron donor to electrolyte. This higher open circuit potential of laser treated relative to initial sample physically implies a delayed corrosion in anodic region. This can be due to the fact that laser radiation has caused an increase in steel austenite percentage. Generally, change in the corrosion potential (E_{corr}) shows a microstructural modification in the metal. In this case, it is shown that E_{corr} of laser treated sample is more positive than the untreated one, i.e., a more noble metal is achieved. Also, it is seen from the curve that the laser treated steel has smoothly reached the passivation region. This effect implies that probably most inclusions, such as sulphides at the surface have been dissolved in the structure due to remelting or alternatively, they are covered by molten material. This is a highly important point to notice with regard to medical implantation inside a body. The XRD analysis indicates a crystallographic changes at the surface of steel due to rapid solidification. The important point

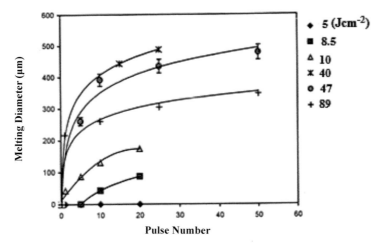

Figure 8.5. Variation of melting diameter as a function of laser pulse number at different fluences.

Table 8.1. Experimental results of potentiodynamic corrosion test for 316L stainless steel.

	I_{corr} (Acm^{-2})	E_{corr} (V)	E_{pit} (mV)
Untreated	2.175	−0.482	−150
Treated	2.135	−0.211	−14

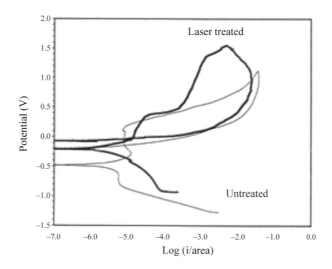

Figure 8.6. Potentiodynamic polarization tests for untreated and treated sample in physiological Hank's solution.

to notice is that relative intensity of $\gamma(111)$ is almost twice as much as the untreated sample. However, the increase of $\gamma(111)$ in treated area shown in Fig. 8.7 confirms the reduction of segregation percentage of these elements in 316L stainless steel under irradiation. Therefore, the laser treated surface is covered by a superaustenite layer, which in effect means the substrate corrosion resistance will be greater due to anodic protection.

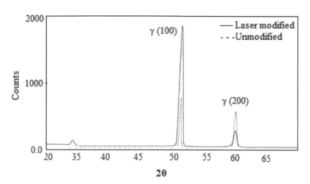

Figure 8.7. XRD results for untreated and treated stainless steel 316 L.

8.3.2 *CO_2 laser surface modification of polyurethane* (Khosroshahi et al. 2004)

This study was undertaken to evaluate and compare the effects of chop-wave (CPW) and super pulse wave (SPW) of CO_2 laser on polyurethane. The results showed that at the threshold fluences of 200 and 400 m Jcm^{-2} for CPW and SPW, the final temperatures would be about 322 and 343 K, justified by their effective absorption coefficients of 1.2×10^3 cm^{-1} and 1.3×10^3 cm^{-1}, respectively. These values are well below the minimum melting temperature (393 K) of polymer. The ATR-FTIR spectral analysis showed four new peaks at 1436, 1370, 1259, and 958 cm^{-1} after laser irradiation indicative of increased hydrogen bonding. The best surface free energy of 50 mNm^{-1} was obtained after 8 pulses of CPW, which corresponds to a contact angle of 75°. Topological studies using SEM evaluation illustrated that a smooth wall crater can be produced by SPW and CPW at higher laser pulse numbers and relatively low input power. Also, the contact angle measurements confirmed the surface free energy of polyurethane has increased from 28 mNm^{-1} to 50 mNm^{-1} after 8 pulses at 0.1 W using CPW mode. This corresponds to an increase of $\approx 56\%$ bioadhesivity, which is a considerable improvement for the purpose of cell attachment. Although SPW produced a narrower zone of thermal degradation, surface free energy of polymer was found to be weaker than CPW mode.

As discussed above, the biomaterials are used in contact with living tissue, so there ought to exist an unavoidable interaction between the material and the tissue. The nature of this interaction, however, determines the degree of biocompatibility of the material with the biological environment in which it is used. A variety of biopolymers have been used for different clinical applications (Bruck 1977, Arenholz et al. 1993). Among them is the use of segmented polyurethane elastomers due to its favourable characteristics and widely varying physical and chemical properties (Lyman et al. 1977, Boretos 1980). A well controlled modification of such materials have been studied, which in general can lead to either a smooth blood contacting surface or a relatively rough surface. In the former case, thrombotic events that can cause deposition, attachment, and organized thrombus growth can be avoided. In the latter case, in contrast, cell adhesion is involved in various natural phenomena such as embryogenesis, maintenance of tissue structure, wound healing, immune response, metastasis, as well as tissue interaction of biomaterial (Grabowski and Didisheim 1977, Wurzberg and Buchman 1990).

The ester-based polyurethane samples with commercial trade mark of Laripur®-7025 were used in film form of 400 thick supplied by Iran Polymer Institute (IPI). A 30W CO_2 laser (SM medical) with 10 ms pulse duration in two modes of chop-wave (CPW) and super pulse wave (SPW). The surface properties of polyurethane before and after laser treatment was studied using ATR-FTIR (Nicolet-Nexus 670) technique, where the sample was brought in to contact with a KRS-5 crystal surface and infrared radiation reflected internally across the surface. The contact angle as a function of time was measured using Ownes-Wendt-Rabel and Kaelble method and Kruss-G 40 model instrument. The test liquids consisted of water (Busscher) and Diiodo-Methane (Busscher) with surface free tension of 72.1 mNm^{-1} and 50 mNm^{-1}, respectively. Since in these experiments the spot size is larger than the heated depth, therefore the characteristic time-scale for cooling of the heated surface by conduction into the bulk of the polymer is assumed one dimensional heat flow approximation. By using the Eq. (8.3), one can determine as to when the polymer begins to vaporize

$$t_v = \frac{\pi}{4D_t}\left[\frac{KT_v}{I}\right] \tag{8.3}$$

where t_v and T_v are the vaporization time and vaporization temperature, respectively, and K is thermal conductivity of material. Assuming the average thermal diffusivity is $< D_t > \approx 7.5 \times 10^{-3}$ cm² s⁻¹ and $T_v \approx 513$ K, it yields $t_v \approx 8.5$ ms at P = 0.4 W, which is just below $\tau_p = 10$ ms. This implies that at power levels higher than 0.4 W, one may expect some thermal damage, as in Fig. 8.11. Figure 8.8 shows the ATR-FTIR spectra of untreated and treated Laripur®-7025 aromatic polyurethane. The most abundant molecular bonds correspond to C = O and C-O-C at wave numbers of 1724 cm⁻¹ and 1167 cm⁻¹. However, after laser treatment with both CPW and SPW modes, the intensity of spectral line (i.e., population) at 1530 cm⁻¹ which corresponds to bending δ (N-H) and stretching ν (C-N) bond is reduced considerably,

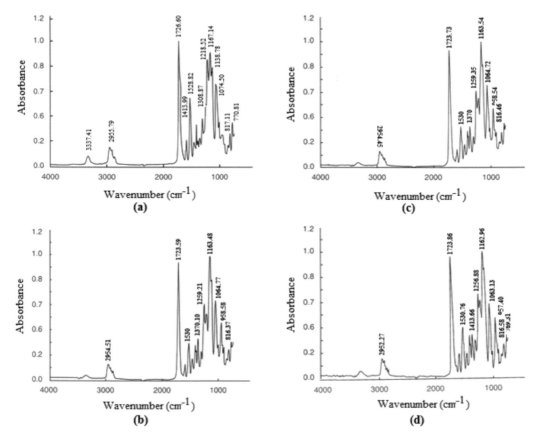

Figure 8.8. ATR-FTIR spectrum of Laripur®-7025 polyurethane: (a) control, (b) 1 SPW at 0.1 W, (C) 1 CPW at 0.1 W, (d) 12 CPW at 0.1 W.

compared to control sample, as seen in Fig. 8.8a. Also, four noticeable peaks at 1463, 1370, 1259, and 958 cm⁻¹ are generated after the laser treatment. It is believed that the increased hydrogen bonding of the urethane occurs when the interfacial region narrows, i.e., when the surface of polyurethane is approached. The resultant hydrogen bonding and chain packing are characteristic of hard-domain crystallization which is seen with highly heat treated polyurethane elastomers.

An analysis of experimental data in Fig. 8.9 indicates that water contact angle decreases from 95 to below 75 after 7 laser pulses, and it increases again up to 87 after 12 pulses. This corresponds to an increase of surface free energy from 28 mNm⁻¹ to 50 mNm⁻¹ after 8 pulses, and a drop of about 15 mNm⁻¹ during subsequent irradiation. The overall results confirm a definite improvement in bioadhesivity.

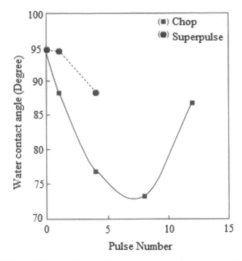

Figure 8.9. Plot of water contact angles as a function of pulse number for CPW and SPW at 0.1 W.

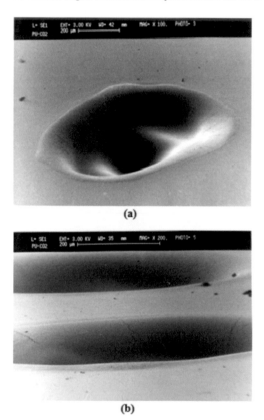

Figure 8.10. Polyurethane surface treated by (a) SPW and (b) CPW at 0.1 W after 12 pulses.

At higher pulse numbers but constant power level (0.1 W) both modes produced a relatively smooth wall craters, as seen in Figs. 8.10a,b. It is also evident from Figs. 8.11a,b that as the power input to the surface of polymer gradually increases, the interaction becomes more rigorous, thus causing the formation of unclean edges due to thermal degradation.

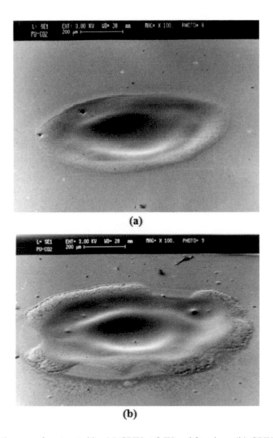

Figure 8.11. Polyurethane surface treated by (a) CPW at 3 W and 2 pulses, (b) CPW at 10 W and 1 pulse.

8.3.3 Photopolymerization of dental resin as restorative material using an argon laser
(Khosroshahi et al. 2008)

The effect of the 488-nm wavelength of argon laser at different power densities and irradiation times on the degree of conversion (DC), temperature rise, water sorption, solubility, flexural strength, flexural modulus, and microhardness of bisphenole A-glycol dimethacrylate and triethylen glycol dimethacrylate with a mass ratio of 75:25 was studied. Camphorquinone and N,N'-dimethyl aminoethyl methacrylate were added to the monomer as a photo initiator system. The DC% of the resin was measured using Fourier transform infrared spectroscopy. The maximum DC% (50%), which was reached in 20 s, and temperature rise because of the reaction (13.5°C) were both higher at 1075 than 700 mWcm^{-2}. Water sorption and solubility were measured according to ISO4049, which in our case were 23.7 and 2.20 µg/mm^3 at 1075 mWcm^{-2}, respectively. A flexural modulus of 1.1 GPa and microhardness of 19.6 kg/mm^2 were achieved above the power density. No significant difference was observed (i.e., $p > 0.05$) for water sorption and flexural strength at 700 and 1075 mWcm^{-2}.

The standard materials used as dental cavity fillings include amalgams, metals, and dental ceramics; however, patients regard most of them as far from being aesthetically attractive, and the use of amalgams is especially harmful because of the presence of mercury. The composite materials containing dimethacrylate monomers are widely used as dental bonding agents, luting agents, restorative dental composites, and fissure sealants simply because of their superior aesthetic and physicomechanical properties (Sideridou et al. 2002). In general, there are two categories of light-induced polymerization systems: UV and visible light, with the latter being safer, i.e., biocompatible and easier to use. Light-cured dental composites are composed of organic monomers, inorganic fillers, a photosensitizer, and a coinitiator. The photosensitizer is one of the most important additions because it initiates the photopolymerization of the resin composite.

One such example is the use of Camphorquinone (CQ) as a diketon photoinitiator, which when exposed to light of correct wavelength and power density, initiates the generation of free radicals that precipitate the polymerization, and finally leads to set material; the possible light source can be improved light-emitting diodes (Mills and Jandt 1998), quartz–tungsten halogen (QTH) (Deb and Sehmi 2003), Xenon-plasma arc, plasma arc curing (PAC) (Peutzfeld et al. 2000, Fano et al. 2002), and argon laser (Powell and Blankenau 1994). All the conventional light sources suffer from serious limitation to induce the so called ideal photoinitiation, such as short lifetime, inadequate energy variability, degradation of lamps, filters, and reflectors with time, broad spectral bandwidth, i.e., polychromatic, fixed high threshold power densities, and incoherency.

On the other hand, the argon laser appeared as a suitable alternative polymerization source of composite resins, particularly for CQ, whose activation is initiated by a hue of blue light covering the range of 400–500 nm with broad peaks at about 468 and 480 nm, depending on the type of diluent (Kelsey et al. 1989, Cassoni et al. 2005). Furthermore, lasers such as argon laser with its inherent optical characteristics like low beam divergence, monochoromacity, collimation, coherency, absorption selectivity because of wavelength tunability, and fiber delivery capability can all make it to be practically a better candidate, which effectively can reduce curing time, provide a larger degree of conversion (DC) of monomers, and enhance physical properties of cured composites (Fleming and Mailet 1999, Conrado et al. 2004). The advantages of Bis-GMA over other small-sized monomers like methyl methacrylate, include less shrinkage, higher modulus, and reduced toxicity because of its lower volatility and diffusivity into the tissue. Furthermore, TEGDMA is added to Bis-GMA to achieve workable viscosity limits because the latter monomer possess very high viscosity because of the intermolecular hydrogen bonding (Sankarapandian and Shobha 1997).

The mass ratio of the mixture was 75:25, supplied by Rohm. This composition is similar to that used in commercial dental resin formulation. The initiator used in this experiment was the visible light-initiating system of CQ (0.5 wt%) and N,N'-dimethyl aminoethyl methacrylate (DMAEMA, 0.5 wt%) were supplied by Fluka. In this experiment 0.5% CQ was used as a photoinitiator for the optimization of the DC. The DC of resins is a major factor influencing their bulk physical properties. In general, the higher the conversion of double bonds, the greater the mechanical strength. The measurement of DC depends on several factors, such as the light source, the light wavelength, the power density, and the resin composition. Thermal effects are also important when characterizing the polymerization behaviour of resins. It is well known that water is absorbed predominantly within the matrix resin, and is most affected by the structure and the amount of this phase. Thus, the study of the water sorption (WS) and solubility (SL) of dimethacrylate resins made from monomers is important in understanding their behaviour in the composite.

The FTIR spectra of uncured and cured specimens with 1075 and 700 mWcm^{-2} with a frequency range of between 1680 and 1580 cm^{-1} are shown in Fig. 8.12. The absorbance peak at 1638 cm^{-1} refers to the aliphatic C = C stretching of the vinyl group, which in fact can be used to quantify the methacrylate double-bond conversion, and the peak at 1608 cm^{-1} assigned to the aromatic C–C bond was used an internal standard. Thus, the decrease in absorbance intensities of bonds and the area peak to peak under the curve effectively indicates the amount of double bond consumed during polymerization.

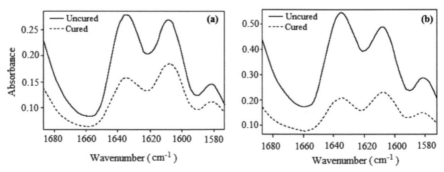

Figure 8.12. (a,b) FTIR spectra of uncured and cured specimens with 1075 and 700 mWcm^{-2}, respectively with a frequency range between 1680 and 1580 cm^{-1}.

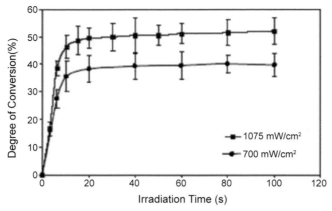

Figure 8.13. Percent degree of conversion vs. irradiation time for cured specimens with different power densities.

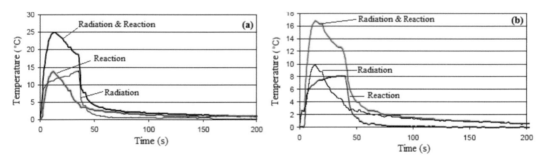

Figure 8.14. Temperature rise vs. time for the specimens. (a) The total maximum temperature produced during the curing process was 25°C at 1075 mWcm⁻², (b) The total maximum rise was about 16°C at 700 mWcm⁻².

As is seen in Fig. 8.12, the DC% reaches its maximum after 20 s, which for 1075 and 700 mWcm⁻² corresponds to about 50 and 38%, respectively. These values remained almost constant over a further irradiation time of 100 s.

The next step vital in any polymerization experiment is to monitor the temperature change during the process. In our case, this was done by following the kinetic behaviour of the process, as it was taking place. As is seen in Fig. 8.14a, the total maximum temperature produced during the curing process was higher at 1075 (25°C) than 700 mWcm⁻² (16°C). Furthermore, because the polymerization is an exothermic reaction, the temperature rise is related to the number of carbon double bonds that react, and thus it is related to the DC% of the dental resin. It is seen in Fig. 8.14a that the completion time for the gel process is after 13 s of irradiation and that the maximum temperature rise because of the reaction is only about 13.5°C. While in the case of 700 mWcm⁻², as seen in Fig. 8.14b, the total maximum rise is about 16°C with 8°C due to the reaction heat only. The maximum temperature rise obained in our work for both mid- and high-power densities were less than the other investigators results reported for the similar material but using different non-laser light sources (Fano et al. 2002, Emami et al. 2003).

Other important parameters affecting the physico-mechanical properties of resin are WS and SL. A rapid increase in WS during the first 3 days was observed, after which the curve reached its plateau. There onwards, both curves remained constant to about 500 h. There is no significant difference ($p > 0.05$) between WS of specimens cured with 1075 (23.7 µg/m³) and 700 mWcm⁻² (25.8 µg/m³). The corresponding values of SL for both power densities are shown in Fig. 8.15. As is seen, a lower value of 2.20 µg/m³ was achieved at 1075 mWcm⁻² compared to 3.40 µg/m³ at 700 mWcm⁻². This can be explained by the fact that the value of SL mainly depends on the DC%, where the higher the DC%, the lower the amount of

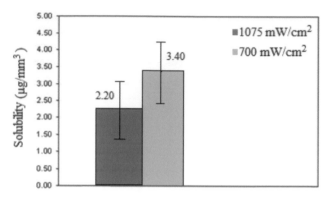

Figure 8.15. The corresponding values of SL for both power densities.

the unreacted monomer and hence the lower the SL value. According to the ISO 9000 standard for dental restorative resins, a resin can be regarded as suitable for clinical applications if they have a WS value lower than 50 $\mu g/m^3$ and SL lower than 5 $\mu g/m^3$.

Knowing that the viscosity is a measure of the resistance of molecules to flow and a high viscosity value is indicative of the presence of intermolecular interactions, therefore, these interactions can cause a decreased mobility of monomer molecules during photopolymerization and also a decreased flexibility of the corresponding polymeric network. As a result of the above argument, a low DC% may give inadequate wear resistance and low bonding stability to the tooth surface, which in effect results in a clinical problem such as marginal shrinkage. Furthermore, our findings from kinetic studies of thermal reaction indicate that by increasing the intensity level, an increase in total temperature rise can be obtained, which is partly due to radiation and partly due to the reaction. Therefore, increasing the intensity and hence the cure temperature can improve the mobility of the reacting media and rate of network formation. Both of these factors can contribute to enhance the polymerization rate observed at evaluated temperatures. According to Fick's law, the equation for diffusion in one dimension (x), i.e., thickness of the specimen when the diffusion coefficient D is constant, is expressed as:

$$\frac{\partial C}{\partial t} = D \frac{\partial^2 C}{\partial x^2} \tag{8.4}$$

where C denotes the concentration of the diffusion species at time t, which in fact is equal to M_t/M_∞, where M_t and M_∞ are the mass of water sorbed (or desorbed) at times t and ∞, respectively. Initially, all the molecules are at the origin at t = 0. As time goes on, the molecules diffuse away from x = 0, while executing their random walks, as t $\rightarrow$ ∞, the concentration approaches zero for all the values of x. The general solution of Eq. 8.5 under consideration is

$$C = \frac{1}{(4\pi Dt)^{1/2}} \cdot e^{-x^2/4Dt} \tag{8.5}$$

Accordingly, for small times when Mt/M∞ is small enough, Eq. 8.6 reduces to a simple well-known Stefan's approximation, i.e.,

$$\frac{M_t}{M_\infty} = \frac{2Dt}{x^2} \tag{8.6}$$

Using the experimental data of x = 2 × 10^{-3}, t = 80 h and D = 3.45 × 10^{-12} m^2 s^{-1} for Bis GMA+TEGDMA mixture (Kalachandra and Kusy 1991), it gives $M_t/M_\infty \approx 0.49$. This is indicative of the fact that the uptake process is diffusion controlled and that it follows the Fickian diffusion until C << 0.5.

8.3.4 *In vitro and in vivo studies of osteoblast cell response to titanium alloy (Ti6Al4V) surface modified by Nd:YAG laser and silicon paper* (Khosroshahi et al. 2009)

The effects of neodymium:yttrium–aluminium–garnet (Nd:YAG) laser and silicon carbide (SiC) paper on the surface micro-topography of titanium-6 aluminium-4 vanadium (Ti6Al4V) alloy were examined in relation to the response of bone cells. The study was performed in three distinct stages: (1) after surface treatment of samples by laser and SiC paper, the surface hardness, surface roughness, corrosion resistance and surface tension were evaluated; (2) the growth of mouse connective tissue fibroblast cells (L-929) on untreated and treated samples was assessed *in vitro*; (3) the response of goat osteoblast cells to untreated and treated implanted samples was assessed *in vivo*. The surface roughness varied between 7 ± 0.02 for laser-treated samples (LTSs) at 140 Jcm^{-2} and 21.8 ± 0.05 for mechanically treated samples (MTSs). The surface hardness was found to vary from 377 Vickers hardness number (VHN) for MTSs to 850 VHN for LTSs. A corrosion potential of -0.21 V was achieved for the LTSs, compared to -0.51 V for the MTSs. The LTSs exhibited a more hydrophilic behaviour (i.e., wettability) than did the MTSs. No cytotoxicity effect, unlike for the MTSs, was observed for the LTSs. The results of *in vivo* tests indicated longitudinal growth of osteoblast cells along the grooves on the samples formed by the SiC paper, and multidirectional spreading of the cells on the LTSs. It is believed that the oxygen content of a material's surface can contribute to the improvement of its wettability characteristics in laser surface modification.

It is generally believed that proteins adsorbed on implant surfaces can play an important role in cell–surface response. Different proteins, such as collagen, fibronectin and vitronectin, which act as ligands, are particularly important in osteoblast interaction with surfaces. Interface reactions between metallic implants and the surrounding tissues play a crucial role in the success of osseointegration. Titanium and its alloys, like some other medical grade metals, are the materials of choice for long-term implants. The effect of implant surface characteristics on bone reactions has thus attracted much attention and is still considered to be an important issue (Albrektsson and Johansson 2001, Buchter et al. 2005). Fibroblasts are spindle shaped or fusiform cells and are responsible for the production of collagen and reticular and elastic fibres. Osteoblasts can be in two states: (a) active, forming bone matrix; (b) resting or bone-maintaining. These make collagen, glycoproteins and proteoglycans of bone the matrix and control the deposition of mineral crystals on the fibrils. An osteoblast becomes an osteocyte by forming a matrix around itself and is buried. Lacunae void of osteocytes indicate dead bone. The osteoclast, a large and multinucleated cell, with a pale acidophilic cytoplasm, lies on the surface of bone, often in an eaten-out hollow Howship's lacuna. Macrophages are irregularly shaped cells that participate in phagocytosis. So far as the surface characteristics of the implants are concerned, two main features that can influence the establishment of osseo-integration are the physico-chemical properties and the surface morphology. Cell behaviour, such as adhesion, morphologic change, and functional alteration, are greatly influenced by surface properties, including texture, roughness, hydrophilicity, and morphology. In extensive investigations of tissue response to implant surfaces, it has been shown that surface treatment of implant materials significantly influences the attachment of cells (Curtis and Wilkinson 1998, Brunette and Cheroudi 1999). Additionally, these modified surfaces must resist both mechanical wear and corrosion (Sighvi and Wang 1998). It is therefore important to evaluate systematically the role of different surface properties and to assess the biological performance of different implant materials.

Sample preparation

Rectangular specimens 20 mm × 10 mm and 2 mm thick, were made from medical grade titanium-6 aluminium-4 vanadium (Ti6Al4V) alloy [American Society for Testing and Materials (ASTM) F136, Friadent, Mannheim, Germany] with the chemical formulation Ti (91.63%) Al (5.12%) V (3.25%). The samples were divided into three groups: untreated (seven samples), laser treated (14 samples), and the last group was gradually wet ground with 300 grit and 800 grit silicon carbide (SiC) papers (14 samples). Prior to treatment, all samples were cleaned with 97% ethanol and subsequently washed twice with distilled water in an ultrasonic bath (Matachana, Barcelona, Spain). They were finally rinsed in deionized water at neutral pH so that a clean surface was obtained. Lastly, an optical microscope with a × 20 magnification was used to ensure that no particles were left on the sample surface.

In vivo tests

Anaesthetization

Before depilation of the operation site, the animal was completely anaesthetized with midazolam (Dormicum®, Roche, Switzerland) 2.5 mg/kg intravenously. If there were any signs of recovery during the operation, the animal was injected slowly with diluted fluanisone/fentanyl (Hypnorm®, India) until adequate effect was achieved, usually 0.2 ml at a time.

Animal implantation

One untreated sample, two MTSs, and two LTSs were implanted on to the femur bone of an 8-months-old male goat weighing 30 kg. Specimens were steam sterilized, before implantation, in an autoclave (Matachana) at 132°C, 2 bar, for 45 min. All the specimens were labelled with separate codes for further studies. The operation site was depilated with soft soap and ethanol before surgery; it was also disinfected with 70% ethanol and covered with a sterile blanket. In order to proceed with implantation, we scraped cortex bone with an osteotome (Matachana) after cutting the limb one-third from the end laterally and elevating it with a self-retaining retractor. Copious irrigation with physiological saline solution was used during the implantation to prevent overheating. To ensure the stable passive fixation of implants during the healing period, we stabilized them with size 4 and size 8 titanium wires (Atila ortoped®, Tehran, Iran) without any external compression forces (Fig. 8.16).

After the operation the animal was protected from infection by the appropriate prescribed uptake of penicillin for the first 4 days and gentamicin for a further 4 days. During the 8 days of recovery, the goat was given multivitamins to help it regain its strength. During this period, the goat was kept in an isolated space at room temperature, under normal humidity, lighting and air conditions, and, before it was returned to its natural environment, radiographs (Fig. 8.17) were taken in order to ensure that the implant had not

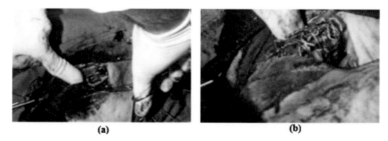

(a)   **(b)**

Figure 8.16. Placement of implants in the femur bone of the goat.

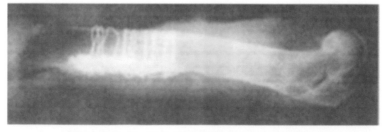

Figure 8.17. The X-ray of the implants wired to the bone.

been displaced during the maintenance period. It was observed that callus bone had grown in the vicinity of the implant.

After 5 months the animal was sacrificed and the implants were removed for further analysis in accordance with the Animal Welfare Act of 20 December 1974 and the Protocol and Regulation on Animal Experimentation of 15 January 1996, approved by the Yazd School of Veterinary Science (Iran) and its animal research authority, as seen in Fig. 8.18.

Histopathology

Surrounding tissues of specimens were retrieved and prepared for histological examination. They were fixed in 4% formalin solution (pH 7.3), dehydrated in a graded series of ethanol (10%, 30%, 50%, 70%, and 90%) and embedded in paraffin after decalcification. Then, 10 µm thick slices were prepared per specimen by a sawing microtome technique. A qualitative evaluation of macrophages, osteoblasts, osteoclasts, polymorphonuclear leukocytes (PMNs), giant cells, fibroblasts, and lymphocytes was carried out by haematoxylin and eosin staining and light microscopy (Zeiss, Gottingen, Germany).

Figure 8.19 indicates the variation of Ti6Al4V surface temperature as a function of laser fluence. Now, if we consider the melting and vaporization points of Ti6Al4V as 1,668°C, and 3,280°C, respectively, and the threshold fluence of ablation as approximately 70 J cm^{-2}, then it would be sensible to choose zone II as the treatment region (i.e., below ablation).

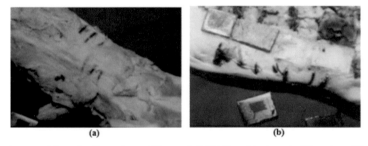

(a)   (b)

Figure 8.18. Implant removal from the femur bone of the goat. (a) Before detachment of the wires, (b) the footprint of the implants on the bone.

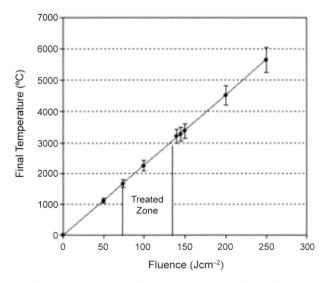

Figure 8.19. Variation of surface temperature with laser fluence.

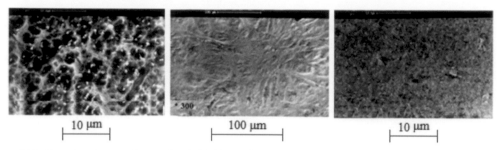

⊢ 10 μm ⊣   ⊢ 100 μm ⊣   ⊢ 10 μm ⊣

Figure 8.20. Scanning electron micrographs of Ti6Al4V surface morphology for (a) untreated and (b) laser-treated samples at 90 J cm^{-2} and (c) at 140 J cm^{-2}, indicating the disappearing of surface scratches by laser surface melting.

Figure 8.20 shows the comparison between three morphologically different areas, i.e., untreated (a) and laser treated at 90 Jcm^{-2}, (b) characterized by random fluctuating dendritic features and 140 Jcm^{-2}, (c) where the inclusions have gradually disappeared and that the scratches from the machining and polishing have been sealed by direct laser surface heating. Ti6Al4V alloy is a ($\alpha + \beta$) two-phase alloy with approximately 6 wt% aluminium stabilizing the α phase and about 4 wt% vanadium stabilizing the β phase. At room temperature, the microstructure at equilibrium consists mainly of primary α phase [hexagonal close-packed (hcp)] with some retained β phase [body-centred cubic (bcc)]. It is also well known that in laser surface melting, steep temperature gradient and thermal cycle lead to some microstructural changes in the heat-affected zone within a very short time, in particular, the $\alpha \rightarrow \beta$ phase transformation during rapid heating and decomposition of the β phase during rapid cooling. The physical and mechanical properties of Ti6Al4V alloy are known to be sensitive to its microstructure. The Ti-β phase has a diffusivity of two orders of magnitude higher than the Ti-α phase, and flow stress is strongly influenced by the ratio of these phases.

The surface hardness measurements presented in Fig. 8.21 clearly indicate that microhardness of the metal increases with laser fluence. Again, a non-linear behaviour was observed, where initially the values of VHN were increased gradually up to approximately 100 J cm^{-2}. Afterwards, there was a sharp increase until a plateau was reached at 140 J cm^{-2}, which corresponds to a roughly 50% improvement in surface hardness. The surface hardness was found to vary from 377 VHN for MTSs to 850 VHN for LTSs.

Change in surface wettability was studied by contact angle measurement for all the specimens (Fig. 8.22). A smoother surface was achieved by laser radiation at 140 J cm^{-2}, which means a reduction in contact angle. This effectively implies an increase in degree of wettability of the metal surface. According to the topology of the primary melting centres, the surface roughness had increased slightly at 100 J cm^{-2}

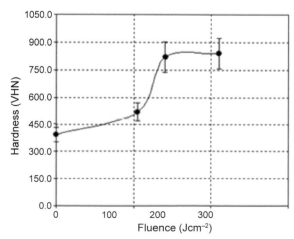

Figure 8.21. Variation of surface hardness with fluence.

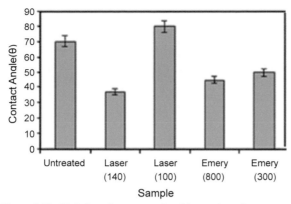

Figure 8.22. Variation of contact angle with sample surface texture.

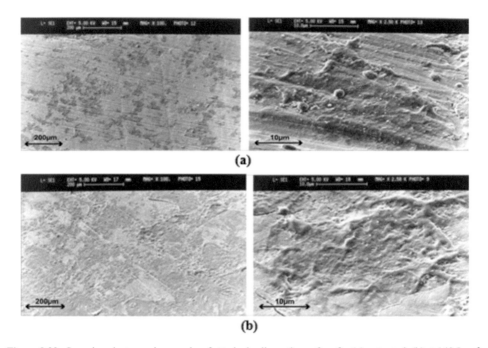

Figure 8.23. Scanning electron micrographs of attached cells on the surface for (a) untreated, (b) at 140 Jcm^{-2}.

(Ra = 14.2 ± 0.29). Thus, an increase in contact angle occurs from 70° to 80°, indicating a lower degree of wettability. Following the laser treatment at 140 J cm^{-2}, the contact angle decreased to 37°, still showing a more acceptable hydrophilic behaviour. Owing to the effects of fine (800 grit) and coarse (300 grit) emery on the surface, the measured contact angle increased from 45° to 50°, respectively.

The SEM analysis of attached cells' morphology (Fig. 8.23) indicated that the density of the cell network is directly dependent on the laser beam fluence and surface topography. The smooth surface produced at 140 J cm^{-2} not only caused a dense cell network but also resulted in a wider area covered by a single cell spreading. The density of the network is due to the change from monolayer attachment (cell–surface) to multilayer attachment (cell–surface and cell–cell). As was seen, no specific directional spread of attached cells was achieved in the laser-treated specimens. However, on the emery-treated surfaces, the orientation of cells was longitudinal and parallel to the lines made by the SiC paper.

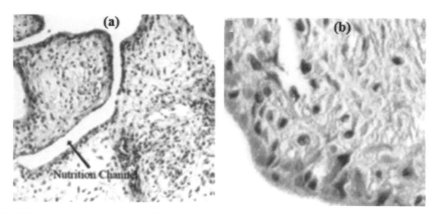

Figure 8.24. Light microscopy evaluation of bone tissue for (a) laser treated sample at 140 J cm⁻², with a nutrition channel shown, and (b) untreated sample without the channel.

Table 8.2. Qualitative evaluation of histology: results of bone tissue around the implants.

Sample	100 J cm^{-2}	140 J cm^{-2}	Emery 800 grit	Emery 300 grit	Untreated
Cells					
Fibroblast	+++	+++	++	++	++
Osteoblast	++	+++	+	++	+
Giant cell	−	−	−	−	−
Osteoclast	−	−	−	−	+
PMN	+	−	−	−	+
Lymphocyte	+++	++	++	++	++
Macrophage	+++	++	+++	+++	++
Healing	+	++	+	+	+

When the implants were retrieved, no inflammatory reaction was observed inside or around the implants. Mineralized matrix deposition and bone cells were observed on the surface of implants, which were formed during the 5 months of implantation. This deposition was found all around the LTS and MTS, and bone formation was characterized by the occurrence of osteocyte embedded in the matrix. Also, the above samples were surrounded by fibroblast and osteoblast cells, and the untreated sample showed not only fewer fibroblast cells, but it also contained osteoclasts and polymorphonuclear leukocytes (PMNs). As can be seen in Fig. 8.24, bone tissue nutrition is carried out through the channel in the LTS, whereas this was not mentioned implant, rather than in all the other evaluated specimens. Fibroblast and osteoblast cells were also numerous at 140 J cm⁻². In Table 8.2, the symbols indicate the presence of cells (+), high (++), very high (+++) and lack of cells (−), respectively.

8.3.5 *Experimental study and modeling of polytetrafluoroethylene (PTFE) and hydroxyapatite biocomposite surface treatment using selective laser sintering* (Khosroshahi et al. 2016)

The selective laser sintering (SLS) is a rapid prototyping (RP) process which uses laser surface treatment to produce consolidation of powder materials. To obtain an efficient SLS, the optical parameters such as laser power, scanning velocity as well as the material properties must be optimized. In this experiment, the SLS of biocomposite of Hydroxyapatite (HA) and poly(tetrafluoroethylene) (PTFE) as secondary polymeric binder is investigated. Microstructural assessments of the samples were conducted using scanning electron microscopy (SEM). To study the effect of laser power on the strength of specimens, pressure test were carried out. Depth of sintering layer and its correlation with laser power numerically is explored. In our case, the best sintering condition was achieved at 3 W and 1 mm/s.

Rapid prototyping (RP) which uses a laser as a heat source to sinter parts is an advanced manufacturing technology commercialized in the middle of 1980s. These methods have great effect in the shorten of design-manufacturing cycle time, therefore reducing the cost of production and increasing competitiveness

(Gibson and Shi 1997, Wiria et al. 2010). SLS is a powder based RP technique where data is created by computer aided design (CAD) from a solid modelling environment to generate 3-D physical objects. RP systems process CAD data by mathematically slicing the computer model of final desired object into thin even layers. During SLS operation, the laser beam is selectively scanned over the powder surface following the cross sectional profiles carried by the slice data. The interaction of the laser beam with the powder increases the powder temperature to melting point and causes the particles to bind together to form a solid mass. Subsequently, the new layers are built directly on top of previously sintered layer (Tan et al. 2003). The importance of SLS is mainly because of its real potential in the production of complex 3-D objects and broad range of material to be used. Generally, it is believed that any material that can be densified by traditional sintering techniques can be processed by SLS. Advantages of SLS over other rapid prototyping methods include high degree of controllability, the use of inexpensive and safe materials with a wide variety form polymers to metals, and no need to support the parts during the fabrication process (Tan et al. 2003, Hu et al. 2002). Interestingly, SLS process have been widely investigated in the biomedical engineering where it enables production of scaffolds in different size and shape (Lima et al. 2014, Chen et al. 2014, Tampieir et al. 1997). One such example is the increasing tendency in the use of polymeric material in SLS operation as substrate with metallic or ceramic materials (Suman 2008, Eosoly et al. 2010). This is due to their low melting temperature, melting flow control, increase of composite toughness, and low rate of degradation as a bioimplant. Polymers, in comparison to metals and ceramics, have much less strength, but their strength will enhance through blending with metals and ceramics. In an investigation (Duan et al. 2010), a bone was used as a model material to described the potential of SLS in fabricating nanocomposite scaffolds for bone tissue engineering. It was found that the mechanical properties of both the polymer and nanocomposite scaffolds decreased gradually after their immersion in PBS at 37°C.

For sintering operation, a 30W CW CO_2 laser (SM MEDICAL Captain 30) with a Gaussian output beam distribution and wavelength of 10.6 μm was used to irradiate the samples. The beam was focused by a 100 mm hand piece manipulator to a desirable spot size. HA has a high absorption coefficient at this wavelength. A home-built XY scanning unit which was used for 1-D and 2-D SLS. For a complete description of SLS process, distribution of heat generated by laser incidence must be taken into account which requires the modelling of laser-material interaction. By assuming a Gaussian laser beam, the laser beam intensity relation is

$$I(r,w) = I_0 e^{-\frac{2r^2}{w^2}} = \frac{2P}{\pi w^2} e^{-\frac{2r^2}{w^2}} \tag{8.7}$$

where I_0 is the initial intensity, r is the radial distance up to centre of beam, w is the radius of laser beam, and P is the laser power which can be approximately calculated by the following equation:

$$\frac{v \times \rho \times D \times h \times [C_p \times (T_m - T_b) + I_f]}{(1-R)} \tag{8.8}$$

where D is the diameter of laser beam on the part bed, T_m is the melting temperature, T_b is the part bed temperature, If is the latent melting heat, and R is the reflectivity fraction of laser beam reflected by the powder surface. Laser fluence is directly proportional to laser power and inversely proportional to scanning velocity (Yagi and Kunii 1957)

$$Fluence = \frac{P \times f}{v \times \gamma} \tag{8.9}$$

where f is the conversion factor and γ is the scanning distance which should not exceed the diameter of laser beam diameter on the sample surface. To model thermal binding of polymer powder grains, analysis of physical characteristics of composite powder is required. The details can of modelling can be found from the paper. A mixture of PTFE/HA was produced by physically blending pure PTFE and HA powders with 20 wt% HA content filled in a mould with 5 × 5 × 1 mm dimension. As PTFE is a bioinert material, the addition of HA particles will improve the bioactivity of the composite. In this study scanning space is 1.3 mm. The surface of samples were studied after treatment for change of texture, discoloring, and possible melting using the optical microscopy. Finer studies of SLS-fabricated parts were carried out using scanning electron microscopy (SEM), LEO 440i, to characterize the individual parts and to analysis the surface morphology and microstructure of the sintered specimens. For analysing the effect of laser power on the strength of specimens, pressure test was carried out. A finite element was used to study the optimal processing parameters for SLS, here the parts are modelled as porous. Strength analysis of samples demonstrated a relation between the strength of SLS built parts, laser power and scanning velocity. Compressive strength is calculated by dividing the maximum load by the original cross-sectional area of a specimen. Surface treatment of samples was accompanied by a color change as they altered from white to brown, as seen in Fig. 8.25. The color change was more significant at lower scanning velocity and higher laser power. However, as power increased, the size of material porosity and its distribution on the surface was significantly decreased. This can be explained by the fact that at higher powers, one expects higher temperatures followed by subsequent PTFE melting which in effect covers the porosities.

Figure 8.26 illustrates the micrograph of a sample processed at 3 W, 2 mms^{-1} velocity, and scanning space of 1.3 mm. For this sample the laser spot diameter was 2 mm and its distance from the arm tip focal point was 100 mm. As it can be seen, PTFE particles are melted and the liquid phase was rapidly cooled and the molten material bound together on the surface. The irregular and brighter particles in the microstructures are HA particles which did not exhibit any change in their shape due to their higher melting point. As it is seen at higher laser power, PTFE particles receives more heat which quickly increases its temperature and this in turn causes the viscosity of liquid phase to decrease hence the coalescence of particles is enhanced leading to less porosity compared to that with lower power (2 W).

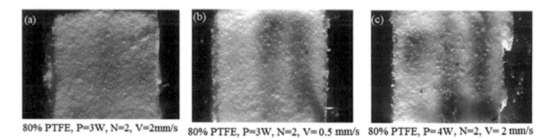

80% PTFE, P=3W, N=2, V=2mm/s   80% PTFE, P=3W, N=2, V=0.5 mm/s   80% PTFE, P=4W, N=2, V= 2 mm/s

Figure 8.25. Optical microscopy of composite surface with 20% HA and 80% PTFE, (a) 3 W, N = 2, V = 2 mm s^{-1}, (b) 3 W, N = 2, V = 0.5 mm s^{-1}, (c) 4 W, N = 2, V = 2 mm s^{-1}.

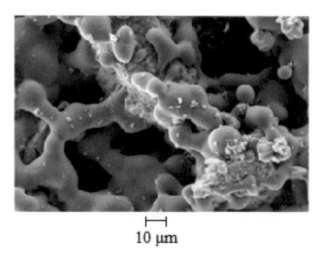

10 μm

Figure 8.26. SEM microstructure of 20% HA and 80% PTFE composite, 3 W, N = 2, V = 2 mm s^{-1} at 600x magnification.

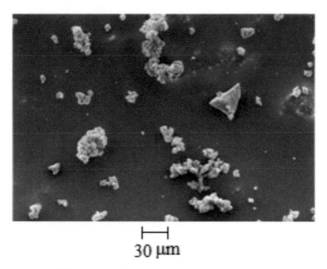

Figure 8.27. SEM microstructure of 20% HA and 80% PTFE composite at 4 W, N = 2, V = 2 mm s⁻¹ at 600x magnification.

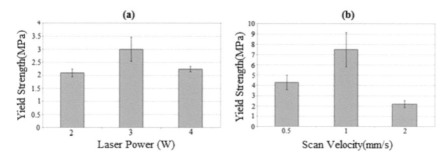

Figure 8.28. Variation of sample yield strength with (a) laser power, N = 2 and (b) scan velocity, N = 2.

Figure 8.27 indicates the microstructure of sample irradiated even higher laser power of 4 W. The SEM micrographs clearly reveals that the porous space is filled more evenly and smoothly, compared to Fig. 8.25. A very smooth surface was produced and the HA particles are completely surrounded by the PTFE pool. This again can be explained on the account of higher temperature gradient which melts greater amount of powder at the surface and depth of sample.

Figure 8.28a indicates the variation of tensile strength with laser power. As it is shown, the strength initially increases with increasing the laser power where it reaches its maximum value of 3 MPa at 3 W. However, beyond this value, the strength decreases to just above 2 MPa at 4 W. In other words, it seems that there is an optimum value of laser power for powder sintering or bonding. Similarly, the tensile strength increases with scan velocity from 4 MPa to maximum value of 8 MPa which from there onwards it declines at higher velocity where it drops to 2 MPa at 3 mm/s, Fig. 8.28b. Low powers or high scan velocity will prevent the powder particles from reaching to a thermal reaction and a required thermal diffusion which effectively implies an untreated area with raw composition hence low yield strength. The maximum difference in the yield strength in Fig. 8.28a is 18%, in comparison to 59% of Fig. 8.28b.

The sintering depth of the composite powder versus time and temperature is illustrated in Fig. 8.29. This diagram shows that at the moment of laser irradiation of the sample surface, it raises its temperature from room temperature to about 350°C, which can easily cause a phase transition from solid to liquid. When the same position is scanned for number of times, the temperature increased to 358°C, which can thermally degrade PTFE. The temperature distribution shows anisotropic porosity and the thermal load

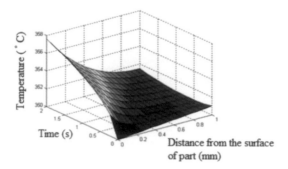

Figure 8.29. Distribution of laser-induced temperature in samples during irradiation.

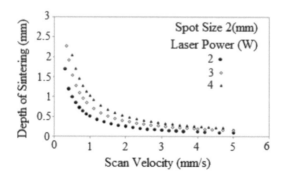

Figure 8.30. Variation of depth of laser sintering with scan velocity and laser power.

vectors is therefore, acting non-uniformly throughout the sample. Because the upper layers absorb more photons, consequently, it produces more heat compared with the lower layers, therefore, the particles are expected to be loosely bound with more porous space between them.

Correlation between the scan velocity and depth of sintering as well as laser power is displayed in Fig. 8.30. It is evident that scanning at constant velocity using higher laser power causes higher degree of sintering, while at constant laser power, the degree of sintering decreases with increase in scan velocity. Thus, based on Figs. 8.28a and 8.30, one can deduce that higher yield strength does not necessarily imply a higher sintering level.

Keywords: Biomaterial, Biocompatibility, Tissue engineering, Regenerative medicine, Biomimic, Biodegradable, Surface modification, Corrosion resistance, Dental resin, Photopolymerization, Bioadhesivity, Fick's law, Contact angle, Wettability, Laser sintering.

References

Albrektsson, T. and C. Johansson. 2001. Osteoinduction, osteoconduction osseointegration. Eur. Spine J. 10: 96–101.

Arenholz, E., J. Heitz and D. Bowerle. 1993. Laser-induced surface modification and structure formation of polymers. Appl. Sur. Sci. 69: 16–19.

Baran, E. 2011. Microchannel-patterned and heparin micro-contact printed biodegradable composite membranes for tissue engineering applications. Tissue Eng. Reg. Med. 5: e108–e114.

Becker, E., S. Landau and A. Manuila. 1986. International dictionary of medicine and biology. Wiley, New York.

Bobbio, A. 1972. The first endosseous alloplastic implant in the history of man. Bull. Hist. Dent. 20: 1–6.

Boch, P. and N. Jean-Claude. 2010. Ceramic Materials: Processes, Properties and Applications. doi: 10.1002/9780470612415. ch12.

Boretos, J. 1980. Past, present, future role of polyurethane for surgical implants. Pure Appl. Chem. 52: 1851–1860.

Bruck, S. 1977. Biological evaluation of biomaterials for cardiovascular application. Med. Tech. 5: 51–56.

Brunette, D. and B. Cheroudi. 1999. The effects of the surface topography of micromachined titanium substrata on cell behavior *in vitro* and *in vivo*. J. Biomech. Eng. 121: 49–57.

Buchter, A., J. Kleinheinz, H. Wiesman, J. Kersken and M. Nienkemper. 2005. Biological and biomechanical evaluation of bone remodelling and implant stability after using an osteotome technique. Clin. Oral. Implants Res. 1: 1–8.

Cassoni, A., M. Youssef and I. Prokopowitsch. 2005. Bond strength of a dentin bonding system using two techniques of polymerization: visible-light and argon laser. Photomed. Laser Surg. 23: 493–497.

Chen, Ch., M. Lee and V. Shyu. 2014. Surface modification of polycaprolactone scaffolds fabricated via selective laser sintering for cartilage tissue engineering, Mat. Sci. Eng. C 40: 389–397.

Chrisey, D., A. Pique and A. McGill. 2003. Laser deposition of polymer and biomaterial films. Chem. Rev. 103: 553–576.

Cotell, C. 1993. Pulsed laser deposition and processing of biocompatible hydroxyapatite thin films. Appl. Surf. Sci. 69: 140–148.

Conrado, L., E. Munin and R. Zangaro. 2004. Root apex sealing with different filling materials photopolymerized with fiber optic delivered argon laser light. Lasers Med. Sci. 19: 9599.

Cristescu, R., A. Doraiswamy, T. Patz and G. Socol. 2007. Matrix assisted pulsed laser evaporation of poly(D,L-Lactide) thin films for controlled-release drug systems. Appl. Surf. Sci. 253: 7702–7706.

Crubezy, E., P. Murail, L. Girard and J. Bernadou. 1998. False teeth of the Roman world. Nature 391: 29–35.

Curtis, A. and C. Wilkinson. 1998. Reaction of cells to topography. J. Biomater. Sci. Polym. Ed. 9: 1311–1324.

Deb, S. and H. Sehmi. 2003. A comparative study of the properties of dental resin composites polymerized with plasma and halogen light. Dent. Mater. 19: 517–522.

Duan, B., M. Wang, W. Zhou and W. Cheung. 2010. Three-dimensional nanocomposite scaffolds fabricated via selective laser sintering for bone tissue engineering. Acta Biomaterialia 6: 4495–4505.

Ducheyne, P. and G. Hastings (eds.). 1984. Metal and Ceramic Biomaterials, Vol. 1.

Emami, N., K. Soderholm and L. Berglund. 2003. Effect of light power density variations on bulk curing properties of dental composites. J. Dent. 31: 189–196.

Eosoly, S., D. Brabazon, S. Lohfeld and L. Looney. 2010. Selective laser sintering of hydroxyapatite/poly-e-caprolactone scaffolds. Acta Biomaterialia 6: 2511–2517.

Fano, L., W. Ma, P. Marcoli and S. Pizzi. 2002. Polymerization of dental composite resins using plasma light. Biomaterials 23: 1011–1015.

Fleming, M. and W. Mailet. 1999. Photopolymerization of composite resin using the argon laser. Clin. Pract. 65: 447–450.

Garrido, C., S. Lobo and F. Turibio. 2011. Biphasic calcium phosphate bioceramics for orthopaedic reconstructions:clinical outcomes. Int. J. Biomat. 2011; 1–10.

Gibson, I. and D. Shi. 1997. Material properties and fabrication parameters in selective laser sintering process. Rapid Prototyping J. 3: 129–136.

Grabowski, E. and P. Didisheim. 1977. Platelet adhesion to foreign surfaces under controlled conditions of whole blood flow. Tran. Am. Soc. for Artificial Int. Organs 23: 141–51.

Hu, J., S. Tosto, Z. Guo and C. Wang. 2002. Functionally graded material by laser sintering. Lasers in Eng. 12: 239–245.

Jackson, C. and J. O'Brien. 1995. Molecular weight distribution of Nephila clavipes dragline silk. Macromolecules 28: 5975–5977.

Kalachandra, S. and R. Kusy. 1991. Composition of water sorption by methacrylate and dimethacrylate monomers and their corresponding polymers. Polymer 32: 2428–2434.

Kaplan, D., S. Mello, S. Arcidiacono and S. Fossey. 1998. pp. 103–131. *In*: Protein Based Materials. McGrath KKD. (ed.). Birkhauser, Boston.

Kelsey, W., R. Blankenau, G. Powell and W. Barkmeier. 1989. Enhancement of physical properties of resin restorative materials by laser polymerization. Lasers Surg. Med. 9: 623–627.

Khosroshahi, M.E., A. Valanezhad and J. Tavakoli. 2004. Evaluation of Mid-IR (HF) radiation effect on 316L stainless steel corrosion resistance in physiological saline. Amirkabir J. Sci. Tech. 15: 107–115.

Khosroshahi, M.E., A. Karkhaneh and F. Orang. 2004. A comparative study of chop wave and super pulse CO_2 laser surface modification of polyurethane. Iran Poly. J. 13: 503–511.

Khosroshahi, M.E., M. Atai and M. Nourbakhsh. 2008. Photopolymerization of dental resin as restrotive material using an argon laser. Laser Med. Sci. 23: 399–406.

Khosroshahi, M.E., M. Mahmoodi and H. Saeedinasab. 2009. An *in vitro* and *in vivo* study of osteoblast cells response to surface modified of Ti6Al4V using Nd:YAG laser and emery paper. Lasers in Med. Sci. 24: 925–939.

Khosroshahi, M.E., H. Safaralizadeh and A. Anzanpour. 2016. Experimental study and modeling of polytetrafluoroethylene (PTFE) and hydroxyapatite biocomposite surface treatment using selective laser sintering. AASCIT J. Mat. 1: 75–82.

Lima, M., V. Correlo and R. Reis. 2014. Micro/nano replication and 3D assembling techniques for scaffold fabrication. Mat. Sci. Eng. C 42: 615–621.

Lyman, D., W. Sear and D. Albo. 1977. Polyurethane elastomers in surgery. Int. J. Polym. Mat. 5: 211–229.

Mills, R. and K. Jandt. 1998. Blue LEDs for curing polymer based dental filling materials. LEOS News 12: 9–10.

Monsees, T., K. Barth and S. Tippelt. 2005. Effects of different titanium alloys and nanosized surface patterning on adhesion, differentiation, and orientation of osteoblast-like cells. Cells Tissues Organs 180: 81–95.

Murr, L., S. Quinones, S. Gaytan, M. Lopez and E. Martinez. 2009. Microstructure and mechanical behavior of Ti-6Al-4V produced by rapid-layer manufacturing, for biomedical applications. J. Mech. Behav. Biomed. Mat. 2: 20–32.

Nakayamay, K., T. Yamamuro and P. Kumar. 1981. *In vitro* measurement of anodic polarization of orthopaedic implants alloys: comparative study of *in vivo* and *in vitro* experiments. Biomat. 10: 420–424.

Park, J. and R. Lakes. 1992. Biomaterials: An Introduction. Plenum Press, New York.

Park, J., J. Bronzino and Y. Kim. 2004. Metallic biomaterials, ceramic biomaterials. pp. 1–45. *In*: Park, J. and J. Bronzino (eds.). Biomaterials Principles and Applications. CRC Press, Boca Raton, USA.

Perera, I., D. Allwood, P. Dyer and G. Oldershaw. 1995. Formation of homo and hetro multimeric ions of large proteins in matrix-assisted UV laser desorption/ionization. J. Mass Spect. S3–S12.

Peutzfeld, A., A. Sahafi and E. Asmussen. 2000. Characterize of resin composites polymerized with plasma arc curing units. Dent. Mater. 1: 330–336.

Ping, L., U. Bakowsky, F. Yu and C. Loehbach. 2003. Laser ablation patterning by interference induces directional cell growth. IEEE Trans. On Nanobiosci. 2: 138–145.

Powell, G. and R. Blankenau. 1994. Argon laser polymerization of composite blue lines vs. multilines. J. Clin. Laser Med. Surg. 12: 325–326.

Sankarpandian, M. and H. Sobha. 1997. Characterization of some aromatic dimethacrylates for dental composite applications. J. Mat. Sci. Mat. Med. 8: 465–468.

Sideridou, I., V. Tserki and G. Papanastasiou. 2002. Effect of chemical structure on degree of conversion in light-cured dimethacrylate based dental resins. Biomaterials 23: 1819–1829.

Sighvi, R. and D. Wang. 1998. Review: effects of substratum morphology on cell physiology. Biotechnol. Bioeng. 43: 764–771.

Singh, A., R. Goel and T. Kaur. 2011. Mechanisms pertaining to arsenic toxicity. Toxicol. Int. 18: 87–93.

Shoorgashti, Z., M. Khorasani and M.E. Khosroshahi. 2010. Plasma-induced grafting of polydimethylsiloxane onto polyurrthane surface: characterization and *in vitro* assay. Rad. Phys. Chem. 79: 947–952.

Stephen, J. 2014. Department of Chemistry, Massachusetts Institute of Technology. http://authors.library.caltech.edu/25052/10/BioinCh_chapter9.pdf.

Suman, Das. 2008. Selective laser sintering of polymers, polymer-ceramic composites. pp. 229–260. *In*: Bidanda, B. and P. Bartolo (eds.). Virtual Prototyping & Bio. Manufacturing in Medical Applications. Springer-Verlag Press.

Tampieir, A., G. Celotti, F. Szontagh and E. Landi. 1997. Sintering and characterization of HA and TCP bioceramics with control of their strength and phase purity. J. Mat. Sci. Mat. In. Med. 8: 29–37.

Tan, K., C. Chua, K. Leong and C. Cheah. 2003. Scaffold development using selective laser sintering of polyetheretherketon-hydroxyapatite biocomposites blends. Biomat. 24: 3115–3123.

Thamaraiselvi, T.V. and S. Rajeswari. 2004. Biological evaluation of bioceramic materials—a review. Carbon 24: 172.

Wiria, F., K. Leong and C. Chua. 2010. Modeling of powder particle heat transfer process in selective laser sintering for fabricating tissue engineering scaffolds. Rapid Prototyping J. 16: 400–410.

Wong, Po Foo and C.D. Kaplan. 2005. Genetic engineering of fibrous proteins: spider dragline silk and collagen. Adv. Drug Deliv. Rev. 54: 1131–1143.

Wurzberg, E. and A. Buchman. 1990. Preadhesion laser surface treatment of polycarbonate and polyetherimide. Int. J. Adhesion and Adhesives 10: 254–262.

Yagi, S. and D. Kunii. 1957. Studies on effective thermal conductivities in packed beds. AIChE Journal 3: 371–381.

Zitter, H. and H. Plank. 1987. The electrochemical behaviour of metallic materials as an indicator of their biocompatibility. J. Biom. Mat. Res. 21: 881–896.

9

Nanomaterials

9.1 Introduction

Perhaps the broadest definition of *nanomaterials* is the materials where the sizes of individual building blocks are less than 100 nm, at least in one dimension, and have properties strongly dependent on the grain size. Figure 9.1 illustrates that to understand the concept of nanomaterials, a sound knowledge of physics, chemistry, biology, and materials is essential depending on the type of application. For example, many applications such as nanomedicine, nanobiotechnology, some knowledge of biology, and medicine is also required.

A bridge between nanomaterials and biomaterials (either biological or non-biological) as discussed in previous chapter, is referred to as '*nanobiomaterials*' with nanoscale materials providing the building blocks for the construction of the nanobiomaterials. It is emphasized once again that within this concept, biomaterial is specifically one which is both biocompatible and non-toxic, thus, magnetite iron-oxide can be considered as non-biological biomaterial. Viruses, on the other hand, are natural nanoparticles which have evolved into a variety of shapes. At pH < 6.5, the virus adopts a compact spherical structure. However, at pH > 6.5 the structure becomes porous, allowing the pH-controlled release of encapsulated content, e.g., drug molecules. One example is delivery of genes in transfection applications. Gene therapy is attracting immense attention as a means to treat diseases by modifying the expression of genetic material. Figure 9.2 indicates the scales of such materials (nanomaterials/nanobiomaterials) where most of the synthesized nanomaterials/nanobiomaterials are within 1–100 nm.

The main difference between nanotechnology and conventional technology is in their approach to nanomaterial synthesis. In the former, the '*bottom-up*' approach (e.g., Collisional dispersion, Pyrolysis inert gas condensation, and Sol-gel fabrication) is preferred where atoms or molecules are used as the building blocks to produce nanoparticles, nanotubes, etc. Generally bottom-up techniques include: chemical, electrochemical, sonochemical, thermal, and photochemical reduction. In the latter the '*Top-down*' is

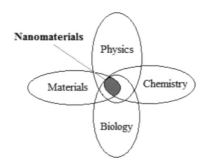

Figure 9.1. Schematic diagram showing interdisciplinary concept of nanomaterials.

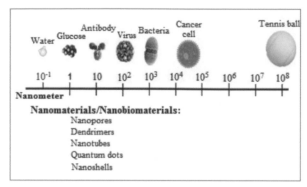

Figure 9.2. Comparison of different material scale. Most nanomaterial devices range between 1–100 nm.

used when starting from large pieces of material for producing the desired structure by mechanical (e.g., crushing or milling) or chemical techniques. As discussed in Chapter 7, one of the major problems with top-down technique is the presence of imperfections in the surface structure which may modify the physical properties of material. Figure 9.3 schematically shows the above concept.

In order for such unique nanomaterials to be used in variety of applications, the translation of the properties of nanoscale components into the different dimensions is required. Nanomaterials may be zero-dimensional (0-D), e.g., nanoparticles, one-dimensional (1-D), e.g., nanorods or nanotubes, two-dimensional (2-D), e.g., thin films, and three-dimensional (3-D), e.g., networks or more complicated hierarchical structures. Examples of some nanostructures are shown in Fig. 9.4.

Research involving nanoparticles or indeed nanoscale materials and structures has created a tremendous interest for scientists and engineers of almost all disciplines. This is mainly because number of physical properties including optical, thermal (e.g., specific heats, melting points) electrical, magnetic are size-dependent. This is believed to be the result of the high surface to volume ratio. In the nanoscale regime, materials like metals and metal oxides can be imagined as neither atomic species which can be represented by molecular orbitals, nor as an ordinary bulk materials which are represented by electronic band structures, but rather exhibit size-dependent broadened energy states. Among these perhaps metal

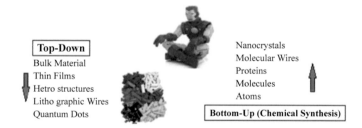

Figure 9.3. Bottom-up and Top-down approaches for synthesis of nanomaterials.

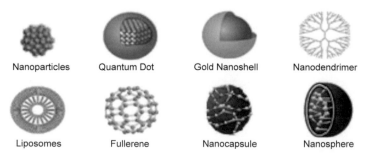

Figure 9.4. Examples of various nanosystems which can be employed for biomedical applications.

nanoparticles as the simplest form of inorganic nanomaterial, which can be used for a wide range of systems and greatly vary in dimension and composition, are the most important because of their wide applications in industry and medicine. Therefore, understanding their properties from an isolated form to different sizes of clusters is an inevitable task for scientists from different disciplines and particularly methods of their preparation for chemists. Thus, because of size and shape dependent properties of these materials, different geometries such as spherical, cylindrical and hollow, or even branched (star shape) with different sizes have all been manufactured. Also, it is believed that the shape of nanoparticles has a direct influence on cell toxicity. Nanoparticles are often dispersed in a colloidal solution. A *colloid* is a finely dispersed substance in an intermediate state between an homogeneous solution and an heterogeneous dispersion. In other words, it consists of a substance of microscopic dimensions (1–1000 nm) dispersed within a continuum phase. *Solution* on the contrary are homogenous systems in which everything is in the same phase, while *suspension* contain particles of larger dimensions and thus, influenced by gravitational forces, which finally sink or sediment to the bottom of the container.

Plasmonic nanoparticles are particles whose electron density can couple with electromagnetic radiation of wavelengths that are far larger than the particle due to the nature of the dielectric-metal interface between the medium and the particles. Plasmonic nanoparticles exhibit interesting scattering, absorbance, and coupling properties based on their geometries and relative positions. These unique properties have made them a focus of research in many applications including solar cells, spectroscopy, signal enhancement for imaging, and cancer treatment. These nanoparticle-based materials have been used for coloring glasses before the Medieval Ages, such as stained glasses in cathedrals, although in those days craftsmen did not surely have the knowledge, nor could understand the physics behind it. One of the oldest plasmonic glass materials is the '*Lycurus*' cup from fourth century AD on display in British museum, as can be seen in Fig. 9.5. It appears red when transilluminated, but shines green when imaged in reflection. The physics of this phenomena which is related to concept of Surface Plasmon Resonance (SPR) is explained in the subsequent sections.

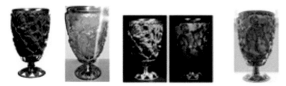

Figure 9.5. 'Lycurgus' cup from the fourth century AD on display in the British museum.

9.1.1 Colloids stability

Two factors which strongly affect a nanoparticle colloidal state or the suspension stability are: (a) Sedimentation in y-direction and (b) Agglomeration occurring in x-direction. In the former, the gravitational force is influenced directly, and in the latter, once the agglomeration and clustering is formed, it becomes a determining parameter in cluster sedimentation at later times. The sedimentation can be avoided as long as the thermal energy, kT, is strong enough to enable the particles to move freely in solution. As we will see in the next chapter, there is a limit for maximum particle diameter, for example for ferrofluids, which ensures the sedimentation stability with the additional problem of avoiding agglomeration. The agglomeration issue can be resolved by using appropriate materials as *surfactant*. Surfactants are usually organic compounds that are amphiphilic, meaning they contain both *hydrophobic* groups (their tails) and *hydrophilic* groups (their heads). Therefore, a surfactant contains both a water-insoluble (or oil-soluble) component and a water-soluble component. Surfactants will diffuse in water and adsorb at interfaces between air and water or at the interface between oil and water, in the case where water is mixed with oil. The water-insoluble hydrophobic group may extend out of the bulk water phase, into the air or into the oil phase, while the water-soluble head group remains in the water phase. Depending on the type of protection used, they can be redispersed in water (hydrosols) or organic solvents (organosols). A large variety of stabilizers, e.g., donor ligands, polymers, and surfactants are used to control the growth of the primarily formed nanoclusters and to prevent them from agglomeration. Nanostructures colloidal metals require protective agents for stabilization and to prevent agglomeration. The two distinguished methods of stabilization are: (a) Electrostatic which involves the coulombic repulsion between the particles caused by electrical double layer formed by ions adsorbed at the particle surface (e.g., sodium citrate) and the corresponding counterions. As an example, we used sodium citrate to prepare gold colloids by reduction of $AuCl_4^-$, as seen in §9.2.2, and (b) Steric where organic molecules act as protective shields on the metallic surface. In this way nanometallic cores are separated from each other, and agglomeration is prevented. The details of these mechanisms are fully explained in Chapter 2, as we can see in §4.2. All in all, lipophilic agents provide metal colloids that are soluble in organic media (organosols) and hydrophilic agents provides water-soluble colloids (hydrosols).

9.2 Iron-oxides

9.2.1 Review of magnetism basics

There are three main categories of materials: (a) *Diamagnetism*, (b) *Paramagnetism*, and (c) *Ferromagnetism*. Magnetization of *diamagnetic* materials is very weak and opposed to the applied field, the permeability $\mu < 1$ and susceptibility $\chi < 0$. The origin of diamagnetism is based on the orbital motion of electrons of the atoms acting like tiny electric current loop, hence producing magnetic fields. In an external field, these current loops align in a way so as to oppose the applied field, thus exposed to a force pushing them out of the magnetic field. Generally, the thermal motions of the atoms will cause the magnetic moments to be oriented purely at random and there will be no resultant magnetization. If, however, a field is applied, each atomic moment will try to set in direction of the field, but thermal motions will prevent a complete alignment. In *paramagnetic* material, the atoms act as tiny magnetic dipoles that can be oriented by an external magnetic field where magnetization develops parallel to the applied field as the field increases from zero, but the strength of the magnetization is small, $\mu > 1$ and $\chi > 0$. Clearly, paramagnetism is temperature dependent. At low temperatures, the thermal motions will be less effective in preventing the alignment of the moments, and so the susceptibility will be larger. At higher temperatures, thermal motions will make the alignment more difficult, and at very high temperatures, the material may become diamagnetic. *Ferromagnetism* is a property of those materials which are intrinsically magnetically ordered and develop spontaneous magnetization without the need to apply a field. The reason for such long range ordering causing to line up the dipoles parallel is due to the interacting dipoles, i.e., quantum mechanical exchange interaction, which are represented by the unpaired spins. Above a critical temperature called *Curie temperature,* ferromagnetics become paramagnetic. The magnetic domains are separated by magnetic walls known as Bloch walls. Bloch walls may connect magnetic domains with orientation differences of 90° or 180°, and the size of the domains and width of walls are determined by thermodynamics. By moving the Bloch walls, the direction of magnetization within grain is changed, as can be seen in Fig. 9.6.

If a magnetic material is placed in a magnetic field of strength H, the individual atomic moments in the material contribute to its overall response, the magnetic flux density B (or magnetic induction) is defined by

$$B = \mu_0 H + M = \mu_0 (H + \chi H) = \mu_r \mu_0 H \qquad (9.1)$$

where $\mu_0 = 4\pi \times 10^{-7}$ Hm^{-1} is the permeability of free space. This gives the horizontal component of the earth's H $\approx$ 16 Am^{-1} and B $\approx$ 20 μT in London, the stray fields from the cerebral cortex are about 10 fT, $\mu_r = (1 + \chi)$ is the relative permeability, χ is the susceptibility of the magnetic material, M is the magnetization (i.e., the magnetic dipole moment μ_m per unit volume V).

$$M = \mu m / V \qquad (9.2)$$

If we take any ferromagnetic and increase the field from zero to a maximum value, and decrease the field back through zero to an equal and opposite value and then return again to the original peak value,

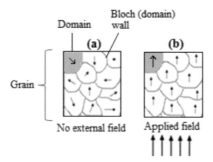

Figure 9.6. In the absence of external magnetic field moments are randomly oriented within a grain Domain (a) and are oriented when the field is applied (b).

we will have a loop known as an '*hysteresis*' (meaning loss in Greek) loop. Thus, energy is dissipated as heat in traversing the loop. A schematic magnetization curve indicating the most characterizing points is shown in Fig. 9.7. As the material approaches saturation, the domains cannot yield much further, and the susceptibility falls to a low value. After the specimen has become saturated, and the field H is reduced to zero, the material is still strongly magnetized, setting up a flux density, B_r known as *remanence*. It is due to the tendency of domains to stay aligned after H becomes zero. However, when the field is reversed, the residual magnetism is opposed. Every increase of field H causes a decrease of flux density B, as domains are twisted farther out of alignment. Eventually, B reduces to zero, while opposing field H has the value H_c. This is called the *coercive force*. Another important property of magnetic material is the energy product which is given by the product of *remanence* and *coercivity*. The shape of these loops are determined by particle size.

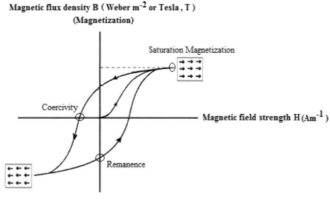

Figure 9.7. A typical B-H hysteresis loop for an iron specimen.

9.2.2 Superparamagnetic iron-oxide nanoparticles (SPION)

When a grain size becomes so small that it is comparable to a magnetic domain, i.e., a single domain, its hysteresis loop will exhibit no area and the material will have zero remanence and coercivity. This commonly is referred to as *superparamagnetism* which approximately applies for particles with dimensions smaller than 15 nm. At this scale ferromagnetism is no longer observed and no permanent magnetization remains after the particles have been subject to external magnetic field. But, the particles will have a considerable degree of paramagnetism with a very large χ, as the name suggests. The underlying physics behind this is found in the material crystal anisotropy. Magnetocrystalline anisotropy is an intrinsic property of any magnetic material, independent of grain size. The energy required to magnetize a ferro or ferromagnetic crystal depends on the direction of the magnetic field relative to the orientation of the crystal. In superparamagnetic material, the magnetization vector fluctuates between different easy magnetic directions, hence overcoming hard directions. The magnetic moment of the particle as a whole is free to fluctuate in response to thermal energy, while the individual atomic moments maintain their ordered state relative to each other. The direct proportionality between the energy barrier to moment reversal ΔE, and particle volume V (i.e., $\Delta E = KV$) where K is the anisotropy energy density.

Magnetite, Fe_3O_4, is a common ferromagnetic iron oxide that has a cubic inverse spinel structure with oxygen forming a face-centered cubic (fcc) crystal system. In magnetite, all tetrahedral sites are occupied by Fe^{3+} and octahedral sites are occupied by both Fe^{3+} and Fe^{2+}. The electrons can hop between Fe^{2+} and Fe^{3+} ions in the octahedral sites at room temperature, rendering magnetite an important class of half-metallic materials. In the recent decades, magnetic nanoparticles (MNPs), especially magnetite (Fe_3O_4) and maghemite (γ-Fe_2O_3), have attracted increasing interest because of their outstanding properties, including superparamagnetism and low toxicity. The major difficulty in the synthesis of ultrafine particles is to control the particle size at the nanometric scale. This difficulty arises as a result of the high surface energy of these systems. With proper surface coating, these magnetic nanoparticles can be dispersed into suitable solvents, forming homogeneous suspensions, called ferrofluids. Some important properties of MNPs include: (1) they have sizes that place them at dimensions comparable to those of a virus (20–500 nm), a protein (5–50 nm), or a gene (2 nm wide and 10–100 nm long), thus, improving the diffusion through tissue and having a long circulation time; (2) they obey Coulomb's law, and can be manipulated by an external magnetic field gradient. This can be helpful in decreasing nanomagnets concentration in blood and therefore diminishing the associated side effects; and (3) they have a large specific surface area that can be properly modified to attach biological agents. Iron oxide nanoparticles with appropriate surface chemistry have been widely used experimentally for numerous *in vivo* applications as contrast enhancement in bioimaging (Enochs et al. 1999, Thomas et al. 2013), tissue engineering (Bock et al. 2010), immunoassay (Mikhaylova et al. 2004), hyperthermia (Piñeirol et al. 2015, Sadat et al. 2014), drug delivery (Jain et al. 2005, Talelli et al. 2009), and in cell separation (Hengyi et al. 2011). Applications can impose strict requirements on the particles physical, chemical, and pharmacological properties, including chemical composition, granulometric uniformity, crystal structure, magnetic behaviour, surface structure, adsorption properties, solubility, and low toxicity. In addition, these applications need special surface coating of the magnetic particles, which has to be not only non-toxic and biocompatible, but also allow a targetable delivery.

Physical basis of SPIONs applications

In all *in vitro* and *in vivo* applications of SPIONs, such as magnetic separation, drug delivery, magnetic resonance imaging (MRI) and hyperthermia, magnetic field is involved to manipulate the particles. A short review of some basic elements would help us to obtain a greater insight. It is known from electromagnetism that a magnetic field gradient is needed in order to exert a force at a distance, a uniform field causes a torque but not linear (i.e., translational). The magnetic force acting on a point-like dipole μ_m is

$$F_m = (\mu_m \cdot \nabla)B \tag{9.3}$$

where $\nabla \equiv i\dfrac{\partial}{\partial x} + j\dfrac{\partial}{\partial y} + k\dfrac{\partial}{\partial z}$ is Laplace (nabla) operator which can act on a scalar or a vector field. Therefore, $\mu_m \cdot \nabla$ can be considered as differentiation with respect to the direction of μ_m, so if $x = 0$, $y = 0$ and $z = \mu_{mz}$, then $m \cdot \nabla = \mu_{mz}(\partial/\partial z)$, and provided there is a field gradient in the z-direction, then magnetic dipole will experience a force acting on it. Using Equations (9.1) and (9.2) we get

$$M = \Delta\chi H \tag{9.4}$$

where $\Delta\chi = \chi_m - \chi_w$ is the effective susceptibility of the particle relative to the water. Substituting Eqs. (9.2) and (9.4) in (9.3), it gives

$$F_m = \frac{V_m \Delta\chi}{\mu_0}(B \cdot \nabla)B \tag{9.5}$$

Assuming there is no time-varying current or electric field, then using one of the four maxwell's equation, $\nabla \times B = \mu_0 J = 0$ in the identity $\nabla(B \cdot B) = 2(B \cdot \nabla)B$, we obtain

$$F_m = \frac{V_m \Delta \chi \nabla}{\mu_0} \left(\frac{B^2}{2\mu_0} \right) \tag{9.6}$$

Substituting $H = B/\mu_0$ from Eq. (9.1) in (9.6), it gives

$$F_m - V_m \Delta \chi \nabla \left(\frac{1}{2} B . H \right) \tag{9.7}$$

Equation (9.7) shows that the magnetic force is related to the differential of the magnetostatic field energy density, 1/2 B . H. Now, in a magnetic separation process, the material is separated from its original solution by passing the fluid through a region where there is a magnetic field gradient, which can immobilize the tagged material via the magnetic force defined by equation (9.7). This force has to overcome the hydrodynamic drag force acting on the magnetic particles in the flowing solution.

$$F_d = 6\pi \, \eta_m R_p \Delta v \tag{9.8}$$

where η_m is the viscosity of the medium surrounding the cell (e.g., water), R_p is the particle radius, and $\Delta v = v_c - v_m$ is the difference in velocities of the cell and water (Zborowski 1997). Writing $V_p = \frac{4}{3}\pi R_p^3$ and equating the equations (9.7) and (9.8), gives the velocity of the particle relative to the carrier fluid

$$\Delta v = \frac{R_p^2 \Delta \chi}{9\mu_0 \eta} \nabla(B^2) = \Delta v = \frac{\xi}{\mu_0} \nabla(B^2) \tag{9.10}$$

where ξ is the magnetophoretic mobility of the particle, i.e., a parameter which describes how the manipulable a magnetic particle can be.

Generally, there are three standard methods for synthesizing magnetic iron oxide nanoparticles:

1) *Physical-based methods*: (a) Gas phase deposition and (b) Electron beam lithography, (c) Laser pyrolysis, and (d) Spray pyrolysis
2) *Chemical-based methods*: (a) Co-precipitation (wet chemical route), (b) Microemulsion, (c) Thermal decomposition, (d) Polyols, and (e) Sol-gel
3) *Biological-based methods*: (a) Magnetosome in magnetostatic bacteria

The summary of some of these methods with the advantages and disadvantages is given in Table (9.1).

9.2.3 Preparation and characterization of silica-coated iron-oxide (Fe_3O_4/SiO_2) bionanoparticles under N_2 gas (Khosroshahi and Ghazanfari 2010)

Controlled co-precipitation technique under N_2 gas was used to prevent undesirable critical oxidation of Fe^{2+}. The synthesized Fe_3O_4 (311) NPs were first coated with trisodium citrate (TSC) to achieve solution stability, and then covered by SiO_2 layer using Stober method. For uncoated Fe_3O_4 NPs, the results showed an octahedral geometry with saturation magnetization range of (82–96) emu/g and coercivity of about (80–120) Oe for particles between (35–96) nm, respectively. The best value of specific surface area (41 m²/g) was obtained at 0.9 M NaOH at 750 rpm. However, it increased to about 81 m²/g for Fe_3O_4/SiO_2 combination with 50 nm as particle size, indicating the presence of about 15 nm SiO_2 layer. Finally, the stable magnetic fluid (nanoferrofluid) contained well dispersed magnetite-silica nanoshells, which showed fast magnetic response.

Synthesis of Fe_3O_4

The synthesis procedure block diagram is shown in Fig. 9.8. Stock solutions of 1.28 M Ferric chloride hexahydrate ($FeCl_3.6H_2O$, 99%), 0.64 M Ferric chloride hexahydrate ($FeCl_2.4H_2O$, 99%) and 0.4 M hydrochloric acid (HCl, 37%) were prepared as a source of iron by dissolving the respective chemicals in milli-Q water (18.2 M, deoxygenated by bubbling N2 gas for 1 h prior to the use) under vigorous

Table 9.1. Summary of some of the methods used for synthesizing magnetic iron oxide nanoparticles.

Synthetic methods	Advantages	Disadvantages	References
Co-precipitation	Rapid synthesis with high yield, low cost	Problem of oxidation aggregation	Gupta and Gupta 2005 Kim and Shimal 2007
Hydrothermal reactions	Narrow size distribution and good control, scalable	Long reaction times	Wang et al. 2005 Wan et al. 2007
High temperature decomposition	Good control of size and shape, high yield, narrow size distribution	Furthers steps needed to obtain water stable suspension	Park et al. 2004 Sun et al. 2004
Microemulsion	Uniform properties and control of particle size	Difficult to remove surfactant, only small amount of nanoparticles can be synthesized and poor yield	Gupta and Gupta 2005 Liu et al. 2004 Dresco and Zeitsev 1999
Aerosol/vapour (pyrolysis) method	High production rate	Large aggregates are formed	Kang and Park 1996 Gupta and Gupta 2005
Gas deposition method	Useful for protective coating and thin film deposition	Require very high temperatures	Gupta and Gupta 2005
Sol-gel method	Particles of desired shape and length can be synthesized, useful making hybrid nanoparticles	Product usually contains sol-gel matrix components at their surfaces	Lu et al. 2001 Gupta and Gupta 2005
Laser pyrolysis	Pure, well-crystallized and uniform nanoparticles in one step, narrow size distribution	A gas is required as absorbent and the carrier to transport the carbonyl vapour to the reaction	Cannon et al. 1982 Veintemillas et al. 2004

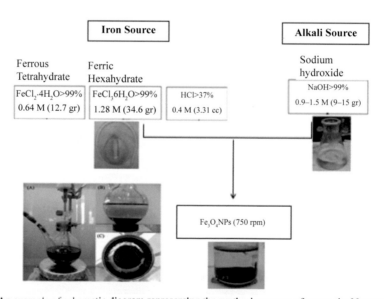

Figure 9.8. An example of schematic diagram representing the synthesis process of magnetite Nanoparticles.

stirring. In the same way, stock solutions of 0.9–1.5 M NaOH were prepared as the alkali sources and the synthesized Fe_3O_4 samples were classified as S1–S4 where each sample were synthesized using different NaOH concentration, i.e., 0.9, 1.1, 1.3 and 1.5 M of NaOH corresponds to S1, S2, S3, and S4, respectively. Aqueous dispersion of magnetic nanoparticles was prepared by alkalinizing an aqueous mixture of ferric and ferrous salts with NaOH at room temperature. Twenty-five mL of iron source was added drop-wise into 250 mL of alkali source under vigorous magnetic stirring (450 and 750 rpm) for 30 min at ambient temperature. A complete precipitation of Fe_3O_4 should be expected between 7.5–14 pH, while maintaining a molar ratio of Fe^{2+}: Fe^{3+} = 1:2 under a non-oxidizing environment, otherwise, Fe_3O_4

might also be oxidized. This would critically affect the physical and chemical properties of the nanosized magnetic particles. The precipitated powder was isolated by applying an external magnetic field, and the supernatant was removed from the precipitate by decantation. The powder was washed and the solution was decanted twice after centrifugation at 5000 rpm for 15 min. Then 0.01M HCl was added to neutralize the anionic charge on the particle surface. The cationic colloidal particles were separated by centrifugation and peptized by watering. The obtained magnetic mud was then redispersed in a 200 mL portion of TSC solution (0.5 M) and heated at 90°C for 30 min under magnetic stirring (750 rpm). All the main synthesis steps were carried out by passing N2 gas through the solution media to avoid possible oxygen contamination during the synthesis. An appropriate amount of acetone was added to remove the excessive citrate groups adsorbed on the nanoparticles and collected with a magnet. After coating, the product was washed to remove the physically adsorbed surfactant on the particle. Centrifugation was done and peptizing the solution twice, then they freeze-dried at –60°C. The obtained powder was suspended in water. Finally, the resultant dispersion was adjusted to 2.0 wt%.

Coating citrate-modified Fe_3O_4 with silica

Following the Stober method, with some modifications, the coating of citrate-modified Fe_3O_4 with silica were carried out in a basic ethanol/water mixture at room temperature using the obtained magnetite dispersion (only sample S1 at 750 rpm as an optimized value) as seeds. Magnetite dispersion (2.0 g) was first diluted with water (40 mL), absolute ethanol (120 mL), and then 3.0 mL ammonia aqueous (25 wt%) was added as suggested in Deng et al. (2005), Du et al. (2006), and Yang et al. (2009). The resultant dispersion was well-dispersed by ultrasonic vibration for 15 min. Finally, 0.9 g of Si $(OC_2H_5)_4$ (tetraethyl orthosilicate, TEOS) diluted in ethanol (20 mL) was added to this dispersion drop-wise under continuous mechanical stirring. All of the analytic reagents were purchased from Merck company. The reaction mechanism is explained as:

$$Si (OC_2H_5)_4 + 4H_2O \rightarrow Si (OH)_4 + 4C_2H_5OH$$
$$Si (OH)_4 \rightarrow SiO_2 + 2H_2O \tag{9.11}$$

After stirring for 12 h, the obtained magnetic product was collected by magnetic separation and washed twice with ethanol. Subsequently, magnetite–silica (M-S) nanoshells was obtained through the sol–gel approach. After coating, the surfactant adsorbed physically on the particle surface was removed by washing, centrifugation and peptizing the solution for three times. For the TEOS concentration used in our case, the induction period was approximately 30 min. The Brunauer-Emmett-Teller (BET) method was utilized to calculate the specific surface areas by Quantachrome TPR Win v1.0 using nitrogen as the sorbate. Transmission electron microscopy (TEM) was performed using a Phillips CM-200-FEGmicroscope operating at 120 kV. Magnetization measurements were carried at 300 K in a magnetic field (H) of up to 20 KOe with a vibrating sample magnetometer (VSM-PAR 155) that can measure magnetic moments as low as 103 emu. For the magnetization measurements, uncoated Fe_3O_4 nanoparticles was obtained in dry powder form by evaporating the water from the solution. X-ray diffraction (XRD) measurements were performed at room temperature using a FK60-04 X-ray diffractometer with Cu radiation. Fourier transform infrared (FT-IR) spectra were recorded by EQUINOX 55 FT-IR spectrometer. Scanning electronic microscopy (SEM) images were recorded by electron microscope at an accelerating voltage of 25 kV.

As shown in Fig. 9.9a, the mean Fe_3O_4 particle size examined by TEM imaging exhibited an almost dispersed state. It is notable that, the particles have an octahedral-like geometry. The influence of the chemical potential on the shape evolution of crystals has been elucidated by Liu et al. (2002). In the case of crystal growth, it would be beneficial to have a higher chemical potential, which is mainly determined by the NaOH concentration. Octahedral Fe_3O_4 with high quality and crystallinity could be obtained in concentrated solution, because higher OH-ion concentration and higher chemical potential in the solution favor the growth of octahedral structures over other possible iron-oxide crystal forms. Figure 9.9b shows the variation of particle size with NaOH concentration. As is seen in this figure, particle size decreases at lower NaOH%, which in our case this corresponds to 35 nm at 0.9 M of NaOH. The reason may be due to the reaction mechanism of magnetite:

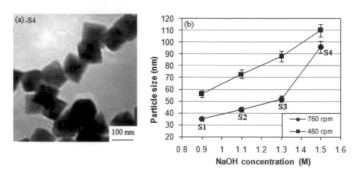

Figure 9.9. TEM micrograph of uncoated Fe_3O_4 nanoparticles (S4) (a) and variation of particle size with NaOH concentration (b).

$$Fe^{3+} + 3OH^- = Fe\,(OH)_3$$

$$Fe\,(OH)_3 = FeO\,(OH) + H_2O \tag{9.12}$$

$$Fe^{2+} + 2OH^- = Fe\,(OH)$$

$$2FeO\,(OH) + Fe\,(OH)_2 = Fe_3O_4 + 2H_2O$$

A decrease in molarity affects the above reactions, and may in turn influence the kinetics of the nucleation and growth of Fe_3O_4 particles. The reduction in particle size creates negative pressure on the lattice which consequently leads to a lattice cell volume expansion. Furthermore, the reduction can also decrease the magnetic transition temperature. The increase in unit cell volume with reduction in particle size of Fe_3O_4 particles perhaps implies an increase in Fe^{2+} content in the sample [ionic radius of Fe^{2+} (0.74A°) is larger than that of Fe^{3+} (0.64A°)]; so, the particle size of magnetite colloidal nanocrystal clusters (CNCs) are influenced by changes in the base molarity.

Saturation magnetization Ms, residual magnetization Mr, and coercivity Hc are the main technical parameters to characterize the magnetism of a ferromagnetic particle sample. A value of 82 emu/g as saturation magnetization was found for these particles, which steadily increased by increasing the particle size, see Fig. 9.10a. This value is slightly higher than the value achieved by Yang et al. (2009) for Fe_3O_4 NPs. The corresponding values of coercivity were measured and plotted in Fig. 9.10b.

These results suggest that coercivity, Hc, is strongly size dependent and bulk samples with sizes greater than the domain wall width can cause magnetization reversal due to domain wall motion. As domain walls move through a sample, they can become pinned at grain boundaries, and additional energy is needed for them to continue moving. Pinning is one of the main sources of the coercivity. Grain size dependence of coercivity and permeability (GSDCP) theory (Xue et al. 2008) predicts:

$$H_c = P_1 \frac{\sqrt{AK}}{M_s D_g} \propto 1/D_g \tag{9.13}$$

here A denotes the exchange constant, K is an magnetocrystalline anisotropy constant, M_s the saturation magnetization, P_1 and P_2 are dimensionless factors. Therefore, reducing the grain size, D_g, creates more pining sites and increases H_c. For ultrafine particles, the modified form of theory predicts:

$$H_c = P_2 \frac{K^4 D_g^6}{M_s A} \propto D_g^6 \tag{9.14}$$

where P_1 and P_2 are dimensionless factors. The difference between equations (1) and (2) is defined by ferromagnetic exchange length as:

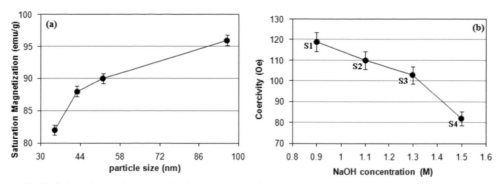

Figure 9.10. Variation of saturation magnetization (a) and coercivity (b) with particle size for uncoated Fe_3O_4 nanoparticles at 750 rpm.

$$L_{ex} = \sqrt{\frac{A}{K}} \tag{9.15}$$

Using the following parameters for magnetite ($K = 1.35 \times 10^4$ J/m³, $A = 10^{-11}$ J/m), the exchange length can be estimated as $L_{ex} = 27$ nm.

Figure 9.11a shows the variation of residual magnetization with NaOH concentration, where it exhibits the lowest value of 20 (emu/g) at 0.9 M and it gradually increases up to 33 (emu/g) as turning point on the curve at 1.1 M. In other words, the smallest nanoparticle has lowest Mr. The size of magnetic particles, D_m, can be calculated from the magnetization data given in Fig. 9.11b using the following equation (Liu et al. 2002):

$$D_m = \left(\frac{18K_B T}{\pi}\frac{\chi_i}{\rho M_s}\right)^{1/3} \tag{9.16}$$

$$\chi_i = \left(\frac{dM}{dH}\right)_{H \to 0} \tag{9.17}$$

Here, χ_i is the initial magnetic susceptibility, $K_B = 1.38 \times 10^{-23}$ Jk⁻¹ is the Boltzmann constant, H is the magnetic field strength, and ρ is the density of Fe_3O_4 (5.18 gr/cm³). As it is expected from Fig. 9.11b, the smaller nanoparticles also possess the lowest magnetic moment, which in this case a value of 1×10^{-20} (emu.m³/g) was determined and increased for larger sizes of particles.

In ferrofluid, stability is maintained by electrostatic and repulsive interactions between counter ions and amphoteric hydroxyl ions (H_3O+ or OH^-). TEOS solution was added and reacted with H_2O adsorbed on the surface of Fe_3O_4 to connect Si–O with NPs. Further hydrolysis of TEOS causes $-OCH_2CH_3$ to transfer into $-OH$. The adjacent $-OH$ group loses a molecule of H_2O to form a cross-linked structure and subsequently under polycondensation process, SiO_2-coating is formed. M-S nanocomposites prepared

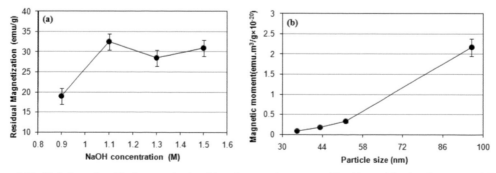

Figure 9.11. Variation of residual magnetization (a) and magnetic moment (b) with particle size for uncoated Fe_3O_4 nanoparticles at 750 rpm.

in this manner can resist corrosion of strong acid or base, indicating that citrate modified Fe_3O_4 NPs are capsulated by SiO_2. Exposing M-S nanocomposites to a magnetic field resulted in removal of all milky material from the liquid. This result indicates that the silica particles must be physically or chemically attached to the magnetite. This attachment is strong enough to cause the suspended silica particles to migrate with the magnetite in a magnetic field. It is worth mentioning that flowing N2 gas not only protects the critical oxidation but also reduces the particle size when compared with methods without removing the oxygen. This is mainly because of generation of bubbles in the reaction solution due to the use of high stirring rates which may cause magnetites to be oxidized. A complete precipitation of Fe_3O_4 should be expected between 7.5–14 pH, while maintaining a molar ratio of $Fe^{2+}:Fe^{3+} = 1:2$.

Each dried sample (0.01–0.02 g) after being accurately weighed was placed in a sample tube (reference an empty tube). Analysis was performed using an automatic five-point adsorption programme. The surface area of all samples was determined by the BET method. Figure 9.12a shows the variation of specific surface area with nanoparticles size. N2 adsorption–desorption isotherms demonstrated that highest specific surface area of 41 m^2/g was achieved for 35 nm particles at 750 rpm using 0.9 M NaOH. According to the BET values, one can calculate the amount of particle size, D_{BET}, considering the following Eq.:

$$D_{BET} = \frac{6}{\rho A_s} \qquad (9.18)$$

There is not any significant difference between these values and the ones which are obtained by other methods.

Figure 9.12b shows the XRD patterns for (b) citrate-modified, and (c) SiO_2-coated Fe_3O_4 NPs with each pattern normalized to its maximum intensity. All of the peaks in the patterns of the Fe_3O_4 NPs can be indexed with the cubic structure corresponding to magnetite phase. The average size of the crystals was estimated using Scherrer's formula,

$$D_{hkl} = \left(\frac{k\lambda}{\sqrt{B_M^2 - B_S^2}\, \cos\theta_{hkl}} \right) \qquad (9.19)$$

where k is the shape factor, λ the X-ray wavelength, B_M the half maximum line width (FWHM) in radians, B_S the half maximum line width of the instrument, y the Bragg angle, and D_{hkl} the mean size of the ordered (crystalline) domains. The dimensionless shape factor has a typical value of about 0.9, but varies with the actual shape of the crystallite. Based on the XRD results, citrate modified Fe_3O_4 NPs that were 8.5 nm in size, were selected for coating treatment. Figure 9.12b shows that the XRD pattern of the SiO_2-coated Fe_3O_4 NPs is very similar to that of the uncoated Fe_3O_4. This indicates that the coated silica is in an amorphous form and possibly their small and wide peaks are dominated by magnetite sharp peaks. The indicated lines are characteristic for spinel magnetite. The pattern of silica-coated magnetite displayed the same lines, especially the most intense one, confirming the existence of magnetite.

The difficulty in the synthesis of ultrafine particles arises from the high surface energy of these systems. The MNPs can be coated with a biocompatible and diamagnetic material to prevent the formation of large

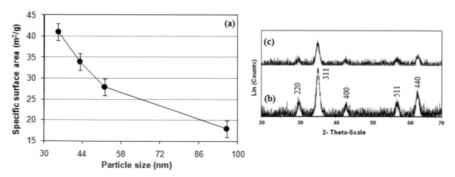

Figure 9.12. Variation of specific surface area with NaOH concentration uncoated Fe_3O_4 nanoparticles at 750 rpm (a) X-ray diffraction pattern for (b) Citrate-modified Fe_3O_4 and (c) Silica-modified Fe_3O_4 nanoparticles. All Miller indices in (b) and (c) correspond to magnetite.

aggregates of MNPs and to functionalize for biological agents attachment. For example, coating of SPIONs with water-soluble synthetic polymer such as polyvinyl alcohol (PVA) prevents their aggregation via steric hindrance mechanism and leads to the formation of monodispersed nanocrystals (Sairam et al. 2006). Considering the importance of nanoparticles physico-chemical properties in biomedical applications, the effect of coating and stirring on the SPIONs size was recently studied at different conditions including: uncoated magnetic nanoparticles (MNPs), MNP + polyvinyl alcohol (PVA), MNP + Au only and MNP + amorphous silica (SiO_2) + gold (Au) (Ghazanfari and Khosroshahi 2015). A systematic study of the formation and characterization of different core-shell nanostructures demonstrated that the particle size of magnetite colloidal nanocrystals are influenced by changes in the base molarity and the stirring speed. Also, it was shown that by optimizing the preparation condition using PVA, silica, and gold as coating materials, an stable magnetic fluid containing well-defined core-shell structures can be achieved. These results provided a conceptual understanding of the structural and magnetic properties for these binary and tertiary nanoparticles. The high saturation magnetization of nanostructures makes them suitable for MRI applications. Additionally, NPs with suitable optothermal and magnetic properties are also frequently used in photo-acoustic imaging of tissues as contrast agent. Furthermore, uniform dispersion would make all the synthesized nanostructures potential candidates for biomedical applications.

9.3 Metallic nanostructures

9.3.1 Introduction

The importance of the metallic nanoparticles originates from their ability to absorb and scatter the incident light in the visible and the infrared (IR) regions. The optical response of NPs depends on their morphology, size, type of metal, and the surrounding medium (Oldenberg et al. 1998). By controlling the morphology of nanoparticles, one can change the way the light can be polarized. Polarization of positive ions and negative charges, i.e., electron cloud is considered a unique way to control the characteristics of plasmonic modes such as band position, band width, and intensity. Orientation of the nanoparticles, however, in the incident field controls the type of the excited of such modes. The unique optical-electronics properties of colloidal gold nanoparticles have been utilized for organic photovoltaics, sensory probes, therapeutic agents bioimaging, drug delivery, and many others. The application of the metallic nanostructures requires the deposition of a densely-packed assembly of particles of different shapes, sizes, and configurations. The optical and electronic properties of gold nanoparticles are tunable by changing the size, shape, surface chemistry, or aggregation state. Therefore, understanding these properties of an isolated particle is the main key for tuning the optical properties of large clusters. Basically, the optical response of metallic clusters can be controlled by the metal type, interparticle distance, polarization state of the incident light.

Nanoshell (NS) particle is a class of nanocomposite which consists of concentric particle, in which particle of one material is coated with a thin layer of another material. They are highly functional materials with significant properties, which are very different to either the core or the shell material alone, and can be prepared in different sizes and shapes (e.g., spherical or rod). As we shall discuss in the next section, gold nanoshells (GNS) are more efficient at converting the electromagnetic wave to energy than nanoparticles due to plasmon resonance along both the inner and outer surface of the shell, as opposed to the surface only in the case of nanoparticles. Therefore, their properties can be modified by changing either the constituting materials or the core-shell ratio. Figure 9.13 illustrates that by decreasing the thickness of the shell (i.e., thinner layer), the peak of plasmon resonance is shifted towards the longer wavelengths.

It is this *tunability* which is the main reason that GNS are preferred to GNP. One major applicability of GNS tunability in biomedicine is based on the optical fact that not all the wavelengths can be transmitted easily through the skin, specially those which show high absorption coefficient for water (e.g., mid-IR, see §6.2.2) and those which may suffer from considerable amount of scattering in the visible spectrum. Thus, GNS can be tuned and functionalized in such a way that can fit within the *therapeutic window* range (i.e., 600–1300 nm) in order to provide a more efficient non-invasive treatment. More on this is discussed in the application section. Finally, NS materials can be synthesized using any material, but usually dielectric materials such as silica and polystyrene are commonly used as core because they are highly stable, chemically inert and water-soluble; therefore, they can be employed in biological applications.

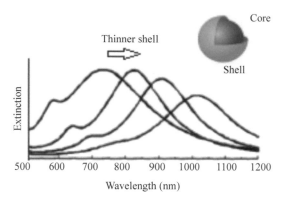

Figure 9.13. Variation of surface SPR with shell thickness.

The possible core-shell combinations of a NS are: dielectric-metal (Oldenberg et al. 1998), dielectric-semiconductor (Hebalkar et al. 2004), dielectric-dielectric (Lu et al. 2004), semiconductor-metal (Kim et al. 2005), semiconductor-semiconductor (Peng et al. 1997), semiconductor-dielectric (Chang et al. 1994), metal-metal (Toshima and Yonezawa 1998), metal-dielectric (Caruso et al. 2001).

9.3.2 Optical properties of metal NPs

(i) Complex refractive index and absorption

The complex refractive index is defined as

$$\tilde{n}(\omega) = n_r(\omega) + ik_e(\omega) \tag{9.20}$$

According to the principle of causality, the real and imaginary parts of the complex refractive index are connected through Kramers-Kronig relations. The real part, $n_r(\omega)$ is the refractive index of NP and the imaginary part, $k_e(\omega)$ is the extinction coefficient, where ω is the angular frequency of the light, λ is the wavelength. The wavenumber k is defined as

$$k = \frac{2\pi n_m}{\lambda} = \frac{n_m \omega}{c} \tag{9.21}$$

where nm is the refractive index of surrounding medium. Substituting (920) in (9.21) we obtain

$$k = \frac{2\pi(n_m + ike)}{\lambda} \tag{9.22}$$

The equation for plane electromagnetic wave is

$$\underline{E}(z,t) = \text{Re}\left[E_0 e^{-i(kz - \omega t)}\right] \tag{9.23}$$

Substituting (9.22) in (9.23) and simplifying it gives

$$\underline{E}(z,t) = e^{-2\pi kz/\lambda}.\text{Re}\left[E_0 e^{i(kz-\omega t)}\right] \tag{9.24}$$

And the absorption coefficient of NP is

$$\alpha = \frac{4\pi k_e}{\lambda} \tag{9.25}$$

(ii) Complex dielectric permittivity constant

Complex dielectric permittivity is defined as

$$\tilde{\epsilon} = \epsilon_R + i\epsilon_i \qquad (9.26)$$
$$(\text{or} \quad \tilde{\epsilon} = \epsilon_1 + i\epsilon_2)$$

where ϵ_R and $i\epsilon_i$ are the real and imaginary parts of permittivity respectively. Also,

$$\tilde{\epsilon} = \tilde{n}^2 \qquad (9.27)$$

Thus, by equating the equations (9.20) and (9.26) and simplifying the expansion we obtain

$$\epsilon_R = n_p^2 - k_e^2 \qquad (9.28a)$$

$$i\epsilon_i = 2n_p k_e = n_p \lambda \alpha / \pi \qquad (9.28b)$$

Since, the permittivity of NP is

$$\epsilon_p = -2\epsilon_m \qquad (9.29)$$

(i.e., $\epsilon_1 = -2\epsilon_2$ where $\epsilon_1 \equiv \epsilon_p$ and $\epsilon_2 \equiv \epsilon_m$, the permittivity of surrounding medium). Therefore, the real part of refractive index becomes

$$k_e = \left[\frac{[-\epsilon_1 + \sqrt{(\epsilon_1^2 + \epsilon_2^2)}]}{2} \right]^{1/2} \qquad (9.30a)$$

and the imaginary,

$$k_e = \left[\frac{[-\epsilon_1 + \sqrt{(\epsilon_1^2 + \epsilon_2^2)}]}{2} \right]^{1/2} \qquad (9.30b)$$

Thus, the complex permittivity of NP becomes

$$\tilde{\epsilon} = (n_p^2 - k_e^2) + 2n_p k_e \qquad (9.31)$$

where $\epsilon_R = n_p^2 - k_e^2$ and $i\epsilon_i = 2n_p k_e^2$

(iii) Efficiency and cross-section

Absorption cross-section σ_α of a NP is defined as the product of absorption efficiency η_α and the NP's cross-sectional area. The scattering and total attenuation coefficient cross-sections are also defined in a similar way. The extinction coefficient is maximum when $\epsilon_p + 2\epsilon_m = 0$ due to dipole-plasmon resonance effects, where ϵ_p is responsible for SPR band (Khlebtsov and Khlebtsov 2007). According to Mie theory, the absorption cross section, σ_α, of a particle embedded in a medium is

$$\sigma_\alpha = \eta_\alpha \cdot \pi R_p^2 \qquad (9.32)$$

$$\sigma_\alpha = \frac{8\pi^2 R_p^3}{\lambda} \left[\frac{\epsilon_p(\omega) - \epsilon_m}{\epsilon_p(\omega) + 2\epsilon_m} \right] \qquad (9.33)$$

where R_p is the radius of a metal nanoparticle. Similarly the scattering cross section is

$$\sigma_\beta = \frac{128\pi^5}{\lambda^4} R_p^6 \left[\frac{\epsilon_p(\omega) - \epsilon_m}{\epsilon_p(\omega) + 2\epsilon_m} \right] \qquad (9.34a)$$

$$\sigma_\beta = \frac{8\pi k^4}{3} R_p^6 |\mu|^2 \qquad (9.34b)$$

where μ is the polarizability of a metallic sphere. The extinction cross section of a spherical particle is a measure of the reduction in intensity of transmitted light for a specific medium, and is defined as $\sigma_{ext} = \sigma_\alpha + \sigma_\beta$. The extinction efficiency, η_{ext}, of a particle is the normalized extinction cross section of an area.

$$\eta_{ext} = \frac{\sigma_{ext}}{\pi R_p^2} \tag{9.35}$$

9.3.3 Physics of surface plasmon resonance (SPR)

(a) Definition

There are three cases where one can deal with plasmon resonance phenomena:

(i) Bulk metal, (ii) Metal surface, and (iii) Localized surface plasmon resonance (LSPR). Here, the last case is considered. Briefly, the conduction band electrons in metals can be considered as essentially free electrons where the presence of the periodic distribution of positively charged core atoms is classified by their effective mass. Upon interaction of electromagnetic field of an incident light, such as laser with a metal nanoparticle, polarization of the conduction electrons is produced with respect to the much heavier positive core ions. This is schematically illustrated in Fig. 9.14.

The polarization can oscillate (i.e., displaced) under the direct influence of oscillating electric field, hence producing plasmonic oscillations. The so-called surface plasmon resonances (SPR) are of great importance at a metal-dielectric interface and the nanoparticle plasmon resonances (NPPR) have a key influential role on the optical spectra of metallic particles. For small (~30 nm) monodisperse GNP the SPR phenomena causes an absorption of light in the blue-green portion of the spectrum (~450 nm), while red light (~700 nm) is reflected, yielding a rich red color. Sometimes it is preferred to use the term NPPR instead of LSPR as it shows some differences to surface plasmons. Strictly speaking, the term palsmonic resonance is not same as plasmon, as the first one originates from electrodynamic discussions (i.e., interaction of light with matter), whereas the second is more related to particle nature from quantum mechanical point of view. Also, it may be argued that a more correct term to use is plasmon-polaritons as they are a combined entity of photons and plasmons. However, for simplicity, it is generally used as just plasmons.

(b) SPR process

In the interaction process of an electromagnetic source such as laser with a nanostructure, SPR occurs in the following steps:

(i) Field coupling, (ii) Displacement of charges, (iii) Dielectric polarization, and (iv) Harmonic oscillator.

Let us assume the total energy U of an electromagnetic field is obtained by integration over the corresponding volume V of spherical nanoparticles,

$$U = \varepsilon_0 \int_V |E(r)|^2 d^3r \tag{9.36}$$

where an oscillating photon with frequency ω has energy $E_p = \hbar\omega$. One can obtain the average field strength

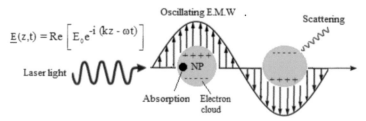

Figure 9.14. Illustration of e.m.w. (e.g., laser) interaction with gold nanoparticle and induced charge polarization followed by its subsequent oscillation.

$$<|\underline{E}|> = \sqrt{h\omega/\varepsilon_0 V} \tag{9.37}$$

that corresponds to one photon. This quantity is important if, for example, we want to describe the coupling of particle to the field oscillation. For monochromatic planar waves the characteristic solution of the Helmholtz equation is

$$(\nabla^2 + k^2)\underline{E}(r) = 0 \tag{9.38}$$

in Cartesian coordinate (x,y,z):

$$(\frac{\partial^2}{\partial x^2} + \frac{\partial^2}{\partial y^2} + \frac{\partial^2}{\partial z^2} + k^2)\underline{E}(r) = 0 \tag{9.39}$$

These waves are vector waves with constant polarization vector and amplitude E_0. Recalling the equation (9.23) where the wave vector is defined by k.z. Now, in conducting materials such as gold (Au), charges can move freely, but under influence of an applied external time varying electric field (e.g., laser) accelerates electrically charged particles, and in doing so it generates polarization and current through displacement of charges. As a result of this polarization, a dipole moment is induced within the particle. Thus by using Maxwell's equation for time varying fields, we get

$$\nabla \times \underline{H} = j + \frac{\partial}{\partial t}D \tag{9.40}$$

where D is dielectric displacement given by

$$D = E\varepsilon_0(1 + \chi_e) \tag{9.41a}$$

$$D = E\varepsilon_0\varepsilon_r = E\varepsilon \tag{9.41b}$$

where ε_r is relative permittivity, and

$$\frac{\partial D}{\partial t} = J_{dis} + J_{pol} \tag{9.42}$$

with J_{dis} and J_{pol} are displacement and polarization currents, respectively. Displacement currents not usually as important as the currents arising due to the motion of free charges, but if J = 0 then the displacement current is the only current present. Dielectrics are classified according to their response to the external field. The polarization may be directly proportional to E, in which case we speak of a *linear* dielectric. If in addition the electrical properties of the dielectric are independent of direction the dielectric is referred to as linear *isotropic* dielectric and

$$P = E\varepsilon_0\chi_e \tag{9.43}$$

where χ_e the electrical susceptibility is a constant. If the polarization is proportional to the electric field, χ_e is *linear* (i.e., χ_e^1), if not then the relation become *non-linear* (i.e., χ_e^2, χ_e^3). When the polarization significantly increases with increasing E, the property is used for special functions such as oscillators. The incident of an electromagnetic field on a nanoparticle surface causes surface polarizability of the charges P′ of the particle free electron conduction electrons. The movement of these charges has a resonance due to equilibrium consideration described by

$$P' = 4\pi\varepsilon_0 R_p^3 \left[\frac{\varepsilon_p(\omega) - \varepsilon_m}{\varepsilon_p(\omega) + 2\varepsilon_m} \right] \tag{9.44}$$

The dielectric response of a metal nanoparticle to electromagnetic radiation is given by the complex dielectric constant defined by Eq. (9.26)

$$k_{SP} = \frac{\omega}{c}\sqrt{\frac{\varepsilon_p\varepsilon_m}{\varepsilon_p + \varepsilon_m}} \tag{9.45}$$

where ksp is the surface plasmon wave vector, ω is the angular frequency of light. If, however, the nanostructure is a nanoshell then the Eq. (9.42) can be rewritten as

$$k_{SP} = \frac{\omega}{c}\sqrt{\frac{\varepsilon_c \varepsilon_s}{\varepsilon_c + \varepsilon_s}} \tag{9.46}$$

and ε_c and ε_s represent the core (e.g., SiO_2) and shell (e.g., Au) dielectric constant, respectively. The real part of complex dielectric constant ε_r, Eq. (9.28a), determines the degree to which the metal polarizes in response to an applied external electric field and determines the SPR spectral peak position. The imaginary part ε_r, Eq. (9.28b), quantifies the relative phase shift $\Delta\phi$ of the induced polarization with respect to the external field, i.e., it determines the bandwidth and includes losses such as ohmic heat loss.

$$\Delta\phi = \Delta\left[\frac{2\pi(n_r - ik_e)}{\lambda}\right]2R_p \tag{9.47}$$

Another important quantity in a metal dielectric response is the plasmon frequency defined as

$$\omega_p^2 = \frac{n_e e^2}{m_{eff}\varepsilon_0} \tag{9.48}$$

where n_e is the density of electrons, e is the electron charge (1.6×10^{-19} C), and ε_0 is the vacuum dielectric constant permittivity (8.85×10^{-12} Fm^{-1}). We know that the dimensions of metallic nanoparticles are so small that light can easily penetrate the whole nanoparticle (unlike the thin-film interface) and grasp at all conduction band electrons. The results in the sea of conduction band electrons that is displaced with respect to positively charged ions from the metallic lattice. Therefore, the electric dipole on the nanoparticle represents a storing force and hence it can be considered as harmonic oscillator, driven by a light wave and damped by some ohmic losses, e.g., heat or as radiative (scattering) losses as mentioned above. The latter is equivalent to the re-emission of photon on the expense of nanoparticle plasmon (NPP) excitation. Since the NPPs are localized, we do not have to worry about the wave vectors in their excitation. We can always excite a spherical metal NPPR regardless of the incident radiation direction. The only required condition is to choose the correct wavelength to satisfy the SPR.

9.3.4 Harmonic oscillators and energy loss

The interaction of e.m.w. radiation with metal nanoparticles results in interparticles forces and torques, hence moving them into new positions. These changes will affect all optical responses of aggregates due to their strong dependence on the interparticle distance. The dynamics of nanoparticles in an optical electromagnetic field can be an important factor, particularly for those without fixed positions, such as nanoparticles in solutions or nanoparticles assembled by organic or biomolecules. It is noteworthy that biological matters are polarizable and indeed the subject of matter polarizable goes back to Loretnz. In his model, electrons that are considered are harmonically bound to an ionic core with a spring (i.e., oscillatory atomic bond) and oscillating at optical frequencies ω. The resulting electric dipole on the nanoparticle represents a restoring force, and hence the nanoparticle can be considered as a harmonic oscillator, driven by light wave and damped by some losses, such as ohmic losses of heat and radiative (scattering) losses. The scattering is equivalent to the re-emission of a photon on the expense of nanoparticle plasmon excitation. The restoring force F_r is

$$F_r = m_p\omega_0^2 x \tag{9.49}$$

where m_p is mass of the nanoparticle, ω_0 is frequency of oscillator, and x is the displacement of nanoparticle in the opposite direction from the origin. Assuming that damping of the oscillator is caused by release of the radiation energy, the damping force given by

$$F_d = -m_p\gamma\left(\frac{dx}{dt}\right) \tag{9.50}$$

where γ is the damping rate and $\gamma \ll \omega$. The polarizability of a harmonic oscillator m_p carrying a total charge Q in an alternating field E of frequency ω is obtained from the equation of motion. The displacement x(t) at time t satisfies the equation

$$m_p \frac{d^2 x(t)}{dt^2} = QE(t) - kx(t) \tag{9.51}$$

where the right hand side is the net force. At any time the induced dipole is Qx(t), which is by definition equal to $P'(\omega)$ E(t). This allows us to substitute for E(t) in terms of x(t) and using Eq. (9.44) we find

$$m_p \frac{d^2 x(t)}{dt^2} = \left[\frac{Q^2}{P'(\omega)} - m\omega_o^2 \right] x(t) \tag{9.52}$$

We assume that $E(t) = E_0\, e^{i\omega t}$ and the solution is in the form of $x(t) = x_0\, e^{i\omega t}$ driven at the same frequency. Substituting in Eq. (9.52) shows that this solution requires the polarizability to be given by

$$P'(\omega) = \frac{Q^2}{m_p\left(\omega_0^2 - \omega^2\right)} \tag{9.53}$$

In this model, the polarizability increases as the frequency increases, as long as $\omega < \omega_0$. We know that an oscillating dipole radiates electromagnetic waves. This damps the oscillation, causing the displacement to become out of phase with driving field and requiring an input of energy to sustain the oscillation. These effects modify the polarizability. If we introduce a damping force to the right hand side of Eq. (9.51), we get

$$P'(\omega) = \frac{Q^2 / m_p}{\omega_0^2 - \omega^2 + i\gamma} \tag{9.54}$$

Therefore, polarizability becomes complex, its imaginary part indicating a component of induced dipole out of phase with the driving field.

Potential and Field due to electric dipole

As it was defined before, an electric dipole in its simplest form consists of equal and opposite electric charges ±q separated by scalar distance d (this in the case of nanoparticle would be the distance from positive nuclei to free electrons of conduction band). The magnitude of the dipole is qd and from the potential due to a point charge, as we can see in Fig. 9.15.
we write

$$V = \frac{q}{4\pi\varepsilon_0} \left[\frac{1}{r+} - \frac{1}{r-} \right] \tag{9.55}$$

Using the cosine rule and assuming that field point is sufficiently far away from the dipole such that $r \gg d$, where r is the distance from the center of d to the field point N (i.e., dN in Fig. 9.15)

$$V = \frac{q}{4\pi\varepsilon_0} \frac{d \cos\theta}{r^2} \tag{9.56}$$

or in terms of the dipole p = qd

$$V = \frac{p.\, r}{4\pi\varepsilon_0} \tag{9.57}$$

Equation (9.57) equally applies for an electric dipole, irrespective of whether p arises from a pair of charges or from a more complex distribution of electric charge when

$$p = \sum q_i r_i + \int r\rho(r)d\tau \tag{9.58}$$

where $\rho(r)$ and $d\tau$ are volume charge density distribution and volume element, respectively, so $dq = \rho(r)\, d\tau$. The electric field E can be found from $E = -\nabla .V$, thus

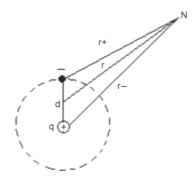

Figure 9.15. Diagram representing the magnitude of a dipole (i.e., qd) and from the field point N such that $r \gg d$, where r is the distance from the centre of d to the field point N.

$$E = -\nabla \left[\frac{p.r}{4\pi\varepsilon_0 r^3} \right] \tag{9.59}$$

After some substitution and simplification we obtain

$$E = \frac{1}{4\pi\varepsilon_0} \left[\frac{3(p.r)r - r^2 p}{r^5} \right] \tag{9.60}$$

Therefore, the electric field due to a dipole decreases faster (r^{-3}) than due to a single point charge or monopole (r^{-2}), because in the dipole case the equal and opposite charges help cancel out each other's effect. There are three cases: (i) Near zone: $d \ll r \ll \lambda$, (ii) Intermediate zone: $d \ll r \sim \lambda$ and (iii) Far zone: $d \ll \lambda \ll r$.

9.3.5 Propagation of dipole moment-induced radiation in a medium

The problem in free space is relatively straight forward compared to when a dipole is placed inside a medium. To appreciate how complicated this situation can be, it suffice to remind the following possibilities: (i) Medium can be homogenous or inhomogeneous, (ii) A dipole can be considered without being subject to an external light source either incoherent or coherent, hence self-generated dynamic equations of motion due to coulombic forces, (iii) A dipole can be subject to any of the above sources, hence the corresponding and appropriate equations of motions, (iv) A single dipole to be considered, (v) Multi-dipoles to be considered, (vi) A single or multi-dipoles can be considered as stationary, linear, or rotating depending on the applied field polarization. Here it is intended to consider a case where a single dipole (i.e., one nanoparticle) is placed inside an inhomogeneous medium (e.g., a biological medium such as tissue or cell), and is subject to external laser field.

This is refers to a condition where the dipole moments are oscillating and the resulting re-emitted e.m.w. is propagating within a medium. In the presence of matter the e.m.w. problem can become very difficult and solving the maxwell's equations when real media are involved is a very complicated problem. In this respect, one major difference between non-conducting and conduction medium is the attenuation which occurs in the latter case. For an isotropic and homogeneous linear conducting medium and obeying Ohm's law, $J = \Upsilon E$, where Υ is conductivity, Maxwell's equations become

$$\nabla^2 E - \mu\Upsilon \frac{\partial E}{\partial t} - \mu\varepsilon \frac{\partial^2 E}{\partial t^2} = 0 \tag{9.61a}$$

$$\nabla^2 H - \mu\Upsilon \frac{\partial H}{\partial t} - \mu\varepsilon \frac{\partial^2 H}{\partial t^2} = 0 \tag{9.61b}$$

The electric and magnetic fields still have the main features but the electric vector varies as follows

$$E = E_0 e^{i(kz-\omega t)} e^{(-Cz)} \tag{9.62}$$

$$C = \sqrt{\frac{\omega\mu\Upsilon}{2}} > 0 \tag{9.63}$$

where μ is permeability of medium and the refractive index of medium is related to complex permittivity by Eq. (9.27). The maximum amplitude of the electric (and magnetic) vector thus decreases as it travels along the z-axis, and this process is called attenuation. It is important to note that a wave cannot propagate in a conduction medium without attenuation. Thus, high frequency e.m.w. propagates only a very small distance in a conducting medium. The electric field is confined to a very small region at the surface and that significant currents will flow only at the surface and the resistance of the medium therefore, increases with frequency. Similarly, to reach the far field position (i.e., $d \ll \lambda \ll r$) within the medium, low frequency oscillations are more appropriate due to lower attenuation.

Now we turn our focus on the importance of metallic nanostructures, which originates from their ability to absorb and scatter the incident light in both the visible and infrared regions. The electromagnetic properties of a material are represented by the relative permittivity ε_r and the relative permeability μ_r both of which are complex. We have

$$n^2 = \varepsilon_r \mu_r \tag{9.64}$$

and we take the solution with Im (n) $\gg$ 0. The interaction of an electromagnetic field of a laser defined by Eq. (9.23) with plasmonic nanoparticles causes the dielectric polarization, P, of surface charges, as a result of which charges oscillate like simple dipole moment. Such dipole is often referred to as a *Hertzian oscillator* and radiates E.M.W. We assume a time harmonic-dependence which allows us to write the current density as

$$j(r,t) = \text{Re}\left[j(r)e^{-i\omega t} \right] \tag{9.65a}$$

and the dipole moment as

$$p(r,t) = \text{Re}\left[p(r)e^{-i\omega t} \right] \tag{9.65b}$$

The equation of motion of a harmonically oscillating dipole in an inhomogeneous medium under external field can be written

$$\frac{d^2}{dt^2}p(t) + \gamma_0 \frac{d}{dt}p(t) + \omega_0^2 p(t) = \frac{q^2}{m_s}E(t) \tag{9.66}$$

where ω_0 is the oscillating frequency and m_s is the mass of system (electrons and nuclei). Note that for homogenous medium the right hand side of the Eq. (9.66) is equal to zero. The trial solutions for dipole moment and driving field when conductivity $\Upsilon > 0$ are

$$p(t) = \text{Re}\left[p_0 e^{-i\omega t} \cdot e^{-i\gamma t/2} \right] \tag{9.67}$$

and

$$E(t) = \text{Re}\left[E_0 e^{-i\omega t} \cdot e^{-i\gamma t/2} \right] \tag{9.68}$$

where γ and ω are the new decay rate and resonance frequency, respectively. It is assumed that $\gamma \ll \omega$ and that

$$\omega^2 p_0 \ll \frac{q^2}{m_s}E_0 \tag{9.69}$$

Rate of energy dissipation of emitted power in an inhomogeneous medium

For an oscillating electric dipole embedded in such a medium, the complex amplitude of the emitted electric and magnetic fields are

$$E_p(r) = -\frac{1}{3\varepsilon_0\varepsilon_r} p\delta(r) + \mu_r \frac{k^3}{4\pi\varepsilon_0}$$

$$\times \left\{ p - (\hat{r}.p)\hat{r} + \left[p - 3(\hat{r}.p)\hat{r} \right] \frac{i}{nq}\left(1 + \frac{i}{nq}\right) \right\} \times \frac{e^{inq}}{q} \tag{9.70}$$

$$B_p(r) = \frac{n\mu_r}{c} \frac{k^3}{4\pi\varepsilon_0}(\hat{r}\times p)\left(1 + \frac{i}{nq}\right)\frac{e^{inq}}{q} \tag{9.71}$$

where $p(t) = \text{Re}\ (p_0\ e^{-i\omega t})$ is electric dipole moment and $p_0 = q_0\ r$ is complex amplitude, $k = \omega/c = 2\pi/\lambda$ is the wavenumber, $\hat{r}$ is radial unit vector, and n is the refractive index. The first term on the right-hand side of (9.70) is the self-field, which only exists inside the point source. The rest of terms represent outgoing spherical waves. The energy flow of wave in a medium is represented by time-averaged Poynting vector is defined as

$$S(r) = \frac{1}{2\mu_0} \text{Re}\left[\frac{1}{\mu_r} E(r)^* \times B(r)\right] \tag{9.72}$$

The factor ½ comes from time averaging the fields. According to Poynting's theorem, the radiated power of any current distribution with a harmonic time dependence in a linear medium has to be identical to the rate of energy dissipation U = dW/dt given by

$$\frac{dW}{dt} = -\frac{1}{2} \int_V \text{Re}\left[j^*.E\right] dV \tag{9.73}$$

where j^* is complex conjugate of current density j and V is the source volume (e.g., NP). The current density $j = j_s + j_c$ where j_s generates the fields, and j_c represents loss of current which is associated with thermal losses. In either way, j represents both energy sources and energy sinks. We can write

$$\frac{dW}{dt} = \frac{\omega}{2} \text{Im}\left[p^*.\ E(r_0)\right] \tag{9.74}$$

where the field E is assessed at the dipole's origin r_0. The importance of equation (9.74) is appreciated when we consider an emitting dipole in an inhomogeneous medium. The rate of energy released can be determined by integrating the pointing vector over a surface enclosing the dipole emitter. To do this, we need to know the electromagnetic field everywhere on the enclosing surface. For an inhomogeneous environment, this field is superposition of the dipole field E_p and the scattered field E_s from the environment. Thus, to determine the energy dissipated by the dipole, one needs to evaluate the electromagnetic field everywhere on the surface. This can be done for the total field at the dipole's origin r_0 by using equation (9.73).

$$E\ (r_0) = E_p(r_0) + E_s(r_0) \tag{9.75}$$

Substituting Eq. (9.75) in (9.74) allows us to separate the rate of energy dissipation U = dW/dt into two parts and the contribution from E_p is

$$U_0 = \frac{n_m p^2 \omega\ k^3}{12\pi\varepsilon_0\varepsilon_p} = \frac{n_m (qd)^2\omega^4}{12\pi\varepsilon_0\varepsilon_p c^3} \tag{9.76}$$

Here n_m is the refractive index of the dipole surrounding medium and ε_p is the permittivity of dipole. The normalized rate of energy dissipation becomes

$$\frac{U}{U_0} = 1 + \frac{6\pi\varepsilon_0\varepsilon_p}{p^3} \frac{1}{k^3} \text{Im}\left[p^* . E_s(r_0)\right] \qquad (9.77)$$

Therefore, the change of energy dissipation depends on the secondary (scattered) field of the dipole. This field corresponds to the dipole's own initial emitted field and arrives at the position of the dipole after it has been scattered in the medium.

To highlight the major points: There is a difference between SPRs and NP resonances (NPPR) in that the excitation of SPR is that the wave vectors of the propagating SPRs and the photons must match. However, in the case of NPPR do not propagate and on the scale of light wavelength they are in fact localized, which is the reason why they are called LPR. One can always excite a metal nanoparticle regardless of the incident light direction, as long as a correct wavelength is used to match the resonance of nanoparticle oscillation. Therefore, thinking in terms of appropriate applications perhaps this accounts a major advantage for biosensors. In the limit of nanoparticles defined by Rayleigh limit, the spectral position of the resonance is independent of the shape of nanoparticles. The only geometrical factor that involves is the volume, but again it determines the scattering and absorption cross sections, and not their spectral position. Normally, the condition for Rayleigh scattering is $R_p \ll \lambda/20$ and size parameter $x = 2\pi Rp/\lambda < 1$, and as the size of nanoparticle increases, it approaches Mie scattering limit, i.e., $Rp \gg \lambda/20$ and that $x > 1$. The plasmonic nanoparticles can act as a dipole source inside either an homogeneous or inhomogeneous medium, where the rate energy flow and radiated power dissipation can be represented by Poynting vector. The biomedical application of such line of analysis together with use thermodynamics and chaos would be to investigate the effects of interaction of such laser-induced plasmonic radiation and its secondary emitted radiation on the cellular contents such as mitochondria or in fact the cell's membrane itself.

9.3.6 *Laser-induced heating effect by gold nanoparticles*

When initially a metal nanoparticle such as gold is illuminated by a pulsed or modulated laser, depending on the wavelength, the optical properties and the size of NP, the beam is partly scattered in the surroundings and partly is absorbed, which is then converted into heat. The heating effect is then quickly equilibrated within the NP ensemble. Subsequently, the heat is transferred from the NPs to the surrounding medium or matrix via non-radiative relaxation within a few ps leading to an elevated temperature of the surrounding medium. Heat generation becomes especially strong in the case of metal NPs in the regime of SPR. The efficiency of each of these processes can be characterized by σ_α and σ_β, as defined by equations (9.33) and (9.34). Normally, scattering processes dominate for NPs with diameters larger than ~ 50 nm. In the absence of phase transformations, the temperature distribution around optically-stimulated plasmonic nanoparticles (i.e., heat transfer) placed in a surrounding medium is described by the paraboloic Fourier's heat conduction equation. However, in a number of cases such as those in biomedical applications where NPa are probably placed inside tissue or cells, it takes some time for absorbed photons to generate heat. In this case, it is more appropriate to use hyperbolic non-Fourier's model to account this delay, see §6.2.

$$\rho_g(r) c_g(r) \frac{\partial T(r,t)}{\partial t} = K_m \nabla^2 T(r,t) + Q_T(r,t) \qquad (9.78)$$

where $T(r,t)$ is local temperature, Q is the heating source, $\rho_g(r)$ and $c_g(r)$ are density, and specific heat of a GNP, respectively, K_m is the thermal conductivity of the surrounding medium. The total amount of heat produced is $Q_T = Q_m + Q_g$, where Q_m and Q_g represent the heat produced by medium and gold NPs, respectively.

For a single GNP exposed to a laser beam the power of heat generation is

$$P = I \sigma_\alpha \qquad (9.80)$$

where σ_α is defined by equation (9.33) and

$$I = \frac{n_m c_0 \varepsilon_0}{2} |E|^2 \qquad (9.81)$$

Substituting (9.33) and (9.81) in (9.80) and simplifying we obtain

$$P = \frac{4\pi^2 R_P^3}{\lambda} \left[\frac{\varepsilon_g(\omega) - \varepsilon_m(\omega)}{\varepsilon_g(\omega) + 2\varepsilon_m(\omega)} \right] \cdot n_m c_0 \varepsilon_0 |E|^2 \qquad (9.82a)$$

$$P = 2\pi\omega R_P^3 \left[\frac{\varepsilon_g(\omega) - \varepsilon_m(\omega)}{\varepsilon_g(\omega) + 2\varepsilon_m(\omega)} \right] \cdot n_m \varepsilon_0 |E|^2 \qquad (9.82b)$$

Also, $Q_g = P/V_g$ where V_g is the volume of the NP. Thus, the heat source is derived from the heat power density as

$$h_\rho(r) = \int_v h_\rho(r) \, d^3r \qquad (9.83)$$

where the integral is over the NP volume V_g. To calculate $Q_g(r,t)$, we assume the size of a NP is smaller than the laser wavelength so that electrons inside the NPs respond collectively to the applied electric field of the laser radiation,

$$E = E_0 \frac{3\varepsilon_m}{\varepsilon_g + 2\varepsilon_m} \qquad (9.84)$$

and

$$Q_g(r,t) = \, <j(r,t) \cdot E(r,t)> = \frac{\omega}{8\pi} |E|^2 \, \mathrm{Im} \, \varepsilon_g \qquad (9.85)$$

Substituting (9.84) in (9.85), it yields

$$Q_g(r,t) = \frac{\omega}{8\pi} \left| E_0 \frac{3\varepsilon_m}{\varepsilon_g + 2\varepsilon_m} \right|^2 \mathrm{Im} \, \varepsilon_g = \frac{\omega}{8\pi} E_0^2 \left| \frac{3\varepsilon_m}{\varepsilon_g + 2\varepsilon_m} \right|^2 \mathrm{Im} \, \varepsilon_g \qquad (9.86)$$

This is valid when the wavelength is much larger than NP radius (i.e., $\lambda \gg R_p$) and $j(r,t)$ is the current density inside the metallic NP and the heat generated is thus directly proportional to the square modulus of the NP electric field (Govorov and Richardson 2007). The temperature distribution $T(r)$ of NPs in an aqueous environment similar to tissue generated by the heating power density distribution $Q_T(r,t)$ is governed by Poission equation

$$K\nabla^2 T(r) = -Q(r,t) \qquad (9.87)$$

Temperature inside the sphere is not really important since we are mainly concerned with the surface temperature. The temperature spatial variation δT throughout the structure,

$$\delta T \approx \frac{d^2 Q}{K_P V_P} \qquad (9.88)$$

where K_P is the thermal conductivity of NP (for gold it is 318 Wm^{-1} K^{-1}), V_p is the volume of NP and is the typical spatial dimension of the structure. Based on the Eq. (9.88), $\delta T \approx 0.1°C$ along the NP which indicates that the thermal diffusion is rapid and remains almost uniform even though the heating undergoes strong spatial variations. The temperature outside the NP when $r > R_p$ where r is the distance from the center of NP, is simply

$$\Delta T = \frac{P_{abs}}{4\pi R_P K_P} = \frac{QV_P}{4\pi R_P K_P} = \frac{I\sigma_{abs}}{4\pi R_P K_P} \qquad (9.89)$$

The heat generation is given by Eq. (9.86). The maximum temperature increase occurs at $r = R_p$ and is given by

$$\Delta T_{max}(I_0) = \frac{R_P^2}{3K_m} \frac{\omega}{8\pi} \left| \frac{3\varepsilon_m}{\varepsilon_g + 2\varepsilon_m} \right|^2 \mathrm{Im} \, \varepsilon_g \frac{8\pi.I_0}{c\sqrt{\varepsilon_m}} \qquad (9.90a)$$

$$\Delta T_{max}(I_0) = \frac{R_p^2}{3K_m} \frac{\omega}{8\pi} \left| \frac{3\varepsilon_m}{\varepsilon_g + 2\varepsilon_m} \right|^2 Im\left(\frac{\varepsilon_g - \varepsilon_m}{\varepsilon_g + 2\varepsilon_m} \right) \frac{8\pi.I_0}{c\sqrt{\varepsilon_m}} \tag{9.90b}$$

Equation (9.90) shows that temperature of the medium containing plasmonic nanoparticles is proportional to the square of the nanoparticle radius, i.e., $\Delta T \propto R_p^2$. There are two factors leading to this dependence:

(i) the total heat generation rate inside the NP is given by $V_p Q$ and is proportional to the NP volume, and (ii) the total heat current from the NP surface is given by $K_m A_p \partial T/\partial t$ where A_p is the NP surface area. Thus, from the energy balance equation and an estimate of $\partial \Delta T/\partial r \approx T/R_p$, one obtains

$$\Delta T_{max} \approx \frac{V_p.R_p}{A_p} \approx R_p^2 \tag{9.91}$$

This implies that the size dependence of the temperature increase is mainly governed by the total rate of heat generation and by heat transfer through the NP surface.

One practical consequence of the above discussion is in nanomedicine, where for example, the gold nanosystems: nanoparticles, nanoshells, and nanorods are selected for photothermal cancer therapy due to their resonance of the heat generation and can be tuned into the temperature spectral window of human tissue. Now, one may argue that for a spherical NP excited at its LSPR, the heating arises mainly from the outer part of the nanoparticles facing the incident laser radiation. Therefore, the major part of the NP can remain unaffected since it is covered by other nanoparticles or tissue, and hence does not contribute to heating. Equally, we may not be allowed to completely neglect the fact that quasiuniform heating of inside a NP can also obtained due to very rapid thermal diffusion, therefore, the inside of the NP heats up because of thermal conductivity of metal. In either way, the point is that this does not occur in the case of other nanostructures such as naorods (NR). First, because the LSPR markedly depends on the NP shape. In the case of NR, the surface plasmon divides into two parts of longitudinal and transverse as the aspect ratio of the ellipsoid is increased. In the former case, plasmon mode is is significantly red-shifted and the transverse plasmon blue-shifted slightly. In the case of NR, the inner part is closer to the outer part, and hence less such shielding effect occurs. Consequently, the whole volume of the structure is thus involved in the heating process.

9.3.7 Synthesis and evaluation of time dependent optical properties of plasmonic–magnetic nanoparticles (Fe₃O₄/Au) (Hassannejad and Khosroshahi 2013)

Magnetic-plasmonic nanostructures were synthesized and their optical properties investigated based on experimental results and theoretical calculations. Magnetite nanoparticles with diameter of 9.5 ± 1.4 nm were fabricated using coprecipitation method and subsequently covered by a thin layer of gold to obtain 15.8 ± 3.5 nm nanoshells measured by TEM micrographs. Crystalinity, surface chemistry, magnetic, and optical properties were also studied by XRD, FT-IR, VSM and UV-Vis spectroscopy, respectively. The plane indices data from XRD and calculated unit cell parameter proved the purity of the prepared magnetite nanoparticles. Magnetic saturation of synthesized magnetite nanoparticles reduced from 46.94 to 11.98 emu/g after coating with a thin layer of 5.8 ± 3.5 nm gold, but still is high enough to be used as contrast agents in magnetic resonance imaging (MRI). FT-IR results showed a successful functionalization of magnetite nanoparticles which was followed by gold coating. The changes of the optical properties of gold nanoshells during the shell growth based on self-assembly were studied by UV-Vis spectroscopy. In our case, a red Doppler shift of about 15% corresponding to 12 nm in surface plasmon resonance wavelength (λ_{SPR}) position was observed within the first minute of growth phase. This was followed by 45% of blue Doppler shift corresponding to 5 nm in two minutes. A good agreement between the UV-Vis spectra and calculated absorption efficiency was observed. The calculated scattering and absorption efficiencies and cross sections of prepared nanoshells have made them an efficient agent for photothermal cancer therapy.

Materials and methods

Chemical and reagents

All analytical reagents were used without further purification. Ferric chloride hexahydrate ($FeCl_3.6H_2O$, 99%), ferrous chloride tetrahydrate ($FeCl_2.4H_2O$, 99%), hydrochloric acid (HCl, 37%), sodium hydroxide, formaldehyde solution (H_2CO, 37%), and absolute ethanol were purchased from Merck. Gold (iii) chloride trihydrate ($HAuCl_4.3H_2O$, ≥ 49% Au basis), and 3-aminopropyltriethoxysilane (APTES) were purchased from sigma. Tetrakis (hydroxymethyl) phosphonim chloride (THPC) was an 80% aqueous solution from Aldrich. Deionized water (18 MΩ) was provided by a Milli-Q system and deoxygenated by vacuum for 1 hour prior to the use.

Magnetite nanoparticles fabrication

Magnetite nanoparticles (MNPs) were fabricated by following a previously reported procedure with some modification (Khosroshahi and Ghazanfari 2010). Briefly, $FeCl_2.4H_2O$ and $FeCl_3.6H_2O$ (3.18 g and 8.65 g, respectively) were added to 25 ml deoxygenated aqueous solution of 0.4 M HCl under vigorous stirring. Subsequently, the brownish yellow solution was added dropwise to 250 ml 1.5 M NaOH in a three naked flask equipped with mechanical stirring (1500 rpm) for 30 min at room temperature. This step generated an instant black precipitate. The synthesized nanoparticles were separated by a permanent magnet while the supernatant was removed out. The isolated precipitate was washed with deionized, deoxygenated H_2O for 5 times and followed by washing twice using absolute ethanol. The final precipitate was dried under vacuum at room temperature for 48 hours. All the synthesis steps were carried out under passing N_2 gas through the solution medium to eliminate oxygen contamination during reaction, and dried powder was stored under vacuum until further characterization.

Functionalization of magnetite nanoparticles

Amino groups were grafted on the nanoparticle surface by silanization reaction. Magnetite nanoparticles (0.074 g) were dispersed in 25 ml ethanol by probe sonicator for 30 min. This suspension was diluted to 150 ml by ethanol and 1 ml H_2O. 35 µl APTES was added to the prepared suspension under vigorous stirring (Ma et al. 2003). One ml H_2O was introduced into the reaction medium to initiate the hydrolysis. The synthesis operation proceeded for 7 hours at room temperature. Subsequently, functionalized magnetite nanoparticles were isolated by applying an external magnetic field and washed for 5 times to remove excess amines and then dried into powder under vacuum at room temperature.

Au nanoshell fabrication

Magnetite/gold nanoshells were prepared by a multistep procedure through electroless plating of Au onto nanoshell precursor particles (i.e., gold-seeded magnetite nanoparticles). A THPC gold solution composed of 2–3 nm gold colloids was produced according to Duff and Baker procedure (Duff and Baiker 1993) and aged for 2–3 weeks. Nanoshell precursor particles was prepared by adding 1 ml of 0.0128 M amine-terminated magnetite nanoparticles in ethanol into 40 ml THPC gold solution and 4 ml 1 M NaCl and left unperturbed for 12 hours at 4°C. This step was followed by washing and redispersion of nanoparticles in 10 ml deionized H_2O. The final concentration of precursor solution was 1.28 mM. A plating solution was prepared by mixing 3 ml $HAuCl_4$ (1%) with 200 ml aqueous solution of K_2CO_3 (1.8 mM) and aged for 2–3 days. A continuous gold shell was grown around the magnetite nanoparticles by adding 1 ml of precursor suspension to 9 ml of plating solution. For reduction of Au^{3+} 50 µl of H_2CO was quickly added into a 10 ml prepared suspension of precursor nanoparticles in plating solution in a glass vial and gently vortexed by hand for 10 s and subsequently aged for 15 min. The excess formaldehyde was removed by washing two times and the obtained gold coated magnetite nanoparticles were collected by centrifuge at 6000 g.

Results and discussion

TEM

The bright field TEM micrographs along with particle size distribution of particles at different steps of nanoshell fabrication are presented in Fig. 9.16. NIH ImageJ software (http://rsb.info.nih.gov/ij/) was used to measure size of particles. Uncoated MNPs show slight agglomeration, which may be due to the magnetic interaction. As seen, the mean average diameter of uncoated-MNPs is 9.5 ± 1.4 nm. The difference between the calculated sizes of nanoparticles from XRD results with TEM micrographs may be due to some disorders at the surface of nanoparticles. Growing of the gold shell increased the particle size to 15.3 ± 3.5 nm. The energy-dispersive X-ray spectroscopy (EDS) (Fig. 9.16d) confirms the formation of gold-seeded MNPs.

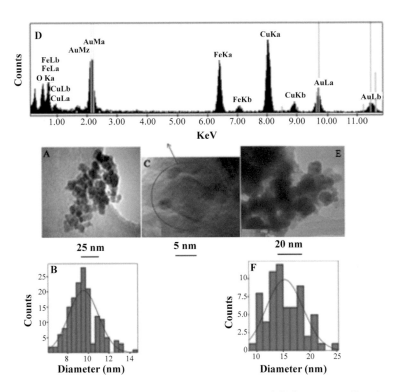

Figure 9.16. TEM images showing (a) MNPs of diameter 9.5 ± 1.4 nm and (b) its corresponding size distribution, (c) precursor nanoparticles and (d) its corresponding EDS pattern, (e) Fe_3O_4/Au nanoshells of diameter 15.3 ± 3.5 nm and (f) its corresponding size distribution.

VSM

The magnetization as a function of applied magnetic field of bare MNPs, precursor nanoparticles and nanoshells at 300 K is shown in Fig. 9.15. No hysteresis loop is observed for magnetite nanoparticle which implies their superparamagnetic behaviour. The saturation magnetization Ms of bare MNPs was determined to be 47.62 emu g^{-1} at 6 kOe which decrease to the 35.3 emu g^{-1} and 12 emu g^{-1} for precursor nanoparticles and nanoshells, respectively. In our case, the Ms value for obtained nanoshells is larger than that reported by (Xu et al. 2007) with the same Fe_3O_4 core size and 3.5 nm Au shell thickness.

Optical properties of Fe_3O_4/Au nanoshells

The critical optical properties of core-shell nanoparticles are—plasmon resonance wavelength, the extinction cross-sections, and the ratio of scattering to absorption efficiency at plasmon wavelength which

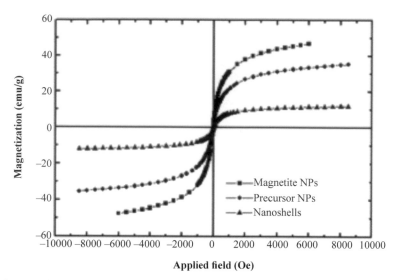

Figure 9.17. The magnetization as function of applied magnetic field of bare MNPs (-■-), precursor nanoparticles (-●-) and Fe$_3$O$_4$/Au nanoshells (-▲-) at 300 K.

determines the applications of any fabricated nanoparticles. In order to observe the changes of the optical properties of gold nanoshells during the shell growth, reaction of gold reduction was carried out in the spectrophotometer quartz cuvette and the absorption measurements recorded at times of 2, 3, 4, 5, and 16 minutes after addition of the formaldehyde to the mixture of precursor nanoparticles and Au^{3+} solution. The UV-Vis absorption spectrum of gold-seeded MNP shows no absorption peak. This is consistent with many literature reports that there is no SPR feature for such small Au particles (~2 nm) on the surface of magnetite nanoparticles (Levin et al. 2009). The change in the position of the surface plasmon resonance wavelength (λ_{SPR}) is presented in the inset of the Fig. 9.18a, where the absorption values of gold nanoshells is measured in terms of wavelength at various time. As shown, after 2 minutes a weak absorption peak appeared at 523 nm, which is the characteristic surface plasmon resonance of gold nanoparticles. Reduction of additional gold ions resulted in the subsequent growth and coalescence of the deposited gold nanoparticles and the formation of a thin Au shell on the surface of the precursor nanoparticles. This can be deduced from the red-shift of the λ_{SPR} to 536 nm as well as the color change of the solution to blue, which is characteristic of the nanoshells formed (Fig. 9.18b). The maximum red-shift of about 12 nm was observed over 3 minutes. As the reaction time progressed, the peak appeared to have a blue-shifted to about 531 nm. This is probably due to the fact that during this time, more Au^{3+} was reduced to Au^0 by formaldehyde on the surface of the precursor nanoparticles to form a thicker shell. The shift is accompanied by SPR peak narrowing, i.e., the full-width at half-maximum (FWHM) of Au nanoshell peak reduced from 0.29 eV after 3 minutes to 0.28 eV after 16 minutes.

The intensity of UV-Vis spectra increased as the shell growth proceeds, except for 16 minutes, where a slight decrease could be observed. Increase in shell thickness is expected to cause a corresponding increase in extinction coefficient due to a larger amount of plasmonic metal per particle. The decrease of the intensity in the last spectrum could be due to the slight aggregation of nanoshells in water. To further investigate this phenomenon, some part of nanoshell solution was refrigerated without washing and removal of formaldehyde for 1 week. The presence of formaldehyde can result in particle aggregation. The absorbance of aged nanoshells in comparison with those washed after 16 minutes is presented in Fig. 9.19. As is seen in the Fig. 9.19, plasmon resonance of obtained nanoshells red-shift to 535 nm as well as decrease in the absorption intensity is clearly observable. This can be attributed to the exciton-coupling of aggregated nanoparticles.

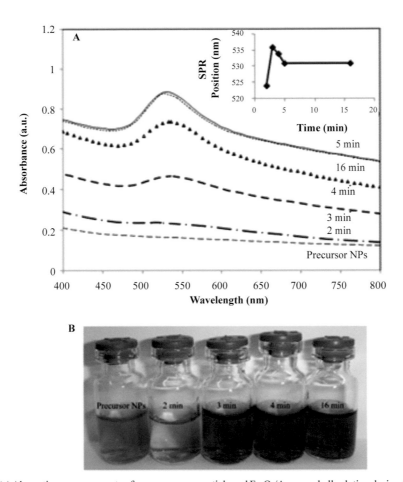

Figure 9.18. (a) Absorption measurements of precursor nanoparticle and Fe_3O_4/Au nanoshell solution during the shell growth until 16 min. The inset is corresponding SPR wavelength position as a function of time. Each spectrum is labeled by the corresponding reaction time. Optical image of nanoparticles is shown in (b).

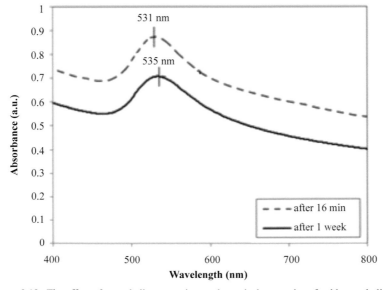

Figure 9.19. The effect of nanoshell aggregation on the optical properties of gold nanoshells.

Surface plasmon resonance induced by electric field of light results in strong electric field confined on the surface of the nanoparticles. The electric field at the surface of a metal nanoparticle in the dipolar mode is given by:

$$E_{surface} = \frac{(1+K)\varepsilon_m}{(\varepsilon_p + K\varepsilon_m)} E_0 \qquad (9.92)$$

where, K is a shape factor (for a sphere, $K = 2$), ε_m is dielectric constant of medium, ε_p is metal dielectric function, and E_0 is the incident field at frequencies corresponding to the LSPR. When two particles are brought together, the near-field at the surface of particles can interact with each other, which result in the red-shift of LSPR. As a result the electric field affects each particle and the total field is summation of the incident light E_0 and the near-field E_{nf} of the neighboring particle,

$$E = E_0 + E_{nf} \qquad (9.93)$$

The extent of the red-shift by self-assembly or aggregation of nanoparticles depends on the number of nanoparticles in ensemble as well as the distance between them (Storhoff et al. 2000). In a larger assembly each particle would be subject to the near-field of a large number of particles, resulting in a much stronger coupling and hence a larger red-shift. It has been shown by Liu et al. (2008) that assembly of three nanoshells make the SPR shifts approximately 8 nm toward the IR wavelength by adding each particle, i.e., 16 nm red shifted from the SPR of the first nanoshell by adding two other particles with the same size. In addition, it is shown that the absorption efficiency significantly decreases when nanoshells are placed closer to each other. If the separation between the nanoshells were long enough, the interaction can be ignored in near field accordingly (Liu et al. 2008). Then, the position of the λ_{SPR} and the absorption efficiency can be monitored to evaluate the stability of gold nanoparticles during storage time.

Pham et al. (2008) could synthesize the polydisperse Au-Fe oxide nanoshells with the size of 15–40 nm, which exhibited a SPR wavelength at 528 nm. The magnetic-plasmonic nanoparticles produced (Lim et al. 2008) had an 18 nm iron oxide core and a gold shell thickness of 5 nm with a SPR peak at 605 nm. Also, Liu et al. (2010) reported a λ_{SPR} of 590 nm for PVP-coated gold nanoshells with a total and core size of 8 nm and 3–6 nm, respectively. In our case, a λ_{SPR} of 531 nm was obtained for nanoshells with a total size of 15.8 ± 3.5 nm and a shell thickness of about 6 nm, which corresponds to 5 nm blue shift. The higher λ_{SPR} reported for some synthesized nanoshells with the same size may be due to the formation of an incomplete shell layer during the reduction of Au^{3+} with different reducing agents (Ma et al. 2003). Some reported TEM micrographs exhibit a discrete Au islands on the nanostructure surface (Lim et al. 2008).

The scattering and absorption efficiencies (Q_{sca} and Q_{abs}) and cross sections (C_{sca} and C_{abs}) for synthesized magnetic-plasmonic nanoshells were calculated using classical Mie scattering theory (Bohren and Huffman 1983). The required parameters were the dimensions of nanoshell, as well as the complex dielectric function of gold and magnetite. The values of complex dielectric functions for gold and magnetite at different wavelengths were obtained from literature (Johnson and Christy 1972, Goossens et al. 2006). The embedding medium was considered to be water with a refractive index n_m of $1.33 + 0i$. The comparison of theoretical calculation with experimental data is depicted in Fig. 9.20. The larger FWHM of experimental curve can be attributed to the polydispersity of particle size as well as reduced mean free path of conduction electrons. There is a good agreement between the experimental and theoretical curves at wavelengths smaller than λ_{SPR}. But in experimental results, the curve tail progressively increased beyond λ_{SPR}. In analyzing this difference, it is intended to assign this observation to the existence of solution-stable agreements of gold nanoshells (Kemal et al. 2008). As described before, coupling of the LSPR of nanoshells can cause a red-shift of λ_{SPR} as well as broadening of the SPR band.

The cross-sections can be converted to the molar coefficients measured by spectrophotometer through the following equation (Brullot et al. 2011):

$$\varepsilon = \frac{C_i}{3.82 \times 10^{-21}} \qquad (9.94)$$

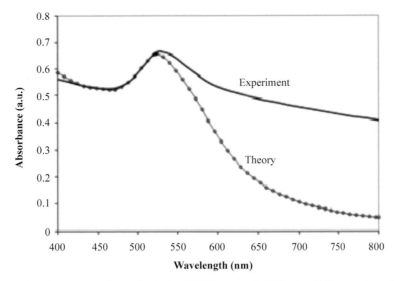

Figure 9.20. Comparison between experimentally obtained UV-Vis spectra (solid line) and Mie scattering calculations (dotted line) for Fe_3O_4/Au nanoshells of core diameter of 9.5 ± 1.5 and shell thickness of 6 ± 3.5.

where, ε is the molar coefficient (in $M^{-1}\ cm^{-1}$) and C_i is the relevant cross-section (in cm^2). The calculated values of extinction, scattering and absorption efficiencies and molar coefficients, as well as their corresponding cross sections of synthesized gold nanoshells for geometrical cross-sectional area of $183.76 \times 10^{-18}\ m^2$ and concentration of 1×10^{16} atom/cm^2 at λ_{SPR} are summarized in Table 9.2.

The calculated value of molar extinction coefficient for our gold nanoshells is $3.22 \times 10^9\ M^{-1}cm^{-1}$ at a λ_{SPR} of 531 nm. This value is 5 orders of magnitude larger than the molar extinction coefficient of indocyanine green ($1.08 \times 10^4\ M^{-1}\ cm^{-1}$), which is a NIR dye commonly used in laser photothermal treatments (Nourbakhsh and Khosroshahi 2011). The cross section is a measure of the effectiveness of the interaction between two particles, i.e., photons and nanoparticles. Nevertheless, the absolute magnitude of the optical cross section does not provide a reliable measure for the optical properties of an ensemble of nanoparticles, because in a given volume greater number of small nanoparticles can be placed than larger particles. Therefore, a more meaningful characteristic for comparison across a range of sizes is the size-normalized cross section or volumetric coefficient C/V where V is the particle volume (Bohren and Huffman 1983). In our case, the volumetric coefficients for absorption μ_a and scattering μ_s are 64 μm^{-1} and 1.2 μm^{-1}, respectively, and the ratio of μ_s/μ_a is 0.02. The higher value of μ_a than μ_s makes our synthesized nanoshell an efficient agent for photothermal therapy.

Under steady-state condition and with the assumption that all the energy absorbed from the incident light is converted to thermal energy, the surface heat flux $\dot{q}$ (W m^{-2}) from a single particle can be calculated from the following equation (Harris et al. 2006):

$$\dot{q} = \frac{1}{4}\int_{\lambda_1}^{\lambda_2} Q_{abs} E_\lambda\, d\lambda \tag{9.95}$$

where Q_{abs} is the absorption coefficient, E_λ is the spectral irradiance of the light source (W $m^{-2}\,nm^{-1}$), and λ is the wavelength of light.

Table 9.2. The calculated values of extinction, scattering and absorption efficiencies and molar coefficients as well as their corresponding cross sections of synthesized gold nanoshells.

	Extinction	Scattering	Absorption
Q	0.669	0.0123	0.656
C (m^2)	1.23×10^{-16}	2.26×10^{-18}	1.2×10^{-16}
ε ($M^{-1}cm^{-1}$)	3.22×10^9	5.92×10^6	3.14×10^9

9.3.8 *Synthesis and functionalization of SiO₂ coated Fe₃O₄ nanoparticles with amine groups based on self-assembly* (Khosroshahi and Ghazanfari 2012)

The purpose of this research was to synthesize amino modified Fe_3O_4/SiO_2 nanoshells for biomedical applications. Magnetic iron-oxide nanoparticles (NPs) were prepared via co-precipitation. The NPs were then modified with a thin layer of amorphous silica as described by Stober. The particle surface was then terminated with amine groups. The results showed that smaller particles can be synthesized by decreasing the NaOH concentration, which in our case this corresponded to 35 nm using 0.9 M of NaOH at 750 rpm with a specific surface area of 41 m^2 g^{-1} for uncoated Fe_3O_4 NPs, and it increased to about 208 m^2 g^{-1} for $Fe_3O_4/SiO_2/APTS$ nanoshells. The total thickness and the structure of core-shell was measured and studied by transmission electron microscopy (TEM). For uncoated Fe_3O_4 NPs, the results showed an octahedral geometry with saturation magnetization range of (80–100) emu g^{-1} and coercivity of (80–120) Oe for particles between (35–96) nm, respectively. The Fe_3O_4/SiO_2 NPs with 50 nm as particle size, demonstrated a magnetization value of 30 emu g^{-1}. The stable magnetic fluid contained well-dispersed $Fe_3O_4/SiO_2/APTS$ nanoshells, which indicated monodispersity and fast magnetic response.

Functionalization of silica NP surfaces with APTS

Synthesis of FeO_3 core coated with SiO_2 was fully described in §9.2.3. Here we only continue with the next step. Silanol groups are the predominant functional groups at the surface of unmodified silica nanoshells. 3-aminopropyltriethoxysilane (APTS) was obtained from Sigma-Aldrich (St. Louis, MO) and the required amount for surface functionalization is estimated according to the approximate concentration and surface area of the silica nanoshells (Pham et al. 2002). Consequently, we added an excess of APTS (65 μl) to a 200 ml of the magnetic NP solution and the mixture has been vigorously stirred for 2 h. The feasibility of functionalization reaction could be confirmed visually by observing the precipitation of APTS functionalized magnetic NPs while remaining a clear ethanolic solution at the top. After that, covalent bonding between the APTS groups and the magnetic NPs was enhanced by refluxing the solution for 1 hour. The magnetic NPs was centrifuged and redispersed in 200 ml of ethanol for future use.

Instrumentation

The analysis of synthesized material was performed by using the followings: pH (EUTECH 510 pH meter), XRD (FK60-04), FTIR (EQUINOX 55), BET (Quantachrome TPR Win v1.0) to calculate the specific surface areas, thermogravimetric analysis-TGA (PL analyzer), TEM (Phillips CM-200-FEG), magnetization measurements (VSM-PAR 155), and particle size analyzer (Malvern Zetasizer).

Results and discussion

Most of the related results are given in §9.2.3 and here only the new results are added. A complete precipitation of Fe_3O_4 should be expected between (7.5–14) pH where it is proved that silica coated magnetite NPs have an excellent biocompatibility and can homogeneously disperse in aqueous solutions with a wide range of pH values. The NH_2 adsorption strongly depends on pH value of the feed solution (Table 9.3). In our case (pH = 8), relatively large number of NH_2 groups exists on the surface of the silica

Table 9.3. pH measurement.

Materials	pH value
Magnetite (at room temperature)	14
Magnetite (after watering)	9
Magnetite (after adding HCl)	6
Magnetite + Ethanol + Ammonia + Water	8
Magnetite + TEOS (MS) {after 12 hours}	9
Magnetite + TEOS + APTS	8

adsorbents. At pH < 10, protonation of the amines may give a positive surface charge which accounts for the high stability of these dispersions.

To observe the agglomeration state, particle size distribution, polycrystalline electron diffraction pattern (EDP) of Fe_3O_4/SiO_2 nanoparticles TEM was used. Figure 9.21 shows a typical TEM image (3a) and EDP of Fe_3O_4/SiO_2 NPs (3b), where the reflection corresponds to diffraction plane (311) characteristic of the magnetite phase. The typical size of core-shell structure was measured about 50 nm which is comparable with the results obtained by (Deng et al. 2005). The uniform dispersion would make them as a suitable candidate for biomedical applications.

Table 9.4 demonstrates that SiO_2 coated NPs have numerous nanopores in the walls, which results in a high BET surface (81 $m^2\,g^{-1}$). The BET value increased to about 208 $m^2\,g^{-1}$ for $Fe_3O_4/SiO_2/APTS$ nanoshells.

Figure 9.22 shows the squareness, SQ = (M_r/M_s) versus particle size. It is worth mentioning that the amount of SQ has a significant impact on the configuration of hysteresis loop in magnetic NPs. The non-linear variation of squareness of particles with their size can be attributed first of all to that fact that there is a non-uniform distribution of particles size within a given sample group (e.g., S1,....S4) which implies a random selection of a particle for TEM purpose, and secondly, some magnetite can be changed into maghemite (γ-Fe_2O_3) due to oxidization.

Figure 9.23 shows the room-temperature magnetization curve of the Fe_3O_4/SiO_2 NPs obtained using a VSM. The M (H) hysteresis loop for the Fe_3O_4/SiO_2 NPs was almost completely reversible. It means the magnetization curve exhibits zero remanence and coercivity, which proves that Fe_3O_4/SiO_2 NPs has superparamagnetic properties. The M_s value for the Fe_3O_4/SiO_2 NPs was 30 emu g^{-1} at an applied magnetic field of 6000 Oe, which is about 3.6% of the M_s for Fe_3O_4. Taking these results together, we conclude that the decrease in M_s is most likely the result of a large volume of SiO_2 in the coated NPs. When the external magnetic field was removed, the particles could redisperse rapidly, which is an advantage to their biomedical applications.

The main absorption peaks around 591 and 3422 cm^{-1} in Fig. 9.24 a corresponds to Fe–O and O–H stretching vibration modes, respectively. The presence of magnetite is evident at 418 and 462 cm^{-1}. The absorption peaks of citrate-modified samples at 1622 cm^{-1} and 1397 cm^{-1} are due to the COO–Fe carboxylate bond (Fig. 9.24b). The band at 1092 cm^{-1} and 802 cm^{-1} are characteristic peaks of the symmetrical and asymmetrical vibrations of Si–O–Si. The band at 466 cm^{-1} is an indication of the presence of Si-O-Fe (Fig. 10c). Figure 10d is the IR spectra of APTS-coated Fe_3O_4 NPs. The broad Band near 1092 cm^{-1} and

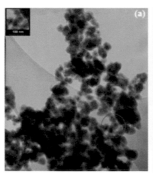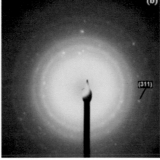

Figure 9.21. (a) TEM micrograph of Fe_3O_4/SiO_2 NPs, (b) polycrystalline electron diffraction pattern of the magnetite phase corresponding to Fe_3O_4/SiO_2 NPs.

Table 9.4. Brunauer-Emmett-Teller (BET) values for $Fe_3O_4/SiO_2/APTS$ nanostructure.

Materials	BET value ($m^2\,g^{-1}$)
Magnetite	41
Magnetite + TSC	112
Magnetite + TSC + TEOS	81
Magnetite + TEOS + APTS	208

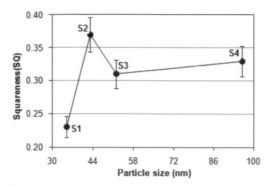

Figure 9.22. Variation of squareness with particle size for uncoated Fe_3O_4 NPs at 750 rpm.

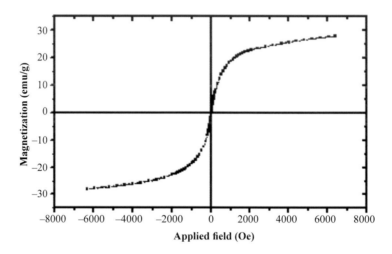

Figure 9.23. Variation of Fe_3O_4/SiO_2 NPs magnetization with applied field.

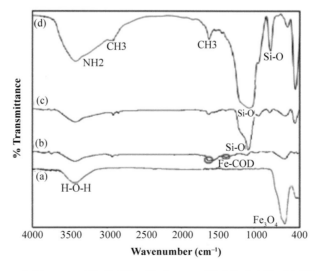

Figure 9.24. FT-IR spectra of: (a) uncoated Fe_3O_4 NPs, (b) citrate-modified Fe_3O_4 NPs, (b) SiO_2 coated Fe_3O_4 NPs, (c) $Fe_3O_4/SiO_2/APTS$ nanoshells.

798 cm^{-1} is the contribution of Si-O. The adsorption bands in 2930 and 2850 cm^{-1} are due to stretching vibration of -CH$_2$. Bands near 3430 and 1633 cm^{-1} exhibit the existence of -NH$_2$.

The heat endurance of Fe$_3$O$_4$/SiO$_2$/APTS nanoshells was evaluated by thermo-gravimetric (Fig. 9.25). Fe$_3$O$_4$/SiO$_2$ NPs indicated three distinct weight loss stages: (i) a small weight loss in the range of 40–180°C mainly due to the evaporation of residual alcohol, physically adsorbed water and slight dehydration of silanol groups, (ii) a large weight loss is in the range of 200–450°C which is attributed to the decomposition of organic substances, (iii) a minor weight loss at the higher temperatures, 500–550°C, due to the complete dehydration of silica species which there after remain to be stable. According to TGA analysis, the residual mass percent of silica coated NPs is 89% at 550°C, while that of SiO$_2$–NH$_2$ is 87%, which indicates the grafting percentage of APTS is approximately 6%. The particle size distribution obtained at room temperature using dynamic light scattering test is shown in Fig. 9.26. As it is seen, the average diameter of the APTS functionalized magnetic NPs is about 60 nm with relative maximum intensity of 35% based on optical density of 1.046 and the refraction index of 1.358.

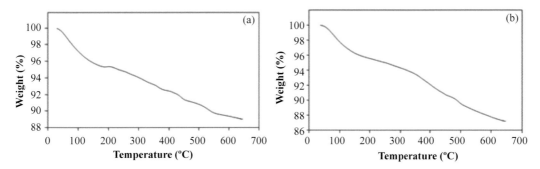

Figure 9.25. TGA graphs of (a) SiO$_2$ coated Fe$_3$O$_4$ NPs, (b) Fe$_3$O$_4$/SiO$_2$/APTS nanoshells.

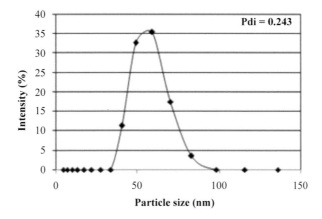

Figure 9.26. Particle size distribution of Fe$_3$O$_4$/SiO$_2$/APTS nanoshells.

9.3.9 *Physicochemical characterization of Fe$_3$O$_4$/SiO$_2$/Au multilayer nanostructure*
(Khosroshahi and Ghazanfari 2012)

The purpose of this research was to synthesize and characterize gold-coated Fe$_3$O$_4$/SiO$_2$ nanoshells for biomedical applications. Magnetite nanoparticles (NPs) were prepared using co-precipitation method. Smaller particles were synthesized by decreasing the NaOH concentration, which in our case this corresponded to 35 nm using 0.9 M of NaOH at 750 rpm with a specific surface area of 41 m^2/g. For uncoated Fe$_3$O$_4$ NPs, the results showed an octahedral geometry with saturation magnetization range of (80–100) emu/g and coercivity of (80–120) Oe for particles between (35–96) nm, respectively.

The magnetic NPs were modified with a thin layer of silica using Stober method. Small gold colloids (1–3 nm) were synthesized using Duff method and covered the amino functionalized particle surface. Magnetic and optical properties of gold nanoshells were assessed using Brunauer–Emmett–Teller (BET), vibrating sample magnetometer (VSM), UV-Vis spectrophotometer, atomic and magnetic force microscope (AFM, MFM), and transmission electron microscope (TEM). Based on the X-ray diffraction (XRD) results, three main peaks of Au (111), (200), and (220) were identified. The formation of each layer of a nanoshell is also demonstrated by Fourier transform infrared (FTIR) results. The $Fe_3O_4/SiO_2/Au$ nanostructures, with 85 nm as particle size, exhibited an absorption peak at ~550 nm with a magnetization value of 1.3 emu g^{-1} with a specific surface area of 71 m^2 g^{-1}.

Coating Fe_3O_4/SiO_2 nanocomposites with gold

At this stage, an excess of APTS (65 μl) to a 200 ml of the magnetic NP solution was added according to the approximate concentration and surface area of the silica nanoshells (Pham et al. 2002), and the mixture was vigorously stirred for 2 hours and refluxed for 1 hour. Then 0.5 ml of 1 M of NaOH and 1 ml of THPC solution was added to a 45 ml aliquot of water as suggested (Ji et al. 2007), and the mixture was stirred for 5 minutes. Then, 2 ml of 1% $HAuCl_4$ in water was added quickly to the stirred solution and the obtained colloidal gold particles were 2–3 nm in size. After that an aliquot of APTS-functionalized silica NPs dispersed in ethanol (1 ml) was placed in a centrifuge tube along with an excess of gold NPs (5 ml of gold colloid solution). This led to the attachment of THPC gold nanocrystals onto the silica surface. The mixture was stored at 4°C overnight to maximize the surface coverage of the THPC gold nanoseeds. The attachment is sufficiently strong so that the gold NPs remain attached to the silica NPs when the silica NPs are centrifuged at 3500 rpm out of solution. Finally, 25 mg of K_2CO_3 was dissolved in 100 ml of water. After 10 minutes of stirring, 1.5 ml of 1% $HAuCl_4$ was added. The solution initially appeared yellow and became colorless in 30 minutes. 200 μl of the solution containing the $Fe_3O_4/SiO_2/Au$ nanocomposites was then added to 4 ml of the colorless solution. The gold nanoshells were prepared by reduction of gold solution with formaldehyde (37%) in the presence of $Fe_3O_4/SiO_2/Au$ nanocomposites. After 2–4 minutes, the solution changed from colorless to purple, which is characteristic of nanoshell formation.

Results and discussion

Figure 9.27 shows the XRD patterns for (a) citrate-modified Fe_3O_4 NPs, (b) Fe_3O_4/SiO_2 nanoshells, (c) $Fe_3O_4/SiO_2/Au$ nanostructures, with each pattern normalized to its maximum intensity. The peaks are indexed with the fcc structure corresponding to magnetite phase. The XRD results showed that the citrate-modified

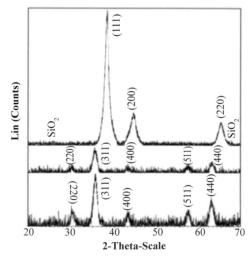

Figure 9.27. X-ray diffraction patterns for (a) citrate-modified Fe_3O_4 NPs, (b) Fe_3O_4/SiO_2 nanoshells, (c) $Fe_3O_4/SiO_2/Au$ nanostructures.

Fe$_3$O$_4$ NPs are about 8 nm. Figure 9.27b shows that the pattern of silica-coated magnetite displayed the same lines as uncoated magnetite. This indicates that the coated silica is in an amorphous form before the step of mixing the Fe$_3$O$_4$-embedded silica solution with the gold solution during the synthesis process. However, it appears that the coating of Au particles on silica could induce small crystallization of silica even at room temperature. For the Fe$_3$O$_4$/SiO$_2$/Au nanostructures, the XRD pattern shown in Fig. 9.27c displays three wide peaks that can be identified as the (111), (200), and (220) reflection lines of the Au fcc-cubic phase, indicating that the gold particles are crystallized. Considering the fact that most of SiO$_2$-coated particles are spherical (see TEM results) and the observation that usually spherical SiO$_2$ particles are in the amorphous form, we believe that most of the silica nanoshells are in the amorphous phase. Interestingly, the Fe$_3$O$_4$ peaks (Fig. 9.27a,b) appearing in the patterns of the SiO$_2$-coated and citrate-modified Fe$_3$O$_4$ NPs are not seen in the pattern of the Au/SiO$_2$ coated particles shown in Fig. 9.27c, which can be explained by the strong absorption of and scattering from the Au-coated particles.

Figure 9.28 shows the magnetization curve for Fe$_3$O$_4$/SiO$_2$ nanoshells obtained by VSM at room temperature. The results indicate that these NPs show no remanence and redisperse rapidly when the applied magnetic field is removed, i.e., the curve passing through the origin. It, therefore, can be deduced that the magnetite NPs have magnetization saturation of about 82 emu/g, and when the TEOS is added, the M$_s$ values of the resultant Fe$_3$O$_4$/SiO$_2$ nanoshells rapidly decreased to 30 emu/g, due to the deposition of nonmagnetic silica on the magnetite NPs. Clearly based on the Fig. 9.28, no hysteresis loop with unmeasurable coercivity and remanence is observed for 50 nm core-shell particles which likely implies their superparamagnetic behaviour. Similarly, Fig. 9.28 shows the room-temperature magnetization curve of the Fe$_3$O$_4$/SiO$_2$/Au nanostructures. The hysteresis loop for the Fe$_3$O$_4$/SiO$_2$/Au nanostructures shows a reversible behaviour, implying that the magnetization curve exhibits zero remanence and coercivity. The M$_s$ value for these nanostructures is 1.3 emu/g, which is about 1.5% of the M$_s$ for Fe$_3$O$_4$. So, the decrease in M$_s$ is most likely the result of a large volume of SiO$_2$/Au in the coated sample. When the external magnetic field (1000 Oe) was removed, the particles could redisperse rapidly, and this relatively fast magnetic response can be an advantage in many applications.

Figure 9.29 shows the UV–Vis spectra for (a) Fe$_3$O$_4$/SiO$_2$/APTS and (b) Fe$_3$O$_4$/SiO$_2$/Au nanostructures, respectively. It is seen from the image of Fig. 9.29a that the Fe$_3$O$_4$/SiO$_2$/APTS nanostructure has a strong absorption peak of about 200 nm with a relatively weaker peak at 230 nm which are mainly due to the presence of amine groups. However, its visible absorption is quite different from Fe$_3$O$_4$/SiO$_2$/Au nanostructure which confirms the effect of surface plasmon resonance played by Au shell (Brown et al. 2000). The optical absorption spectrum range of Fe$_3$O$_4$/SiO$_2$/Au nanostructures (Fig. 9.29b) is relatively

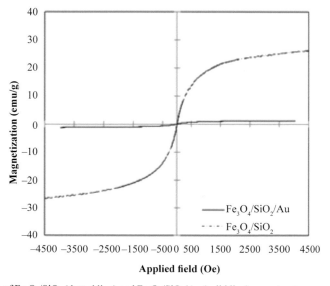

Figure 9.28. Variation of Fe$_3$O$_4$/SiO$_2$ (dotted line) and Fe$_3$O$_4$/SiO$_2$/Au (solid line) nanostructures magnetization with applied field.

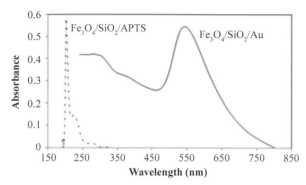

Figure 9.29. UV-vis spectra of (a) Fe$_3$O$_4$/SiO$_2$/APTS (dotted line) nanostructure, (b) Fe$_3$O$_4$/SiO$_2$/Au (solid line) nanostructures.

broad compared to that of pure gold colloid. In addition, the plasmon line-width is dominated by electron surface scattering. According to Mie's theory, the broadening of resonance absorption is related to the size, shape, and aggregation of the gold nanoshells. When gold particles aggregate on the surface of amino-modified silica, the peak plasmon resonance wavelength will shift to the near-infrared range. Furthermore, the silica layer provides a dielectric interface for red-shifting the plasma resonance in electromagnetic spectrum resulting from the charge variation of the gold NPs within the core/shell structure.

To observe the agglomeration state, particle size distribution, and morphology of Fe$_3$O$_4$/SiO$_2$ nanoshells, TEM was used. The gold layer can stabilize the magnetic particles by sheltering the magnetic dipole interaction. Meanwhile, upon the increase of the particle size, their shape become more regular and spherical, as shown in their TEM images. Amine-functionalized silica NPs (treated with APTS) exhibited heavy coverage of gold NPs, as shown in Fig. 9.30a, which is comparable to that reported (Westcott et al. 1998). TEM image shows clusters of small gold NPs assembled on the surfaces of larger silica NPs. Figure 9.30b shows the polycrystalline electron diffraction pattern of the Au as the metal phase. The self-assembled aggregates consist of tens of gold NPs.

TEM is still the most commonly used microscopy technique for visualizing colloidal particles, though AFM and MFM are serious alternatives which provide some different information about particles, such as the variation in particle surface irregularities (morphology and surface texture). The typical SPM forces are mechanical contact force, Van der Waals force, capillary forces, electrostatic forces, magnetic force (MF), etc. AFM relies on the interaction between the specimen and a nanometric tip attached to a cantilever, which scans the sample surface. The force constants were 0.1 N/m for contact-mode imaging. AFM images of nanoshells as shown in Fig. 9.31, and were expected to show a considerable surface roughness due to the agglomeration of the nanoshells. In addition, the agglomeration of NPs is evident in the topography image because the powders were confined directly on the copper tape. Both height (Fig. 9.31a) and phase (Fig. 9.31d) images are useful for visualizing the morphology (Fig. 9.31c) and size (Fig. 9.31b) of the Fe$_3$O$_4$/SiO$_2$/Au nanostructures, but the cluster composition is better seen in the phase

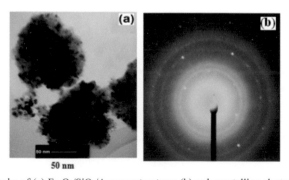

Figure 9.30. TEM micrographs of (a) Fe$_3$O$_4$/SiO$_2$/Au nanostructures (b) polycrystalline electron diffraction pattern of the metal phase corresponding to Fe$_3$O$_4$/SiO$_2$/Au nanostructure.

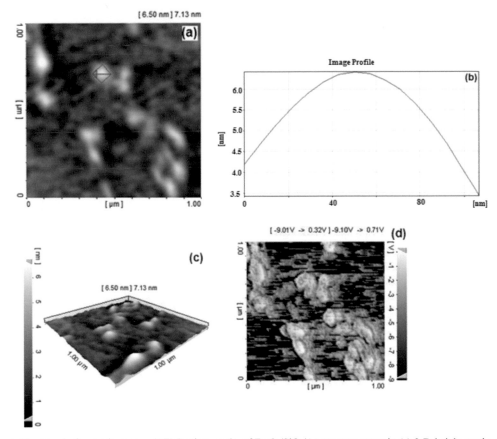

Figure 9.31. Atomic force microscopy (AFM) micrographs of $Fe_3O_4/SiO_2/Au$ nanostructures in (a) 2-D-height mode, (b) image profile, (c) 3-D-height mode, and (d) phase mode.

image. Clusters of few particles are mainly formed during drying due to the capillary forces even when highly diluted samples were used.

An AFM microscope has the capacity to be used in different operating modes in such a way that one can study the roughness or morphology of surface in different scales. In the application of this approach, the displacements of the surface points from the reference plane are modeled as a random surface and characterized by appropriate distribution of the height function (roughness) values z (Rice 2007). The normal distribution is often used as a model for the surface roughness description. The density function of the normal distribution depends on two parameters, mean, (μ) and standard deviation, (σ)

$$f(z) = \frac{1}{\sigma\sqrt{2\pi}} \exp\left[\frac{-(z-\mu)^2}{2\sigma^2}\right] \tag{9.96}$$

Departures from normality often take the form of asymmetry. For a normal distribution, the third central moment equals zero:

$$\int_{-\infty}^{\infty} (z-\mu)^3 f(z)dz = 0 \tag{9.97}$$

Asymmetry of the roughness distribution can therefore be tested by using the sample coefficient of R_{sk} (Narayan and Hancock 2003):

$$R_{sk} = \frac{\sum_{i=1}^{n}\left(z_i - \bar{z}\right)^3}{ns^3} = -0.24 \tag{9.98}$$

where R_{sk} is skewness, or measure of symmetry over the surface profile, n is the number of height function values, z is the sample mean, and s is the sample standard deviation and is defined as follows:

$$s = \sqrt{\iint (f(x,y))^2 \, dxdy} = 778\text{pm} \tag{9.99}$$

Large values of $|R_{sk}|$ implicate deformation of the roughness distribution shape. Symmetric distributions can depart from normality by being heavily- or light-tailed or too peaked or flat in the center. Negative skewness indicates the predominance of valleys and positive skewness denotes a ripple type surface. MFM (Fig. 9.32) is a variant of AFM, in which a probe with a magnetic coating is used, conferring sensitivity to the magnetic fields of the sample. In order to obtain useful information, it is necessary to separate the magnetic forces acting on the probe from short and long range non-magnetic forces.

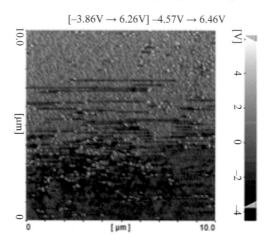

Figure 9.32. Magnetic force microscopy (MFM) micrograph of $Fe_3O_4/SiO_2/Au$ nanostructures.

9.4 Polymeric

9.4.1 Introduction

In the recent years, biodegradable nanoparticles have been widely used as drug delivery vehicles due to their good biocompatibility, easy design and preparation, better encapsulation, control release, and less toxic properties. Polymeric nanoparticles with a size in the nanometer range protect drugs against *in vitro* and *in vivo* degradation and play a significant role because they can deliver therapeutic agents directly into the intended site of action, with superior efficacy (Prasad and Geckelera 2011). It releases the drug in a controlled manner and also offers the possibility of drug targeting. The use of polymeric drug nanoparticles is a universal approach to increase the therapeutic performance of poorly soluble drugs in any route of administration. Two types of polymers can be used in nanodelivery, which are natural and synthetic. Natural polymers or biopolymers may be naturally occurring materials which are formed in nature during the life cycles of green plants, animals, bacteria, and fungi are polymers or polymer matrix composites. Natural polymers occur in nature and can be extracted. They are often water-based. Examples of naturally occurring polymers are silk, wool, DNA, cellulose, and proteins. The biodegradable polymeric nanoparticles are commonly prepared by five different techniques such as emulsification-solvent evaporation, solvent displacement, salting-out, emulsification-solvent diffusion, and double emulsion solvent evaporation. The choice of method depends on a number of factors, such as, particle size, particle size distribution, area of application, etc. Biopolymers are polymers produced by living organisms; in other words, they are polymeric biomolecules. Since they are polymers, biopolymers contain monomeric units that are covalently bonded to form larger structures. There are three main classes of biopolymers, classified according to the monomeric units used and the structure of the biopolymer formed: polynucleotides (RNA and DNA), which are long polymers composed of 13 or more nucleotide monomers; polypeptides, which are short polymers of amino acids; and polysaccharides, which are often linear bonded polymeric carbohydrate structures. Synthetic polymers are human-made polymers. From the utility point of view, they can be classified into four main categories: thermoplastics, thermosets, elastomers, and synthetic fibers. A wide variety of synthetic polymers are available with variations in main chain as well as side chains. The back bones of common synthetic polymers such as polythene, polystyrene and poly acrylates are made up of carbon-carbon bonds, whereas hetero chain polymers such as polyamides, polyesters, polyurethanes, polysulfides, and polycarbonates have other elements (e.g., oxygen, sulfur, nitrogen) inserted along the backbone. The synthesizing methods include salting-out method (Allemann et al. 1992); it is based on the separation of a water miscible solvent from aqueous solution through the salting out effect, solvent displacement method (Allemann et al. 1993), phase separation method (Niwa et al. 1995), evaporation precipitation (Chen et al. 2002), antisolvent precipitation and electrospray methods (Gomez et al. 1998).

Depending upon the method of preparation nanoparticles, nanospheres, or nanocapsules can be obtained. Nanocapsules are systems in which the drug is confined to a cavity surrounded by a unique polymer membrane, while nanospheres are matrix systems in which the drug is physically and uniformly dispersed.

Many polymers can be applied for biomedical applications, such as natural polymers including polysaccharide (starch, alginate, chitin/chitosan) or proteins (collagen, fibrin gels) and synthetic polymers such as poly(lactic acid) (PLA), and poly(ε-caprolactone) (PLC), and poly(glycolic acid) (PGA). They are biocompatible and degradable into non-toxic components with a controllable degradable rate. Also, the soluble polymers in water such as poly(Vinyle alcohol) (PVA), poly(acrylic acid) (PAA), poly(vinyl acetate) (PVA), poly(ethylene glycol) (PEG) are used in this field. Other polymers are also extensively been used in biomedical applications including: polyurethane (PU), polypropylene (PP), and polyethylene (PE).

Advantages of polymeric nanoparticles

- Increases the stability of any volatile pharmaceutical agents, easily and cheaply fabricated in large quantities by a multitude of methods.
- They offer a significant improvement over traditional oral and intravenous methods of administration in terms of efficiency and effectiveness.
- Delivers a higher concentration of pharmaceutical agent to a desired location.
- The choice of polymer and the ability to modify drug release from polymeric nanoparticles have made them ideal candidates for cancer therapy, delivery of vaccines, contraceptives, and delivery of targeted antibiotics.
- Polymeric nanoparticles can be easily incorporated into other activities related to drug delivery, such as tissue engineering.

9.4.2 *Preparation and rheological studies of uncoated and PVA-coated magnetite nanofluid* (Khosroshahi and Ghazanfari 2012)

Experimental studies of rheological behaviour of uncoated magnetite nanoparticles (MNPs)$_U$ and polyvinyl alcohol (PVA) coated magnetite nanoparticles (MNPs)$_C$ were performed. Co-precipitation technique under N2 gas was used to prevent undesirable critical oxidation of Fe^{2+}. The results showed that smaller particles can be synthesized in both cases by decreasing the NaOH concentration, which in our case corresponded to 35 nm and 7 nm, using 0.9 M NaOH at 750 rpm for (MNPs)$_U$ and (MNPs)$_C$, respectively. The stable magnetic fluid contained well-dispersed Fe_3O_4/PVA nanocomposites which indicated fast magnetic response. The rheological measurement of magnetic fluid indicated an apparent viscosity range of (0.1–1.2) pa.s at constant shear rate of 20 s^{-1} with a minimum value in the case of (MNPs)$_U$ at 0 Tesla and a maximum value for (MNPs)C at 0.5 Tesla. Also, as the shear rate increased from 20 s^{-1} to 150 s^{-1} at constant magnetic field, the apparent viscosity also decreased correspondingly. The water-based ferrofluid exhibited the non-Newtonian behaviour of shear thinning under magnetic field.

Introduction

Magnetic field-responsive materials are specific subsets of smart materials that can adaptively change their physical properties due to external magnetic field. Magnetic liquids or ferrofluids (FFs) are colloidal system of single domain magnetic nanoparticles that are dispersed either in aqueous or organic liquids. Usually solid particles in these fluids are about 10 nm in size and a surfactant is used for stabilization. The most important advantage of these fluids over conventional mechanical interfaces is their ability to achieve a wide range of viscosity (several orders of magnitude) in a fraction of millisecond. This has been a source of various technical and clinical applications (Ohmori et al. 2000, Park et al. 2007). Based on the mesoscopic physical, tribological, thermal and mechanical properties of superparamagnetic iron oxide nanoparticles (SPION), they offer a variety of applications in different areas such as FFs, color imaging, and magnetic recording (Popplewell and Sakhini 1995, Palma et al. 2007). Various approaches have been explored for synthesis and characterization of high-quality magnetic iron oxide NPs (Kim et al. 2001, Khosroshahi and Ghazanfari 2010, Khosroshahi and Ghazanfari 2011, Khosroshahi and Ghazanfari 2012). Applying an appropriate amount of polyvinyl alcohol (PVA) on SPIONs prevents their aggregation mostly via steric hindrance mechanism and gives rise to mono-dispersed NPs (Chastellain et al. 2004, Sairam et al. 2006). The measurement of the suspension's viscosity can be used to characterize the microstructural state of a dispersion. The rheology of a magnetic particle dispersion is very complicated because such dispersions are multi-component systems consisting of magnetic particles and polymers. Moreover, the polymer is not only present in the solvent, but is also adsorbed onto the particle surface (Gleissle 1980, Borin et al. 2011). Rheology is a major subject of investigating the flow and deformation of materials can be monitored by the application of a field, either magnetic or electric. Most studies have been focused on measurement of field-induced effects in FFs under shear flow (Pop and Odenbach 2006, Borin and Odenbach 2009) and shear stress versus shear rate (Vlaev et al. 2007, Welch et al. 2006). Focusing on the change of fluid's viscous behaviour due to the action of an appropriate magnetic field seems to be the most prominent effect and accounts as a challenging topic in FF research. The aim of the research is to investigate the rheological properties of uncoated and PVA-coated Fe_3O_4 NPs synthesized in an oxidative environment and its possible impact in clinical applications.

Synthesis

All samples S1–S4 were prepared as described previously. Aqueous dispersion of magnetite NPs (MNPs) was prepared by alkalinizing an aqueous mixture of ferric and ferrous salts with NaOH at room temperature. 25 ml of iron source was added drop-wise into 250 ml of alkali source under vigorous magnetic stirring (750 rpm) for 30 min at ambient temperature. A complete precipitation of Fe_3O_4 should be expected between 7.5–14 pH, while maintaining a molar ratio of $Fe^{2+}:Fe^{3+} = 1:2$ under a non-oxidizing environment. The precipitated black powder was isolated by applying an external magnetic field, and the supernatant was removed from the precipitate by decantation. The powder was washed and the solution was decanted twice after centrifugation at 5000 rpm for 15 min. Then 0.01 M HCl was added to neutralize the anionic charge on the particle surface. The cationic colloidal particles were separated by centrifugation and peptized by watering. In order to prevent them from possible oxidation in air as well as from agglomeration, Fe_3O_4 NPs were coated with PVA shell. 4 gr of PVA was dissolved in water and added to the magnetic solution, then it was heated at 90°C for 30 min under magnetic stirring (750 rpm). The samples were classified as S5–S8 where each sample were synthesized using different NaOH concentration, i.e., 0.9, 1.1, 1.3, and 1.5 M of NaOH corresponds to S5, S6, S7, and S8, respectively. The obtained magnetic product was collected by magnetic separation. After coating, the surfactant adsorbed physically on the particle surface was removed by washing, centrifugation and peptizing the solution for three times, then they were freeze-dried at –60°C.

Rheological property of magnetic fluid

For the successful application of magnetic fluid, it is very important to obtain its rheological property. Assuming a suspension of MNPs under the influence of a shear flow, the particles will rotate in the flow with their axis of rotation parallel to the vorticity of the flow. If the magnetic moment of the particles is fixed within the particle, then the Brownian relaxation time is shorter than the Neel time, and thus the particles are magnetically hard. An anisotropic change of viscosity of the fluid depends on the strength and the direction of the field relative to the flow. The magnetic field can be applied in perpendicular or collinear direction. In the former case, the magnetic field will tend to align the magnetic moment with the field direction. Thus, viscous torque exerted by the flow tries to rotate the particle, whereas in the second case, the magnetic moment will be aligned in the direction of the field. However, since this is identical with the axis of rotation of the particles, no field influence will appear on the rotation of the particle. As a result no change of viscosity of the fluid will be observed. For perpendicular alignment of field and vorticity an absolute maximum of the relative change of viscosity is given by

$$R_{max} = \frac{3}{2}\varphi' \tag{9.100}$$

where φ denotes the volume fraction of the particles including the surfactant. Thus, in a suspension of diluted solution, magnetically hard particles with a volume fraction of magnetic material about 7 vol.%, mean particle diameter of about 7 nm, the relative change of viscosity in a field cannot exceed about 40%. The viscosity of the fluid should be a function of the shear ratio (SR) of viscous to magnetic stress

$$SR = \frac{\dot{\gamma}\eta_0}{\mu_0 M_0 H} \tag{9.101}$$

Here $\dot{\gamma}$ denotes the shear rate, η_0 the viscosity of the solvent, μ_0 is the susceptibility of vacuum, M_0 the spontaneous magnetization of the magnetic material, H the magnetic field strength. In diluted solutions, the ratio of the fluid's viscosity under influence of H to that of the fluid for $H = 0$ is only a function of the stress parameter SR

$$\frac{\eta}{\eta_{(H=0)}} = \wp\left(\frac{\dot{\gamma}\eta_0}{\mu_0 M_0 H}\right) \tag{9.102}$$

The viscous behaviour should be at a constant minimum level for large values of the stress parameter. In the intermediate range the viscosity is assumed to depend on shear and field.

Einstein proposed a simple equation to calculate the viscosity of particles suspension, $\eta = (1+2.5cs)$ ηL where, cs is the solid content of FFs and ηL is the viscosity of carrier liquid. The Bingham model takes account of the yield stress of fluids, $\tau = \tau_0 + \dot{\gamma}\eta$: when the shear stress is less than the yield stress τ_0, there is no fluid motion. But the Bingham model could not predict the shear-thinning/thickening behaviours of some fluids. The Carson model taking account of both the yield stress threshold and the shear-thinning behaviour, adopts a relatively simple form, $\sqrt{\tau} = \sqrt{\tau_c} + \sqrt{\eta_c}\,\dot{\gamma}$. The H–B model also takes account of both the yield stress threshold and the shear-thinning phenomenon, but takes a relatively complicated form of:

$$\tau = \tau_0 + k\left[\dot{\gamma}^n - (\tau_0/\mu_0)^n\right] \tag{9.103}$$

and

$$\eta = k\,\dot{\gamma}\,n\text{-}1 \tag{9.104}$$

For most of the fluids, the H–B equation can be simplified as:

$$\tau = \tau_0 + k\,\dot{\gamma}\,n \tag{9.105}$$

The consistency index (k) and the shear-thinning exponent (n) are influenced by the intensity of applied magnetic field, particle content in FFs, magnetic properties of MNPs and the dosages of surfactants (Welch et al. 2006). There are two kinds of viscosity variations for FFs when the shear rate increases: Newtonian and shear-thinning behaviour. Figure 9.33 shows that the viscosity of both uncoated and PVA coated Fe_3O_4 solution increases with decreasing the shear rate for a given magnetic field. However, at constant shear rate the viscosity increases with increase in the magnetic field (Fig. 9.37) until it reaches a saturation point which is in agreement with the findings of Pop et al. (2004).

For FF, the viscosity is determined by the viscosity of carrier liquid (water) and the interaction of MNPs. The viscosity of water is not affected by applied magnetic field, while the MNPs were polarized by magnetic field and arranged their orientation along the direction of magnetic field. The viscosity of magnetic fluid shows the tendency to increase because of the magneto-viscous effect of magnetic solution. As it can be seen in Fig. 9.34, increasing the magnetic field causes an increase in apparent viscosity which is more significant at lower shear rate. It is also known that under an applied magnetic field orderly microstructures are formed. As the shear rate increases, these microstructures are disoriented under the shear stress, thus, the viscosity of high-concentration FFs diminishes rapidly. Shulman et al. (1986) suggested that magnetorheological suspensions under applied magnetic field could be described using the Bingham model. Our results showed that the characteristics of FFs gradually deviated from the Bingham model when the intensity of applied magnetic field increased. Figures 9.33 and 9.34 demonstrate the shear-thinning behaviour of FFs under different magnetic fields and without magnetic field. It is seen that the viscosity and shear stress of FFs increases gradually as the intensity of applied magnetic field increases. This is due to the fact that the MNPs are arranged to form a chaining structure along the applied magnetic field, and hence the attraction among these micro-chains increases with the intensity of applied magnetic field, and the viscosity. This results in an increase of yield stress of FFs compared with the case without magnetic field. The shear-thinning exponent (n) and viscous coefficient (or called consistency index, k) were correlated from the experimental data, while the yield stress was derived theoretically. It was reported by Hong et al. (2007) that chaining microstructures are formed in FFs when the intensity of applied magnetic field is strong enough.

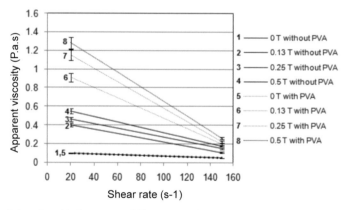

Figure 9.33. Variation of viscosity with shear rate at different applied magnetic field for uncoated (S1) and PVA-coated (S5) Fe_3O_4 NPs.

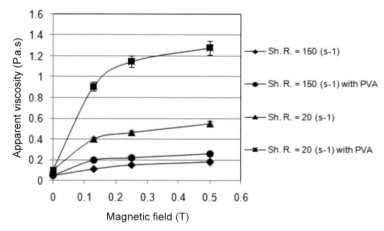

Figure 9.34. Viscosity versus applied magnetic field at different shear rate for uncoated (S1) and PVA-coated (S5) Fe_3O_4 NPs.

The H–B model takes account of both the yield stress and the shear-thinning behaviour of FFs. Therefore, this model is currently used for describing the rheological properties FFs with or without applied magnetic field. The results corresponding to the relationship between shear stress and shear rate in different magnetic fields are shown in Fig. 9.35a,b for without and with PVA, respectively when the ratio of solid concentration of magnetite/PVA is 7%. Similar rheological properties were obtained in the case of PEG-coated Fe_3O_4 NPs as reported by Hong et al. (2007).

The PVA not only acted as an outer surfactant shell but also enhanced the viscosity of the carrier fluid, which led to a remarkable reduction of sedimentation velocity. The sedimentation velocity of the particles/ aggregates in FF (S5) was about 6.0 mm/month obtained from Stokes law:

$$v = \frac{(\rho_1 - \rho_2)gd^2}{18\eta} \tag{9.106}$$

where $\rho 1$ is the density of solid particles (5.18 g/cm³), ρ_2 is density of carrier fluid (0.998 g/ml), g is the gravitational acceleration (9.81 m/s²), d is the diameter of aggregates (31.8 nm for S5), and η is the viscosity of the carrier fluid (1.00 mPa s). The density of aggregates is much less than that of the magnetite particles. That is to say, the Stokes equation (9.106) over predicted sedimentation rate of aggregates.

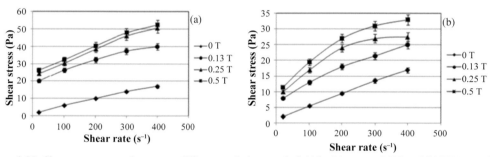

Figure 9.35. Shear stress versus shear rate at different applied magnetic field for (a) uncoated (S1) and (b) PVA coated (S5) Fe_3O_4 NPs.

9.5 Dendrimers

9.5.1 Introduction

As it is illustrated in Fig. 9.36, dendrimers can be resembled to a tree, where the main bulk of the body consists of large number of branches, which in turn are subdivided into further smaller branches. In a similar way, dendrimers are a class of well-defined nanostructured macromolecules with a three-dimensional structure composed of three architectural components: a core (I), an interior of shells (generations) consisting of repeating branch-cell units (II), and terminal functional groups (the outer shell or periphery) (III) (Tomalia 2005, Peng et al. 2008). Functional groups play an important role in the production of organic shell around inorganic core to prepare uniform and stable suspension (Peng et al. 2008, Antharjanam et al. 2009).

They are synthesized from a polyfunctional core by adding branched monomers that react with the functional groups of the core, in turn leaving end groups that can react again (Menjoge et al. 2010, Klajnert and Bryszewska 2002). One such example is poly (amidoamine) (PAMAM), which acts as a template or stabilizer for preparation of inorganic nanocomposites. Some important properties of these structures include a large number of end groups, the functionable cores, the nanoporous nature of the interior at higher generations (Peng et al. 2008, Antharjanam et al. 2009). These mentioned properties, resulted in finding a noticeable situation in energy transfer, molecular recognition, catalysis, tissue targeting applications, and drug delivery systems (Malik et al. 2000, Grabchev et al. 2003). The dendrimer-nanoparticle structure can be obtained via two approaches: (i) the physical encapsulation of particles in the internal cavity of a dendrimer, and (ii) the chemical formation of dendrimer branches around inorganic core, i.e., conjugation (Peng et al. 2008, Shen and Shi 2010). The resultant nanocomposites have much applicable potential such as gen vector, catalysis, resonance imaging agents, and nanocapsules (Stemmler et al. 2009, Thompson

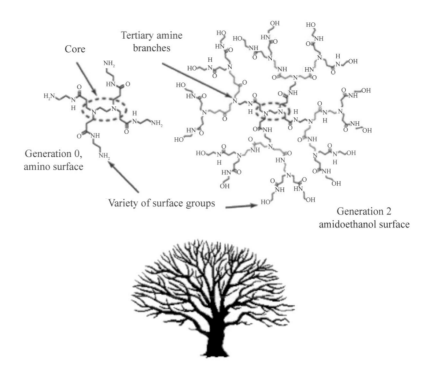

Figure 9.36. Schematic illustration of nanodendrimer consisting a core and variety of surface groups.

et al. 2012, Shen and Shi 2010). Since dendrimers have unique chemical structures, molecular weight, and molecular size which can provide special type of functionality, they received privileged attention in developing fields of materials science (Majoros et al. 2006, Syahir et al. 2009, Al-Jamal et al. 2013). Considering a large number of terminal groups on the exterior of the molecule and interior voids, dendrimers introduce an attractive platform for metal ion celates (Venditto et al. 2005). Indeed, dendrimer-entraped inorganic nanoparticles (DENP) include a nanostructure where one or more inorganic nanoparticles with the diameter of less than 5 nm are entrapped within an individual dendrimer molecule. In the case of dendrimer-stabilized inorganic nanoparticles (DSNP), one inorganic nanoparticle, which usually has the diameter larger than 5 nm, is stabilized by multiple dendrimer molecules (Bronstein and Shifrina 2011). Evaluation of formation of both DENP and DSNP in the presence of amine-terminated PAMAM dendrimers with and without addition of reducing agents has been the subject of several studies over the past few years (Shi et al. 2009, Hoffman et al. 2011).

9.5.2 *An efficient method of SPION synthesis coated with third generation PAMAM dendrimer*
(Tajabadi et al. 2013)

In this study, superparamagnetic iron oxide nanoparticles were synthesized by coprecipitation of $FeSO_4.7H_2O$ and $FeCl_3.6H_2O$ with NH_4OH at different temperatures and iron salt concentrations. The results showed that magnetite nanoparticles synthesized at higher temperature (70°C) and moderate salt concentration (0.012 M for $FeCl_3$) had the highest saturation magnetization (67.8 emu/gr) with the size of about 9 nm. The optimal magnetite nanoparticles with the lowest aggregation and highest magnetic behaviour were coated by polyamidoamine (PAMAM) dendrimer. The samples were characterized with X-ray diffractometry (XRD), transmission electron microscopy (TEM), Fourier transform infrared (FTIR) spectroscopy, UV-Visible spectroscopy, fluorescent spectroscopy, and magnetization measurements (VSM). The coated materials illustrated strong magnetic behaviour and XRD pattern like magnetite. The presence of Fe-O-Si bond in FTIR spectra confirmed the formation of thin APTS layer on the surface of magnetite nanoparticles. Energy-dispersive X-ray spectroscopy (EDS) and Thermo-Gravimetric Analysis

(TGA) indicated that the modification of core synthesis technique can raise the efficiency of aminosilane coating reaction (as an initiator for PAMAM dendrimer) up to 98% with the production of about 610 dendritic arms. TGA and FTIR spectra of PAMAM-grafted nanoparticles also verified the perfection of repetitive Michael addition and amidation reactions. The fluorescence spectrum displayed the excitation and emission peaks around 298 and 328 nm, respectively for PAMAM-grafted nanoparticles. We believe the resultant material showed the fluorescent properties which could be an applicable and powerful tool for biomedical diagnostic applications.

Materials and methods

Synthesis of magnetite nanoparticles

Different solutions of ferrous chloride hexahydrate ($FeCl_3.6H_2O$, 99%, Merck) and ferric sulfate heptahydrate ($FeSO_4.7H_2O$, 99%, Merck) were prepared as iron sources in double distilled water. The ratio of Fe^{2+}/Fe^{3+} was set to 0.5. Ammonia solution (0.9 M) was used as alkaline source and vigorously stirred under N_2 bubbling at room temperature. The mixture of ferric and ferrous solutions was deoxygenated by bubbling N_2 gas following sonication for 30 minutes. This solution was added drop wise to the stirring ammonia solution. The color of this reaction mixture immediately turned to black. In this experiment, two different temperature programs were applied to the samples. In the first group, the reaction temperature was kept constant at 25°C for 1 hour in a water bath before the mixture purified. The samples in the second group were mixed at the same condition (25°C for 1 hour) and then transferred to 70°C water bath under vigorous stirring for 30 minutes before purification. For both groups, the black precipitation was purified using magnetic separation five times and sedimented by centrifugation. The resultant material was dried by freeze dryer (Unicryo MC-4L) for 24 hours. Table 9.5 shows detailed description of each sample. After precise characterization, the optimal sample (having the lowest aggregation and highest magnetic behaviour) was chosen to perform modification processes.

Table 9.5. Parameters affecting the Fe_3O_4 synthesis and calculated particle size.

Sample	FeCl$_3$ concentration (M)	NH$_4$OH concentration (M)	Temperature (°C)	TEM-particle size (nm)	VSM-particle size (nm)
Fe-A1	0.006	0.9	25	7.84	10.48
Fe-A2	0.006	0.9	70	5.31	8.42
Fe-B1	0.012	0.9	25	10.12	9.44
Fe-B2	0.012	0.9	70	9.76	7.67
Fe-C1	0.018	0.9	25	12.34	12.18
Fe-C2	0.018	0.9	70	12	11.66

Coating of magnetite nanoparticles by aminosilane

A solution of optimal iron oxide sample with concentration of 2.13 mM was prepared in ethanol (149 mL): double distilled water (1 mL) and sonicated for 30 minutes. The amount of 35 μL of aminopropyle triethoxysilane (APTS, 99%, Sigma-Aldrich) was added to the mixture with vigorous stirring for 7 hours. It was then washed with ethanol five times using magnetic separation and finally sedimented by centrifugation. In order to remove the solvent, precipitated material was placed in freeze dryer for 24 hours. The obtained materials act as G0 in the synthesis procedure of PAMAM-grafted magnetite nanoparticles.

Fabrication of dendrimer functionalized magnetite nanoparticles

Formation of PAMAM dendrimer on the surface of amine-functionalized magnetite nanoparticles was done according to the methods of Liu et al. (2008) and Pan et al. (2005) with some modifications. Dendritic polymer synthesis involves iteration of two main reactions which consist of alkylation of primary amines using MA (Methyl Acrylate, 99%, Aldrich), namely Michael addition, and amidation of the ester groups with Ethylene diamine (EDA, 99%, Sigma-Aldrich). Each Michael addition reaction produces a half generation of PAMAM dendrimer and amidation reaction creates the full generation.

Step 1. (Michael addition of MA to amine groups): For this reaction, 50 mL of 5 wt% full generation ethanol solution was sonicated for 30 minutes in order to produce finely dispersed material, and the solution was then vigorously stirred by magnetic stirrer under N_2 atmosphere. The amount of 200 mL of MA solution (20% v/v) was added drop wise to the stirring full generation solution at 0°C. Afterwards the flask was sealed and the mixture stirred at 25°C. After 48 hours, the resulting material was precipitated by applying magnetic field, washed with ethanol five times repeatedly and sedimented by centrifugation.

Step 2. (Amidation of terminal ester groups): After rinsing the half generation material, 40 mL of EDA solution in ethanol (50% v/v) was added to the flask. Subsequently, the flask was sealed and immersed in an ultrasonicating water bath at 25°C for 3 hours. The particles were rinsed with ethanol five times using magnetic separation. These two steps were repeated for different number of cycles until the specified generation of dendrimer was obtained.

Characterization

Crystalline phase of nanoparticles was confirmed using X ray diffraction with radiation of Cu Kα (XRD, λ = 1.5406 Å, FK60-40 X-ray diffractometer). Magnetic properties of prepared samples were measured using vibrating sample magnetometer (VSM-PAR 155) at 300 K under magnetic field up to 8 KOe. The presence of silane and PAMAM typical bonds on the surface of magnetite nanoparticles was proved by Fourier transform infrared (FTIR) spectroscopy (BOMEM, Canada). Particle size and morphology of magnetite nanoparticles were determined by transmission electron microscopy (TEM, Philips CM-200-FEG microscope, 120 KV). The amount of APTS and PAMAM molecules covered the surface of magnetite nanoparticles was estimated using Energy-dispersive X-ray spectroscopy (SEM-EDS) and Thermogravimetric analysis (TGA50, Shimadzu, Japan). The fluorescent properties of PAMAM-grafted magnetite nanoparticle were determined using fluorescence measured by SpectroFluorophotometer (RF–1510, Shimadzu, Japan).

Results and discussion

Uncoated magnetite nanoparticles

XRD analysis

Crystalline structure of magnetite nanoparticles were analyzed by XRD (Fig. 9.37). The results confirmed the formation of highly purified magnetite phase of iron oxide. The diffraction peaks at (111), (220), (311), (400), (422), (511), (440), (533) are the characteristic peaks of the Fe_3O_4 inverse spinel structure (JCPDS file no. 19-0629) without any interference with other phases of Fe_xO_y. Among Fe^{2+} and Fe^{3+}, ferric is the most stable iron form, thus ferrous ions (Fe^{3+}) could easily change into ferric ones. This process depends on many factors like pH of iron salt solution, initial temperature of reaction, and dissolved oxygen. It is reported by Gnanaprakash et al. (2007) that lower pH slows down the oxidation reaction. Therefore, in coprecipitation reaction, iron salt solution must be kept at lower pH and temperature prior to precipitation by alkaline media. In this study, the initial pH and temperature of salt solution were adjusted to 1.7 and 25°C, respectively to obtain a pure magnetite phase. The inter-planar space (d-value) of synthesized nanoparticles can be calculated using Bragg equation for the reflection peaks, as shown in Table 9.6. This can be used to distinguish between γ-Fe_2O_3 and Fe_3O_4 crystallographic structure. Broadening of the dominant intense peak in XRD graph (311) confirms the small size of the resultant particles. The crystalline size of Fe-B1 synthesized at 25°C and Fe-B2 at 70°C was calculated as 10.10 nm and 9.98 nm, respectively using Debay-Sherrer's equation (9.107) (Faiyas et al. 2010).

$$D = \frac{K\lambda}{\beta\cos\theta} \tag{9.107}$$

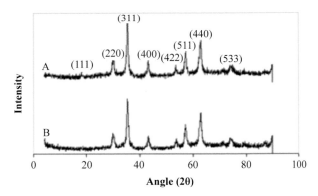

Figure 9.37. XRD pattern of synthesized magnetite nanoparticles at (a) 25°C (b) 70°C.

Table 9.6. Comparison between theoretical and calculated amount of d-value.

Angle (2θ)	Calculated d-value (Å)	Theoretical d-value of Fe_3O_4 (Å)	Theoretical d-value of γ-Fe_2O_3 (Å)	Crystalline plane (hlk)
18.28	4.84	4.85	4.82	(111)
30.155	2.961	2.96	2.95	(220)
35.395	2.534	2.532	2.51	(311)
43.075	2.098	2.099	2.089	(400)
53.705	1.709	1.71	1.70	(422)
57.020	1.614	1.615	1.61	(511)
62.820	1.478	1.48	1.47	(440)

In this equation, D, λ, and β represent the mean diameter of particles, the wavelength of incident X-ray, and the full width at half height (FWHM), respectively and constant K is equal to 0.9. Table 9.6 shows the details of theoretical and calculated values for crystalline plane.

As described above, in order to prevent oxidation of ferrous ions, the initial reaction temperature was set to 25°C. As Nyirokosa et al. (2009) reported, at constant ionic strength, increasing temperature from 25 to 90°C had no effect on crystal size, but Hosono et al. (2009) showed that at reaction temperatures above 50°C, a single phase magnetite can be obtained. Also, Guang et al. (2007) reported that as the reaction time increased to 4 hours, the size of magnetite nanoparticles decreased. It was asserted that unreacted $Fe(OH)_3$ in the samples synthesized at shorter times make sample sizes larger than those synthesized in prolonged times (particles reach their smallest diameter at prolonged times when the $Fe(OH)_3$ was completely reacted into magnetite). In this study all samples, similar to previous works (Tao et al. 2008, Khosroshahi and Ghazanfari 2011), showed magnetite phase with an added finding that smaller grain size was obtained by increasing time and temperature of the reaction.

TEM analysis

Morphology and mean size of quasi spherical particles prepared at 25°C and 70°C were studied by TEM.

Depending on the synthesis conditions, their sizes varied from 7 to 12 nm, as seen in Table 9.4. The samples prepared at room temperature possessed more polydispersity and aggregation in comparison with those at higher temperature. The nanoparticles can be aggregated due to the high surface/volume ratio, thus leading tp augmentation of magnetic dipole-dipole interactions. Fe-A1 and Fe-A2 showed the smallest size and the highest aggregation. Increasing the concentration of Fe salts causes the increase in particle size, likely due to the nucleation and growth phenomena that happens in supersaturation state (Nyirokosa et al. 2009, Yu et al. 2009). This means that in supersaturation state more nuclei are produced. Therefore, with reduction in ingredient concentration, the nuclei tend to grow using the available ions (i.e., the more ingredient concentration, the higher the particle size) (Yu et al. 2009). Figure 9.38 illustrates the variation

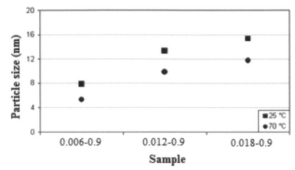

Figure 9.38. Variation of particle size with Fe salt concentration and temperature measured by TEM.

of particle size regarding the Fe salt concentration at two distinct temperatures. As it can be seen, increasing in iron salt concentration at constant temperature results in larger particles. However, when the temperature increases a similar behaviour is observed, but at a smaller scale.

Magnetic measurements

Magnetic properties of nanoparticles were determined by VSM at room temperature. The results show that the saturation magnetization can reach up to 63 emu/gr at 25°C and 68 emu/gr at 70°C. The VSM results confirm the superparamagnetic behaviour of these nanoparticles where the particles have sizes around magnetic monodomain, as seen in Fig. 9.39. Saturation magnetization, Ms, of nanoparticles is reduced compared to bulk material (92 emu/gr) possibly because of the presence of non-magnetic layer at the particle surface, cation distribution, and spin effects (Guang et al. 2007, Faiyas et al. 2010, Hosono et al. 2009). Early models interpreted the reduction of Ms based on the existence of a dead magnetic layer originated by the demagnetization of the surface spin, with paramagnetic behaviour. Figure 9.39 shows that increasing the iron salt concentration at constant temperature increases Ms value from 42 to 64 emu/g due to growth of particle size (Yu et al. 2009).

As is also seen from Fig. 9.40, at constant temperature (25°C) the Ms value increases by increasing the salt concentration until it reaches a plateau at about 60 emu/g. A similar behaviour is also observed when the samples reacted at higher temperature (70°C). It should be noted that magnetization saturation of the samples prepared at higher temperature was higher than the other ones. Using Langevin's equation and magnetic experimental data, the average magnetic particle diameter were calculated (Racuciu 2009):

$$a_M^3 = \frac{18K_B T}{\pi\mu_0 M_b M_s}(\frac{dM}{dH})_{H\to 0}$$

(9.108)

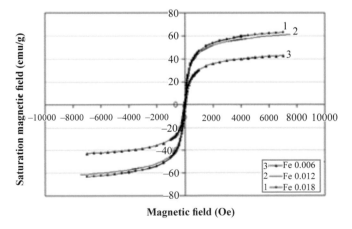

Figure 9.39. VSM diagrams of (Fe-A1, Fe-B1, and Fe-C1) prepared at 25°C.

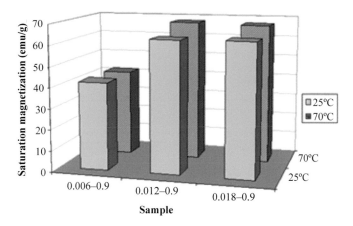

Figure 9.40. Variation of Ms with Fe salts concentration and temperature.

where a_M is the magnetic particle diameter, k_B is Boltzmann's constant, μ_0 is the vacuum magnetic permeability, and M_b is the magnetization of bulk magnetite. The results of particle size calculation using the above equation are given in Table 9.5. According to these results, magnetite nanoparticles synthesized at elevated temperature and moderate iron salt concentration showed improved magnetic properties and finer particle size distribution compared to lower temperature. Therefore, based on these results, the rest of experiment was carried out using the finer nanoparticles synthesized at higher temperature.

Coated magnetite nanoparticles

One of the most important aspects in production of stable ferrofluid is the prohibition against aggregation especially in biological medium. Stabilization of such materials could be achieved by the equilibrium between attractive and repulsive forces. There are several forces which act in relationship in nanomaterials, Van de Waals forces and repulsive forces. In a system consisting magnetic materials, magnetic dipolar forces must be considered. Most of the researches in the area of stabilization of magnetic nanoparticles are focused on the development of two important kinds of repulsive forces: i.e., electrostatic and steric repulsive forces (Laurent et al. 2008). Because of high surface-to-volume ratio, surface activity of nanoparticle and pendent surface functional groups, superficial atoms of these nanoparticles are apt to absorb ions and atoms existed in solution. Therefore magnetite can make covalent bonds with atoms of solution. Many studies indicated that magnetite surface hydroxyl can undergo chemical and physical reactions to functionalize surface with desired molecules (Nakanishi et al. 2004, Laurent et al. 2008). One of the most interesting and noble material which could be used for surface coating of magnetite is dendrimer. There have been two fundamental synthesis roots developed for the production of dendrimer construction: namely, divergent and convergent methods. Most researchers followed the early attempt of PAMAM dendrimer synthesis in which Tomalia (2005) reported the divergent strategy for production of this kind of dendritic structure. This technique begins with focal point or core and the final peripheral groups is generated by reiterated synthesis steps. Schematic modification reaction of magnetite with PAMAM dendrimer, which could enhance both electrostatic and steric repulsive forces, is illustrated in Fig. 9.41.

FTIR spectroscopy

In order to technically assert the formation of APTS layer and also PAMAM dendritic polymer on the surface of magnetite, FTIR spectroscopy was performed (Fig. 9.42). The absorption bands at 420 and 446 cm^{-1} and strong peaks around 581 and 629 cm^{-1} confirm the existence of magnetite nanoparticles (these peaks represent that initial ones at 370 and 570 cm^{-1} were split and shifted towards shorter wavelengths because of small size of particles) (Feng et al. 2008). The peak at 993 cm^{-1} (in G-0 curve) is related to

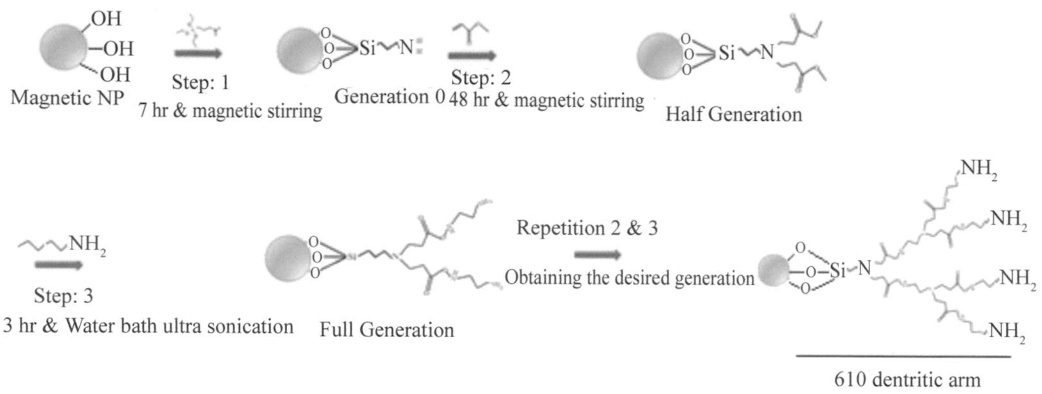

Figure 9.41. Schematic reaction of magnetite surface coating with PAMAM dendrimer.

Si-O-Fe bonds and the stretching vibration of C-N bond which overlaps with stretching vibration of Si-O observed at 1048 cm^{-1} (Launer 1987). Peaks at 1148 cm^{-1} and 1544 cm^{-1} show Si-CH$_2$(CH)xCH$_3$ and SiO3(CH$_2$)3NH$_2$ bonds, respectively which confirms the binding of APTS molecules at the surface of magnetite (Launer 1987). Moreover, bands at 2855 and 2922 cm^{-1} illustrate the presence of CH$_2$ bonds on aminopropyl group. The broad peak at 3444 cm^{-1} shows the bending mode of free NH$_2$ groups existed at APTS (Yamaura et al. 2004, Ma et al. 2003). The peak at 1151 cm^{-1} (in PAMAM-grafted magnetite nanoparticles) indicates the presence of C=O bond in ester groups and may overlap with the band related to Si-CH$_2$(CH)$_x$CH$_3$ group. In these spectra two intense peaks at 1570 cm^{-1} and 1631 cm^{-1} are observed that can be assigned to the N-H bending/C-N stretching (amide II) and C-O stretching (amide I) vibration of PAMAM dendrimer, respectively (Baykal et al. 2012). Evidently, the results revealed that with increasing the dendrimer generation, the corresponding signal intensity of these two peaks also increases. This effectively indicates a successful repetitive formation of amide bonds on the surface of magnetite nanoparticles. The band at 1718 cm^{-1} which appears in the FTIR spectra of ester terminated PAMAM dendrimers (half generations: G0.5 and G2.5) affirms the presence of ester groups (-CO$_2$CH$_3$) (Li et al. 2010). This band was not observed in the amino terminated products (full generations: G1 and G3), which implies the perfection of amidation reaction in this procedure. The incompletion of amidation reaction during the synthesis of PAMAM dendrimer is counted as a drawback of divergent method, which was omitted in present investigation by performing the synthesis reaction under N$_2$ atmosphere. The band at 1480 cm^{-1} was related to methylene group (Tsubokawa and Takayama 2000) and also the bands at 2861 cm^{-1} and 2935 cm^{-1} contributed to the symmetrical and anti-symmetrical stretching vibration of C-H groups, respectively (Ma et al. 2003, Tsubokawa and Takayama 2000). In addition, the peak at 3418 cm^{-1} is related to bending vibration of secondary amine groups.

EDS and TGA

As mentioned above, the mean diameter of optimal magnetite nanoparticles is about 9 nm, and in an ideal case, one can calculate the number of Fe atoms in every Fe$_3$O$_4$ particle using the following formula:

$$N_{Fe} = \frac{\frac{4}{3}\pi R^3 N_a}{\overline{V}_{Fe_3O_4}} \times 3 = 19677 \qquad (9.109)$$

where $\overline{V}_{Fe_3O_4}$ refers to the molar volume of bulk Fe$_3$O$_4$, R is the mean radius of Fe$_3$O$_4$ nanoparticles, and Na is Avogadro's number. If there is a monolayer of APTS molecules coated on the Fe$_3$O$_4$ particle, then the total number of APTS molecules on the surface of every Fe$_3$O$_4$ nanoparticle can be calculated by following formula:

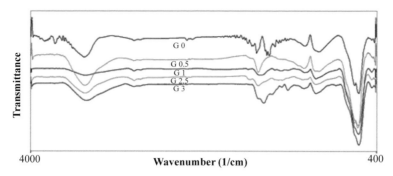

Figure 9.42. FTIR spectra of APTS and dendrimer-grafted magnetite nanoparticles.

$$N_{APTS} = \frac{S_{Fe_3O_4}}{S_{APTS}} = \frac{4\pi R^2}{S_{APTS}} = 748 \tag{9.110}$$

In this equation, SFe_3O_4 is the surface area of Fe_3O_4 particle and SAPTS is the surface coverage area of about 0.40 nm^2 per APTS molecule according to the literature (Boerio et al. 1980). So the atomic ratio of Fe/Si is = 26.30. From the peak area of Fe and Si in SEM-EDS elemental analysis graph of APTS-magnetite nanoparticles (Fig. 9.43), the atomic ratio of Fe/Si is calculated as $40.02/1.55 = 25.81$. This demonstrates that the atomic percent of Si is close to the expected value, which confirms the formation of layer with a thickness of about one APTS molecule on the surface of magnetite nanoparticles.

One trustworthy way of quantifying the number of coated molecules on the surface of nanoparticles is TGA. Figure 9.44 presents TGA curve of magnetite nanoparticles modified with APTS and PAMAM dendrimer. As can be seen in this figure, the APTS-coated compound lost 8 percent of its mass at 700°C while the mass lost began at about 300°C. This may be explained by vaporization and carbonization of organic component. Since the mean diameter of the magnetite nanoparticles was known and there was no mass loss for unmodified magnetite nanoparticle, so the number of APTS molecules calculated according to the following formula (Fu et al. 2001):

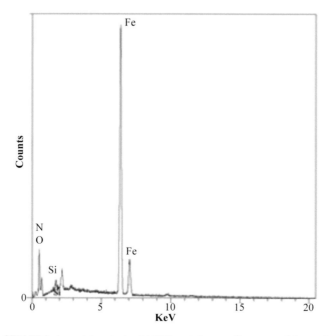

Figure 9.43. SEM-EDS elemental analysis of APTS-coated magnetite nanoparticles on Au substrate.

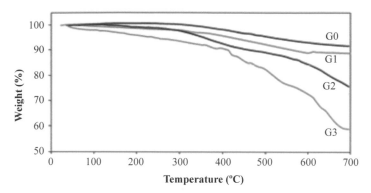

Figure 9.44. TGA curve of magnetite nanoparticles modified with different generation of dendrimer.

$$N_{APTS} = \frac{\omega N_a \rho \frac{4}{3} \pi R^3}{(1-\omega)M_{APTS}} \tag{9.111}$$

Here N_{APTS} is the APTS number on each particle, ω is the mass loss, ρ is the density of magnetite, and M_{APTS} is the relative molecular weight of APTS. As a result, it can be estimated that 610 APTS molecules attend to form a layer on the surface of each magnetite nanoparticle. Using the EDS and TGA data, it can be concluded that there are about 610 amine groups available on the surface of each coated particle which effectively could participate in the reaction leading to the formation of dendritic arms for PAMAM dendrimer coating on the surface of magnetite nanoparticles.

The TGA results are similar to previous studies related to synthesis of PAMAM dendrimer (Baykal et al. 2012, Shi et al. 2009). The percent of mass loss was increased with increasing the dendrimer generation number, which is expected due to the increase in chain length of C-backbone and molecular weight of dendrimers (compared to the lower generations). The remaining quantities may manifest the residual inorganic content due to the existence of iron oxide phase. Our findings are in good agreement with Niu et al. (2011), who reported ester terminated products (half generation) are thermally stable under 200°C. However, decomposition of amino-terminated products began at the start of heating, and thus the full generation dendrimers had relatively low thermal stability. Clearly, the TGA curves of PAMAM dendrimer have two stages of mass loss which was observed and reported before (Zheng et al. 2009). At the first stage, the formation of hydrogen bonds between the amine groups leads to the increase in viscosity of G1, G2, and G3, which made the complete removal of amine groups difficult at first stage. The second stage accounts for the decomposition of the dendrimer structure. As mentioned above there are 610 dendritic arms on each particle, and mass loss of G1–G3 dendrimer-grafted magnetite nanoparticles were theoretically calculated by the following formula:

$$W = \frac{610 \frac{M_{den}}{N_a}}{\rho \frac{4}{3} \pi R^3 + 610 \frac{M_{den}}{N_a}} \times 100 \tag{9.112}$$

Here, W is the mass loss of PAMAM-grafted magnetite nanoparticles and M_{den} is the relative molecular weight of dendritic arms calculated according to their chemical structure. TGA graphs show the average mass loss of about 8%, 11.58%, 24.32%, and 41.01% for different generations of dendrimer grafted magnetite nanoparticles (generation 0 to 3, respectively). The theoretical and experimental values of mass losses are represented in Table 9.7, which indicates a high efficiency and accuracy of synthesis method for production of PAMAM-grafted magnetite nanoparticles.

Table 9.7. Theoretical and experimental mass loss of G0-G3 dendrimers-grafted magnetite.

Material	Weight loss %	
	Theoretical	**Experimental**
G_0	----	8.19
G_1	11.08	11.58
G_2	23.431	24.32
G_3	40.071	41.01

XRD and TEM analysis

The XRD graph of APTS-coated magnetite nanoparticles shows no dramatic change in crystalline structure (Fig. 9.48b). The XRD pattern of PAMAM-grafted magnetite nanoparticles (Fig. 9.45c), reveals a noteworthy intensity decrease of Bragg peaks which may show the amorphous nature of coating material (PAMAM dendrimer) on the surface of inorganic core with the magnetite phase. According to Eq. 9.125, the particle sizes of coated samples are about 11.2 nm and 13.5 nm for APTS-coated and PAMAM-grafted magnetite nanoparticles, respectively. Figure 9.46 shows a relatively uniform distribution and less aggregation of nanoparticles in the presence of APTS and PAMAM molecules on the surface of magnetite particles.

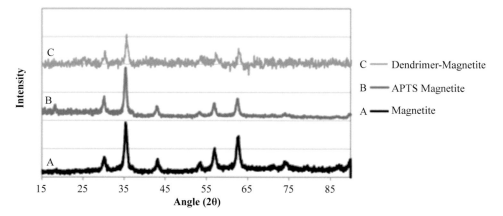

Figure 9.45. XRD graph of (a) APTS-coated and (b) PAMAM-grafted magnetite nanoparticles.

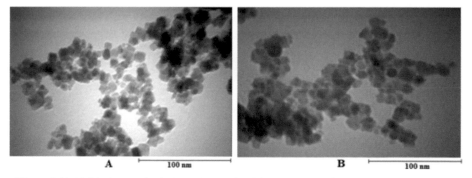

Figure 9.46. TEM micrograph of (a) APTS-coated and (b) PAMAM-grafted magnetite nanoparticles.

Magnetic measurements

As it is observed from VSM results in Fig. 9.47, the APTS-coated and PAMAM-grafted magnetite nanoparticles exhibited a strong magnetization of 65.4 and 62.1 emu/gr, respectively with no hysteresis loop at 300 K and that the magnetization process was reversible. Also, due to lack of any measurable coersivity and remanance, materials are superparamagnetic. It should be, however, noted that the magnetization of APTS-coated and PAMAM-grafted magnetite is slightly lower than the magnetite nanoparticles which is because of the presence of non-magnetic material (Herea and Chiriac 2008).

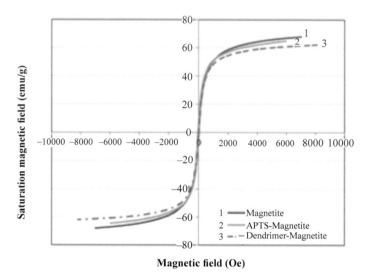

Figure 9.47. VSM result of (1) magnetite nanoparticles synthesized at 70°C and (2) APTS-coated (3) PAMAM-grafted magnetite nanoparticles.

UV-Vis and fluorescence spectroscopy

The absence of absorption peak in the UV-Vis spectra with the presence of fluorescent illumination at the same time is an important feature of PAMAM dendrimer (Majoros et al. 2006, Wang et al. 2007). This property could be considered as an excellent way to recognize the formation of PAMAM moieties on the surface of magnetite nanoparticle cores. Figure 9.48 shows the absorption peaks for the UV-Vis spectrum of magnetite nanoparticles in the range of 340–380 nm. With formation of polymeric layer on the surface of this inorganic material, the intensity of the peaks reduces at higher generation order.

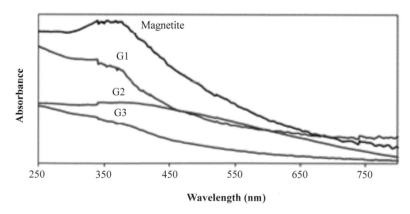

Figure 9.48. UV-Vis spectra of pure magnetite nanoparticles G1, G2, G3-modified magnetite nanoparticles.

Figure 9.49 shows the fluorescent properties of the resultant PAMAM-grafted magnetite nanoparticles (generation 3). This material has an excitation at 298 nm and a corresponding emission band ranging between 305 nm and 335 nm with a maximum peak around 328 nm. These results are found to be in good agreement with the finding of Divsar et al. (2009). The emission band is thought to be related to the creation of amine rich nanocluster and electron-hole recombination processes involving correlated electron-hole excitation states between localized states of electrons and holes within PAMAM (Pastor-Perez et al. 2007).

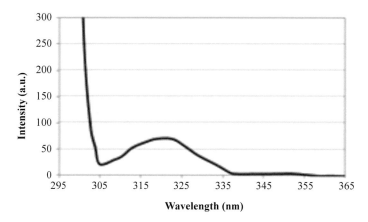

Figure 9.49. Fluorescent spectrum of PAMAM-grafted magnetite nanoparticles.

9.5.3 The effect of pH and magnetic field on the fluorescence spectra of fluorescein isothiocyanate (FITC) conjugated SPION-dendrimer nanocomposites (Rezvani Alanagh et al. 2014)

In this study, fluorescent dendro-nized magnetic nanoparticles (FDMNPs) with their unique pH sensitive nature were synthesized for biomedical applications. First, superparamagnetic iron oxide nanoparticles (SPIONs) were prepared by coprecipitation of Fe^{+2} and Fe^{+3} with NH_4OH, and then modified by amino silane. Polyamidoamine (PAMAM) dendrimer were coated on the SPIONAPTS surface using Michel addition method and grew from generation 0.5 to 3. In the final step of synthesis, the reaction between isoslulfosyanic groups of fluorescein isothiocyanate (FITC), and amine terminal groups of DMNPs was lead to the formation of magnetic fluorescent nanocomposites. The FDMNPs were studied using Fourier transform infrared spectrometer (FT-IR), X-ray diffraction (XRD), transmission electron microscopy (TEM), UV-visible spectroscopy, fluorescence spectroscopy, vibrating-sample magnetometery (VSM), zeta potential, and Dynamic Light Scattering (DLS). The size of SPIONs and FDMNPs were about 10 nm and 14 nm, respectively. The possibility of conjugating a large number of fluorescein isothiocyanate (FITC) molecules on the SPIONs together with high amount of magnetization saturation, Ms (52 emu/g in our case) and other unique characteristics have nominated FDMNPs as a suitable candidate for biomedical applications.

Materials and methods

All analytic reagents were of analytical grade and were used without further purification. FITC was purchased from Aldrich Chemical Co. Ferric chloride ($FeCl_3.6H_2O$), ferrous sulfate ($FeSO_4.7H_2O$), amine propyl trimethoxy silane (APTS), ethylenediamine, and methylacrylate were obtained from Merck.

Preparation of fluorescent magnetodendrimer

Synthesis procedure for SPION (MNPs) and PAMAM-functionalized SPION nanoparticles (DMNPs) was same as those described in the previous section. FDMNPs could be obtained by the reaction between the isosulfocyanic group of FITC and the amino groups of the DMNs. 0.002 g/ml of ethanol solution of FITC (large excess of the amino groups) was added to 0.02 g/ml aqueous solution of magnetic particles grafted by third generation PAMAM. After 24 h of stirring in the dark at room temperature, the products were washed through four cycles of centrifugation/ethanol and centrifugation/deionized water.

Characterization of FDMNPs

The purity of the FITC-DMNPs conjugates were evaluated by thin layer chromatography (TLC) (data has not been shown). The average size was estimated using a transmission electron microscope (Model CM120, PHILIPS). Fourier transformation-IR (FT-IR) spectra of samples were obtained using a FT-IR spectrophotometer (NEXUS 670, Nicolet). X-ray diffraction studies were performed using EQUINOX (3000, INEL) with monochromated $Cu K\alpha 1$ ($\lambda = 1.5406A°$, 40 kV, 40 mA), the extent of FITC conjugation was measured in a UV visible spectrophotometer (Sunnyvale, CA). Magnetization measurement was performed at room temperature using a vibrating sample magnetometer (VSM) device. Magnetisation measurements were carried at 300K in a magnetic field (H) up to 8.5 k Oe with a vibrating sample magnetometer (VSM-PAR 155). Zeta potential of DMNP and FDMNP along with hydrodynamic diameter of FDMNP were determined through zeta sizer (Malvern, Nano ZS). Fluorescence spectroscopy (Perkin Elmer, Ls55) was used to evaluate the pH and external magnetic field sensibility of FDMNPs. Before the measurements, the samples were dried at 15°C in a vacuum for 6 h.

Results and discussion

FTIR spectroscopy

The formation of FDMNPs in Fig. 9.53 was confirmed by comparing the FT-IR spectra of MNPs-APTS, DMNPs, and FITC. All the samples exhibited the characteristic peaks of Fe_3O_4 nanoparticles which are including: Fe_{2+}–Fe_{2-} band, observed at 590 cm^{-1} and Fe_{3+}–Fe_{2-} band observed at 445 cm^{-1} (Larson and Tucker 2001). The peaks at 995 cm^{-1} and 1049 cm^{-1} are due to presence of Si-O and C-N bonds, respectively (Jia and Song 2012). However, their frequencies are shifted to lower values, indicating strong Si bonding. These peaks apparently confirm the accuracy of the second stage of our synthesis where the stretching vibration of Si–O at the surface of aminosilane–MNP is at 995 cm^{-1} which shifts to about 1038 cm^{-1} of the DMNPs due to the presence of highly electronegative –CO–NH groups (Cole et al. 1990), as shown in Fig. 9.50a. This provides further evidence to confirm that the aminosilanization reaction was successfully achieved during the preparation.

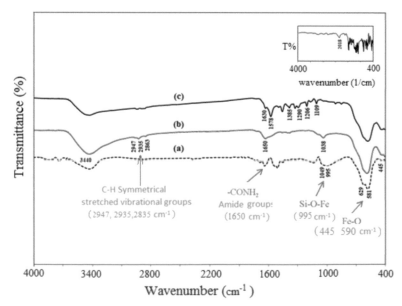

Figure 9.50. FT-IR spectra of (a) MNPs-APTS, (b) DMNPs, (c) FDMNPs; inset: FT-IR spectra of FITC.

The bending vibration of –NH₂ group is at 3440 cm⁻¹ and for –CO–NH– group is at 1650 cm⁻¹ which is in agreement with previous studies (Pelliccioli and Wirz 2002, Mchedlov-Petrossyan and Mayorga 1992). Also, it can be seen from Fig. 9.50b that compared to the G0 sample, the G3 DMNPs exhibits absorption bands at 2863, 2935, and 2947 cm⁻¹ due to stretching vibration of the C–H bond. These observations reveal the presence of PAMAM dendrimer (Zhang 2009). The formation of the FITC-DMNP conjugate in Fig. 9.53c is evident from the disappearance of the characteristic isothiocyanate stretching band of FITC at 2018 cm⁻¹ (Zhang 2009) (inset Fig. 9.50). This indicates that FDMNP does not have free FITC in its combination. The weakened absorbance band of NH₂ at 3400 ~ 3250 cm⁻¹ compared to DMNPs spectrum and the disappearance of the absorbance band at 2000–2280 cm⁻¹ of N=C=S may all indicate the formation of a thiourea bond that could be confirmed by the absorption peaks at 1150–1450 cm⁻¹ (Veronesi et al. 2002). The 1150–1450 cm⁻¹ bands are assigned to the reaction between the primary amine of the dendrimer surface and the isothiocyanate group of FITC. The absorption peaks of functional groups of FDMNPs are shown in Table 9.8.

Table 9.8. Absorption peaks of functional groups of FDMNPs.

Peak (cm⁻¹)	Functional group	Peak (cm⁻¹)	Functional group
3400–3250	Primary amide	3000–2500	O-H
1630	C=O (stretching)	1578	C-N-H
1385, 1549	Secondary amide	1206	C=S
1290	C-N (stretching)	1109	C-O-C

UV-Vis Spectroscopy

The results of absorption spectroscopy for MNPs, DMNPs, FDMNPs, and FITC are shown in Fig. 9.51 where no significant absorption is observed for MNPs and DMNPs as expected (Jia and Song 2012, Yang et al. 2009). However, when DMNPs were conjugated with FITC, the peak at 490 nm (for FITC) was shifted towards a longer wavelength at 504 nm showing about 14 nm red shift which corresponds to thiourea bond in FDMNPs. The average number of FITC molecules conjugated to each DMNP was 58 per a DMNP determined by the standard calibration curve of free FITC. Considering the large number of amino terminal groups on DMNPs surface, this is a significant amount (Liu et al. 2011).

VSM

Figure 9.52 illustrates the magnetization curve recorded at room temperature. A saturation magnetization (Ms) of 67.4 emu/g and 52.1 emu/g were determined for MNPs and FDMNPs, respectively (data for MNPs

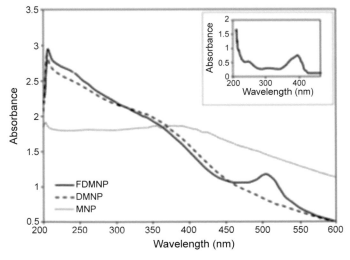

Figure 9.51. UV spectra of MNPs, DMNPs and FDMNPs; inset: UV spectra of FITC.

is not shown). The reduced Ms of magnetite nanoparticles may be explained by the fact that a PAMAM dendrimer coating lead to the formation of a nonmagnetic layer on top of the magnetic core which can substantially decrease the magnetization of the nanoparticles (Baykal et al. 2012). Also, the spins of the oxygen atoms close to the surface are pinned and this weakens the super exchange interaction between Fe-O-Fe atoms, causing the overall magnetization of the nanocomposite to decrease (Neuberger et al. 2005). The decrease in Ms is further enhanced by the presence of FITC on the surface of DMNPs. However, the Ms of these superparamagnetic nanocomposites is still high enough to be used for magnetic resonance imaging (MRI) and magnetic drug targeting (MDT) (Hadjipanayis et al. 2008).

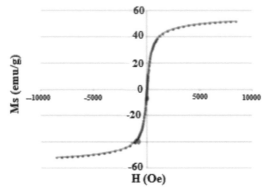

Figure 9.52. Magnetization curve of FDMNPs at 300 K.

Fluorescence spectroscopy

FITC conjugation

Various works have been done for evaluation of dendrimers fluorescence emission for different application (Liu et al. 2007, Jia and Song 2012). In our case, 0.25 mg/ml concentration of FITC conjugated DMNPs was excited at 495 nm. As is clearly seen in Fig. 9.53, there is a strong fluorescence emission at wavelength 520 nm for FDMNPs with no emission associated with MNPs and DMNPs. However, it should be noted that observing the fluorescence of dendrimers requires higher concentrations and an absorption wavelength in the range of 380–440 nm (Larson and Tucker 2001).

Evaluation of pH sensitivity of FDMNPs

The variation of FDMNPs fluorescence intensity with pH is shown in Fig. 9.54, where the output signal increases with increasing the pH value. It appears that by increasing the pH, not only the intensity amplitude

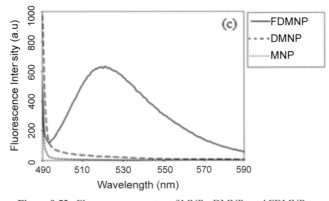

Figure 9.53. Fluorescence spectra of MNPs, DMNPs and FDMNPs.

increases, but also the peaks gradually shift towards longer wavelengths showing a red Doppler shift and covering a range between 520–524 nm. It is interesting to note that the corresponding FWHM increases by about 5 nm when pH increases from 5 to 9. This characteristic is attributed to protropic forms of FITC which have different fluorescence intensities (Cole et al. 1990). As pH increases, the dianion form of FITC which is more fluorescent than the other protropic types becomes the dominant absorber in solution (Pelliccioli and Wirz 2002, Mchedlov-Petrossyan and Mayorga 1992). Three other protropic forms of mono-anion, natural, and cation with some overlapping pK are produced as pH decreases (Zhang 2009).

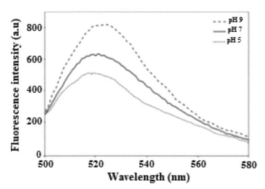

Figure 9.54. Fluorescence spectra of FDMNPs at different pH values of 4,6,8 and excitation wavelength of 495 nm.

Evaluation of fluorescence sensitivity to external magnetic field

One way to evaluate the effect of external magnetic field on the rate of sedimentation of nanoparticles is to study the fluorescence emission as a function of time. In Fig. 9.55, a vessel containing the FDMNPs suspended in ID water was placed on a magnet and the fluorescence was recorded at different times. As it is seen, the fluorescence amplitude decreases with time, indicating a progressively diminishing available nanoparticles concentration, but at the same time the width of curves at FWHM increases. Generally, In terms of spectroscopy, the width itself arises essentially because energy levels of atomic and molecular system (e.g., fluorophores) are not accurately determined and exhibits some degree of "fuzziness" causing broadening effect. As for the intensity, it can be explained by considering three important factors: (i) Transition probability, (ii) Population of states which tells us the most intense spectral line will arise from the level which initially has the greater population, and (iii) Path length of sample which relates the concentration of sample to amount of absorbed energy. It can be explained in terms of quenching rate that the decrease of observed intensity as a result of interaction of the ground or excited states of a fluorophore with other species in the medium, and is expressed as follows:

$$\phi = \frac{k_f}{k_f + K_i + k_x} \tag{9.113}$$

where ϕ is the efficiency of emission or quantum yield and k_f is the rate constant for fluorescence emission, k_i the rate constant for radiationless energy loss, and k_x the rate constant for intersystem crossing. The term k_f also relates to the average life time of the excited state τ_a by the equation $k_f = (\tau_a)^{-1}$. It is noted that the brightness (B) of a fluorophore is proportional to the ability of a substance to absorb light and fluorescence quantum yield; it is defined as $B = \phi$. Hence, highly fluorescent molecules have high values of both molar attenuation coefficient and fluorescence quantum yield, thus high absorbance and efficient emission. Thus, changes seen in the fluorescence spectrum can be attributed to the changes in number of factors including chromophores density, the physical structure, and chemical composition.

The FDMNPs nanocomposites are synthesized and characterized. Their appropriate size, magnetic saturation (Ms), the large number of conjugated FITC, pH sensitive, and the fluorescence nature are the key features for biomaterial applications, including multimodal imaging, theranostic, and drug delivery. In our case, a fluorescence range between 500–560 nm was observed and was shown that the intensity peak

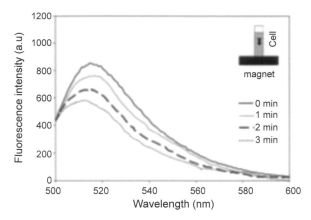

Figure 9.55. Fluorescence spectra of FDMNP at constant pH of 7 and excitation wavelength of 495 nm under magnetic field in 3 minutes.

increases with increasing pH, but it decreases as a function of time, which confirms that the path length of sample which relates the concentration to the absorbed energy gradually diminishes due to sedimentation under the external magnetic field. Moreover, since the appropriate range of hydrodynamic diameter of FDMNPs nanocomposites is between 30–150 nm, and sense some external triggers as pH and magnetic field so we believe they can be effectively utilized in biological sensing and diagnostics applications.

9.6 Quantum dots (QDs)

Quantum dots are essentially fluorescent-emitting semiconductor nanocrystals and have in recent years been used for bioimaging (Michalet et al. 2005, Xing and Rao 2008, Barroso 2011). They have broad excitation spectra, narrow emission spectra, tunable emission peaks due to tunable core size between (1–10 nm), long fluorescence life-times, and ability to be conjugated to proteins and negligible photobleaching. The optical properties of QDs are because of quantum confinement of valence electrons at nanometers. The fluorescent emission wavelength is defined by the energy band gap determined by the particle size and composition. The emission peak redshifts as the particle size increases. QDs have narrow emission band and the absorption spectra ranges from UV to visible wavelengths, hence providing multicolor fluorescence.

However, QDs are also subject to blinking, a random, intermittent loss of fluorescence intensity that disrupts particle tracking. Blinking originates from enhanced nonradiative decay resulting from additional charges on the nanoparticle surface, and defects. Blinking kinetics are stochastic, so when large number of QDs aggregate and form due to colloidal instability, they do not exhibit blinking. Since blinking kinetics of individual QDs in aggregate are out of phase, it produces a continuous fluorescent signal. Small clusters (e.g., $< 10^{15}$) can exhibit discernable blinking responses because of individual blinking within cluster. Therefore, this can be utilized to discern aggregation status of stationary particles (Nirmal et al. 1996, Yum et al. 2009). Most QDs are composed of binary alloys of II-VI, such as CdSe or III-V, such as InP semiconductor materials. To improve the quantum yield, DQDs are encapsulated in an insulating inorganic shell, e.g., ZnS. QDs are normally synthesized using an organometallic approach in which they are stabilized by hydrophobic surfactant and are therefore, soluble in non-polar media. It is critical to provide QDs water-soluble through modification of their surface in preparation for biological applications. Before using QDs in cellular imaging, one should consider the following: (a) stability and solubility in biological media, (b) high resistance to photobleaching and photophysical properties in aqueous media, (c) functional groups to conjugate to biomolecules, and (d) minimal overall hydrodynamic size. It should be noted that electrostatically stabilized QDs can increase the possibility of non-specific binding. Although coating with polymers can reduce these problems, the hydrodynamic size can indeed increase due to creating a steric barrier around the nanocrystal (see §4.2.7).

9.7 Upconversion nanoparticles

Photon upconversion is a process in which absorption of two or more photons leads to the emission of light at shorter wavelength than the excitation wavelength. It is an anti-Stokes type emission. Materials which can be used for upconversion are Ln3+, Ti2+, Ni2+, Mo3+, Re4+, Os4+, and so on. Unlike QDs, upconversion nanoparticles can absorb infrared radiation, e.g., 980 nm of commercial InGaAs diode lasers, and emit photons at visible spectra, e.g., 600 nm. Since this IR wavelength has a high penetration depth in biological tissues, it thus has the potential to be used for bioimaging applications. The upconversion process is achieved through continuous excitation of valence electrons of lanthanide ions by photon absorption or energy transfer from nearby lanthanide ions. The particles are composed of a host material doped with lanthanide ions that are sensitizers (Yb^+) and activators (Er^{3+}, Tm^{3+} and Ho^{3+}). The absorption and emission peaks of upconversion nanoparticles have an emission spectrum that can be tuned wide range by changing host materials and doping density.

9.8 Nanotoxicity

Nanomedicine is rapidly growing and advancing in different areas, generating a large number of potential diagnostic and therapeutic applications of nanosystems with variety of sizes (1–100 nm) and shapes in recent years. For example, nanoparticles less than 12 nm in diameter may cross the blood-brain barrier (Oberdorster et al. 2004) and objects of 30 nm or less can be endocytosed by cells (Conner and Schmid 2003). Thus, obtaining a knowledge about them and their impact on health, which may raise an issue seems to be essential. Safety issues of nanomaterials in any clinical applications are a major concern. The nanotoxicity of different nanomaterials has been studied extensively and are available in literature (Colvin 2003, Maynard et al. 2006, Helmus 2007, Pisanic et al. 2007, Lewinski et al. 2008, Alkiany and Murphy 2010, Lesniak et al. 2012, Seabra and Duran 2015, Liu et al. 2015, Khosroshahi and Tajabadi 2016).

Let us begin by reminding ourselves that when nanoparticles are injected into biological medium, either *in vivo* or *in vitro*, as in cell culture medium where it consists of mixture of electrolytes, proteins, nutrients and metabolites, they are rapidly coated with plasma proteins, such as immunoglobulins and fibronectin called protein corona and consequently build aggregates known as opsonization. The high surface area to volume ration makes nanoparticles particularly a potential candidate as catalysts and such particles can readily adhere to biological molecules. Therefore, in either case various components could interact with nanoparticles and change their physio-chemical properties including size, aggregation state, surface charge, and surface chemistry. In the case of *in vivo*, the opsonized particles are recognized by the reticuloendothelial system (RES) or mononuclear phagocytic system (MPS), which is comprised of macrophages acting as foreign bodies scavengers and are related to liver (Kupffer cells), spleen, lymph nodes, nervous system (microglia), and bones (osteoclasts). The RES is a defense system and comprises highly phagocytotic cells derived from bone marrow. These cells travel in the vascular system as monocytes and reside in their particular tissues. These macrophages internalize the opsonized nanoparticles through phagocytosis and deliver them to the liver, kidney, lymph node, and bone marrow (Lenaerts et al. 1984). This process occurs within 0.5–5 min (Couvreeur et al. 1980), thus removing the active nanoparticles from the circulation and prevent their access to the tumor tissue. Anyway, the size and surface charge of nanoparticles enable them to access places where larger particles may be blocked, such as passage through cellular membranes. The unfiltered nanoparticles by body's defense system due to their small size may cause inflammatory or toxic response. Thus, it is not the question of preventing the nanoparticles from entering the cells via a particular route as many biomedical applications relies on this process, but the fate of nanoparticles once they are entered and populated within cells, and if so what adverse effects can they impose internally if at all, and when? How can they be assessed?

It is well established that the presence of physiological medium and high ionic strength of the biological media can cause nanoparticle aggregation via electrostatic screening. On the other hand, the nanoparticles have a surface charge which tends to stabilize them against such aggregation via electrostatic repulsion. The importance of nanoparticles aggregation or clustering is in their influence on the cells during interaction process or may even enter the cells which can introduce new complexity to the system. Also, the protein corona can mediate the uptake of nanoparticles via receptor-mediated endocytosis. Therefore, different media with different protein compositions can cause various toxicity and uptake results. To this end, one can see how hard it is to reach one solid general conclusion regarding the nanoparticles' safety and toxicity despite large number of studies. This is mainly due to variability of the physical and chemical properties of particles, different experiment conditions, different methods of nanoparticle preparation, cell type, dosing parameters, the type of biochemical assay used, and lack of standard protocol for assessment. The cytotoxicity of a nanomaterial is influenced by number of parameters including: How the nanoparticles with regard to surface charge (pH, zeta potential), type of cell line, cell culture medium conditions, how to introduce particles for studies, nanoparticles concentration, size, and exposure time.

a) Cell lines: It is possible that the degree of cytotoxicity of two sets of the same cell lines be different when prepared by different protocols.

b) Testing method: This is an influential factor as some discrepancies between the results of toxicity assays can be observed. Generally, viability assays evaluate the overall dose-dependent toxicity of nanoparticles on the cultured cells including cell survival and proliferation after nanoparticles exposure. There are many assays which can be used, for example, the gold standard is the metabolic assay MTT. This is a colorimetric assay for assessing cell metabolic activity. NAD(P)H-dependent cellular oxidoreductase enzymes may, under defined conditions, reflect the number of viable cells present. These enzymes are capable of reducing the tetrazolium dye MTT 3-(4,5-dimethylthiazol-2-yl)-2,5-diphenyltetrazolium bromide to its insoluble formazan, which has a purple color. Another method is ROS (reactive oxygen species) assay which monitors the oxidative stress by measuring the level of ROS, and real-time polymerase chain reaction enhancement and DNA micro-array analysis to examine the expression levels of genes that are related to stress in the cell. It is noteworthy that measurement of cell response is one thing, and to find out where the nanoparticles are localized within the cell and what is their fate in future is something else. In many *in vitro* cytotoxicity analysis, cell death is studied by colorimetric assays, such as shift of absorption or emission of markers. One serious problem here is that nanoparticles can absorb and emit light which can be mixed with the marker hence producing a false or mixed signal. Since, cytotoxicity tests are primarily used to measure the effect of compound after it has been diffused into target cell, thus it is sensible to do the measurement within a limited time frame but long enough for nanoparticles to settle in as they are less mobile. Such tests cannot run for few days.

c) Characterization: The physical and chemical characterization methods are very crucial for cytotoxicity assessments. Typically, there are two distinct methods by which the assessment can be done: Dynamic light scattering (DLS) and Transmission electron microscopy (TEM). There are some discrepancies between these two methods which is due to differences in preparation, the nanoparticle sizing methods in polydisperse batches or samples. TEM serves as a means of determining of particles size and as its limitation it can only do it after the particles have been suspended and dried. Many different regions of particles should be measured in order to represent a true picture of sample geometry. On the other hand, DLS is performed in solutions and the suspending medium and the way the nanoparticle sample was mixed, e.g., by sonication can affect the nanoparticle hydrodynamic size.

d) Surface chemistry: This is important in cytotoxicity assay since citrate is the conjugate base of citric acid, which is used as reducing agent. It provides a negatively charged surface moiety that stabilizes nanoparticle colloids through Columbic repulsion. Such stabilized nanoparticles suspended in water have a considerable negative charge which acidifies the aqueous solution.

e) Protein corona: This affects the biocompatibility of nanoparticles by coating them and changing their surface properties.

As it was explained above, once the nanoparticles are introduced into a biological system, they confront complicated situation where they suffer number of problems such as corona effect, can be degraded because of neighboring biomolecules or even encapsulated by phagocytic cells or misdirected from the main target by lymphatic system. It is for these reasons that the results of an *in vitro* assay may not be possibly apply to an *in vivo* case. Also, an *in vivo* cytotoxicity assay should include inflammatory response, though these assays are subject to error because cells can behave differently depending on the type of assay used. The major limitations of current cytotoxicity assay are: (a) limited time-dependent monitoring of cell's activity because after a single assay, the cells cannot be recovered to their original state, (b) a single cell's response to the nanoparticles cannot be recorded individually because the assay's data are averaged over all the cells present, (c) the resident nanoparticles inside a cell may interfere with the dye fluorescence signal. In addition, protein corona is quite possible in a cell culture medium, thus affecting the nanoparticles normal interactions with cells. Furthermore, the assay's true positive signal can be influenced when the nanoparticles are bound to cytokines released from the cells.

Gold nanoparticles (Au-NPs)

Generally, AuNPs are considered inert and biocompatible, however, some contradictory results concerning their toxicity are reported (Alkiany et al. 2010, Dreaden et al. 2012). Smaller particles exhibit greater surface to volume ratio, thus providing a larger surface for interaction with cellular or intercellular components. The toxic effects of bare AuNPs include membrane injury, inflammatory responses, DNA damage, and apoptosis in mammalian cells (Pan et al. 2009, Kang et al. 2010). The toxicity originates from the generation of ROS that is essential for the signal transduction pathways that regulate cell growth and redox status. Excess ROS is linked to DNA damage and cellular apoptosis, which can activate mitogen-activated protein kinase (MAPK) pathways. These are signal transduction mediators, which regulate many cellular processes (Torres 2003). However, it is well known that suitably coating the AuNPs with polymers or silica can greatly reduce the toxic effects (Shi et al. 2007). Multiplexed analysis of nanoparticles in the same well with single cells can be used as new strategy in safety studies of various nanoparticles. Zhu et al. (2003) used this technique to study the AuNPs uptake by cells using mass spectrometry. They showed that the cellular uptake of functionalized AuNPs with cationic or neutral surface ligands can be readily determined using laser desorption/ionization mass spectrometry. The technique allowed different nanoparticles to be simultaneously identified and quantified at levels as low as 30 pmol. Vujacic et al. (2011) investigated the concentration and size dependent cytotoxic effects of Au-NPs, using two *in vitro* human cells model system: proliferating lymphocytes and connective tissue fibroblasts. Treatment of lymphocytes cultures including nanoparticles caused cytotoxic effects as revealed by significant enhancement of cell proliferation potential when compared to the control. The enhancement of micronuclei incidence and proliferation index depend not only on concentration but also the size of the nanoparticles. In a work, Soenen et al. (2012) evaluated the effects of polymethacrylate acid (PMA) coated 4 nm diameter Au-NPs on variety of cells: C17.2 neural progenitor cells, human vein endothelial cells, and PC12 rat pheochromocytoma cells, using a multiparametric approach. They used various concentrations and incubation times and performed a stepwise analysis of the NP effects on cell viability, ROS, cell morphology, cytoskeleton structure, and cell functionality. The data showed that higher NP concentration (200 nM) reduce cell viability mainly through induction of ROS, which was significantly induced at concentration of 50 nM or higher. At 10 nM, no significant effects on any cellular parameter could be observed. They suggested that multiple assay is able to cover the broad spectrum of cell-NP interactions. Recently, Liu et al. (2015) reported that results of cytotoxicity assay using various gold-mesoporous silica nanoparticles for breast cancer cells. All AuNPs showed little cytotoxicity below 6.25 µg/mL. Time-dependent toxicity was also investigated at 12.5 µg/mL. Janus Au@mSiO$_2$ showed lowest toxicity than other nanoparticles with more potential biomedical applications.

Magnetic nanoparticles (MNPs)

MNPs offer some attractive possibilities in biomedicine, and similar to other nanoparticles, their size can vary from few nanometers to tens of nanometers. MNPs possess unique magnetic properties enabling them to offer a range of interesting applications such as enhanced quality of magnetic resonance imaging (MRI), hyperthermia treatment of malignant cells, targeted drug delivery. Although iron oxide are relatively less toxic compared to other transition metal or semiconductor nanomaterials, recent studies have shown these particles can affect normal cell functionalities, instead of only being carriers (Lewinski et al. 2008, Jiang et al. 2008). Uncoated MNPs can cause significant cell death after cellular internalization. The cytotoxicity is greatly reduced by coating the particles by hydrophilic and biocompatible substances. It has been suggested that the adverse effect of MNPs is due to ROS and cellular internalization (Lewinski et al. 2008). Transition metal oxide nanoparticles can produce ROS as catalysts in a Fenton-type reaction, in which hydrogen peroxide is reduced by ferrous ions to form very active hydroxyl-free radicals and lead to biological damage within the diffusion range (Lewinski et al. 2008). The ultimate intercellular target of MNPs is important as far as the safety at such scale is concerned. It is for this reason that nanoparticles are coated and specifically functionalized for receptor-mediated internalization and the endocytic pathway. Parameters which affect this include shape, size, chemical composition, aspect ratio, and surface charges. In a research by Pisanic et al. (2007), the specific effects of anionic dimercaptosuccinic acid (DMSA)-coated MNPs on cultured PC12 cells were investigated. Enhanced endocytosis via anionic DMSA coating is simple, efficient, and well-characterized method of intracellular delivery of Fe_3O_4 nanoparticles due to nonspecific adsorption to the cell surface followed by endocytosis into the cell. It was shown that even intercellular delivery of even moderate levels of Fe_3O_4 nanoparticles may have adverse effects on cell function. The most obvious effect that MNPs had on the cells was their ability to generate mature neurites. Of the live cells evaluated, those exposed to 0.15, 1.5, and 15 mM AMNP iron concentrations on average produced 2.67, 1.9, and 0.97 neurites per cell, respectively, as compared to 2.79 in the control (Pisanic et al. 2007). Recently Sabareeswaran et al. (2016) investigated the acute changes in cell morphology and function following intravenous administration of surface-modified SPIONS in a rat model. Dextran-coated (DEX) and polyethylene glycol-coated (PEG) SPIONS were synthesized and characterized, and cytocompatibility was evaluated *in vitro*. Haematological, histopathological, ultrastructural, and oxidative stress analyses were carried out 24 h post intravenous administration *in vivo*. They concluded that, although surface modification of SPIONS improved biocompatibility *in vitro*, they affected anti-oxidant and tissue nitrite levels, which greatly influenced mast cell infiltration *in vivo*.

Keywords: Nanobiomaterial, Magnetite, Iron-oxide, Superparamagnetism, Curie temperature, Ferrofluid, Rheology, Gold nanoparticle, Surface plasmon resonance, Nanoshell, Aggregation, Dendrimers, Cytotoxicity.

Refferrence

Al-Jamal, K., W. Al-Jamal, J. Wang, N. Rubio and J. Buddle. 2013. Cationic poly-l-lysine dendrimer complexes doxorubicin and delays tumor growth *in vitro* and *in vivo*. ACS Nano. 7: 1905–1917.

Alkiany, A., R. Frerry and C. Murphy. 2010. Gold nanorods as nanomicelles: 1-naphthol partitioning into a nanorod-bound surfactant bilayer. Langmuir. 24: 10235–10139.

Alkiany, A. and C. Murphy. 2010. Toxicity and cellular uptake of gold nanoparticles: what we have learned so far? J. Nanopart. Res. 12: 2313–2333.

Allemann, E., R. Gurny and E. Doelker. 1992. Preparation of aqueous polymeric nanodispersions by a reversible salting-out Process: Influence of process parameters on particle size. Int. J. Pharm. 87: 247–253.

Allemann, E., R. Gurny and E. Doelker. 1993. Drug-loaded nanoparticles: Preparation methods and drug targeting issues. Europ. J. Pharm. Biopharm. 39: 173–191.

Antharjanam, P., M. Jaseer, K. Ragi and E. Prasad. 2009. Intrinsic luminescence properties of ionic liquid crystals based on PAMAM and PPI dendrimers. J. Photoch. Photobio. A 203: 50–55.

Barroso, M. 2011. Quantum dots in cell biology. J. Histo. Cytochem. 59: 237–251.

Baykal, A., M. Toprak, Z. Durmus, M. Senel, H. Sozeri and A. Demir. 2012. Synthesis and characterization of dendrimer-encapsulated iron and iron-oxide nanoparticles. J. Supercond. Nov. Magn. 25: 1541–1549.

Bock, N., A. Riminucci, C. Dionigi and A. Russo. 2010. A novel route bone tissue engineering: magnetic biomimetic scaffolds. Acta Biomat. 6: 786–796.

Boerio, F., L. Armogan and S. Cheng. 1980. The structure of γ-aminopropyltriethoxysilane films on iron mirrors. J. Colloid Interf. Sci. 73: 416–424.

Bohren, C. and D. Huffman. 1983. Absorption and Scattering of Light by Small Particles. John Wiley & Sons, New York.

Borin, D. and S. Odenbach. 2009. Magnetic measurements on frozen ferrofluids as a method for estimating the magnetoviscous effect. J. Phys. Condens. Matter 21: 246002.

Borin, D., A. Zubarev, D. Chirikov, R. Muller and S. Odenbach. 2011. Ferrofluid with clustered iron nanoparticles: slow relaxation of rheological properties under joint action of shear flow and magnetic field. J. Mag. Mag. Mater. 323: 1273–1277.

Bronstein, L. and L. Shifrina. 2011. Dendrimers as encapsulating, stabilizing, or directing agents for inorganic nanoparticles. Chemical Rev. 111: 5301–5344.

Brown, K., D. Walter and M. Natan. 2000. Seeding of colloidal Au nanoparticle solutions. 2. improved control of particle size and shape. J. Chem. Mater. 12: 306–313.

Brullot, W., V. Valev and T. Verbiest. 2011. Magnetic-plasmonic nanoparticles for the life sciences: calculated optical properties of hybrid structures. Nanomedicine 8: 559–568.

Caruso, F., M. Spasova and V. Salgueirino. 2001. Multilayer assemblies of silica-encapsulated gold nanoparticles on decomposable colloid templates. Adv. Mater. 13: 1090–1094.

Cannon, W., S. Danforth, J. Flint, J. Haggerty and R. Marra. 1982. The CO_2 laser pyrolysis of gas- and vapor-phase reactants offers an alternative approach for the synthesis of uniform nanoparticles. J. Am. Ceram. Soc. 65: 324–401.

Chang, S., L. Liu and S. Asher. 1994. Preparation and properties of tailored morphology, monodisperse colloidal silica-cadmium sulphide nanocomposites. J. Am. Chem. Soc. 116: 6739–6744.

Chastellain, A., A. Petri and H. Hofmann. 2004. Particle size investigations of a multistep synthesis of PVA coated superparamagnetic nanoparticles. J. Colloid Interf. Sci. 278: 353–360.

Chen, X., T. Young, M. Sarkari and R. Williams. 2002. Preparation of cyclosporine a nanoparticle by evaporative precipitation into aqueous solution. Int. J. Pharm. 242: 3–14.

Cole, L., J. Coleman, D. Evans and C. Hawes. 1990. Internalisation of fluorescein isothiocyanate and fluorescein isothiocyanatedextran by suspension-cultured plant cells. J. Cell Sci. 96: 721–730.

Colvin, V. 2003. The potential environment impact of engineering nanomaterials. Nat. Biotech. 21: 1165.

Conner, S. and S. Schmid. 2003. Regulated portals of entry into the cell. Nature 422: 37.

Couvreur, P., B. Kante and V. Lenaerts. 1980. Tissue distribution of antitumor drugs associated with polyyalkylcyanoacrylate nanoparticles. J. Pharm. Sci. 69-199-2012.

Deng, Y., Ch. Wang, J. Hu, W. Yang and S. Fu. 2005. Colloids Surfaces A: investigation of formation of silica-coated magnetite nanoparticles via sol–gel approach. Physicochem. Eng. Aspects 262: 87–93.

Divsar, F., A. Nomani and M. Chaloosi. 2009. Synthesis and characterization of gold nanocomposites with modified and intact polyamidoamine dendrimers. Microchim. Acta. 165: 421–426.

Dreaden, E., A., X. Huang, A. Alkilany and C. Murphy. The golden age: gold nanoparticles for biomedicine. Chem. Soc. Rev. 41: 2740–2779.

Dresco, P. and V. Zaitsev. 1999. Preparation and properties of magnetite and polymer magnetite nanoparticles. Langmuir. 15: 1945–1951.

Du, G., Z. Liu, X. Xia, Q. Chu and S. Zhang. 2006. Characterization and application of Fe_3O_4/SiO_2 nanocomposites. J. Sol–Gel Sci. Tech. 39: 285–291.

Duff, D. and A. Baiker. 1993. A new hydrosol of gold clusters. 1. Formation and particle size variation. Langmuir 9: 2301–2309.

Enochs, W., G. Harsh, F. Hochberg and R. Weissleder. 1999. Improved delination of human brain tumors on MR images using a long circulating SPION agent. J. Mag. Reson. Imag. 9: 228–232.

Faiyas, A.P., E. Vinod, J. Joseph, R. Ganesan and R.K. Pandey. 2010. Dependence of pH and surfactant effect in the synthesis of magnetite (Fe_3O_4) nanoparticles and its properties. J. Magn. Magn. Mater 322: 400–404.

Feng, B., R. Hong, L.Wang, L. Guo, H. Li, J. Ding and Y. Zheng. 2008. Synthesis of Fe_3O_4/APTES/PEG diacid functionalized magnetic nanoparticles for MR imaging. Colloids Surf. A 328: 52–59.

Fu, L., V. Dravid and D. Johnson. 2001. Self-assembled (SA) bilayer molecular coating on magnetic nanoparticles. Appl. Surf. Sci. 181: 173–178.

Ghazanfari, L. and M.E. Khosroshahi. 2015. Effects of coating and stirring on superparamagnetic iron oxide nanoparticles size and magnetic characteristics. Int. J. Innov. Res. Sci. Eng. Tech. 4: 6659–6666.

Gleissle, S., W. Gleissle, H. McKinley and H. Buggisch. 1980. The normal stress behaviour of suspensions with viscoelastic matrix fluids. 2: 554–555. *In*: G. Astarita, G. Marrucci and L. Nicolais (eds.). Rheology, Proceedings of the 8th International Congress on Rheology. Plenum, New York.

Gnanaprakash, G., S. Mahadevan, T. Jayakumar, P. Kalyanasundaram and J. Philip. 2007. Effect of initial pH and temperature of iron salt solutions on formation of magnetite nanoparticles. Mater. Chem. Phys. 103: 168–175.

Gomez, A., D. Bingham, L. de Juan and K. Tang. 1998. Production of protein nanoparticles by electrospray drying. J. Aerosol Sci. 29: 561–574.

Govorov, A. and H. Richardson. 2007. Generating heat with metal nanoparticles. Nanotoday 2: 30–38.

Goossens, V., J. Wielant, S. Gils, R. Finsy and H. Terryn. 2006. Optical properties of thin iron oxide films on steel. Surf. Interface Anal. 38: 489–493.

Grabchev, I., V. Bojinov and J. Chovelon. 2003. Synthesis, photophysical and photochemical properties of fluorescent poly(amidoamine) dendrimers. Polymer 44: 4421–4428.

Gupta, K. and M. Gupta. 2005. Synthesis and surface engineering of iron oxide nanoparticles for biomedical applications. Biomaterials 26: 3995–4021.

Guang, Y., Z.T. Lai, Q.X. Jing, Z.J. Guo and Y. Li. 2007. Effects of synthetical conditions on octahedral magnetite nanoparticles. Mater. Sci. Eng. B. 136: 101–105.

Hadjipanayis, C., M. Bonder, S. Balakrishnan, X. Wang and H. Mao. 2008. Metallic iron nanoparticles for MRI contrast enhancement and local hyperthermia. Small. 4: 1925–1929.

Harris, N., M. Ford and M. Cortie. 2006. Optimization of plasmonic heating by gold nanospheres and nanoshells. J. Phys. Chem. B 110: 10701–10707.

Hassannejad, Z. and M.E. Khosroshahi. 2013. Synthesis and evaluation of time dependent optical properties of plasmonic–magnetic nanoparticles. Optical Materials 35: 644–651.

Hengyi, X., P. Zoraida, L. Yang and K. Kuang. 2011. Antibody conjugated magnetic iron oxide nanoparticles for cancer cell separation in fresh whole blood. Biomaterials 32: 9758–9765.

Hebalkar, N., S. Kharrazi, A. Ethiraj and R. Fink. 2004. Structural and optical investigations of SiO_2-CdS core-shell particles. J. Colloid Interface Sci. 278: 107–114.

Helmus, M. 2007. The need for rules and regulations. Nat. Nanotechnol. 2: 333–334.

Herea, D. and H. Chiriac. 2008. One-step preparation and surface activation of magnetic iron oxide nanoparticles for biomedical applications. Optoelect. Adv. Mat. Rapid Commun. 2: 549–552.

Hoffman, L., G. Andersson, A. Sharma, S. Clarke and N. Voelcker. 2011. New insight into the structure of PAMAM dendrimer/gold nanoparticle nanocomposites. Langmuir 27: 6759–6767.

Hong, R., Z. Ren, Y. Han, H. Li, Y. Zheng and J. Ding. 2007. Rheological properties of water-based $Fe_3O_4Fe_3O_4$ ferrofluids. Chem. Eng. Sci. 62: 5912–5924.

Hosono, T., H. Takahashi, A. Fujita, R.J. Joseyphus, K. Tohji and B. Jeyadevan. 2009. Synthesis of magnetite nanoparticles for AC magnetic heating. J. Magn. Magn. Mater. 321: 3019–3023.

Jain, T., M. Morales, S. Sahoo and L. Diandra. 2005. Iron oxide nanoparticles for sustained delivery of anticancer agents. Mol. Pharm. 2: 194–205.

Jain, P. and M.A. El-Sayed. 2010. Plasmonic coupling in noble metal nanostructures. Chem. Phys. Lett. 487: 153–164.

Ji, X., R. Shao, A. Elliott, R. Stafford and E. Esparza-Coss. 2007. Bifunctional gold nanoshells with a superparamagnetic iron oxide-silica core suitable for both MR imaging and photothermal therapy. J. Phys. Chem. C 111: 6245–6251.

Jia, X. and H. Song. 2012. Facile synthesis of monodispersed-Fe_2O_3 microspheres through template-free hydrothermal route. J. Nanopart. Res. 14: 1–8.

Jiang, W., B. Kim and J. Rutka. 2008. Nanoparticle-mediated cellular response is size-dependent. Nat. Nanotech. 3: 145–50.

Johnson, P. and R. Christy. 1972. Optical Constants of the Noble Metals. Phys. Rev. B 6: 4370–4379.

Kang, Y. and S. Park. 1996. Preparation of nanometre size oxide particles using filter expansion aerosol generator. J. Mater. Sci. 31: 2409–2416.

Kang, B., M. Mackey and M. El-sayed. 2010. Nuclear targeting of gold nanoparticles in cancer cells induces DNA damage, causing cytokinesis arrest and apoptosis. J. Am. Chem. Soc. 132: 1517–1519.

Kemal, L., X. Jiang and K. Wong. 2008. Experiment and theoretical study of poly(vinyl pyrrolidone)-controlled gold nanoparticles. J. Phys. Chem. C 112: 15656–15664.

Khlebtsov, B. and N. Khlebtsov. 2007. Biosensing potential of silica/gold nanoshells: sensitivity of plasmon resonance to the local dielectric environment. J. Quant. Spect. 106: 154–169.

Khosroshahi, M.E. and L. Ghazanfari. 2010. Preparation and characterization of silica-coated iron-oxide bionanoparticles under N2 gas. Physica E 42: 1824–1829.

Khosroshahi, M.E. and L. Ghazanfari. 2011. Amino surface modification of Fe_3O_4/SiO_2 nanoparticles for bioengineering applications. Surf. Eng. 27: 573–580.

Khosroshahi, M.E. and L. Ghazanfari. 2012. Synthesis and functionalization of SiO_2 coated Fe_3O_4 nanoparticles with amine groups based on self-assembly. Mat. Sci. Eng. C 32: 1043–1049.

Khosroshahi, M.E. and L. Ghazanfari. 2012. Preparation and rheological studies of uncoated and PVA-coated magnetite nanofluid. J. Mag. Mag. Mat. 324: 4143–4146.

Khosroshahi, M.E. and L. Ghazanfari. 2012. Physicochemical characterization of $Fe_3O_4/SiO_2/Au$ multilayer nanostructure. Materials Chemistry and Physics 133: 55–62.

Khosroshahi, M.E. and A. Mandelis. 2015. Combined photoacoustic ultrasound and beam deflection signal monitoring of gold nanoparticle agglomerate concentrations in tissue phantoms using a pulsed Nd:YAG laser. Int. J. Thermophys. 36: 880–890.

Khosroshai, M.E. and M. Tajabadi. 2016. Characterization and cellular fluorescence microscopy of superparamagnetic nanoparticles functionalized with third generation nanomolecular dendrimers: *In vitro* Cytotoxicity and uptake study. J. Nanomater. Mol. Nanotechnol. 5: 1–11.

Kim, H., M. Achermann and L. Balet. 2005. Synthesis and characterization of Co/CdSe core/shell nanocomposites. J. Am. Chem. Soc. 127: 544–546.

Kim, T. and M. Shima1. 2007. Reduced magnetization in magnetic oxide nanoparticles. J. Appl. Phys. 101.

Kim, D., Y. Zhang, W. Voit, K. Rao and M. Muhammed. 2001. Synthesis and characterization of surfactant-coated superparamagnetic monodispersed iron oxide nanoparticles. J. Magn. Magn. Mater. 225: 30–36.

Klajnert, B. and M. Bryszewska. 2002. Fluorescence studies on PAMAM dendrimers interactions. Bioelectrochemistry 55: 33–5.

Larson, C.L. and S. Tucker. 2001. Intrinsic fluorescence of carboxylate-terminated polyamido amine dendrimers. Appl. Spect. 55: 679–683.

Launer, P. 1987. Infrared Analysis of Organosilicon Compounds: Spectra-Structure Correlations, Laboratory for Materials, Inc. Burnt Hills, New York.

Laurent, S., D. Forge, M. Port, A. Roch, C. Robic, L.V. Elst and R.N. Muller. 2008. Magnetic iron oxide nanoparticles: synthesis, stabilization, vectorization, physicochemical characterizations, and biological applications. Chem. Rev. 108: 2064–2110.

Lenaerts, V., J. Nagelkerke and T. Van Berkel. 1984. *In vivo* uptake polyisobutyl cyanoacrylate nanoparticles by rat liver kupffer endothelial, and parenchymal cells. J. Pharm. Sci. 73: 980–982.

Lesniak, A., F. Fenaroli and M. Monopoli. 2012. Effects of the presence or absence of a protein corona on silica nanoparticle uptake and impact on cells. ACS Nano. 6: 5845–5857.

Levin, C., C. Hofmann, T. Ali, A. Kelly and E. Morosan. 2009. Magnetic-plasmonic core-shell nanoparticles. ACS Nano. 3: 1379–1388.

Lewinski, N., V. Colvin and R. Drezek. 2008. Cytotoxicity of nanoparticles. Small. 4: 26–49.

Li, J., Q. Chen and L. Yang. 2010. The synthesis of dendrimer based on the dielectric barrier discharge plasma grafting amino group film. Surf. Coat. Tech. 205: S257–S260.

Lim, J., A. Eggeman, F. Lanni and R.D. Tilton. 2008. Synthesis and single-particle optical detection of low-polydispersity plasmonic-superparamagnetic nanoparticles. Adv. Mater. 20: 1721–1726.

Liu, Z., Y. Liu, K. Yao, Z. Ding, J. Tao and X. Wang. 2002. Synthesis and magnetic properties of Fe_3O_4 nanoparticles. J. Mater. Syn. Proc. 10: 83–87.

Liu, Z., X. Wang, K. Yao and G. Du. 2004. Synthesis of magnetite nanoparticles in W/O microemulsion. J. Mat. Sci. 39: 2633–26.

Liu, R., Y. Ren, Y. Shi, F. Zhang and L. Zhang. 2007. Controlled synthesis of ordered mesoporous $C-TiO_2$ nanocomposites with crystalline titania frameworks from organicinorganicamphiphilic coassembly. Chem. Mater. 20: 1140–1146.

Liu, C., C. Mi and B. Li. 2008. Energy absorption of gold nanoshells in hyperthermia therapy. IEEE Trans. Nanobioscience 7: 206–214.

Liu, H., J. Guo, L. Jin and W. Yang. 2008. Fabrication, Functionalization of dendritic poly(amidoamine)-immobilized magnetic polymer composite microspheres. J. Phys. Chem. B 112: 3315–3321.

Liu, H., P. Hou and W. Zhang. 2010. Synthesis of monosized core–shell Fe_3O_4/Au multifunctional nanoparticles by PVP-assisted nanoemulsion process. Colloids and Surf. A: Physicochem. Eng. Asp. 356: 21–27.

Liu, J., L. Chu, Y. Wang, Y. Duan, L. Feng, C. Yang, L.Wang and D. Kong. 2011. Novel peptidedendrimer conjugates as drug carriers for targeting nonsmall cell lung cancer. Int. J. nanomedicine. 6: 59–69.

Liu, G., Q. Li, W. Ni and N. Zheng. 2015. Cytotoxicity of various types of gold-mesoporous silica nanoparticles in human breast cancer cells. Int. J. Nanomed. 10: 6075–6087.

Lu, Y., Y. Yadong, T. Mayers and X. Younan. 2001. Modifying the surface properties of SPIONs through a sol-gel approach. Nano Let. 2: 183–186.

Lu, Y., J. McLellan and Y. Xia. 2004. Synthesis and crystallization of of hybrid spherical colloids composed of polystyrene cores and silica shell. Langmuir. 20: 3464–3470.

Ma, M., Y. Zhang, W. Yu and H. Shen. 2003. Preparation and characterization of magnetite nanoparticles coated by amino silane. Colloids Surf. A Physicochem. Eng. Asp. 212: 219–226.

Malik, N., R. Wiwattanapatapee, R. Klopsch, K. Lorenz and H. Frey. 2000. Dendrimers: relationship between structure and biocompatibility *in vitro*, and preliminary studies on the biodistribution of 125I-labelled polyamidoamine dendrimers *in vivo*. J. Control. Release 65: 133–148.

Majoros, I., A. Myc, T. Thomas, C. Mehta and J. Baker. 2006. PAMAM dendrimer-based multifunctional conjugate for cancer therapy: synthesis, characterization, and functionality. Biomacromolecules 7: 572–579.

Maynard, A., R. Aitken and T. Butz. 2006. Safe handeling of nanotechnology. Nature 444: 267–269.

Mchedlov-Petrossyan, N. and R. Mayorga. 1992. Extraordinary character of the solvent influence on protolytic equilibria: inversion of the fluorescein ionization constants in H_2O-DMSO mixtures. J. Chem. Soc. 88: 3025–3032.

Menjoge, A., R. Kannan and D. Tomalia. 2010. Dendrimer-based drug and imaging conjugates: design considerations for nanomedical applications. Drug discovery today. 15: 171–85.

Michalet, X., F. Pinaud, L. Bentolila and J. Tsay. 2005. Quantum dots live *in vivo* imaging diagnostics. Science 307: 538–544.

Mikhaylova, M., D. Kyung Kim, C. Catherine and A. Zagorodni. 2004. BSA immobilization on amine-functionalized superparamagnetic iron oxide nanoparticles. Chem. Mater. 16: 2344–2354.

Nakanishi, T., Y. Masuda and K. Koumoto. 2004. Site-selective deposition of magnetite particulate thin films on patterned self-assembled monolayers. Chem. Mater. 16: 3484–3488.

Narayan, P. and B. Hancock. 2003. The relationship between the particle properties, mechanical behaviour, and surface roughness of some pharmaceutical excipient compacts. Mater. Sci. Eng. A 355: 24–36.

Neuberger, T., B. Schpf, H. Hofmann, M. Hofmann and B. Von Rechenberg. 2005. Superparamagnetic nanoparticles for biomedical applications: possibilities and limitations of a new drug delivery system. J. Magn. Magn. Mater. 293: 483–496.

Nirmal, M., B. Dabbousi and M. Bawendi. 1996. Fluorescence Intermittency in Single Cadmium Selenide Nanocrystals 383: 802–804.

Niu,Y., H. Lu, D. Wang, Y. Yue and S. Feng. 2011. Synthesis of siloxane-based PAMAM dendrimers and luminescent properties of their lanthanide complexes. J. Organomet. Chem. 696: 544–550.

Niwa, T., H. Takeuchi, T. Hino, M. Nohara and Y. Kawashima. 1995. Biodegradable submicron carriers for peptide drugs: Preparation of Dl-lactide/glycolide copolymer (PLGA) nanospheres with nafarelin acetate by a novel emulsion-phase separation method in an oil system. Int. J. Pharm. 121: 45–54.

Nourbakhsh, M.S. and M.E. Khosroshahi. 2011. An *in-vitro* investigation of skin tissue soldering using gold nanoshells and diode laser Lasers Med. Sci. 26: 49–55.

Nyirokosa, I., D.C. Nagy and M. Posfai. 2009. Size and shape control of precipitated magnetite nanoparticles. Eur. J. Mineral. 21: 293–302.

Oberdorster, G., Z. Sharp and V. Atudorei. 2004. Translocation of inhaled ultrafine particles to the brain. Inhal. Toxicol. 16: 437.

Oldenberg, S., R. Averitt, S. Westcott and N. Halas. 1998. Nanoengineering of optical resonances. Chem. Phys. Lett. 288: 243–247.

Ohmori, T., H. Takahashi, H. Mametsuka and E. Suzuki. 2000. Photocatalytic oxygen evolution on α-Fe_2O_3 films using Fe3+ ion as a sacrificial oxidizing agent. Phy. Chem. 2(2000): 3519–3522.

Palma, R. De, C. Liu, F. Barbagini, G. Reekmans and K. Bonroy. 2007. Magnetic particles as labels in bioassays: interactions between a biotinylated gold substrate and streptavidin magnetic particles. J. Phys. Chem. C 111: 12227–12235.

Pan, B., F. Gao and H. Gu. 2005. Dendrimer modified magnetite nanoparticles for protein immobilization. J. Colloid. Interf. Sci. 284: 1–6.

Pan, Y., A. Leifert and D. Ruau. 2009. Gold nanoparticles of diameter 1.4 nm trigger necrosis by oxidative stress and mitochondrial damage: Small. 5: 2067–2076.

Park, H., M. Schadt, L. Wang, I. Lim, P. Njoki and S.H. Kim. 2007. Fabrication of magnetic core@shell Fe oxide@Au nanoparticles for interfacial bioactivity and bio-separation. Langmuir 23: 9050–9056.

Park, J., K. An and Y. Hawang. 2004. Ultra-Large Scale Synthesis of Monodisperse in Medicine 3: 891–895.

Pastor-Perez, L., Y. Chen, Z. Shen and A. Lahoz. 2007. Unprecedented blue intrinsic photoluminescence from hyper branched and linear polyethylen-imines: polymer architectures and pH-effect. Rapid Commun. 28: 1404–1409.

Pelliccioli, A. and J. Wirz. 2002. Photoremovable protecting groups: reaction mechanisms and applications. Photochem. Photobiol. Sci. 1: 441–458.

Peng, X., M. Schlamp and A. Kadavnchi. 1997. Epitaxial growth of highly luminescent CdSe/CdS core/shell nanocrystals with photostability and electronic accessibility. J. Am. Chem. Soc. 119: 7019–7029.

Peng, X., Q. Pan and G. Rempel. 2008. Bimetallic dendrimer-encapsulated nanoparticles as catalysts: a review of the research advances. Chem. Soc. Rev. 37: 1619–1628.

Pham, T., J. Jackson, N.J. Halas and T. Lee. 2002. Preparation and characterization of gold nanoshells coated with self-assembled monolayers. Langmuir 18: 4915–4920.

Pham, T., C. Cao and S. Sim. 2008. Electrochemical analysis of gold-coated magnetic nanoparticles for detecting immunological interaction. J. Magn. Magn. Mater. 320: 2049–2055.

Pisanic, T., J. Blackwell and V. Shubayev. 2007. Nanotoxicity of iron oxide nanoparticle internalization in growing neurons. Biomaterials 28: 2572–2581.

Piñeirol, P., Z. Vargas, J. Rivas and M. López-Quintela. 2015. Iron oxide based nanoparticles for magnetic hyperthermia strategies in biological applications. Eur. J. Inorg. Chem. 2015: 4495–4509.

Pop, L., J. Hilljegerdes, S. Odenbach and A. Wiedenmann. 2004. The microstructure of ferrofluids and their rheological properties. Appl. Organomet. Chem. 18: 523–529.

Pop, L. and S. Odenbach. 2006. Investigation of the microscopic reason for the magnetoviscous effect in ferrofluids studied by small angle neutron scattering. J. Phys. Condens. Matter 18: S2785.

Popplewell, J. and L. Sakhini. 1995. The dependence of the physical and magnetic properties of magnetic fluids on particle size. J. Magn. Magn. Mater. 149: 72–78.

Prasad Raoa, J. and K. Geckelera. 2011. Polymer nanoparticles: preparation techniques and size-control parameters. Progress in Polym. Sci. 36: 887–913.

Racuciu, M. 2009. Synthesis protocol influence on aqueous magnetic fluid properties. Curr. Appl. Phys. 9: 1062–1066.

Rezvani Alanagh, H., M.E. Khosroshahi, M. Tajabadi and H. Keshvari. 2014. The effect of pH and magnetic field on the fluorescence spectra of fluorescein isothiocyanate conjugated SPION-dendrimer nanocomposites. J. Supercond. Nov. Magn. 27: 2337–2345.

Rice, J. 2007. Mathematical statistics and data analysis. Thomson Books/Cole, Belmont, USA.

Sabareeswaran, A., E. Beeran Ansar, P. Varma, H. Varma and P. Mohanan. 2016. Effect of surface-modified superparamagnetic iron oxide nanoparticles (SPIONS) on mast cell infiltration: An acute *in vivo* study. Nanomedicine 12: 1523–1533.

Sadat, M., R. Patel, J. Sookoor, S. Budko and R. Ewing. 2014. Effect of spatial confinement on magnetic hyperthermia via dipolar interaction in Fe_3O_4 nanoparticles for biomedical applications. Mat. Sci. Eng. C. 42: 52–63.

Sairam, M., B. Naidu, S. Nataraj, B. Sreedhar and T. Aminabhavi. 2006. Poly(vinyl alcohol)-iron oxide nanocomposite membranes for pervaporation dehydration of isopropanol, 1,4-dioxane and tetrahydrofuran. J. Membr. Sci. 283: 65–73.

Seabra, A. and N. Duran. 2015. Nanotoxicology of metal oxide nanoparticles. Metals. 5: 934–975.

Shah, J., S. Park, S. Aglyamov and T. Larson. 2008. Photoacoustic and ultrasound imaging to guide photothermal therapy: *Ex vivo* study. SPIE 6856, 68560U-1.

Shen, M. and X. Shi. 2010. Dendrimer-based organic/inorganic hybrid nanoparticles in biomedical applications. Nanoscale 2: 1596–1610.

Shi, X., Sh. Wang, H. Sun and J. Baker. 2007. Improved biocompatibility of surface functionalized dendrimer entrapped gold nanoparticles. Soft Matter. 3: 71–74.

Shi, X., K. Sun and J. Baker. 2009. Spontaneous formation of functionalized dendrimer-stabilized gold nanoparticles. J. Phy. Chem. C Nanomat. Interf. 112: 8251–8258.

Shulman, Z., V. Kordonsky and E. Zaltsgendler. 1986. Insight into magnetorheological shock absorbers. Int. J. Multiphase Flow 12: 935–955.

Soenen, S., B. Manshian, J. Montenegro and A. Fahim. 2012. Cytotoxic effects of gold nanoparticles: A multiparametric study. ACS Nano. 5767–5783.

Stemmler, M., F. Stefani, S. Bernhardt, R. Bauer and M. Kreiter. 2009. One-pot preparation of dendrimer-gold nanoparticle hybrids in a dipolar aprotic solvent. Langmuir. 25: 12425–12428.

Storhoff, J., A. Lazarides, R. Mucic, C. Mirkim, R. Letsinger and G. Schatz. 2000. What controls the optical properties of DNA-linked gold nanoparticle assemblies? Am. Chem. Soc. 122: 4640–4650.

Sun, S., H. Zeng and D. Robinson. 2004. Monodisperse MFe_2O_4 nanoparticles. J. Am. Chem. Soc. 14: 273–279.

Syahir, A., K. Tomizaki, K. Kajikawa and H. Mihara. 2009. Poly(amidoamine)-dendrimer modified gold surfaces for anomalous reflection of gold to detect biomolecular interactions. Langmuir. 25: 3667–3674.

Talelli, M., C. Rijcken, T. Lammers and P. Seevinck. 2009. Superparamagnetic iron oxide nanoparticles encapsulated in biodegradable thermosensitive polymeric micelles: toward a targeted nanomedicine suitable for image-guided drug delivery. Langmuir 25: 2060–2067.

Tajabadi, M., M.E. Khosroshahi and Sh. Bonakdar. 2013. An efficient method of SPION synthesis coated with third generation PAMAM dendrimer. Colloids and Surf. A: Physicochem. Eng. Aspects 431: 18–26.

Tao, K., H. Dou and K. Sun. 2008. Interfacial coprecipitation to prepare magnetite nanoparticles: Concentration and temperature dependence. Colloids Surf. A 320: 115–122.

Thomas, R., I. Park and Y. Jeong. 2013. Magnetic iron oxide nanoparticles for multimodal imaging anf therapy of cancer. Mol. Sci. 14: 15910–15930.

Thompson, J., J. Vasquez, J. Hill and P. Pereira-Almao. 2008. The synthesis and evaluation of up-scalable molybdenum based ultra dispersed catalysts: effect of temperature on particle size. Indust. Eng. Chem. Fund. 123: 1623.

Thompson, D., J. Hermes, A. Quinn and M. Mayor. 2012. Scanning the potential energy surface for synthesis of dendrimer-wrapped gold clusters: Design rules for true single-molecule nanostructures. ACS Nano 6: 3007–3017.

Tomalia, D. 2005. Birth of a new macromolecular architecture: dendrimers as quantized building blocks for nanoscale synthetic polymer chemistry. Prog. Polym. Sci. 30: 294–324.

Torres, M. 2003. Mitogen-activated protein kinase pathways in redox signaling. Front Biosci. 8: d639–d391.

Toshima, N. and T. Yonezawa. 1998. Bimetallic nanoparticles-novel materials for chemical and physical applications. New J. Chem. 22: 1179–1202.

Tsubokawa, N. and T. Takayama. 2000. Surface modification of chitosan powder by grafting of 'dendrimer-like' hyperbranched polymer onto the surface. React. Funct. Polym. 43: 341–350.

Venditto, V., C. Regino and M. Brechbiel. 2005. PAMAM dendrimer-based macromolecules as improved contrast agents. Molecul. Pharm. 2: 302–311.

Veintemillas, S., M. Morales and O. Bomati-Miguel. 2004. Colloidal dispersions of maghemite nanoparticles produced by laser pyrolysis with application as NMR contrast agents. J. Phys. D: Appl. Phys. 37: 2054–2059.

Veronesi, B., C. Haar, L. Lee and M. Oortgiesen. 2002. The surface charge of visible particulate matter predicts biological activation in human bronchial epithelial cells. Toxicol. Appl. Pharm. 178: 144–154.

Vlaev, D., I. Nikov and M. Martinov. 2007. The CFD approach for shear analysis of mixing reactor. Verification and examples of use. Chem. Eng. Sci. 61: 5455–5467.

Vujacic, A., V. Vodnik, R. Antic and V. Vasic. 2011. Particle size and concentration dependent cytotoxicity of citrate capped gold nanoparticles. Digest. J. Nanomat. Biostr. 6: 1367–1373.

Wan, J., Y. Yao and G. Tang. 2007. Controlled-synthesis, characterization and magnetic properties of Fe_3O_4 nanoparticles. Appl. Phys. A. 89: 529–532.

Wang, X., J. Zheng and J. Pemg. 2005. A general strategy for nanocrystal synthesis. Nature 437: 121–124.

Wang, D., T. Imae and M. Miki. 2007. Fluorescence emission from PAMAM and PPI dendrimers. J. Colloid Int. Sci. 306: 222–2209.

Welch, C., G. Rose, D. Malotky and S. Eckersley. 2006. Rheology of high internal phase emulsions. Langmuir 22: 1544–1550.

Westcott, S., S. Oldenburg, T. Randall Lee, J. Naomi and J. Halas. 1998. Formation and adsorption of gold nanoparticle-clusters on functionalized silica nanoparticle surfaces. Langmuir 14: 5396–5401.

Xing, Y. and J. Rao. 2008. Quantum dot bioconjugates for *in vitro* diagnostic and *in vivo* imaging. Cancer Biomarkers 4: 307–319.

Xu, Z., Y. Hou and S. Sun. 2007. Magnetic core/shell Fe_3O_4/Au and Fe_3O_4/Au/Ag nanoparticles with tunable plasmonic properties. J. Am. Chem. Soc. 129: 8698–8699.

Xue, D., G. Chai, X. Li and X. Fan. 2008. Effects of grain size distribution on coercivity and permeability of ferromagnets. J. Magn. Magn. Mater. 320: 1541–1543.

Yamaura, M., R. Camilo, L. Sampaio, M. Macedo and M. Nakamura. 2004. Preparation and characterization of (3-aminopropyl) triethoxysilane-coated magnetite nanoparticles. J. Magn. Magn. Mater. 279: 210–217.

Yang, D., J. Hu and S. Fu. 2009. Synthesis and study of structural and magnetic properties of superparamagnetic Fe_3O_4@SiO_2 core/shell nanocomposite for biomedical applications. J. Phys. Chem. C 113: 7646–7675.

Yang, W., Y. Cheng, T. Xu, X. Wang and L. Wen. 2009. Targeting cancer cells with biotindendrimer conjugates. Eur. J. Med. Chem. 44: 862–868.

Yu, C., K. Tam and E. Tsang. 2009. Chemical methods for preparation of nanoparticles in solution. pp. 113–141. *In*: Handbook of Metal Physics. Elsevier B.V.

Yum, K., S. Na, Y. Xiang and N. Wang. 2009. Mechanochemical delivery and dynamic tracking of fluorescent quantum dots in the cytoplasm and nucleus of living cells. 9: 2193–2198.

Zborowski, M. 1997. Physics of magnetic cell sorting. pp. 205–31. *In*: M. Zborowski (ed.). Scientific and Clinical Applications of Magnetic Carriers. Plenum Press, New York, USA.

Zhang, X. 2009. Study of novel nanoparticle sensors for food pH and water activity. Rutgers University-Graduate School-New Brunswick.

Zheng, P., L. Gao, X. Sun and S. Mei. 2009. The thermolysis behaviours of the first generation dendritic polyamidoamine. Iran. Polym. J. 18: 257–264.

Zhu, Z., S. Ghosh, R. Miranda and R. Vachet. 2003. Multiplexed screening of cellular uptake of gold nanoparticles using laser desorption/ionization mass spectroscopy. J. Am. Chem. Soc. 130: 14139–14143.

Part V

Nanomedicine: Applications of Biophotonics and Nanobiomaterials

10

Laser-Tissue Soldering

10.1 Introduction

Wound healing is the process by which skin or other body tissue repairs itself after trauma. In undamaged skin, the epidermis (surface layer) and dermis (deeper layer) form a protective barrier against the external environment. Whether wounds are left to be closed naturally or by laser welding or laser soldering, the wound healing process is a dynamic one which can be divided into three phases. It is critical to remember that wound healing is not linear, and often wounds can progress both forwards and back through the phases depending upon intrinsic and extrinsic forces at work within the patient. Figure 10.1 shows the phases of wound healing:

a) Hemostasis (blood clotting): Within the first few minutes of injury, platelets in the blood begin to stick to the injured site. This activates the platelets, causing a few things to happen. They change into an amorphous shape, more suitable for clotting, and they release chemical signals to promote clotting. This results in the activation of fibrin, which forms a mesh and acts as *"glue"* to bind platelets to each other. This makes a clot that serves to plug the break in the blood vessel, slowing/preventing further bleeding.

b) The *inflammatory phase* is the body's natural response to injury. During this phase, damaged and dead cells are cleared out, along with bacteria and other pathogens or debris. This happens through

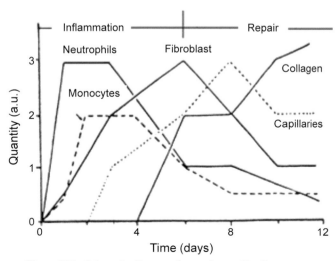

Figure 10.1. Schematic diagram of normal wound healing process.

the process of phagocytosis. After initial wounding, the blood vessels in the wound bed contract and a clot is formed. Once hemostasis has been achieved, blood vessels then dilate to allow essential cells; antibodies, white blood cells, growth factors, enzymes, and nutrients to reach the wounded area. At this stage the characteristic signs of inflammation can be seen, i.e., erythema, heat, oedema, pain, and functional disturbance. The predominant cells at work here are the phagocytic cells; 'neutrophils', and macrophages.

c) During *proliferation* (growth of new tissue): The wound is 'rebuilt' with new granulation tissue, which is comprised of collagen and extracellular matrix and into which a new network of blood vessels develop, a process known as 'angiogenesis'. In fibroplasia and granulation tissue formation, fibroblasts grow and form a new, provisional extracellular matrix (ECM) by excreting collagen and fibronectin. Healthy granulation tissue is dependent upon the fibroblast receiving sufficient levels of oxygen and nutrients supplied by the blood vessels. Healthy granulation tissue is granular and uneven in texture; it does not bleed easily, and is pink/red in color. The color and condition of the granulation tissue is often an indicator of how the wound is healing. Dark granulation tissue can be indicative of poor perfusion, ischaemia, and/or infection. Epithelial cells finally resurface the wound, a process known as 'epithelialisation'. In wound contraction, myofibroblasts decrease the size of the wound by gripping the wound edges and contracting using a mechanism that resembles that in smooth muscle cells. When the cells' roles are close to completion, unneeded cells undergo apoptosis.

d) *Maturation* (remodeling): It is the final phase, and occurs once the wound has closed. This phase involves remodelling of collagen from type III to type I. Cellular activity reduces and the number of blood vessels in the wounded area regress and decrease.

Since the early work on laser-assisted sutureless microvascular anastomosis (Jain and Gorish 1979), considerable amount of research has been done to find a way to introduce laser-based techniques of sutureless wound closure into clinical practice. Lasers have been shown to have significant potential experimentally and clinically for welding and soldering of different types of tissues using various materials (Lemole et al. 1992, Sorg et al. 2000, Capon et al. 2001, Gulsoy et al. 2006). Laser welding is defined as heating the approximated edges of cuts in tissue by a laser beam and can cause immediate irreversible thermal damage of the structural proteins of the tissue through necrosis and denaturation. Denaturation is a rate process of governed by the local temperature-time response, which can be approximated by Arrhenius model (Stewart et al. 1996). The extent of the reaction is linearly proportional to time and exponential function of temperature. Laser soldering, on the other hand, involves heating a biological solder placed between the edges of tissue acting as a bridge after being cured by laser. Both laser welding and laser soldering are very promising surgical techniques since they are in principle faster and easier to master than standard suturing. The primary advantages are (i) immediate water tight seal, (ii) are non-contact which do not introduce foreign materials, and (iii) reduced inflammation (Sorg et al. 2000, Capon et al. 2001, Ditkoff and Perrault 2002). There are three main drawbacks to laser welding: (a) the immediate tensile strength, during the first few days is low; (b) there is often a noticeable thermal damage; (c) the results are frequently inconsistent (McNally et al. 1999, Simhon et al. 2004). Thermal damage to tissue is a major hurdle to overcome in laser soldering. When laser energy is delivered onto tissue without any temperature control, it may cause sloughing of wound edges. This may contribute to a poor wound healing process and low long-term tensile strength (Fried et al. 2000).

Two advances have been useful in reducing the problems of low strength and thermal damage associated with laser tissue welding; (a) the addition of endogenous and exogenous materials to be used as solders, and (b) the application of laser wavelength-specific chromophores. The addition of endogenous and exogenous materials at the tissue junction helps to maintain edge alignment and to strengthen the wound, particularly during the postoperative healing phase and simultaneously protecting the underlying tissue from excessive thermal damage caused by directing absorption of the laser light. The addition of chromophore-enhanced protein solders to augment laser repair procedures significantly reduces the problems of low strength and thermal damage associated with laser tissue welding techniques.

The most notable of these is an indocyanine green (ICG)—doped albumin protein solder used in conjunction with an 808 nm diode laser to repair tissue (Savage et al. 2003, Hoffman et al. 2003).

The advantage of this technique is that the energy is selectively absorbed by the target area. Hence, the requirement for precise focusing and aiming of the laser beam may be neglected. Also due to increased absorption characteristics of the dyed tissue, lower irradiances may be used to achieve the required effect. Laser soldering has been carried out using various types of solders. In some cases a coloring dye was added to the solder, to increase the absorption of the laser irradiation in the solder (Sorg et al. 2000, Gulsoy et al. 2006). McNally et al. (2000) used laser soldering with dye enhanced protein solder of different concentrations of ICG and bovine serum albumin. They found that the highest immediate tensile strength (measured by weight bearing system) was achieved with 60% bovine serum albumin when surface was heated to 85°C. Poppas et al. (1996) investigated the effect of temperature on tensile strength of photo thermal wound closure, and found that the maximum strength was achieved at the surface temperature of 75°C. Advanced systems are currently being evaluated for real time monitoring and control in medical procedures involving laser (Brosh et al. 2004). These systems generally consist of a sensor capable of rapidly measuring a tissue parameters coupled to a feedback loop that adjusts the laser parameters. The response time of this type of system can usually be significantly fast. Sensors can be used to monitor tissue parameters which are not visually discernible. One such parameter being studied for feedback control is surface temperature since it is very important for surgery involving laser induced photocoagulation (Pohl et al. 1998). In these procedures a laser is used as a source of heat to cause thermal denaturation of the illuminated tissue proteins. In the case of tissue photocoagulation, several variables can influence the clinical results. Since the thermal damage to the irradiated tissue is strongly dependent on the evaluated temperature achieved during the laser soldering process, hence the resultant surgical outcome is highly variable (Pohl et al. 1998).

As it was discussed in detail in chapter nine, nanoshells are a class of nanoparticles consisting of a dielectric core surrounded by a thin metal shell. The plasmon resonance of these nanoparticles can be tailored by varying the ratio of the diameter of the core to the thickness of the shell. Through design and control of the particle geometry, nanoshells can be tuned to absorb at a wide range of wavelengths from the visible into the NIR allowing the material's optical properties to be tuned to match the output of a desired laser. Gold nanoshells are currently being used for a variety of biomedical applications and have been shown to be non-toxic and highly biocompatible. The use of nanoshells has several advantages over ICG. The average diameter of nanoshells is about 100 nm, so that reduced diffusion from the site of treatment and concentrating heating at the interface is avoided, which should in effect minimize damage to surrounding tissue (Malicka et al. 2003). ICG chromophore is hydrolytically sensitive and susceptible to photo bleaching in the presence of light (Zhou et al. 1994, Weissleder 2001, Hirsch et al. 2003). Hence, another advantage of nanoshells is that they are more photo-stable, since their absorption properties are determined by their physical structure. Additionally, nanoshells are stronger absorbers than ICG on a per particle or molecule basis. ICG has an absorption cross-section on the order of $\sim 10^{-20}$ m^2, while nanoshells have absorption cross-section on the order of $\sim 10^{-14}$ m^2, so nanoshells are approximately a million-fold more effective absorbers (Ntziachristos et al. 2000).

10.2 Application of albumin protein and indocyanine green chromophore for tissue soldering using IR diode laser: *Ex vivo* and *in vivo* studies (Khosroshahi et al. 2010)

In *ex vivo* studies, the temperature rise, number of scan (Ns), and scan velocity (Vs) were investigated. In *ex vivo* studies, four skin incisions were made over rat dorsa and were closed using two different methods: (a) wound closure by suture (b) closure, using an automated temperature controlled system. An automated soldering system was developed based on a diode laser, IR detector, photodiode, digital thermocouple, and camera, the true temperature of heated tissue was determined using a calibration software method. The results showed that at each laser irradiance (I), the tensile strength (σ) of incisions repaired in static mode is higher than dynamic mode. It must also be noted that the tensile strength of repaired skin wound was increased by increasing the irradiance in both static and dynamic modes. However, in parallel, on increase in corresponding temperature was observed. The tensile strength was measured for sutured and laser soldered tissue after 2–10 days postoperatively. Histopathological studies showed a better healing and less inflammatory reaction than that caused by standard sutures after 7th day. It is demonstrated that automated laser soldering technique can be practical, provided the optothermal properties of tissue is carefully optimized.

Ex vivo experiments

A 40 × 50 cm² fresh piece of sheep skin was obtained from a slaughter house in Tehran and depilated suitably, using a depilation cream (Nair) and cut into 100 pieces of 4 × 5 cm². The prepared samples were stored in refrigerator until required. For experiment, a full thickness 2 × 20 mm² cut was made on the middle of skin, using 11" blades. Protein solder solution was prepared from 25% BSA (Sigma Chemical Co.) and 0.25 mg/ml ICG dye (Sigma Chemical Co.) mixed in deionized water. The protein solder was stored in a light-proof plastic vial in a refrigerator prior to its use.

The setup of laser soldering system is shown in Fig. 10.2. The system includes the following: (a) a tunable CW 1.5–6 W diode laser with an emission at 810 nm with a linear beam profile with dimensions of 1 × 7 mm², (b) a stepper motor that scans the laser probe on the skin surface with variable speed, (c) a digital thermometer (CHY502A1, Taiwan) that measures the skin surface temperature during laser soldering, (d) computer analysis of thermometer signals and recording system, (e) a CCD (Dynamic wv-CP450) camera to observe and record the skin changes during the laser soldering.

The protein solder solution was placed in the incision for 2 min and then irradiated with different power densities in the static and dynamic modes. In the static mode the incision was same as the laser output profile and the laser head was positioned statically at the surface of incision, and irradiated the tissue three times edge-to-edge to fill the full gap at different power densities for 4 minutes. In the dynamic mode, however, the laser probe was located perpendicularly to the incision and scanned the surface with a predefined speed until the soldering was finished set by upper temperature limit. The temperature rise at the skin during the irradiation was measured with a digital thermometer. The laser beam moved from one place to the next, along the cut line, so that each line slightly overlapped the previous one. Tensile strength measurements were performed to test the integrity of the resultant repairs immediately following the laser procedure using a gravity-based instrument. The repaired specimen was then mounted between two metal grips, of which one was fixed and the other was allowed to move. The defined weights were added to moving grip until the first rupture occurred in the repaired skin.

Table 10.1. Physical properties of ICG.

Symbol	Variable	Unit	Values
ρ	Density	gm^{-3}	1.07
K	Thermal Conductivity	$Wcm^{-1o}C^{-1}$	0.0056
C	Special heat	$Jg^{-1o}C^{-1}$	3.4

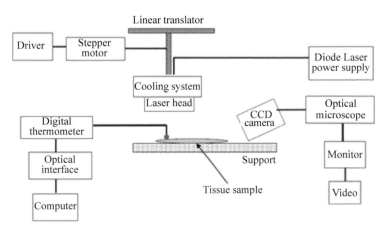

Figure 10.2. *In vitro* experimental setup.

In vivo experiments

We developed a system for real time monitoring and control of the temperature of spot in tissue surface (Fig. 10.3). The heated spot emits an infrared radiation whose intensity (I) is determined by temperature (T). The intensity is monitored and a feedback loop controls the laser power so that the surface temperature is stabilized at some set value. The system includes the following parts: (1) a diode laser with an emission at ≈ 810 nm, (2) a pyroelectric IR detector (EG&G-PA 18936) which converts the emitted intensity to an electrical signal. This signal is proportional to the tissue surface temperature, (3) a photodiode, (4) a computer which analyses the signal and determines the correct surface temperature. The temperature control is based on the feedback algorithm which sends a signal defined and varies correspondingly by the laser power. The detection of the soldering completion is realized by the microprocessor unit. This device first measures the initial reflectance value R_i directly after laser onset. The final reflectance value R_f is immediately calculated. The reflectance signal is then sampled continuously and compared with R_f. If the signal is equal or lower than R_f, the laser irradiation is stopped. The R_f value is calculated according to:

$$R_f = \frac{R_i(100\text{-}x)}{100} \qquad (10.1)$$

where x is a user defined decrease of reflectance in percent. Before the procedure is started, the user adjusts the laser power and x parameter. The experimental setup is shown in Fig. 10.2.

Temperature dynamics during the soldering was studied, and an example of using feedback control system is illustrated in Fig. 10.4. As soon as the laser is switched on, the reflectance, temperature, and the emissivity from tissue surface gradually increases with time. When the temperature reaches to a preset value, e.g., 70°C, the laser is switched off and the cooling cycle takes place until it reaches to the room temperature defined as base line.

Eight male Sprague/Dawley rats weighing 250–300 g were selected for this study. The study was done in accordance with the "guide for the care and use of laboratory animals" published by the U.S. National Institute of Health (NIH publication, No. 85-23, revised 1996), which were divided into two groups of laser and suture as control, each consisting of four rats. They were first anesthetized with Ketamine (50 mg/kg) + Xylazin (5 mg/Kg) interperitoneally (IP), and then their dorsal skin was shaved and depilated. Four longitudinal incisions, each 2 cm long, were made on the dorsum of each rat using 11" blades. Two of the cuts were laser soldered and the other two, which served as a control group, were sutured with 3/0 Prolene suture (Ethicon). Therefore, each rat had 4 incisions, 2 for laser treatment, and 2 for suturing as control, giving overall 32 incisions (i.e., 16 lasers, 16 sutured). For laser soldering, the incision edges were

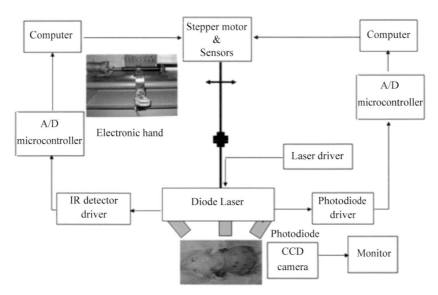

Figure 10.3. Block diagram of *in vivo* experimental setup using a feedback control system.

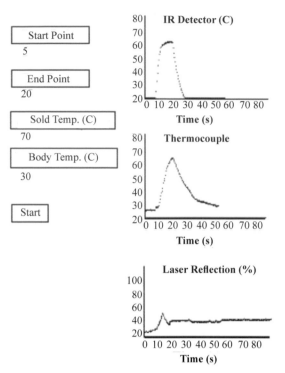

Figure 10.4. Example of output signals displayed during the experiment by a closed feedback-control system.

brought close together using a small clamp on the mid portion of the incision. A drop of solder (1.25 mg/cc ICG + 1.25 gr/cc albumin) was then placed on the incision line and the temperature control was set to 70°C.

The animals were sacrificed with overdose of sodium thiopental (100 mg/Kg) after 2, 5, 7, and 10 days postoperatively. An area of the skin with the repaired (soldered or sutured) incision in the middle was harvested. Four incisions were used for biomechanical measurement, and four for histological evaluations at each time point. The total of 16 repaired skin specimen were tested using a load machine (Zwick/Roell, HCT 25/400 series). Strips were inserted into the head of loading machine and tensile strength measurement was carried out at a rate of 5 mm/min. In order to evaluate the biomechanical properties of repaired wounds, it was attempted to measure the yield stress as a function of healing time for lasered skin (Y_{ls}) and sutured skin (Y_{ss}). For this purpose the average value of yield stress of four scars on each rat, denoted by R, was plotted for both Y_{ls} and Y_{ss}. Another parameter which affects the life time or resistance of scar to rupture is the amount of energy required to induce a physical rupture, E_r. The rupture energy is simply defined as, $E_r = \int_0^t F dt$ where F is the applied force (N). The stiffness (γ) of a body is a measure of the resistance offered by an elastic body to deformation (bending, stretching, or compression). It is defined as $\gamma = P/\delta$, where P is a steady force applied on the body and δ is the displacement produced by the force. For histological evaluation, sections of the soldered tissue were first fixed in 10% formaldehyde solution and then stained by hematoxyline and eosine. The exact general histological evaluating method was performed as described by Simhon et al. (2004). The parameters studied were as follows:

1. Epidermal changes: these include the presence of thermal injury with signs of carbonization or necrosis, the presence of surface albumin as compared to sutured (none irradiated) scars, and the type of re-epithelialization, ulcers or atrophy;
2. Dermal changes: these include the degree of inflammation (classified as mild, moderate, or severe reaction) and the different types of inflammatory cells such as neutrophils, lymphomononuclear cells;
3. Presence or absence of granulation tissue and dermal appendage were examined;
4. The hypodermal parameters.

For lymphomononuclear cells and polymorphonuclears (PMN) the scoring system is based on cell numbers in high-power field (HPF) (magnification $\times 100$), as shown in Table 10.2.

Table 10.2. Grading of the inflammation process.

Degree	Number of cells per high power field (HPF)
+10	< 2
+5	2–3
++++	4–7
+++	8–15
++	15–25
+	25–50
0	50–75
−5	> 75

Statistical measurements

For comparison of methods, the P-values for the differences between methods—static and dynamics in *ex vivo* and suturing and soldering in *in vivo*—were calculated using the one-way analysis of variance (ANOVA) test. Statistically significant differences were considered as $P < 0.05$.

RESULTS

Ex vivo experiments

Tensile strength of repaired specimens were measured as a function of laser irradiance and mode of soldering, as seen in Fig. 10.5. Each σ value of laser treated samples was determined from the mean of 4 wound heals. As it is seen from the Fig. 10.5, the values of σ at corresponding irradiance in static mode is higher than dynamic mode, and the tensile strength of resulting repairs increased significantly with increasing irradiance.

An example of the temperature rise of skin during the laser soldering at 36 Wcm^{-2} is shown in Fig. 10.6a, where each peak was achieved when the laser beam was coincided with the tip of thermometer. Tissue surface temperature rise as a function of irradiance is shown in Fig. 10.6b.

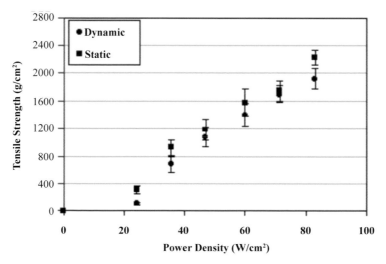

Figure 10.5. The variation of tensile strength of soldered skin with irradiance (p = 0.72).

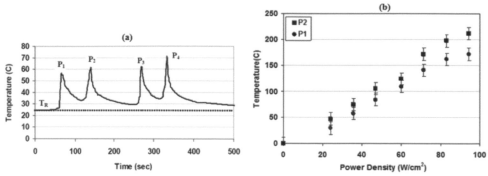

Figure 10.6. Tissue surface temperature rise (a) as a function of time where two consecutives peaks represents a complete round trip at 36 W/cm² and (b) as a function of irradiance (P-value = 0.53).

The effect of number of scan on the tensile strength of repaired skin for two different power densities is illustrated in Fig. 10.7. For the given irradiance, tensile strength increases by increasing the number of scans which may be explained by the fact that not only does the depth of thermal denaturation increase with temperature rise, but also by overlapping tales of thermal signals before the complete cooling of scanned spot. Figure 10.8 indicates that by increasing the scan velocity (Vs), the corresponding value of σ decreases at a given irradiance.

Figure 10.9 indicates the examples of tissue before and after suturing and laser soldering in static (Fig. 10.9a,b) and dynamic (Fig. 10.9c,d) modes. It should be noted that in the former case, the direction of treatment was parallel to the direction of stained incision, whereas in the latter case it was perpendicular. It is clearly seen that the incision is completely closed and thereafter, it is expected that the process of wound healing will take place.

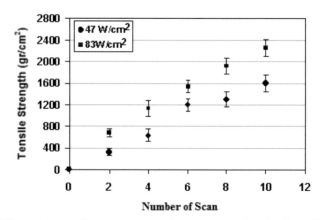

Figure 10.7. Effect of number of scans on tissue tensile strength at a given irradiance (P-value = 0.35).

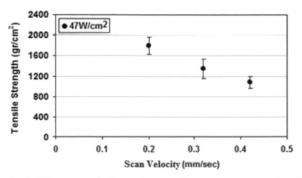

Figure 10.8. Effect scan velocity on tissue tensile strength at a given irradiance.

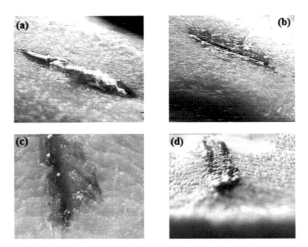

Figure 10.9. Some examples of wound stained by ICG before and after laser tissue soldering in (a,b) static and (c,d) dynamic mode.

In vivo experiments

Yield stress as a function of healing time for lasered skin (Y_{ls}) and sutured skin (Y_{ss}) is shown in Fig. 10.10a. Clearly until day 5, both cases indicated a constant trend, with Y_{ss} being slightly higher. After that Y_{ss} showed a sharp rise, which then reached a plateau at day 7. However the LS sites showed a rapid rise at day 7, and increased up to 400 KPa at day 10, as can be seen from Fig. 10.10b, rupture energy increases for both cases until day 5, with SS being higher by about 200 J. But they equalize at day 7, and

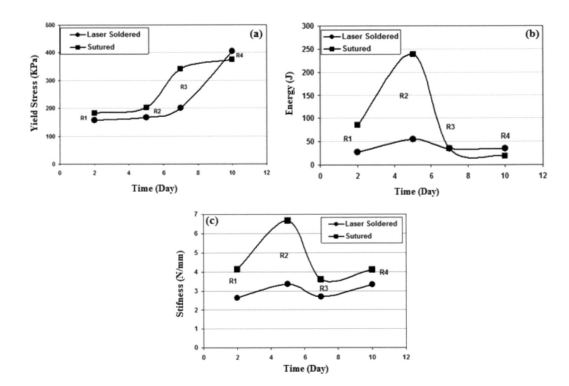

Figure 10.10. Variation of biomechanical parameters for lasered and sutured skin (a) yield stress (P-value = 0.59), (b) rupture energy (P-value = 0.31), and (c) stiffness (P-value = 0.06).

after that LS exceeds SS, and continued until day 10. Although it appears as though this trend would have continued in a saturated and parallel state, the main reason for $E_r(SS) \ll E_r(LS)$ is the increase in so-called tenacity of skin, i.e., at this stage the ratio of residual young modulus of soft tissue with respect to scar has increased. The change of stiffness (γ) for both cases is shown in Fig. 10.9c, where despite a similar oscillatory or non-linear behaviour, $\gamma_{LS} \ll \gamma_{SS}$ for all observed post operation time.

The pathological images of lasered and sutured skin after day 2, 5, 7, and 10 days are illustrated in Fig. 10.11(a–h). Pathological results showed a significant difference between collagen structural formations. Minimal (or none) thermal injury and less inflammation was seen in the soldered wounds after day 5. The degree of re-epithelialization was similar in both soldered and sutured scars, and it reached its maximum on day 7 postoperatively.

Tables (10.3) and (10.4) indicate all the effective histological parameters in a wound healing process. The indices of each factor are obtained from pathological observations. The formation of collagen is the most significant difference between the healing parameters of soldered and sutured cuts. Overall, in the

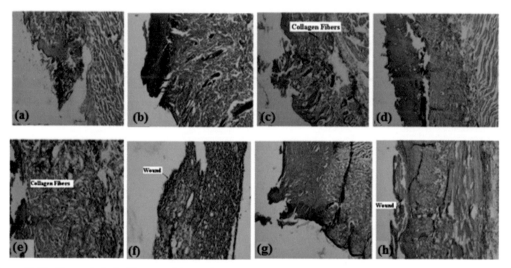

Figure 10.11. Histopathological images of tissue after postoperative day 2 (a: control; b: laser soldered), day 5 (c: control; d: laser soldered), day 7 (e: control; f: laser soldered) and day 10 (g: control; h: laser soldered) (4×) (H&E).

Table 10.3. Effective histologic parameters in a wound healing process of sutured repairs.

Code	Day	Epi	Ulcer	PMN	Lympho Mononuclear Cells	Collagen	Total
2C1	2	A	+5	+5	+10	0	+20
2C2	2	A	+5	+10	+10	0	+25
2C3	2	A	+5	+10	+15	0	+30
2C4	2	A	+5	+10	+15	+10	+40
5C1	5	N	0	+5	0	+20	+25
5C2	5	A	+5	+10	+10	0	+25
5C3	5	A	+0.5	+5	+10	+15	+30.5
5C4	5	A	+5	+10	+10	+0	+25
7C3	7	N	−5	+5	+20	+15	+35
7C4	7	N	−5	+5	+20	+15	+35
10C1	10	N	−5	−5	+10	+20	+20
10C2	10	N	−5	−5	+15	+25	+30
Total							340.5

Table 10.4. Effective histological parameters in the wound healing process for laser soldered repairs.

Code	Day	Epi	Ulcer	PMN	Lympho Mononuclear Cells	Collagen	Total
2L3	2	N	−5	0	+10	+20	+25
2L5	2	N	−5	+5	+10	+15	+25
5L1	5	A	+10	+10	+10	+5.5	+35.5
5L2	5	A	+10	+10	+10	+10	+40
5L3	5	A	+5	+10	+20	+10	+45
5L4	5	N	0	0	0	+20	+20
5L5	5	A	+10	+10	+15	+15	+50
7L1	7	N	0	+0.5	+15	+20	+35
7L2	7	T	+0.5	+5	+20	+15	+40.5
7L3	7	A	+5	+10	+15	+15	+45
7L4	7	N	0	+15	+10	+10	+35
10L1	10	N	0	0	+10	+20	+30
Total							+426

soldered wounds, the process of wound healing is faster and more effective, which is one of the many advantages of this technique (P-value = 0.036). In Tables 10.3 and 10.4, parameters stands for, A: Abnormal, N: Normal, and T: Tanned epidermis.

Discussion

The concepts of wavelength-dependent tissue absorption, optical penetration depth, and thermal relaxation time allow a rational selection of laser wavelengths and define the exposure condition. These parameters can be chosen in such a way that maximum strength with minimum tissue injury is provided. This briefly is the concept of selective photothermolysis introduced by Anderson and Parish (1983). The objects of this research was to study the effect of ICG as the light absorbing dye for enhancement of selective photo thermal interaction on thermal and biomechanical properties of tissue in static and dynamic modes *ex vivo* and *in vivo* operation. The *ex vivo* results showed that the tensile strength of repaired skin wound was increased by increasing the irradiance in both static and dynamic mode. But in doing so, the corresponding temperature also increased. What the preferred tissue temperature should be, at least during an *ex vivo* operation, remains controversial, varying along the above parameters with apposition pressure, tissue type, and chemical composition, and likely age of the tissue. All in all, in our experiment an optimized soldering condition for *ex-vivo* case was obtained by using a low concentration ICG solder (0.25 mg/ml), $I = 47$ W cm^{-2}, $\sigma = 1500$ gr/cm^2, $N_s = 8$, and $V_s = 0.3$ mm/s.

As the laser beam moves away from the treated spot, it cools down by conduction and convection until the beam returns and passes over the previous treated region again. Therefore, each two consecutive peaks (e.g., P_1 and P_2) represent a complete round trip of probe beam. Clearly each scan can contribute to temperature rise by an increment acting as residual heat which accumulates on the previous scan effect. This, in turn, implies that by varying the scanning velocity the distance between peaks and their amplitude can change, hence governing the control of the final temperature rise between two set limits.

Thermal damage kinetic model

Tissue coagulation including collagen denaturation can be described as a rate process using kinetic models. In thermal damage process, the endpoint damage, Ω inside the irradiated tissue can be estimated by solving the Arrhenius integral, assuming that damage is due to thermal denaturation of proteins. Hence,

$$\Omega(t) = \ln\left[\frac{C_0}{C_t}\right] = \int_{t_i}^{t_f} A\exp\left[-\frac{E}{RT(t)}\right] dt \tag{10.2}$$

where t is the time duration of heating treatment, C_0 is the initial concentration of undamaged tissue, C_t is concentration of undamaged tissue after time (t), R is the gas constant (8.31 Jmol^{-1}K^{-1}), E_a is the activation energy (6.28 × 10^5 Jmol^{-1}), A is the frequency factor which is in fact an empirically valued coefficient (3.1 × 10^{98} s^{-1}) (Moritz and Henriques 1947), t_i and t_f are initial (on) and final (off) exposure time, respectively (i.e., $\Delta t_e = t_f - t_i$). Conventionally, $\Omega(t) = 0$ implies no tissue damage at all, $\Omega(t) = 1$ means that most (i.e., 63%) of tissue is damaged, and $\Omega(t) > 1$ indicates a complete tissue necrosis and irreversible damage. Normally, for damage threshold it is assumed ln $\Omega = 2$ (i.e., $\Omega = 0.693$), which is equivalent to 50% tissue damage. A and E are usually found by exposing the tissue to a constant temperature, identifying the experiments in which the damage is threshold, $\Omega = 1$. A is then obtained from the intercept and E from the slope on a plot of ln (t) versus 1/T for the threshold experiments.

Closed loop feedback

At this stage it was intended to omit or reduce the error due to manual measurement of tissue temperature. Feedback control involves a set of sensors to measure some physical characteristic in tissue that is related to the degree of completion of the soldering process (see material and methods). According to Beer-Lambert's law, and assuming the scattering coefficient of ICG at ≈ 810 nm is negligible compared to its absorption coefficient (i.e., $\alpha \gg \beta$), then 85% of incident laser energy is absorbed within twice the optical penetration depth, d_0, of material. For 0.25 mg/ml ICG at 810 nm, $\alpha \approx 117$ cm^{-1} which gives $d_0 \approx 85$ µm (McNally et al. 2000). Based on the values given in Table 10.1 by Crochet et al. (2006), thermal diffusivity can be calculated by $D_t = K/\rho C$, which gives a value of k = 1.53 × 10^{-3} cm^{2}s^{-1}. Thus, the thermal relaxation time within ICG is defined and given by using $\tau_r \approx d_0^2/4$ k ≈ 1.2 µs. Consequently, the thermal penetration depth, $d_t \approx (4$ kt$)^{1/2}$ can be calculated for different exposure time. Using the above argument we obtained $d_t \approx (2.5-4.5)$ mm for (10–30) seconds of exposure time. Final temperature protocol will be a function of tissue configuration, beam size, dye concentration, and exposure time. Heat transfer is proportional to the temperature gradient across the solder, as described by Fourier law.

Tissue biomechanical properties

While varying the irradiance in dynamic and static modes resulted in slight rise of σ and temperature profile, it may be suggested that Ns, and hence Vs, affect the σ as well as the quality of soldered tissue more significantly. This can be argued by the fact that by increasing the Vs, less time is given to tissue to have temperature rise for intertwining tissue fibrillar collagen matrix and subsequent melting transition and fusion. Assuming 75°C as an upper temperature limit during the laser soldering, values of 38 and 47 Wcm^{-2} satisfied the above condition for static and dynamic modes in *in vitro* experiment respectively, as seen in Fig. 10.5b. The corresponding σ values, Fig. 10.5, which were achieved on the same day, are about 100 and 1250 gcm^{-2}. An additional point to remember is that in the dynamic mode, the probability of thermal collateral damage is reduced due to cooling time between consecutive scanning numbers. One other important observation at this stage was the color of solder soon after laser activation, e.g., green, tan, brown, as seen in Fig. 10.8. Green represented no appreciable change, tan showed gradual drying of the solder, and brown represented a gritty drying of the solder. *In vivo* tensile strength of wounds repaired with suture and laser in closed-feedback control experiment indicated a significant difference compared with *in vitro*. The turning point (Fig. 10.9) for both suture and laser was 200 KPa (or 2000 gcm^{-2}) began at 5 and 7 days, respectively postoperatively. However, sutured cuts reached its plateau of about 350 KPa after 8 days, whereas the sutured cuts showed an increasing trend even at 10 days with a value of 400 KPa showing a further increasing rate of collagen synthesis. Studies by Decoste et al. (1992), using ICG dye alone showed that at temperatures above 60°C, a significant reduction of ICG and a steep increase in the temperature occurred. This presumably resulted from the release of ICG from collagen ads the molecules reached its fibrillar melting transition temperature. Previous studies by Kirsch et al.

(1997), using a diode laser with an ICG/albumin solder at a irradiance of 32 Wcm^{-2} indicate that superior immediate tensile strength is obtained in soldered versus sutured skin with a soldered wound, gaining the equivalent immediate tensile strength of a 7 day repaired wound. Also, studies by Cooper et al., using ICG concentration of 0.31, 2.5, and 20 mg/ml and irradiance ranging from 8 to 64 Wcm^{-2} indicated that increasing irradiance has a direct effect on immediate tensile strength up to 24 Wcm^{-2} at a concentration of 0.31 mg/ml and 16 Wcm^{-2} at a concentration of 2.5 mg/ml. Optimal laser wound closure occurred with an ICG of 2.5 mg/ml at a irradiance between 16–24 Wcm^{-2} (i.e., 2000 gr/cm^{-2}) (Cooper et al. 2001). In our case (i.e., 025 mg/ml) this value was obtained for LS using 47 Wcm^{-2} at day 3 and increased to 4000 gr/cm^{-2} at day 10 with an immediate temperature of $\approx$ 80°C. Variation in different research result is largely dependent on reliability factors, such as ICG concentration, response time, sampling errors, tissue type, temperature, and laser treating mode.

Histopathology

The inflammation mainly composed of lymphomononuclear cells and neutrophils in the suture cuts which needed a longer time to resolve. The role of lymphomononuclear cells in the order lines of wound repair has been emphasized before (Nwomeh et al. 1998). The faster disappearance of lymphomononuclear cells from soldered scars indicated more efficient response to the inflammatory phase, giving place to the intermediate and late wound healing. Albumin was seen on day 2 in about 40% of the soldered cuts, but from day 7 on, there was no evidence of its presence. The pathologic micrographs of sutured cuts demonstrated thermally denatured collagen on both sides of the incision, measuring up to 750 μm in thickness. Fibroblasts were seen to the same degree in both types of scars. The appearance of skin appendage inside the scar matrix is an indication of almost full regeneration of normal structures. Starting from day 5, we saw more of this phenomenon in soldered scars.

When studying the hypodermis area, it was found that on day 5, 60% of the soldered scars and 40% of the sutured scars showed good apposition. From day 5 to day 10, we saw faster organization of the soldered scars compare with suture scars (Fig. 10.10). The hypodermis recovered normal structure. Cosmetically the scars formed using laser soldering looked better, both macroscopically and microscopically. Other studies have shown that wounds closed by laser tissue soldering have superior healing characteristics with minimal foreign body reaction and inflammatory response in comparison to wounds closed by suture repair (Gobin et al. 2005) that confirms our results. However, the degree and the depth of tissue damage that is done when using the laser is related to power, spot size, and the absorption/scattering properties of tissue. The incision gap that had been subjected to the laser soldering process exhibited a complete epidermal-dermal wound sealing by forming an immediate matrix coagulum. Franz et al. (2000) suggested a typical trajectory concept (curve pattern) for the evaluation of wound healing processes. The normal average wound healing process is demonstrated by a curve made of dots that integrate the relevant wound healing information as a function of elapsed time intervals. The information includes physical features, such as tensile strength, as well as qualitative and quantitative histological parameters for each time interval. Laser soldering seems to induce and enhance clean and smooth healing. Nonetheless, thermal damage can also be generated by this method (even when using temperature control), which may interfere with the healing process. The denatured albumin adheres to the epidermal and dermal skin layers (Fig. 10.10) and forms a bond that contributes both to the immediate and the long term tensile strength. Moreover, it reduces the amount of thermal damage by the formation of a coagulum dressing that finally disappears during the healing process via biodegradation. Therefore, special attention was paid in this study to the accurate monitoring and control of the laser soldering process.

The inflammation phase is proceeded by an anabolic phase of fibroblast proliferation. Here again, the minimal scar size and the most organized-condensed matrices were obtained in laser-soldered incisions, while an excessively swollen scar, with overproduction of fibroblasts and their disorganized extracellular matrices, typified the sutured wound outcome. In extreme cases of sutured wounds, the inflammation phase fails to terminate, since the suture material inside the reparative tissue behaves as a foreign body and contributes to a characteristic foreign-body reaction and accumulation of lymphomononuclear cells in the healing granulation tissue. The overall healing result in laser soldered wounds includes an arranged anatomical architecture of the epidermis, dermis, and hypodermis, and a reparative tissue with elements resembling the scarless fetal wound healing. The descriptive aesthetic reparative results support the conclusions of the detailed indices. However, the detailed analysis of the healing trajectories, using the suggested histological index of healing, is the most solid reproducible analysis tool.

10.3 An *in vitro* investigation of skin tissue soldering using gold nanoshells and diode laser (Nourbakhsh and Khosroshahi 2011)

Gold coated silica core nanoparticles have an optical response dictated by the plasmon resonance (PR). The wavelength at which the resonance occurs depends on the core and shell sizes, allowing nanoshells to be tailored for particular applications. The purposes of this study was to synthesize and use different concentration of gold nanoshells as exogenous material for *in vitro* skin tissue soldering and also to examine the effect of laser soldering parameters on the properties of repaired skin. Two mixtures of albumin solder and different concentration of gold nanoshells were prepared. A full thickness incision of 2×20 mm^2 was made on the surface and after addition of mixtures it was irradiated by an 810 nm diode laser at different power densities. The changes of tensile strength σ_t due to temperature rise, number of scan (N_s), and scan velocity (Vs) were investigated. The results showed at constant laser power density (I), σ_t of repaired incisions increases by increasing the concentration of gold nanoshells, Ns and decreasing Vs. It is therefore important to consider the trade off between the scan velocity and the skin temperature for achieving an optimum operating condition. In our case this corresponds to $\sigma_t = 1610$ g/cm^2 at I ~ 60 Wcm^{-2}, T ~ 65°C, Ns = 10, and Vs = 0.2 mms^{-1}.

Gold nanoshell synthesis and characterization

Silica cores were first grown using the Stober method, based on reduction of tetraethyl orthosilicate (TEOS) (Sigma-Aldrich, St. Louis, MO). The resultant silica nanoparticles were sized using atomic force microscopy (Dual scope/Raster scope C26, DME, Denmark). Addition of 3-aminopropyl trimethoxysilane (APTMS, Sigma-Aldrich, St. Louis, MO) to silica core provided amine groups on the surface of the core for deposition of gold colloid. Figure 10.12a shows an AFM example of functionalized silica nanoparticles. Gold colloid was prepared with a size range of 2–4 nm using the method described by Duff et al. (1993). The colloid was then concentrated and mixed with the aminated silica particles, allowing small gold colloid to attach to the larger silica nanoparticles surface in order to act as nucleation sites in the subsequent reduction step. The gold shell was then grown by the reduction of gold from HAuCl$_4$ in the presence of formaldehyde. The gold is reduced around the initial colloid sites, coalescing to form a complete shell. An AFM example of Au coated SiO$_2$ nanoshell is illustrated in Fig. 10.12b. Absorption characteristics of the nanoshells were determined using a UV-Vis spectrophotometer (Philips UV/Vis-spectrophotometer PU 8620, Pye Unicam Ltd., Cambridge, UK).

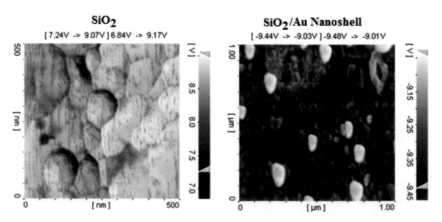

Figure 10.12. AFM photographs of surface topography of SiO$_2$ (a) and SiO$_2$/Au (b).

In vitro skin soldering

A 40 × 50 cm^2 fresh piece of sheep skin was obtained from slaughter house, depilated suitably, and cut into pieces of 4 × 5 cm^2. The thickness of the skin samples was about 2 mm. The prepared samples were then stored in refrigerator in a closed container for maximum 6 hours. After preparation, a full thickness cut of 2 × 20 mm^2 was made on the skin surface using 11" blades. Protein solder solution was prepared using 25% BSA (Sigma Chemical Co.) and two different concentrations of gold nanoshells mixed in HPLC grade water. The setup of laser soldering system is shown in Fig. 10.2. For each concentration of nanoshells, the mixture of nanoshells and BSA Solder (50 μl) was applied to the cut edges, and the edges were brought into contact with one another and then irradiated with different power densities in the dynamic mode. In this procedure, the laser probe was located perpendicularly to the incision and scanning system scanned the surface with a predefined speed until the soldering was completed. The temperature rise at the skin during the irradiation was measured with a digital thermometer. The laser beam moved from one place to the next along the cut line, so that each line slightly overlapped the previous one. Tensile strength measurements were performed to test the integrity of the resultant repairs immediately following the laser procedure using a load machine (HCT 25/400 series, Zwick/Roell Co., Germany). Strips were inserted into the head of loading machine and tensile strength measurement was carried out at a rate of 2 mm/min. For each nanoshell concentration and laser parameter the experiment was repeated five times.

Statistical measurements

For comparison of results, the P-values for the differences between different concentrations were calculated using the one-way analysis of variance (ANOVA) test. Each final data point represents an average of five readings. Statistically significant differences were considered as P < 0.05.

Results

Tensile strength of repaired specimens were measured as a function of laser irradiance and the concentration of gold nanoshells, as seen in Fig. 10.13. Each tensile strength (σ) value of laser treated samples was determined from the mean of 5 repaired cuts. As is seen from the Fig. 10.13, not only does the value of σ increase with power density, but it also increases by increasing the concentration of nanoshells. But for the latter case, the difference is not statistically significant (P-value = 0.52).

Tissue temperature rise as a function of laser power density for different nanoshell concentrations is shown in Fig. 10.14a, and an example of the thermal signal received from the skin during the laser soldering at 60 W/cm^2 is shown in Fig. 10.14b, where each peak was observed when the laser beam was coincided with the tip of thermometer.

The effect of number of scans (Ns) on the tensile strength of repaired skin for two different concentration at constant irradiance (83 W/cm^2) is illustrated in Fig. 10.15. For the given irradiance, tensile strength

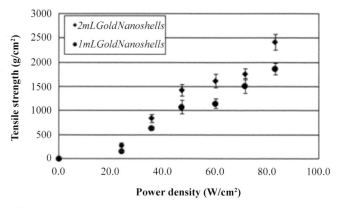

Figure 10.13. Variation of tissue tensile strength with laser power density at constant nanoshells concentration (mean ± SD).

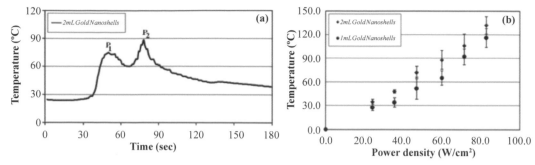

Figure 10.14. Tissue temperature rise (a) as a function of time where two consecutives peaks represents a complete round trip at 60 W/cm² and (b) as a function of laser power density.

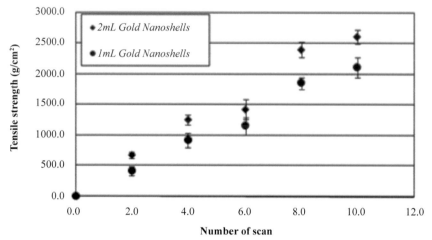

Figure 10.15. Effect of number of laser scans and nanoshells concentration on tissue tensile strength at a given power density (mean ± SD).

increases by increasing the number of scans, which may be explained by the fact that not only does the depth of thermal denaturation increase with temperature rise, but also by overlapping tales of thermal signals before the complete cooling of scanned region. Figure 10.16 indicates that at constant I, increasing Vs cause the corresponding value of σ to decrease due to lower temperature rise.

Examples of tissue before and after soldering at 60 W/cm² are shown in Fig. 10.17. It is clearly seen that the incision is completely closed, and thereafter it is expected that the process of wound healing will take place. Histological images of laser soldered incisions by 60 Wcm⁻² is illustrated in Fig. 10.18. The laser-soldered gap is filled with immediate collagen coagulum, thus sealing the wound from the outside hostile environment. The albumin remnants adhered to the wound surface (either to the epithelial or to the collagen coagulum). A very mild burn was observed on the right margin of the bonded wound, represented by a basophilic stain (H&E, original magnification × 10).

Discussion

Using lasers with wavelengths in the NIR for tissue soldering has distinct advantages. Higher laser power and deep penetration can be achieved because hemoglobin, melanin, and water have low absorption coefficients in the region between 650 and 900 nm (Hirsch et al. 2003). Thermal penetration depths of several centimeters in the above range have been demonstrated in breast tissue as well as brain (Ntziachristos et al. 2000, O'Neal et al. 2004). For achieving better results, use of exogenous absorbers such as ICG can be helpful. Studies by DeCoste et al. (1992) using ICG dye alone showed that at temperatures above 60°C a significant release of ICG and a steep increase in the temperature occurred. This presumably resulted from the release of ICG from collagen, as the molecule reached its fibrillar melting transition temperature. In a study by

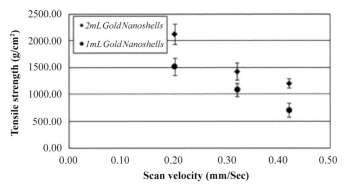

Figure 10.16. Effect of laser scans velocity on tissue tensile strength at a given power density (mean ± SD).

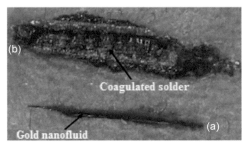

Figure 10.17. An example of skin tissue before and after laser soldering at 60 Wcm^{-2}. (a) Incision plus nanofluid before soldering (b) incision and nanofluid after soldering.

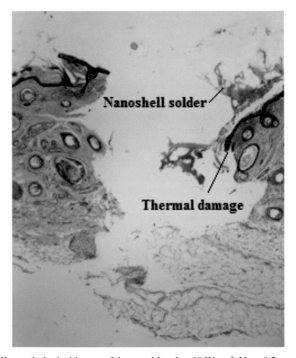

Figure 10.18. Histopathological image of tissue soldered at 60 Wcm^{-2}, Vs = 0.2 mms^{-1}, and Ns = 10.

Kirsch et al. (1997), temperatures during laser activation with an ICG/albumin solder were determined within the solder and underlying dermis over 1 minute of activation. The results showed temperature within the solder reached 101.1°C, while temperature in the superficial and deep skin was 69.9 and 65°C, respectively.

Dew postulated that a denatured coagulum forms at approximately 70°C and serves as "biological glue" that holds the vessel edges together (Dew et al. 1983). Also, our previous work (Khosroshahi et al. 2010) showed that maximum tensile strength of repaired tissue achieved by ICG was ~ 2000 gcm^{-2} which is less than the value obtained by gold nanoshells ~2500 gcm^{-2}.

In the current study, we have synthesized and used gold nanoshells as an exogenous near infrared absorber for laser-tissue soldering. The cores used in our experiments had a diameter of ~100 nm covered with a shell thickness of ~10 nm. The optical properties of nanoshells are well predicted by Mie scattering theory (Alvarez-Puebla et al. 2005), thus allowing one to calculate the dimensions of core and shell required to fabricate nanoshells with strong absorption at a given wavelength. This allows facile tuning to match the output of a desired laser source for a given application. The objects of this research was to study the effect of gold nanoshells as the light absorbing dye for enhancement of selective photo thermal interaction on thermal and biomechanical properties of skin tissue. Our results indicate that laser power density is an important parameter during the laser tissue soldering, affecting the extend of wound healing where temperature plays a crucial role. The results showed that the tensile strength of healed skin wound was increased by increasing the irradiance in both concentrations of gold nanoshells. But in doing so, the corresponding temperature was also increased. What the preferred tissue temperature should be, at least during an *in vitro* operation, remain controversial, varying along the above parameters with apposition pressure, tissue type and chemical composition, and likely age of the tissue. All in all, in our experiment an optimized soldering condition was obtained by using a high concentration of gold nanoshells, $I = 60$ Wcm^{-2}, $\sigma = 1610$ gr/cm^2, $N_s = 10$, and $v_s = 0.2$ mm/s. As the laser beam moves away from the treated spot, it cools down by conduction and convection until the beam returns and passes over the previous treated region again. Therefore, each two consecutive peaks (e.g., P_1 and P_2) represent a complete round trip of probe beam. Clearly, each scan can contribute to temperature rise by an increment acting as residual heat, which accumulates on the previous scan effect. This, in turn, implies that by varying the scanning velocity, the distance between peaks and their amplitude can change, hence governing the control of the final temperature rise between two set limits. Tissue coagulation, including collagen denaturation, can be described as a rate process using kinetic models. In thermal damage process, the endpoint damage, Ω inside the irradiated tissue can be estimated by solving the Arrhenius integral, using Eq. (10.22). The study by Simhon et al. (2004) showed that the tensile strength of soldered skin obtained in temperatures below 40°C were too weak to withstand the manipulations before mechanical testing, and the irreversible thermal damage occurred when temperature was about 90°C. Nevertheless, it is possible to quantitatively evaluate the degree of thermal damage as a function of different temperature settings, as reported by Cohen et al. (2003). Therefore, the optimal temperature for soldering was established at 65 ± 5C. While varying the irradiance on nanoshells result in slight rise of σ and temperature profile, it may be suggested that Ns, and hence Vs, affect the σ as well as the quality of soldered tissue more significantly. This can be argued by the fact while Vs controls the temperature rise for intertwining tissue fibrillar collagen matrix and subsequent melting transition and fusion, Ns influences the thermal accumulation effect on the tissue.

10.4 Enhanced laser tissue soldering using indocyanine green chromophore and gold nanoshells combination (Khosroshahi and Nourbakhsh 2011b)

Gold nanoshells (GNs) are new materials which have an optical response dictated by the plasmon resonance. The wavelength at which the resonance occurs depends on the core and shell sizes. The purposes of this study were to use the combination of indocyanine green (ICG) and different concentration of gold nanoshells for skin tissue soldering and also to examine the effect of laser soldering parameters on the properties of repaired skin. Two mixtures of albumin solder and different combinations of ICG and gold nanoshells were prepared. A full thickness incision of 2×20 mm^2 was made on the surface and after addition of mixtures it was irradiated by an 810 nm diode laser at different power densities. The changes of tensile strength (σ_t) due to temperature rise, number of scan (Ns), and scan velocity (Vs) were investigated. The results showed at constant laser power density (I), σ_t of repaired incisions increases by increasing the concentration of gold nanoshells in solder, Ns and decreasing Vs. It was demonstrated that laser soldering using combination of

ICG + GNs could be practical provided the optothermal properties of the tissue are carefully optimized. Also the tensile strength of soldered skin is higher than skins which soldered with ICG or GNs only. In our case this corresponds to $\sigma_t = 1800$ g/cm^2 at I ~ 47 Wcm^{-2}, T ~ 85°C, Ns = 10, and Vs = 0.3 mms^{-1}.

Material and methods

Refer to sections 10.2 and 10.3.

Results

UV-visible spectrum recorded for gold nanoshells is shown in Fig. 10.19. The resonance peak position depends on the plasmon interaction between separate inner and outer gold layers. The optical absorption spectra shown in Fig. 10.18 are relatively broad compared to that of pure gold colloid. According to the Mie scattering theory, the nanoshells geometry can quantitatively account for the observed plasmon resonance shifts and line-widths. In addition, the plasmon line-width is dominated by surface electron scattering.

Transmission electron microscopy (TEM; PHILIPS CM120) image of the gold nanoshell is shown in Fig. 10.20a, and selected area electron diffraction pattern of gold nanoparticles is shown in Fig. 10.20b, which illustrates the crystalline nature of gold particle. An example of Au-coated SiO$_2$ nanoshells and their 3-D images taken by AFM are shown in Figs. 10.21a and 10.21b, respectively (Khosroshahi et al. 2010).

The tensile strength (σ) of the repaired specimens determined from the mean of five cuts was measured as a function of laser power density and solders combination, and is shown in Fig. 10.22. As it is shown in Fig. 10.22, the value of σ_t increased with increasing power density and nanoshell concentration in the solder. However, for the latter case, the difference is not statistically significant.

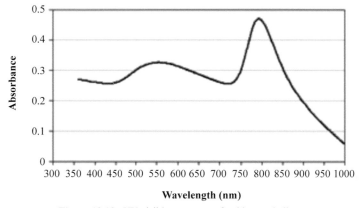

Figure 10.19. UV-visible spectrum of gold nanoshells.

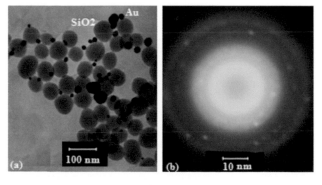

Figure 10.20. TEM photographs (a) and SAED pattern of gold nanoshells formation.

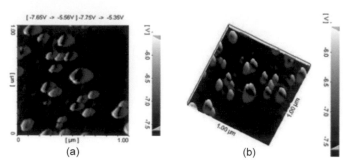

Figure 10.21. AFM photographs of surface topography of SiO$_2$/Au nanoshells 2-D (a) and 3-D (b).

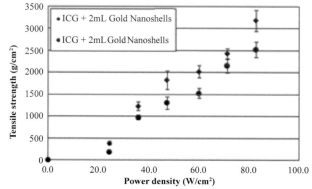

Figure 10.22. Variation of tissue tensile strength with laser power density at constant solder combination.

An example of the thermal signal received from the skin surface during the laser soldering process with I = 60 W/cm^2 is shown in Fig. 10.23a, where each peak was observed when the laser beam was coincident with the tip of the thermometer. The variation in the tissue temperature (T) with laser power density for different solder combination is shown in Fig. 10.23b.

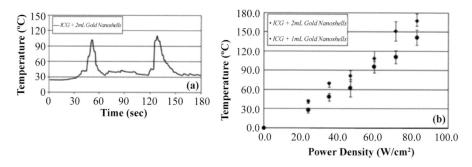

Figure 10.23. Tissue temperature rise (a) as a function of time where two consecutives peaks represents a complete round trip at 60 W/cm^2 and (b) as a function of laser power density.

The effect of the number of scans (Ns) on the tensile strength of the repaired skin for two different solder combinations at a constant power density is illustrated in Fig. 10.24. For a given constant power density, the tensile strength increased with the increasing number of scans. This may be explained by the fact that a higher number of scans cause a greater temperature rise, and hence, more thermal denaturation occurs. Moreover, overlap between sections of a region that was heated during the first round and the heat produced during the second scan can enhance this effect. Figure 10.25 indicates that, at a constant I, an increase in the scan velocity cause the corresponding value of σ to decrease due to a smaller temperature rise.

Histological images of laser soldered incisions by 47 Wcm^{-2} are illustrated in Fig. 10.26 (a and b). A very mild burn was observed on the right margin of the bonded wound, represented by a basophilic stain (H&E, original magnification × 10).

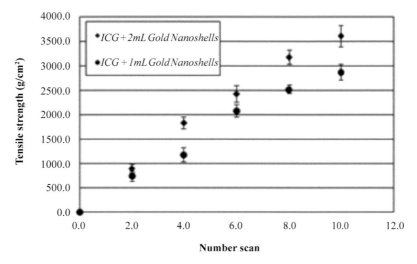

Figure 10.24. Effect of number of laser scans and solder combination on tissue tensile strength at a given power density.

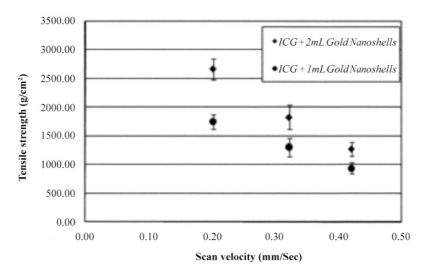

Figure 10.25. Effect of laser scans velocity on tissue tensile strength at a given power density.

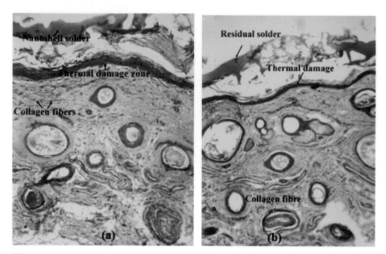

Figure 10.26. Histological images of laser soldered incisions at 47 W/cm² (a and b).

Discussion

In the current study, we have reported the use of combination of ICG and SiO₂/Au nanoshells (ICG + GNs) as an exogenous near infrared absorber and focused on the laser parameters necessary for effective LTS with different concentration of nanoshells. The nanoshells used in these experiments had a diameter of ~110 nm and a shell thickness of ~10 nm. As it can be seen from Fig. 10.19, the absorption peak of gold nanoshells is ~795 nm, and that for ICG is ~800 nm, both of which are close to the wavelength of the diode laser (810 nm). Of course, there always will be some colloidal contamination in synthesis process. However in our case since the maximum absorption peak is at ~800 nm, it indicates the majority of the nanoparticles are gold nanoshells and not just gold colloid (i.e., the second peak at ~ 550 nm). Also the presence of ICG with maximum absorption peak at ~810 nm would help to reduce or even prevent from further effect of contamination on the results. Hence in principle, the combination of gold nanoshells and ICG can be suitable for LTS using a diode laser. Nanoshells are also intense absorbers. Conventional NIR dyes like ICG possess an absorption cross-section of 2.9×10^{-20} m² at 800 nm. In contrast, Mie scattering theory predicts the metal nanoshells possess absorption cross-section on the order of 3.8×10^{-14} m², which is greater by a factor of 106 compared to that of ICG. However, it is clearly demonstrated that gold nanoshells display much stronger absorptive compared to ICG molecules (Hirsch et al. 2003).

In the current study, we have used the combination of ICG and gold nanoshells, as an exogenous near infrared absorbers for enhancement of selective photo thermal interaction on thermal and biomechanical properties of skin tissue and LTS. The nanoshells used in our experiments had an average diameter of ~100 nm (85–115 nm) and a shell thickness of ~10 nm (7–12 nm) measured by TEM. The optical properties of nanoshells are well predicted by Mie scattering theory (Alvarez-Puebla et al. 2005, Gellner et al. 2009), thus allowing one to calculate the dimensions of core and shell required to fabricate nanoshells with strong absorption at a given wavelength. This allows facile tuning to match the output of a desired laser source for a given application. Extinction cross section includes both absorption and scattering:

$$C_{ext} = C_\alpha + C_\beta \tag{10.3}$$

The extinction cross section for a small core-shell particle is:

$$C_{ext} = k \, Im(\alpha) \tag{10.4}$$

where $k = 2\pi \sqrt{\varepsilon_m} / \lambda$, λ is the wavelength of the incident light in vacuum and Im (α) is the imaginary part of complex polarizability of the particle:

$$a = \varepsilon_0 \frac{(\varepsilon_s-\varepsilon_m)(\varepsilon_c+2\varepsilon_s)+(R_c/R_s)^3(\varepsilon_c-\varepsilon_s)(\varepsilon_m+2\varepsilon_s)}{(\varepsilon_s+2\varepsilon_m)(\varepsilon_c+2\varepsilon_s)+(R_c/R_s)^3(\varepsilon_c-\varepsilon_s)(2\varepsilon_s-\varepsilon_m)} 4\pi R_s^3 \tag{10.5}$$

$\varepsilon_0 = 8.85 \times 10^{-12}$F/m is the permittivity of free space, R_c is the radius of core, Rs is the total particle size including shell thickness, and $\varepsilon_c, \varepsilon_s$, and ε_m are the dielectric function of core, shell, and embedding media, respectively.

Laser-bonding was proposed as a preferred method for sealing wounds, which include tissue incisions in general and skin incisions in particular (Tang et al. 1997, Khosroshahi et al. 2010). The rationale behind the tissue laser-bonding procedure is that this technological platform may offer minimal inflammation traits with only minimal scar formation (Kirsch et al. 2001). Laser-soldering temperatures below 60°C generated a weak bond (Brosh et al. 2004), while laser soldering at temperatures exceeding 80°C induced thermal damage. Since one of the objectives of this work was to select an optimal temperature setting that will not induce thermal damage, therefore, the optimal temperature for soldering was 65°C. As is shown in Fig. 10.23, the temperature rise of skin increases with increasing laser power density and the concentration of gold nanoshell in dye combination. For power density above 47 Wcm^{-2} the temperature exceeds 90°C, and it is not suitable for *in vivo* application. In comparison to our previous results with gold nanoshells alone, this condition occurs above 60 Wcm^{-2} (Khosroshahi et al. 2011a, Nourbakhsh and Khosroshahi 2011), so we can conclude that by adding of ICG in albumin solder one may use lower power densities for LTS with acceptable results. Varying the power density on ICG + GNs solder resulted in slight rise of temperature and tensile strength, it may be, however suggested that Ns and hence Vs affect significantly the σ as well as the quality of soldered tissue. This can be argued by the fact while Vs controls the temperature rise for intertwining tissue fibrillar collagen matrix and subsequent melting transition and fusion, N_s influences the thermal accumulation effect on the tissue.

Our results indicate that laser power density is the most important parameter affecting solder temperature during the process of laser tissue soldering. Also, varying the gold nanoshells concentration within the solder resulted in similar thermal behaviour with insignificant changes of temperature. The findings of this study show that temperatures recorded in the beneath of the skin can reach up to 80°C or even higher considering the thermocouple limitation. However, it is important to notice that the thermocouple properties can directly affect the temperature measurements. As it was shown by Verdaasdonk et al. (1991) tissue temperature rise can be influenced by number of parameters mainly, direct absorption of radiation by probe, and also by their geometry. Also a thermal gradient was observed both laterally and in front of the probe. On the other hand, the limitations of such digital thermometer including the size or diameter of thermocouple head, as well as its position relative to the center of exposure should be taken into account. Therefore, we believe that for more accurate conclusions, the above issues must be considered. Needless to mention the use of digital thermal camera for such investigations seems to be more appropriate as it will be used in our further research.

Increasing tensile strength with power density has a same trend in comparison with nanoshells and ICG alone, but in each power density the tensile strength in the case of ICG + GNs is higher. For example, the tensile strengths of repaired skin at power destiny of 47 Wcm^{-2} are 1190 ± 90, 1422 ± 120, and 1830 ± 215 gcm^{-2} for ICG, gold nanoshells, and ICG + GNs, respectively. Studies by DeCoste et al. (1992) using ICG dye alone showed that at temperatures above 60°C a significant release of ICG and a steep increase in the temperature. This presumably resulted from the release of ICG from collagen as the molecule reached its fibrillar melting transition temperature. In a study by Kirsch et al. (2001), temperatures during laser activation with an ICG/albumin solder were determined within the solder and underlying dermis over 1 minute of activation. Their results showed temperature within the solder reached 101°C, while temperature in the superficial and deep skin was 70 and 65°C, respectively. Fung et al. (1999) results showed that wounds repaired at higher temperatures (85 and 95°C) were observed to have lower mea wound strength than wounds repaired at lower temperatures (65 and 75°C). The effect of number of scan on tensile strength of repaired skin is also studied. At eight scans and power density of 83 Wcm^{-2}, the tensile strength of soldered skin with ICG alone is 1920 ± 80 gcm^{-2}, which at the same condition this value is 2407 ± 124 and 3189 ± 139 grcm^{-2} for gold nanoshells and combination of ICG and gold nanoshells, respectively. Also, with combination of these light absorbers we can achieve the acceptable tensile strength in compare with previous studies with lower number of scans. For example, using four scans the tensile strength reached to 1840 ± 122 gcm^{-2} which is comparable to tensile strength of soldered skin with ICG using eight scans. This finding can be important for clinical applications if less operation time to be considered. As is shown in Fig. 10.25, by decreasing the scan velocity, the tensile strength of repaired skin increased for different concentration of gold nanoshells in combination of solder. For a constant scan velocity, for example 0.3 mmsec^{-1}, tensile strength of skin soldered with ICG, gold nanoshells, and combination of ICG and gold nanoshells was 1350 ± 120, 1422 ± 160, and 1830 ± 210 gcm^{-2}, respectively. The latter value is same as the tensile strength achieved by Vs of 0.2 mmsec^{-1} for ICG alone. The comparison of the LTS results is given in Table 10.5.

Table 10.5. Comparison of LTS results with different solder and laser parameters. Column (1) from ref. (Khosroshahi 2010), column (2) from ref. (Khosroshahi 2011b).

	ICG	Gold nanoshell (GNS)	ICG + GNS
1(47 Wcm^{-2})	1075 ± 90	1422 ± 120	1830 ± 210
1(60 Wcm^{-2})	1400 ± 120	1610 ± 110	2022 ± 140
1(83 Wcm^{-2})	1920 ± 110	2407 ± 162	3189 ± 240
Ns = 4	630 ± 80	930 ± 80	1180 ± 122
Ns = 8	1300 ± 75	1860 ± 95	2530 ± 90
Vs = 0.2 mm s^{-1}	1800 ± 140	2120 ± 190	2670 ± 180
Vs = 0.3 mm s^{-1}	1350 ± 190	1422 ± 160	1830 ± 210
Vs = 0.4 mm s^{-1}	1080 ± 90	1200 ± 125	1280 ± 120

Keywords: Tissue soldering, Diode laser, Indocyanine green, Tensile strength, Gold nanoshells, Mie theory, Thermal damage, UV-vis spectroscopy, Atomic force microscopy.

References

Alvarez-Puebla, R.A., D. Ross, G. Nazri and R. Aroca. 2005. Surface-enhanced Raman scattering on nanoshells with tunable surface plasmon resonance. Langmuir 21: 10504–10508.

Anderson, R. and J. Parish. 1983. Selective photothermolysis: precise microsurgery by selective absorption of pulsed radiation. Science 220: 524–527.

Brosh, T., D. Simhon, M. Halpern, A. Ravid, T. Vasilyev and N. Kariv. 2004. Closure of skin incisions in rabbits by laser soldering II: Tensile strength. Lasers Surg. Med. 35: 12–7.

Capon, A., E. Souil and B. Gauthier. 2001. Laser assisted skin closure (LASC) by using a 815-nm diode-laser system accelerates and improves wound healing. Lasers Surg. Med. 28: 168–175.

Cohen, M., A. Ravid, V. Scharf, D. Hauben and A. Katzir. 2003. Temperature controlled burn generation system based on a CO$_2$ laser and a silver halide fiber optic radiometer. Lasers Surg. Med. 32: 413–416.

Cooper, C., Z. Schwartz and D. Soh. 2001. Optimal solder and irradiance for diode laser tissue soldering. Lasers Surg. Med. 29: 53–61.

Crochet, J., S. Gnyawali, C. Yichao, V. Wanl and R. Chen. 2006. Temperature distribution in selective laser-tissue interaction. J. Biomed. Optics. 11: 034031.

DeCoste, S., F. William and T. Flotte. 1992. Dye-enhanced laser welding skin closure. Laser Surg. Med. 25–32.

Dew, D., R. Serbent, W. Hart, G. Boynton et al. 1983. Laser-assisted microsurgical vessel anastomosis techniques: the use of argon and CO$_2$ lasers. Lasers Surg. Med. 3: 135–142.

Ditkoff, M. and D. Perrault. 2002. Potential use of diode laser soldering in middle ear reconstruction. Lasers Surg. Med. 31: 242–246.

Duff, D., A. Baiker and P. Edwards. 1993. A new hydrogel of gold cluster: formation and particle size variation. Langmuir 9: 2301–2309.

Gellner, M., B. Kustner and S. Schlucker. 2009. Optical properties and SERS efficiency of tunable gold/silver nanoshells. Vib. Spec. 50: 43–47.

Gobin, A., P. O'Neal, M. Watkins, J. Halas, A. Drezek and L. West. 2005. Near infrared laser-tissue welding using nanoshells as an exogenous absorber. Lasers Surg. Med. 37: 123–129.

Gulsoy, M., Z. Dereli and H. Tabakogh. 2006. Closure of skin incisions by 980 nm diode laser welding. Lasers Med. Sci. 21: 5–10.

Franz, M., M. Kuhn, T. Wright, T. Wachtel and M. Robson. 2000. Use of the wound healing trajectory as an outcome determinant for acute wound healing. Wound Repair Regen. 8: 511–516.

Fried, N.M. and J.T. Walsh. 2000. Laser skin welding: *In vivo* tensile strength and wound healing results. Lasers Surg. Med. 27: 55–65.

Fung, L., G. Mingin, M. Massicotte, D. Felsen and D. Poppas. 1999. Effects of temperature on tissue thermal injury and wound strength after photothemal wound closure. Lasers Surg. Med. 25: 285–290.

Hirsch, L., R. Stafford, A. Bankson, S. Sershen and B. Rivera. 2003. Nanoshell-mediated near-infrared thermal therapy of tumors under magnetic resonance guidance. Proc. Natl. Acad. Sci. 100: 13549–13554.

Hoffman, G., B. Byrd, E. Soller and D. Heintzelman. 2003. Effect of varying chromophores used in light-activated protein solders on tensile strength and thermal damage profile of repairs. Biomed. Sci. Instrum. 39: 12–7.

Jain, K. and W. Gorish. 1979. Repair of small blood vessels with the Nd:YAG laser: a preliminary report. Surgery 85: 684–688.

Kirsch, A., J. Duckett and H. Snyder. 1997. Skin flap closure by dermal laser tissue soldering: a wound healing model for sutureless hypospadias repair. Urology 50: 263–272.

Kirsch, A., C. Cooper, J. Gatti, H. Scherz, D. Canning, S. Zderic and H. Snyder. 2001. Laser tissue soldering for hypospadias repair: results of a controlled prospective clinical trial. J. Urol. 65: 574–577.

Khosroshahi, M.E., M.S. Nourbakhsh, S. Saremi, A. Hooshyar, Sh. Rabbani, F. Tabatabai and M. Sotudeh Anvari. 2010. Application of albumin protein and indocyanine green chromophore for tissue soldering using IR diode laser: *ex vivo* and *in vivo* Studies 28: 723–733.

Khosroshahi, M.E., M.S. Nourbakhsh and L. Ghazanfari. 2011a. Synthesis and biomedical application of SiO_2/Au nanofluid based on laser-induced surface plasmon resonance thermal effect. J. Modern Phys. 2: 944–953.

Khosroshahi, M.E. and M.S. Nourbakhsh. 2011b. Enhanced laser tissue soldering using indocyanine green chromophore and gold nanoshells combination. J. Biomed. Opt. 16:088002–7.

Lemole, J., J. Ashton and O. Arikan. 1992. Effect of additives on laser assisted fibrinogen bonding. SPIE 1643: 43–44.

Lobel, B., O. Eyal, N. Kariv and A. Katzir. 2000. Temperature controlled CO_2 laser welding of soft tissues: urinary bladder welding in different animal models (rats, rabbits, and cats). Lasers Surg. Med. 26: 4–12.

Malicka, J., I. Gryczynski, C. Geddes and J. Lakowicz. 2003. Metal enhanced emission from indocyanine green: a new approach to *in vivo* imaging. J. Biomed. Opt. 8: 472–478.

McNally, K., B. Sorg, A. Welch and E. Owen. 1999. Photo thermal effects of laser tissue soldering. Phys. Med. Biol. 44: 983–1002.

McNally, M., B. Sorg, E. Chan and A. Welch. 2000. Optimal parameters for laser tissue soldering. Part I: tensile strength and scanning electron microscopy analysis. Lasers Surg. Med. 26: 346–356.

Nourbakhsh, M.S. and M.E. Khosroshahi. 2011. An *in vitro* investigation of skin tissue soldering using gold nanoshells and diode laser. Laser Med. Sci. 26: 49–55.

Ntziachristos, V., A. Yodh, M. Schnall and B. Chance. 2000. Concurrent MRI and diffuse optical tomography of breast after indocyanine green enhancement. Proc. Natl. Acad. Sci. USA 97 6: 2767–2772.

Nwomeh, B.C., D. Yager and I. Cohen. 1998. Physiology of the chronic wound. Clin. Plast. Surg. 25: 341–356.

Moritz, A. and F. Henriques. 1947. Studies of thermal injury: II. The relative importance of time and surface temperatures in the causation of cutaneous burns. American Journal of Pathology 23: 695–720.

O'Neal, D., L. Hirsch, N. Halas and J. Payne. 2004. Photothermal tumor ablation in mice using near infrared-absorbing nanoparticles. Cancer Lett. 209: 171–176.

Poppas, D., R. Stewart and M. Massicotte. 1996. Temperature-controlled laser photocoagulation of soft tissue: *in vivo* evaluation using a tissue welding model. Lasers Surg. Med. 18: 335–344.

Pohl, D., L. Bass, R. Stewart and D. Chiu. 1998. Effect of optical temperature feedback control on patency in laser-soldered micro vascular anastomosis. J. Reconstr. Microsurg. 14: 23–29.

Simhon, D., T. Brosh, M. Halpern, A. Ravid and T. Vasilyev. 2004. Closure of skin incisions in rabbits by laser soldering: I: Wound healing pattern. Lasers Surg. Med. 35: 1–11.

Sorg, B., K. Mcnally and A. Welch. 2000. Biodegradable polymer film reinforcement of an ICG doped liquid albumin solder for laser assisted incision closure. Lasers Surg. Med. 27: 73–81.

Stewart, R., A. Benbrahim, G. LaMuraglia and M. Rosenberg. 1996. Laser assisted vascular welding with real time temperature control. Lasers Surg. Med. 19: 9–16.

Savage, E., J. Lee, G. McCormick and A. Steven. 2003. Near-infrared laser welding of aortic and skin tissues and microscopic investigation of welding efficacy. SPIE – Int. Soc. Opt. Eng. 49: 182–185.

Tang, J., G. Godlewski, S. Rouy and G. Delacretaz. 1997. Morphologic changes in collagen fibers after 830 nm diode laser welding. Lasers Surg. Med. 2: 438–443.

Verdaasdonk, M., F. Holstege, E. Jansen and C. Borst. 1991. Temperature along the surface of modified fiber tips for Nd:YAG laser angioplasty. Lasers Surg. Med. 11: 213–222.

Weissleder, R. 2001. A clearer vision for *in vivo* imaging. Nat. Biotechnol. 19: 316–317.

Zhou, J., M. Chin and S. Schafer. 1994. Aggregation and degradation of indocyanine green. Proc. SPIE 2128: 495–508.

11

Drug Delivery

11.1 Introduction

Nowadays, the application of nanomaterials and nanotechnology to biomedical research (i.e., nanomedicine) has become an emerging field with major impact on the development of new types of diagnostic, imaging, therapeutic agents and drug delivery. Important factors for *in vivo* applications of nanoparticles (NPs) are: biocompatibility (non-toxicity), biodegradability (for carriers), particle size (absorption, scatttering), immunogenicity, surface properties, drug loading capacities/release, drug stability, storage of NP. By definition, drug delivery systems are supramolecular assemblies incorporating agents intended to treat a disease. They are used to overcome the shortcomings of the conventional drugs, such as unfavorable pharmacokinetics, poor solubility, instability, high toxicity, drug resistance, and low cellular uptake. Drug delivery is becoming an increasingly important aspect for medicine field, as more potent and specific drugs are being developed. With the incorporation of nanotechnology, so-called drug-delivery systems integrate biosensing functionalities, which support unaided *in vivo* feedback control that play an essential role in modern nanomedicine. Many biomaterials, primarily polymer- or lipid-based, can be used for this task, offering extensive chemical diversity and the potential for further modification using nanoparticles. The large surface area of the nanoparticles enables us to have opportunities to place functional groups on the surface. A wide range of new types of polymer particles could be designed with the recent advances in chemistry, processing techniques, and analytical instrumentation. For example, there are particles that are hollow, multilobed, conductive, thermo responsive, magnetic, functionalized with reactive groups on the surface, and pH responsive, each with high potential applications.

Traditional drug delivery methods include oral and intravenous routes of administration. These methods are still the most widely used today, yet each has its disadvantages. Oral delivery via tablets or capsules is largely inefficient due to exposure of the pharmaceutical agent to the metabolic processes of the body (Willams et al. 2003). Therefore, a larger than necessary dose is often required and the maximum effectiveness of the drug is limited. Traditional intravenous (IV) administration is much more problematic. Effectiveness, specifically for IV injectable drugs is often low, necessitating large amounts of a drug to be injected into a patent, creating a high concentration of the drug in the blood stream that could potentially lead to toxic side effects (Leroux et al. 1996). Nanoparticle drug delivery, utilizing degradable and absorbable polymers, provides a more efficient, less risky solution to many drug delivery challenges. There are many advantages of using polymeric nanoparticles (PNP) in drug delivery. Perhaps the main advantages are that they generally increase the stability of any volatile pharmaceutical agents and that they are easily fabricated at low cost. Additionally, the use of absorbable or degradable polymers, such as polyesters, provides a high degree of biocompatibility for PNP delivery systems (Leroux et al. 1996, Soppimath et al. 2001).

Efficient, rational drug/gene delivery and targeting of pharmaceutical, therapeutic and diagnostic agents is undoubtedly the projects in the forefront in nanomedicine. Recent advances in cell biology and molecular biology have provided a vast amount of information regarding the structure, properties, and signaling functions of a variety of cell receptors. Thus, targeted drug delivery involves: (a) the ability to target specific location in the body by recognizing the precise targets such as cells and receptors, (b) use of appropriate drug nanocarriers to achieve required goals with minimum side effects. Drug delivery systems (DDS) can not only enhance the efficacy of various pharmaceutical payloads, but they also have the advantages to improve poor solubility, limited stability, biodistributions, pharmacokinetics of drugs, and the reduction of the concentration of drug at nonspecific sites, hence reducing the possible side effects. DDS are categorized into two main groups: (a) capsule-like systems such as micelles and liposomes with a great advantage of carrying relatively large amount of drug, hence maximizing the ratio of drug to carrier, (b) covalent attachment of the drug to the carrier molecule to produce conjugates. One of the most important characteristics of nanoparticles is their ability to encapsulate drugs. This feature can reduce unnecessary exposure and deliver an effective concentration of drugs to the target. Normally, the cancer drugs are administrated systematically at high dosage to ensure a therapeutically effective concentration at the tumor site. Dosage of chemotherapeutics are in the 100-μg range; sometimes they are as high as 1 g a day. However, in recent years a number of drug delivery devices have been developed ranging from macro-sized (1 mm) to micro (100–0.1 μm) and nano-sized (Moghimi et al. 2001, LaVan et al. 2003).

Some common routes of administration are non-invasive per oral, skin (topical), trans-mucosal, and inhalation. Drugs released in the form of degradation, swelling, affinity based interactions and diffusion. The drug is either taken orally or injected in the body. A wide range of materials can be used as drug carriers: biodegradable polymers, dendrimers, liposomes, nanotubes, and nanorods. Examples of polymers includes: poly(lactic acid) (PLA), poly(glycolic acid) (PGA), poly(lactic co-glycolic acid) (PLGA) and polyanhydride. PGA and PLGA and their co-polymers are common biocompatible polymers that are used for fabricating nanoparticles. Gold-based core in mixed monolayer-protected clusters are also promising candidates, essentially due to being inert and nontoxic, and secondly because monodisperse NPs can be fabricated with tunable core size between 1.5–10 nm, thus providing a large surface area for efficient drug targeting and ligand conjugation. The attachment of payload can be achieved by either (i) noncovalent interaction such as DNA, siRNA, or enzymes via electrostatic interaction, or (ii) covalent chemical conjugation of small-molecule drugs. There can be two types of drug delivery methods: (a) Passive targeting and (b) Active targeting.

11.1.1 Drug delivery carriers

The primary objectives of nanoparticle-mediated delivery of anticancer drugs with therapeutic formulation such as doxorubicine, danorubicine, and paclitaxel are: (1) to resolve the problems of delivery to targets prevented by biological barriers, (2) to enhance the carriers blood circulation lifetime, (3) to improve poor targeting selectivity. Clearly, these goals can be achieved by both improving and optimizing the physico-chemical properties of the drug carriers, as well as by conjugation of the drug carriers to biomolecular targeting ligands. Ligands together with drugs can be covalently attached to carrier's coating surface for targeting. This strategy is normally referred to '*multifunctional nanoparticles*' where the carrier is comprised of delivery, imaging, and therapeutic agents. Drug-carrying NPs can be synthesized using a variety of materials and techniques. Commonly used techniques are: precipitation, emulsion, and lipid extrusion. Similarly, the widely used materials based on their biocompatibility and biodegradability include: (a) lipids (liposomes) and (b) polymers (micelles, nanoparticles, and dendrimers). Drugs can be loaded in different ways: (a) dispersed in a matrix, (b) encapsulated by a NP or in a vesicle, (c) dissolved in a hydrophilic or hydrophobic core, and (d) attached covalently to the surface of a NP.

a) *Liposomes*: These are self-assembled structures that are composed of spherical phospholipid bilayers in which the outer layer surrounds a central aqueous core. Water-soluble drug compounds are trapped in the interior part of the liposome-enclosed core. A hydrophobic drug can then be delivered by the encapsulating bilayer. Improvements in *in vivo* stability of the carrier have been made after development of PEG modified liposomes and the circulation half-life of PEGylated liposomes has increased due to changes in the rate of uptake by phagocytic cells.

b) *Polymeric micelles*: These are the core-shell-type nanoparticle formed through the self-assembly of block copolymers or graft copolymers in the selective solvents and are introduced to minimize inherent instability and degradation associated with liposome formulation. Amphiphiles consist of hydrophilic and hydrophobic segments, and the self-assembly in aqueous phase leads to formation of nano-sized particles with hydrophobic core/hydrophilic exterior. The core serves as reservoirs for hydrophobic drugs, whereas the exterior enhances the stability of carrier in an aqueous medium. Basically, these pharmaceutical carriers are colloidal dispersions with particles size between 5 and 100 nm, which can entrap water-soluble anti-cancer drugs, such as paclitaxel, camptotheein, and tamoxifen with the loading capacities between 5 and 25% wt% of drug. Depending on the preparation method, the drug can be chemically, physically, and electrostatically entrapped *in situ* during particle formation or alternatively, covalently attach to the polymer assemblies. Compared to liposomes and surfactant micelles, the polymeric micelles possess high loading capacity, longer circulation time due to higher stability *in vivo*, and lower rates of dissociation, hence longer retention period of loaded drug (Kataoka et al. 2001, Adams et al. 2003, Shuai et al. 2004).

c) *Degradable polymers*: As it is discussed in the following sections, polymeric carriers are interesting because they can be readily modified in a number of different ways to enhance drug delivery and targeting. One such example, which is covered in this chapter, is PLGA. These FDA approved biomaterials are one of most commonly used polymers for drug delivery, mainly due to their unique properties including the ability to breakdown into naturally occurring metabolites, lactic, and glycolic acid. One widely used method for producing biodegradable polymer is liquid emulsion. The spontaneous emulsification-solvent evaporation technique has been employed to prepare drug, loaded PLGA micro and nanoparticles. The main idea of this technique is to produce droplets of polymer solution in a aqueous phase, which then solidifies to form particles by polymer precipitation and organic solvent removal at the air/water interphase (Yeh et al. 1993).

Generally, drug carriers can be externally guided to the target (e.g., magnetically as in MRI), tracked, and once they have reached the target be activated externally by magnetic field, focused ultrasound, radiofrequency, and laser light.

11.1.2 Characteristics of tumor tissues

Neoplasm is an ancient Greek word meaning "New Plasma", i.e., formation or creation, which denotes the formation of abnormal growth (i.e., neoplasia) of tissue commonly referred to as a tumor. Usually, but not always, neoplasia forms a mass. According to World Health Organization (WHO) neoplasms is classified into four main groups: (a) benign neoplasms, (b) *in situ* neoplasms, (c) malignant neoplasms (or cancers), and (d) neoplasms of uncertain or unknown behaviour. Prior to the abnormal growth of tissue, as neoplasia, cells often undergo an abnormal pattern of growth, such as metaplasia or dysplasia. However, metaplasia or dysplasia does not always progress to neoplasia (Birbrair et al. 2014). Tumor cells consist of various structures and areas, of which the actual cancer cells occupy less than 50%, the vasculature 1–10%. The remaining structure consists of a collagen-rich matrix. As it was mentioned in §5.5, tumors develop a chaotic capillary network that distinguishes them from normal vasculature and they follow a branching pattern. The capillary vasculature in tumors is normally accompanied by occlusions caused by rapidly proliferating cancer cells. Hypoxia is produced as a result of compression of vasculature and finally necrosis of viable tumor cells occurs. Unlike normal tissue, tumors often lack a functional lymphatic system. Another characteristic of tumor is the high proportion of proliferating endothelial cells and aberrant basement membranes of tumor vasculature. Tumor blood vessels are up to 3–10 times more permeable to counterbalance the high oxygen and nutrient requirements of the growing tumor (Weindel et al. 1994, Olesen 1986). The interstitial compartment of tumor contains a network of collagen and elastic fibre, which is immersed by hyaluronate and proteoglycan-containing fluid. The interstitial pressure and rapid aberrant cell growth are thought to be the main reasons for the compression and occlusion of blood and lymphatic vessels in solid tumors (Murray and Carmichael 1995). It is crucial to appreciate the fact that any transport of drug into the tumor is dependent on the interstitial pressure as well as on its composition, charge, and the characteristic of the drug. Also, the dense packing of tumor cells limits the movement of molecules from the vessel into the interstitial compartment. Macromolecules and drugs are transported into the tumor cells through interendothelial junctions and vesicular vacuolar organelles. The range of pore cut-off size in tumor tissue has been reported between 100–780 nm (Hobbs et al. 1998, Yuan et al. 1995) and can be increased up to 800 nm, for example in human colon tumors by perfusion with low dosage (10 µg/mL) of vascular endothelial growth factor (VEGF) (Monsky et al. 1999). The process of entering colloidal NPs into interstitial compartment through leaky vessels and accumulation in tumor due to poor lymphatic drainage system is called "Enhanced Permeability Enhancement-EPR" effect.

11.1.3 Surface coating of nanoparticles

It was explained in §9.6 that as soon as NPs are entered into biological system, they are rapidly covered with plasma proteins such as immunoglobulins and fibronectin, and hence build aggregates. This is called opsonization or corona effect. In order to avoid or minimize this effect, nanoparticles are suitably coated by biodegradable matrices so that they become undetected by macrophages. *Hydrophilic* coating prevents interaction of NPs with macrophages of the RES, reducing their chance of being removed from circulation and thus, increasing their circulation life-time. Such coatings are for example: Dextran, Poly(ethylene glycole) (PEG), poly(ethylene oxide) (PEO), poloxamers, poloexamins, and silicones. *Hydrophobic* coating on the other hand, are applied to increase opsonization, leading to copious interaction with macrophages and the nanoparticles are therefore rapidly removed from the circulation. The latter case is applied for targeted delivery of nanoparticles to the RES of liver and spleen. The concept of NPs coating is well established now and the choice of the coating polymers can determine the life-time of the circulation.

11.1.4 Uptake mechanism

Nanoparticles can act at the tissular or cellular level. The latter implies that they can be endocytosed or phagocytosed by, for example, dendritic cells, macrophages, as is illustrated in Fig. 11.1. In this process, the NPs can reach beyond the cytoplasmatic membrane and in some cases, beyond the nuclear membrane (i.e., transfection applications). Cellular uptake mechanism for nanoparticles and macromolecules are: pinocytosis (Weissleder et al. 1997), endocytosis (Yeh et al. 1993), and receptor-mediated endocytosis (Moore et al. 1998). Macromolecules and DNA, which are susceptible to lysosomal degradation can be delivered by nanoparticles which escape lysosomal degradation. Polymeric NPs such as PLGA can be non-specifically (i.e., passive targeting) transported into the cells by clathrin-mediated process known as fluid phase pinocytosis. At physiological pH (7–7.5), negatively charged PLGA nanoparticles are transported to primary endosomes and become positively charged where they enter the acidic secondary endosomes and lysosomes, from which they are transferred to cystol. Those NPs transferred to primary endosomes and then entered to secondary endosomes become cationic and the local interaction with cell membrane releases the NPs into the cytoplasm, hence escaping the lysosomal compartment (Panyam et al. 2002).

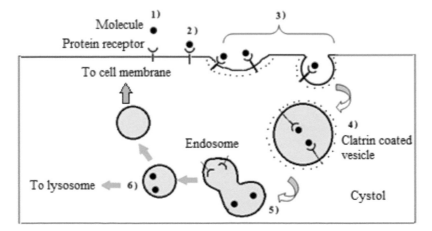

Figure 11.1. Mechanism of cellular uptake indicating. (1) Molecule binds to protein receptor, (2) Receptor-molecule move to clathrin pit, (3) Cell membrane folds inwards, (4) Formation of a coated vesicle, (5) Vesicle fuses with an endosome, (6) Receptors and molecules separate.

11.1.5 Targeting methods

(i) Passive targeting: The NPs are coated but not functionalized. Targeting lymphatic systems can be achieved by using different routes of administration: intramuscular, subcutaneous, intraperitoneal, or oral. Coating NPs is advantageous to enhance circulation time and avoid removal by the MPS, hence increasing their uptake and accumulation in tumor. Generally, passive targeting occurs as a result of extravasation of the NPs at the diseased site (e.g., tumor) where the microvasculature is hyperpermeable and leaky due to tumor poor lymphatic drainage. Thus, NPs accumulate in the interstitial part of the tumor via EPR process. From delivery point of view, there is practically no limitation as the diameters of typical NPs are much smaller than the narrowest capillaries. However, the main limitation is the residence time of NPs in the bloodstream. Thus, the use of conventional NPS for drug delivery by passive targeting would be limited to tumors in MPS (see §9.6) organs (liver, spleen, and bone marrow). Addressing other tumoral tissues does not seem to be feasible without active targeting due to the short circulation time and the low concentration of NPs.

(ii) Active targeting: This is based on the (a) functionalization of different moieties, for example: NPs, dendrimers, liposomes, and micelles by different agents for specific purpose, (b) exclusive or over expression of various receptors in tumoral cells, and (c) specific physical characteristics, as seen in Fig. 11.2. Vectors sensitive to physical stimuli (e.g., temperature, pH, electric charge, light, sound, magnetism) have been developed and conjugated to drugs. Also, active targeting can be achieved by over-expressed species: (a) low molecular weight ligands (e.g., thiamine, fluorescin isothiocyanate (FITC), folic acid, sugers), (b) peptides (RGD, LHRD), (c) proteins (transferrin, antibodies, lectins), and (d) polysaccharides (hyaluronic acid-HA, polysaturated fatty acid, DNA, etc.). Moeities must be designed and fabricated with specific characteristics in such a way so as to not only reach a given target, but also meet the biosafety issues (i.e., the nanotoxicity), which implies attaining a suitable combination of material properties, size, way of conjugating (covalent attachment, encapsulation, etc.) the drug to the nanosystem (i.e., moiety), surface chemistry, hydrophilicity or hydrophobicity, biodegradability and physical response properties (e.g., temperature, pH, electric charge, light, sound, magnetism).

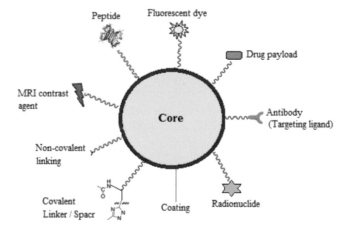

Figure 11.2. Schematic representation of a nanosystem (i.e., a moiety) functionalization of by various receptors.

11.2 Evaluation of drug release from PLGA nanospheres containing betamethasone
(Khosroshahi et al. 2007)

In this research, poly(d,l-lactide-coglycolide acid) (PLGA) as polymeric nanospheres, poly(vinyl alcohol) (PVA) with 87–89% hydrolysis degree as surfactant and distilled water as suspending medium were used. The nanospheres containing Betametasone as drug were prepared by an emulsion–solvent evaporation method and characterized by photon correlation spectroscopy (PCS) and scanning electron microscopy

(SEM). The amount of drug release was determined by HPLC. In emulsion–solvent evaporation technique, time of ultrasound exposure, surfactant content in the formulation and evaporation rate of organic solvents were considered as formulation variables.

Introduction

Biodegradable colloidal particles have received considerable attention as a possible means of delivering drugs and genes by several routes of administration. Special interest has been focused on the use of particles prepared from polyesters like PLGA, due to their biocompatibility and to their resorbability through natural pathways (Kost and Langer 2001, Saltzman and Olbricht 2002). Various methods have been reported for making nanoparticles viz., emulsion-evaporation (Brannon-Peppas 1995), salting-out technique, nanoprecipitation, cross-flow filtration, or emulsion-diffusion technique (Matsumoto et al. 1999). Nanoparticle is a collective name for nanospheres and nanocapsules. Nanospheres have a matrix type structure, where active compounds can be adsorbed at their surface, entrapped or dissolved in the matrix. Nanocapsules have a polymeric shell and an inner core. In this case, the active substances are usually dissolved in the core, but may also be adsorbed at their surface. Nanoparticles or colloidal carriers have been extensively investigated in biomedical and biotechnological areas, especially in drug delivery systems for drug targeting, because their particle size (ranging from 10 to 1000 nm) is acceptable for intravenous injection (Williams et al. 2003). Depending on the desired administration way, the size of the carriers should be optimized. Thus, if the carrier size is under 1 µm, an intravenous injection (the diameter of the smallest blood capillaries is 4 µm) is enabled and this carrier size is also desirable for intramuscular and subcutaneous administration, minimizing any possible irritant reactions. Although a number of different polymers have been investigated for formulating biodegradable nanoparticles, poly(l-lactic-acid) (PLA) and its copolymers with glycolic acid (PLGA) have been extensively used for controlled drug delivery systems (Hickey et al. 2005, Mastsumoto et al. 2005, Garinol et al. 2007) and gene delivery (Wieland et al. 2007, Kakimoto et al. 2007). The lactide/glycolide polymers chains are cleaved by hydrolysis into natural metabolites (lactic and glycolic acids), which are eliminated from the body by the citric acid cycle. PLGA provides a wide range of degradation rates, from months to years, depending on its composition and molecular weight (Leroux et al. 1996, Soppimath et al. 2001, Chawla and Amiji 2002). Indeed PLGA particles are extensively investigated for drug and gene delivery, but still improvements in the existing methods are needed to overcome the difficulties in terms of reproducibility, size, and shape. The size and shape of the colloidal particles are influenced by the stabilizer and the solvent used. Most investigated stabilizers for PLGA lead to negatively charged particles and the plasmid incorporation is achieved via double emulsion technique during particle preparation. This could pose problems in the stability and biological activity of the plasmid due to the involvement of organic solvents during the preparation process. This can be overcome by using cationically modified particles that can bind and condense negatively charged plasmids by simply adding nanoparticles to plasmid or vice versa. Literature suggests PVA as the most popular stabilizer for the production of PLGA nanoparticles leading to negatively charged particles, nevertheless, investigations have been carried out using other stabilizers as well (Bodmeier and McGinity 1998). Thus, the goal of our study was to design a nanoparticulate drug system with a drug controlled delivery, based on the biodegradable polymer PLGA.

Materials

The polymer studied was poly(d,l-lactide-coglycolide acid) (PLGA), with a copolymer ratio of dl-lactide to glycolide of 50:50 (Mw 100,000 g/mol as indicated by the supplier, Sigma Chemical CO, USA). The surfactant used in the emulsification process was poly (vinylalcohol) (PVA) (87–89% hydrolysis degree and molecular mass 72,000 g/mol, Mo Wiol, Germany). As a suspending medium, purified water (Milli-Q, Millipore Corporation, Billerica, MA) was used. The encapsulated drug was Betamethazon (Tolidaru, Iran). Acetonitrile (Mallinkrodt, HPLC grade) was used in the analytical method.

Preparation of polymeric nanospheres

The PLGA nanospheres containing Betamethasone were prepared as follows: 40 mg of PLGA and 2 mg of Betamethasone were dissolved in 4 cc DCM. Aqueous solution with PVA, used as emulsifier, was stirred at 2400 rpm by high-speed homogenizer. The PVA disperses the phase which is not dissolved very well and stabilizes the emulsion. The mixture of drug and polymer is then gradually emulsified into an aqueous solution to make an oil (O) in water (W), i.e., O/W emulsion. The oil in water emulsion was then stirred for 24 hours at room temperature with the magnetic stirrer to evaporate DCM. The produced nanospheres were collected by centrifugation (1200, 15 min) and washed with de-ionized water three times to remove excessive emulsifiers. Freeze-drier was used to remove excessive water to get fine powders. This procedure was applied to make nanospheres with various PVA percentages as emulsifier.

In vitro release of betamethasone

1 mg of each nanoparticle's sample were dispersed in 3cc of phosphorous buffer solution (PBS), in which the pH ws maintained at 7.4. The solution were kept in an orbital incubator at 37.2°C. At defined intervals, the samples were taken out and centrifuged at 12000 rpm for 10 minutes. The amount of drug release was determined by HPLC by UV detection set at 227 nm (150 × 4.6 mm ID, pore size 5 μm, GL Science, Tokyo, Japan). The mobile phase consisted of acetonitrile:water (1:1) and the flow rate was set at 1 ml/min. Separation was achieved using a C18 column (240 mm × 4 mm, 5 μm). The amount of Betametasone entrapped in the nanoparticles was determined after their dissolution in 100 mL phosphate buffer saline (PBS) with pH = 7.4. The solutions were passed through a membrane filter (pore size 0.42 μm, Millipore) before HPLC measurements. All the samples were incubated in 37°C for different times and were centrifuged for 2 min before HPLC injection. Injection volume was 100 μL and the measurements were performed twice for each batch.

Encapsulation efficiency (EE)

The encapsulation efficiency of Betamethasone in nanospheres was determined as the mass ratio of the entrapped Betamethasone in nanosphere to the theoretical amount of Betametasone used in the preparation. 3 mg of nanospheres containing Betamethasone were dissolved in 1 ml DCM and 9 ml mobile phase (acetonitrile) was added to solution. In order to obtain a clear solution, a nitrogen stream was introduced to evaporate DCM at ambient temperature. The resulting solution was analyzed by HPLC in the similar condition illustrated above.

Nanoparticles characterization

The nanoparticles size distribution was determined in bidistilled water at 30°C by photon correlation spectroscopy (PCS) using a particle size analyzer (Brookhaven Instruments Corp.). For the measurements, 1 mL of the nanoparticles suspension was dispersed in 5 mL of distilled water and sonicated during 1 min. The analyses were performed at a scattering angle of 90° and at a temperature of 25°C. For each sample, the mean diameter and the standard deviation of ten determinations were calculated using multimodal analysis.

Results

In order to study the influence of PVA content on the nanoparticles properties, some batches were prepared by using an external aqueous phase consisting of PVA at different concentrations varied by 0.5, 1, 2, and 3 percent (w/v). Figure 11.3 shows a decrease in particle size from 500 to 200 nm when the PVA concentration in the external aqueous phase was increased from 0.5 to 0.3% (w/v).

The betamethasone release from nanoparticles containing different PVA concentration was studied as a function of time. The results over 300 hr are shown in Fig. 11.4, where considerable release difference between nanosphere with 3% PVA concentration and other samples is observed. As a result, the release rate

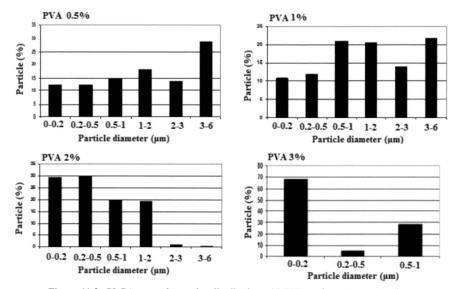

Figure 11.3. PLGA nanospheres size distribution with PVA surfactant concentration.

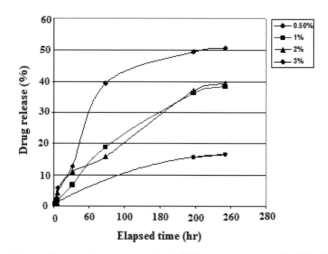

Figure 11.4. SEM morphology of betamethasone encapsulated PLGA nanospheres at (a) 0.5%, (b) 1%, (c) 2% and (d) 3% of PVA concentration.

can be increased by decreasing the particle size and increasing amount of emulsifier used in the formulation. While about 55% of drug from 3% PVA concentrated nanoparticles were found after approximately 250 h, only 17% and 35% of betamethasone were released from nanoparticles with 0.5 and 1% PVA containing particles. The rate of drug release can be controlled by adjusting the type and amount of emulsifier used, as well as entrapment efficiency of drug. The difference in the release behaviour can be related to particle size, for example, for nanospheres with smaller size distribution, the water penetration into the nanosphere is more significant leading to more drug diffusion for release. This may be explained by the fact that smaller nanospheres have larger specific surface area, which could cause more water penetration I to the bulk area.

Table 11.1 shows the encapsulation efficiency (EE) of betamethasone for nanosphere 0.5%, 1%, 2%, and 3%. It can be seen that lowest (11.35%) and highest (78.67%) EE were achieved using 0.5% and 3% w/v PVA nanosphere formulation, respectively. Clearly, the value of EE is directly dependent on the size of nanospheres. In addition, when the PLGA solution precipitate to form nanosphere, the surfactant could promote capability between the betamethasone and PLGA solution network which enhanced the entrapment

Table 11.1. The encapsulation efficiency of PLGA nanospheres with varied emulsifier concentrations.

PVA (Wt%)	EE (%)
0.5	11.35
1	26.11
2	40.78
3	78.67

of drug by polymer. Generally, it can be concluded that, in this case, 3% concentration is more effective formulation for producing smaller size particles with higher EE.

The morphology of PLGA NPs was investigated by SEM, as seen in Fig. 11.5. The results indicated a uniform, rounded particles with relatively smooth surface. PVA as emulsifier dominantly stayed at interface to separate the two phases (the oil and the water). It can also be concluded that the betamethasone loaded nanoparticles with higher PVA concentration were more spherical in shape with lower degree of agglomeration due to higher globules stabilization.

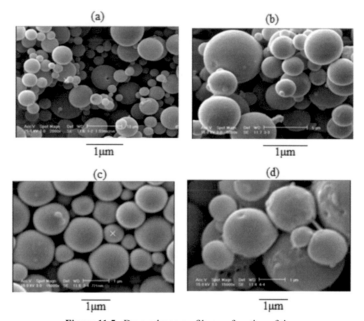

Figure 11.5. Drug release profile as a function of time.

11.3 Dynamic study of PLGA/CS nanoparticles delivery containing drug model into phantom tissue using CO_2 laser for clinical applications
(Mahmoodi et al. 2011)

In this study, cationic nanoparticles (NPs) were prepared by coating chitosan (CS) on the surface of PLGA NPs. To our knowledge most of the work in the field of drug delivery systems using lasers has been performed using short pulses with micron and submicron durations. We carried out an experiment using superlong PLS-R (10 ms) and CW CO2 laser modes on simulated drug biogelatin model where drug was encapsulated by PLGA/CS NPs. Maximum depth of drug containing cavitation was achieved faster at higher powers and shorter irradiation time in CWC mode. We believe that the main mechanism at work with superlong pulses is both photothermal due to vaporization, and photomechanical due to photophoresis and cavitation collapse. In the case of CW, however, it is purely photothermal. Thus, drug molecules can be transported into tissue bulk by thermal waves which can be described by the Fick's law in 3-D model for a given cavity geometry and the mechanical waves, unlike only by pure photomechanical waves (i.e., photoacoustically) as with short pulses. Therefore, our studies could offer an alternative for currently existing method for drug delivery.

Introduction

To date, most of the advanced nanoparticulate (NPs) drug carriers have been developed by utilizing either synthetic or natural polymers or by their combination. For example, PLGA (Poly lactide-co-glycolide acid) is extensively used in biomedical and pharmaceutical applications. PLGA is hydrolytically unstable and insoluble in water; it degrades by hydrolytic attack of ester bonds (Loo et al. 2004). Among the various natural polymers available, CS is perhaps one of the most widely used biopolymers for the preparation of NPs (Xu and Du 2003, Guan et al. 2008). CS is a weak base and is insoluble in water and organic solvents, however, it is soluble in dilute aqueous acidic solution with pH < 6.5. Particle size, density, viscosity, degree of deacetylation, and molecular weight are important characteristics of CS which influence the properties of pharmaceutical formulations based on CS. Drug delivery systems (DDS) are an area of study in which researchers from almost every scientific discipline can make a significant contribution. Understanding the fate of drugs inside the human body is a high standard classical endeavor, where basic and mathematical analysis can be used to achieve an important practical end. No doubt the effectiveness of drug therapy is closely related to biophysics and physiology of drug movement through tissue. Therefore, DDS requires an understanding of the characteristics of the system, the molecular mechanisms of drug transport and elimination, particularly at the site of delivery. In chemical methods, cationic lipids, polymers, and liposomes can be used as a drug carrier (Konan et al. 2002, Pjanovic et al. 2010) while physical methods such as high voltage electric pulse (Riviere and Heit 1997), CW ultrasound (Tachibana and Tachibana 1999), extra corporeal shock wave (Gambihler et al. 1992, Kodama and Tomita 2000), laser induced shock wave (Ogura et al. 2003, Hellman et al. 2008) have been used as a driving force for drug delivery. In transcutaneous laser injection, drug solution is applied onto skin surface topically and then it is irradiated by a laser pulse. Strong absorption of IR lasers (e.g., Er:YAG or CO_2) irradiation by water leads to perforation of both drug solution and skin tissue (Chung and Mazur 2009, Andersson-Engels and Stepp 2010). In our first report on laser induced cavitation and the role of photoacoustic effects (Dyer et al. 1993), we showed that hot, high-pressure vapor cavity produced at 2.6–3 mm can lead to energy being transported well beyond the laser beam penetration depth as a direct result of the bubble expansion following the pulse and large amplitude acoustic waves associated with bubble formation and decay.

Since then many efforts have been reported on the optical cavitation dynamics (Asshauer and Delacretz 1994, Palanker et al. 1997, Frenz et al. 1998, Bremond et al. 2006) and potential use of cavitation and photoacoustic (Galanzha et al. 2009) as a means of delivering drug into tissue (Shangguan et al. 1998, Coussios et al. 2008, Khosroshahi et al. 2006, Kodama et al. 2008) and generally on a solid boundary (Zhao et al. 2007, Gregorcic et al. 2008, Liu et al. 2009). However, for more accurate and localized delivery, controlled drug release based on nanotechnology has been one of the recent developments in this field. To our knowledge no specific work was found in the literature regarding the dynamic studies of long chopped pulse ($\tau_p \gg$ ms) and CW CO_2 laser interaction with drug NPs-biogelatin model as a method of drug delivery. With this view we have used fast photography and photothermal deflection technique to gain an insight into the mechanism of mass transfer into the bulk medium. Also, in this study, Direct Red-encapsulated PLGA and PLGA/CS were fabricated and NPs have been characterized in terms of particle size and encapsulation efficiency and photomechanical drug delivery.

Materials and method

PLGA-encapsulated Direct Red NPs

Nanoparticles were fabricated via the W/O/W double emulsion solvent evaporation surface coating method, as previously described (Chung et al. 2008). Briefly, 3 ml of deionized aqueous 0.18% Direct Red 81 (drug model) (Sigma Alderich-USA) was poured into 15 ml of dichloromethane solution (DCM) (Merck, Germany) containing 300 mg of PLGA (50:50, Resomer RG 504 H, Mw 48000, Bohringer Ingelheim, Germany), and then emulsified using a sonicator (Tecna6-Tecno-GA2-S.P.A.) to form a W/O emulsion. The W/O suspension was added to 30 ml of 1 wt% of polyvinyl alcohol (PVA; Mw 22000, Merck), and emulsified using the same sonicator to produce W/O/W emulsion. 300 ml of 0.5 wt% of PVA was added to the emulsion which was mechanically stirred. The suspension was evaporated for 18 h and stirred at 250 rpm to remove the solvent from the emulsified suspensions. The suspension that contained PLGA-encapsulated Direct Red NPs was centrifuged (Sigma, 3K30, RCF 25568, speed 16500 with rotor 12150 H, Germany) for 20 min to separate the NPs from the suspension. The NPs were rinsed with distilled water and then centrifuged several times to remove PVA and residual solvent. The NPs were further filtered through membrane filters to remove large sub-micron particles. Then, the NPS dried at a freeze dryer (Chaist, Alpha 1–2 LD plus, Germany) for storage.

CS-coated PLGA-encapsulated direct red NPs

To prepare the CS solution (low molecular, 80–85% deacetylation, Merck) for this work, 300 mg CS was dissolved in 150 ml of 1% acetic acid solution and similarly PLGA NPs was followed, except that 150 ml of the 0.1 wt% CS solution and 150 ml of 0.5 wt% PVA solution were added, instead of 300 ml PVA 0.5% solution, to the aforementioned W/O/W emulsion with continuously stirring. The pH value of the emulsion was adjusted to 6–7 during solvent evaporation to enhance CS coating onto PLGA NPs to yield PLGA/CS NPs.

Preparation of biogelatin

In this study, the tissue was modeled using commercial biogelatin (3.5% Gelatin-175 Bloom-Sigma Chemical, Type A) mixed with de-ionized water. The mixture was prepared by adding 20 ml of de-ionized water to 2 g of the biogelatin and then heated to 60°C with a magnetic stirrer until it became clear. The drug was simulated by encapsulating Direct Red by CS coated PLGA NPs, denoted as DRN. The liquid biogelatin was then poured into $10 \times 10 \times 30$ mm cuvettes and covered by 1mm thick DRN solution to model drug on tissue. The experiments were performed using a 30 W CO_2 laser (SM medical) operating in continuous (CWC), single pulse (CWS), and chopped pulse repetition (PLS-R) with 10 ms pulse duration and 5 Hz.

Characterization of PLGA and PLGA/CS NPs

Morphology and zeta potential

The hydrodynamic size of NPs in aqueous solution was determined at 25°C using laser light scattering with zeta potential measurement (Zetasizer ZS, Malvern, UK). The zeta potential of various NPs in deionized water was determined using the same analyzer. The samples were prepared by suspending the freeze-dried NPs in 5 ml deionized water. Scanning electron microscopy (SEM, Vega 2, Tescan, Chek) was employed to determine the shape and surface morphology of the produced NPs. To examine the morphology of NPs, a small amount of NPs was stuck on a double-sided tape attached on a metallic sample stand, then coated under vacuum with a thin layer of gold before SEM. The experiment was repeated three times and results were presented as means and standard deviations from the triplicate (n = 3). Significance in data between different process variables was assessed using all data points obtained over multiple batches via student's t-test and one way ANOVA with post-test. P value < 0.05 was considered significant.

TEM microscopy

Transmission electron microscopy (TEM, Philips CM 10, HT 100 k) was used to determine the shape and study surface morphology of the NPs. This was done by placing the solution of NPs on a 200 mesh size copper grid that had been coated with carbon. Then, 2 wt% phosphotangstic acid was used to stain the NPs on the copper grid. After the NPs were air-dried at room temperature, the morphology of the stained NPs was observed.

FTIR spectroscopy

The FTIR absorption spectra of the PLGA and PLGA/CS NPs were obtained using an FTIR spectrum analyzer at 4 cm^{-1} resolution (Nicolet, Magna-IR Spec. 550, USA). To identify CS in PLGA/CS NPs, 5 mg of the NPs was mixed with KBr and then their spectra were obtained using the analyzer. The absorption spectra were recorded in the range 1000–4000 cm^{-1}.

AFM topographical analysis

A Dualscope/Rasterscope system (C26, DME, Denmark) was used for all imaging by AFM. The micro scope was equipped with a scanner that had a maximum XY scan range of 50 by 50 mm and a Z range of 2.7 mm and was operated by means of a Scan Master (95–50E), a real-time closed-loop scanning control system that allows for the accurate measurement, repositioning, and zooming in on selected features. The images were acquired by using silicon nitride cantilevers with high-aspect-ratio conical silicon tips; the force constants were 0.1 N/m for contact-mode imaging. AFM was used to study the surface morphology and shape of the PLGA/CS NPs.

Optical set up

Figure 11.6 shows the output of the laser was focused by a 100 mm hand piece manipulator into a 500 mm spot size on drug-biogelatin model (D-G) surface. The removal rate and absorption coefficient α (cm^{-1}) measurements of D-G were first made separately using CWS mode by exposing the sample to predetermined number of pulses, n, at pulse repetition frequency of 1 Hz and the depth of material removal, D, was measured by a resolution optical microscope (Euromex ± 2 µm). The average etch depth was calculated from D/n and the slope provided the value of α. The interaction monitoring system mainly included a fast photography (time-resolved) and PTD technique to study the dynamics of laser-induced cavitation and the ablation process at different stages. Time-resolved studies were done by a fast CCD camera (Panasonic Super Dynamic WV-CP450) connected to an optical microscope (Prior-UK). In the PTD experiment the probe beam was a He-Ne laser of 3 mW power which after being expanded was focused by a lens of 100 mm focal length to a spot diameter of ≤ 500 mm. Deflection of the probe beam was measured as a function of pulse fluence by a fast rising time of 1 ns PIN photodiode. The output signal was then recorded by 150 MHz digital oscilloscope (Hitachi VC-7102). The PTD is based on the rapid heating of a sample as a result of absorption of laser radiation, which consequently generates heat due to various non-radiative excitation processes occurring in the sample which then acts as a "thermal piston" driven wave at sound

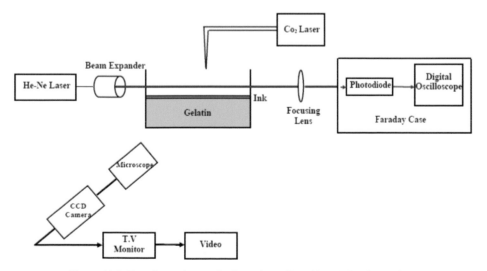

Figure 11.6. Experimental set up for dynamic studies of laser-DGM interaction.

speed. The origin of this wave lies in the heating of air molecules close to the target surface. The heat thus is transferred to the air in the close vicinity of the irradiated surface, resulting in a temperature rise in the surrounding medium. Such a rise in temperature leads to density variations, which create a refractive index gradient in the medium adjacent to the surface. A probe beam propagation through this refractive index gradient perpendicular to the direction of the pump beam will suffer refraction and consequently will deviate from its original path.

Results and discussion

Characterization of nanoparticles

In this study, the Direct Red encapsulated PLGA and PLGA/CS were fabricated by double emulsion solvent evaporation (W/O/W). Table 11.2 presents some of the characteristics of the NPs. The positive zeta potential (+8.47 ± 0.008 mV) of PLGA/CS NPs confirms the presence of CS on the surface of the NPs. The hydrodynamic size of Direct Red loaded PLGA/CS NPs is larger than that of PLGA NPs (290 ± 1.41 nm), and the polydispersion index (PDI) of particles of Direct Red encapsulated PLGA and PLGA/CS NPs are 0.211 and 0.419, respectively, indicating an acceptable distribution. The encapsulation efficiency of Direct Red NPs is 51.21% ± 0.778. The SEM micrographs of Direct Red encapsulated PLGA and PLGA/CS NPs clearly indicate their spherical shape and morphology (Fig. 11.7).

The spherical shape of Direct Red encapsulated PLGA and PLGA/CS NPs are shown by TEM micrographs (Fig. 11.8). As can be seen from Fig. 11.8b, the CS layer is illustrated by a thin dark layer surrounding the PLGA core. The increased particle size of PLGA/CS NPs is mainly due to increased viscosity of CS and its increased adsorption on the PLGA surface. Figure 11.9 illustrates a comparison between the FTIR spectra of PLGA and PLGA/CS NPs. FTIR measurements results confirmed the presence of the CS on the surface PLGA/CS NPs. The characteristic absorption bands of amine group (NH) and OH, NH_3, CH, CN of CS at 3431, 2923, 2853, and 1629 cm^{-1}, respectively were observed. The peaks at 714, 1095, 1176, 2846 cm^{-1} and peaks around 3000 cm^{-1} are attributed to PLGA. The strong peak at 1759 cm^{-1} is due to the O-C = O. The peaks at 3413 cm^{-1} corresponds to stretching and vibrational modes of hydroxyl. The increase of NPs size and the spectra of NPs with peaks at 1629, 2924, 2853, and 3431 cm^{-1} confirm the formation of the CS on the PLGA NPs surface.

Table 11.2. The hydrodynamic size, zeta potential and polydispersion index of the nanoparticles.

Sample	Hydrodynamic size (nm)	Zeta potential	PDI
Dr-PLGA NPs	290 ± 1.91	−1.42 ± 0.021	0.211
DR-PLGA/CS NPs	373 ± 0.816	−8.47 ± 0.008	0.419

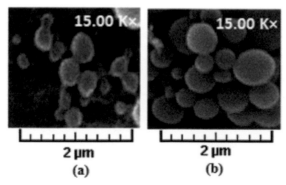

Figure 11.7. SEM micrographs (a) DR-PLGA NPs, and (b) DR-PLGA/CS NPs.

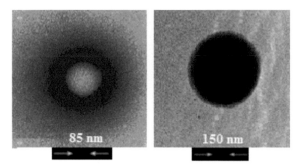

Figure 11.8. TEM micrographs (a) DR-PLGA NPs, and (b) DR-PLGA/CS NPs.

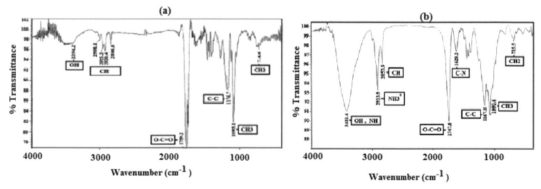

Figure 11.9. FTIR spectroscopy for (a) DR-PLGA NPs, and (b) DR-PLGA/CS NPs.

Figure 11.10 shows 2-D and 3-D images of Direct Red encapsulated PLGA/CS NPs. AFM images show their spherical shape and acceptable dispersion. CS has been shown to possess mucoadhesive properties due to molecular attractive force formed by electrostatic interaction between positively charged CS and negatively charged surfaces. These properties may be attributed to: (1) strong hydrogen bonding groups like –OH, –COOH, (2) strong charges, (3) high molecular weight, (4) sufficient chain flexibility, and (5) surface energy properties. The electrostatic attraction is likely the predominant driving force, especially in the formation of the first monomolecular adsorption layer (Guo and Gemeinhart 2008). The adsorption of CS continues even though a positively charged surface has been achieved, in which hydrogen bond (N–H) or van der Waal's force can be involved. At high concentration of CS, it is possible that the subsequent layer of CS could be adsorbed on the first layer and has no direct contact with the surface. With more layers added, CS chains would repel each other due to the same charge, but be attracted and interact through hydrophobic interactions, van der Waal's forces, and hydrogen bonds. Sinha et al. (2004) and

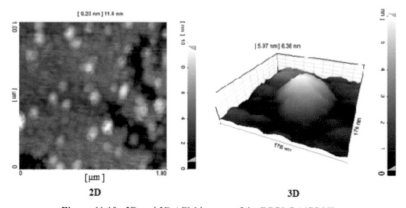

Figure 11.10. 2D and 3D AFM images of the DRPLGA/CS NPs.

Guo and Gemeinhart (2008) reported that the continued adsorption of CS on PLGA NPs does not affect the apparent zeta potential at high concentration (greater than 0.4–0.6 g/l). The zeta potential of PLGA/CS NPs increases with initial CS concentration until it reaches the saturation point where the potential value remains constant. The small size and the high surface energy of PLGA NPs play an important role for multilayer adsorption of CS (Guo and Gemeinhart 2008). The hydrodynamic diameter of CS coated PLGA NPs increases gradually with initial CS concentration. The increased particle size can be attributed to the increased viscosity of CS and the increased amount of adsorbed CS on the surface of PLGA NPs.

Material removal

For optically opaque and strongly absorbing liquids over an infrared wavelength and laser fluences below the optical breakdown threshold, the interaction process is mainly dominated by the thermoelastic effect and gradually approaches to vaporization when the laser fluence increases. The thermal field in such media can be described by the heat transfer equation:

$$\rho c \, \partial T / \partial t = K \left[\partial^2 t / \partial z^2 + 1/r \, \partial / \partial r \, (r \partial T / \partial r) \right] + \alpha \, I_0 e^{-\alpha z} . f(t) . \Psi(r) \tag{11.1}$$

where, ρ is the density, c is the specific heat, K is the thermal conductivity, α is the absorption coefficient of the given medium, I_0 is the peak intensity of the laser radiation, f(t) describes its time dependence and $\Psi(r) = \exp(-r^2/a^2)$ is its Gaussian distribution over the beam cross section. Figure 11.11 shows the etch depth per pulse of D-G as a function of fluence for the CO_2 laser. It is assumed: (i) the absorption coefficient dominates scattering coefficient (i.e., $\alpha_g \gg \beta_g$), (ii) ablation commences instantaneously once a threshold fluence F_t is exceeded, and (iii) if the plume retains the same absorption coefficient as the condensed phase, then based on Fig. 11.11, one can use the well-known Beer Lambert's law to describe the etch depth rate fluence dependences.

$$h = \alpha^{-1} \ln (F / F_t) \tag{11.2}$$

where h and F are etch depth per pulse and fluence, respectively. A fit to the data using Eq. (11.2) yields F_t 32 J cm^{-2} (i.e., 6 W), which is in agreement with the theoretical value given by the energy balance for threshold evaporation intensity, $I_t \approx 3$ kWcm^{-2}, defined by Eq. (11.3).

$$I_t = \frac{(\rho_g . L_v . d_0)}{\tau_p} \tag{11.3}$$

where $\rho_g \approx 1.2$ g cm^{-3} is the density of biogelatin, LV ≈ 2.260 kJ/g is the latent heat of vaporization of water, $d_0 \approx \alpha^{-1} \approx 116$ μm is the optical penetration depth of CO_2 laser radiation in biogelatin, where α_g is determined from the inverse slope in Fig. 11.11 as 86 cm^{-1} and $\tau_p = 10$ ms is the pulse duration. For the maximum pulsed heating of the surface, we have $\alpha^{-1} k \tau_p \ll 1$ where $k = K/\rho_g C_g$ is the thermal diffusivity

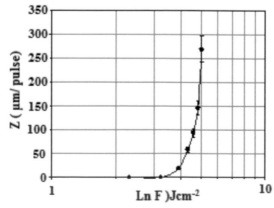

Figure 11.11. Ablation depth per pulse of biogelatin versus fluence.

and K is thermal conductivity of the medium. Since in our experiment the pulse duration is smaller than the thermal relaxation time (i.e., $\tau_p = 10$ ms $\leq \tau_r = d_0^2/k \approx 33$ ms) where $k \approx 1 \times 10^{-3}$ cm^2 s^{-1} and that d_0 is greater than the thermal diffusion depth, d_t (i.e., $d_0 \approx 116$ μm $\geq d_t \approx (4k\tau_p)^{1/2} \approx 63$ μm), thus, a diabetic condition or heat confinement is achieved. At low frequency, e.g., 1 Hz, this physically implies that the heat has already left the absorption region before the arrival of the next pulse, and therefore there will be no time for heat to accumulate and diffuse within tissue model. As a result of the above argument, we may assume that in the surface heat flux model, the heat is deposited at the surface by the laser pulse and is mainly conserved in the material and flows in the axial direction. Of course at 5 Hz this effect was markedly enhanced, as is seen in Fig. 11.12. This results in an exponential spreading of the temperature profile in time, hence implying a strongly decreasing cooling rate with time.

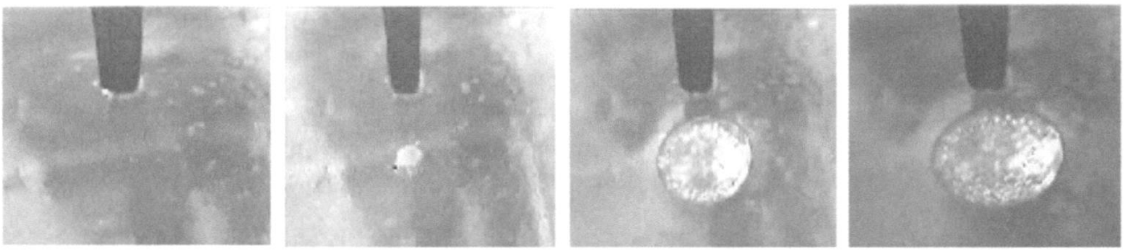

20 mW-10 ms

| $t = 0S$ | 2 | 8 | 20 |

Figure 11.12. Surface radial receding of biogelatin due to vaporization as a function of time.

The experimental effect of this view (i.e., axial heat flow) was observed as spreading surface area of the gelatin heated zone which can be described as follows:

Let S_c be the surface area of the cone,

$$S_c = \pi r^2 + \pi r \left(r^2 + z^2 \right)^{1/2} \tag{11.4}$$

$$\partial S_c / \partial r = 2\pi r + \pi r^2 / \left(r^2 + z^2 \right)^{1/2} + \pi \left(r^2 + z^2 \right)^{1/2} \tag{11.5}$$

$$\partial S_c / \partial z = \pi r z / \left(r^2 + z^2 \right)^{1/2} \tag{11.6}$$

By using Eqs. (11.5) and (11.6), the variation of $\partial S_c/\partial r$ and $\partial S_c/\partial z$ for different values of radial distance, r and depth, z are plotted as a function of pulse numbers, which are shown in Figs. 11.13a and 11.13b. Clearly, as it was expected the inverted logarithm behaviour of the curves shows that the variations of $\partial S_c/\partial r \gg \partial S_c/\partial z$. Also, the maximum value of these variations can be determined by the curve equation $y = a (1-e^{-x})$ where in this case, y and x represent $\partial S_c/\partial r$ (or $\partial S_c/\partial z$) and pulse number respectively. Therefore, as $x \to \infty$, $y = a$, as it is shown in Fig. 11.13a.

The temperature rise at the end of laser pulse on the surface of biogelatin is given by

$$T_f - T_i = \frac{(1-R)\,\alpha_g F}{\rho_g C_g} \tag{11.7}$$

where T_f, T_i are the final and initial temperature (°C) respectively, R is the surface reflectivity (0.1), and C_g is the specific heat capacity (4.98 J g^{-1} K^{-1}). Hence, using the above equation it yields a value of 100°C at 5 J cm^{-2} (or = 1 W). However, when the pulse repetition frequency increases gradually, generated heat accumulates at the surface and slowly diffuses into bulk too. All in all, we can imagine that in the case of PLS where $\tau_p \gg \tau_r$ and low frequency, biogelatin surface acts as a viscoelastic switch, thereby allowing a certain amount of DRN to enter the tissue. But when the pulse repetition frequency increases, the surface appears to be continuously open and hence more amount of DRN can get inside and diffuse similar to a CW operation. By assuming a Gaussian profile for the probe beam, one can write the dependence of the photodiode response ΔV on the beam deflection as follows (Diaci and Mozina 1992):

$$\Delta V = V_0 \; \text{erf} \left[\sqrt{2}\varphi / \theta \right] \tag{11.8}$$

With φ and θ being the beam angular deflection due to change in index of refraction and angular divergence respectively, V_0 is the photodiode output voltage at $\varphi = 0$, erf is the complementary error function, i.e.,

$$\text{erf}(x) = \frac{2}{\sqrt{\pi} \int \exp(-t^2) dt} \tag{11.9}$$

Therefore, only for $\varphi \ll \theta$, ΔV is linear. Figure 11.14 shows the output voltage (hence deflection) as a function of laser fluence. It can be seen that the voltage amplitude increases linearly with fluence which defines the origin of the signals observed. Figure 11.15a indicates that below the ablation threshold the bipolar deflection is mainly caused by thermal piston effect (i.e., a pressure wave) which is generated by hot surface. Since the refractive index of the gelatin increases with density, so that the probe deflects towards the higher or positive density region, and later times it is followed by a negative lobe which is thought to be produced by the mixture of convective plume of the gaseous air and relaxation of the probe beam. In our experiment the probe-surface distance was ≈ 1 mm, which gives a velocity profile of (0.5–2.5) m/s at

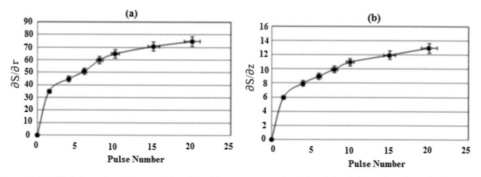

Figure 11.13. Variation of surface area of cavity with respect to radius (a) and depth (b) as function of pulse number.

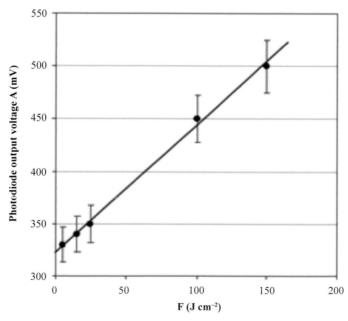

Figure 11.14. Photodiode output signal as a function of fluence.

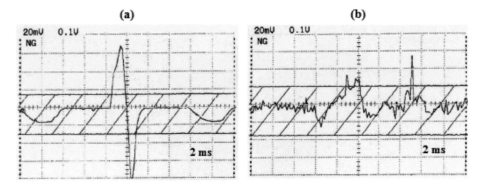

Figure 11.15. Photothermal deflection signals below (a) and above (b) ablation threshold of biogelatin.

30 Jcm^{-2}, whereas in Fig. 11.15b this corresponds to (0.4–10) m/s at 125 J cm^{-2}. It must be noted that at fluences well above threshold, the compressive uni-polar deflection is due to the ablated hot particulates from the target surface.

Therefore, the distribution of heat and mass transfer in Fig. 11.15b shows a hybrid multimode structure or hotspots which is an irregular beam profile resulting in inhomogeneous heating and vaporization of gelatin volume. To visualize these irregularities in two-dimension profile, the He-Ne laser was scanned above the surface (Fig. 11.16a) and just below the gelatin surface (Fig. 11.16b), in an ablative regime. The nature of the bubble motion (photophoresis) is explained by the temperature gradient in irradiated liquid. The propulsion force acting on the bubble arises from the difference in the surface tension on the irradiated and non-irradiated side of the bubble. It is the tendency of the liquid to flow into the region with higher tension coefficient, making the bubbles move towards the source of heating. It is believed that the Archimedes force tends to drive the bubbles from the laser heated zone to somewhat above the probe beam. The pattern of the scattered beam changes as the probe beam suffers total internal reflection on the spherical bubbles surface, and thus is deflected downwards. Brighter portions of the cavity represent the greater bubble density which trap the light as bubbles move upwards just beneath the surface. The time resolved studies related to these phenomena are discussed in the next section.

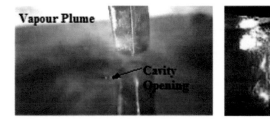

Figure 11.16. Vaporized material visualized above the D–G surface at P ¼ 15 W (a) and trapped probe beam by the bubbles of the cavity at P ¼ 30 W (b).

Cavity dynamics

In order to obtain more information about the cavity formation and possible delivery of DRN into tissue using pulse and CW modes, the ablation process of DGM at different laser power was photographed by a CCD camera, then suitably captured and processed. As can be seen from Fig. 11.17a, at 3 W (15.5 J cm^{-2}) in PLS mode, it takes roughly about 3 seconds for vapor pressure front and thermal wave to traverse the whole DRN layer in order to reach the top of biogelatin. From there onwards, as time passes by, the cavity depth and diameter increases with increasing fluence until it saturates, as similarly observed in other works reported and referred here. The total cavity depth due to vaporization and the hydrodynamic flow resulting from the bubbles which act as a driving thermo-mechanical force can be studied in terms of laser pulse numbers. Almost a similar behaviour was observed in CW case, as seen in Fig. 11.17b.

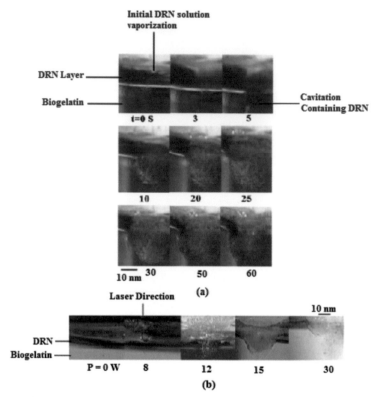

Figure 11.17. Time resolved laser induced cavitation at 3 W and 5 Hz (a) and as a function of laser power (b).

It is interesting as well as important to notice the difference between thermal wave front position with actual DRN position, which clearly explains the heat transfer Eq. (11.1) can act differently to mass transfer and that can affect the understanding about laser delivery of drug. The mass flow per unit time through the surface $r = w_0/z$ due to the pressure gradient is estimated, where w_0 is Gaussian beam radius, z is the depth, and V_0 is the initial velocity of mass:

$$\frac{\delta_m}{\delta_t} = \pi \omega \rho_g d_z V_0(z) \tag{11.10}$$

Figure 11.18 indicates that the drilled cavity (i.e., drug transported depth) increases with pulse number, hence with time, and its maximum occurs after 125 pulse, i.e., 25 seconds. Beyond this point it was observed that the depth gradually decreased and at the same time it increases axially. This explains why there is a transition or kind of non-linearity at this point where the cone volume slowly increases. In other words, the cavity bubbles tend to be transported axially rather than vertically for a longer time.

Similarly for CW mode, as seen in Fig. 11.19, the transported depth also increases with time, but with higher rate for higher powers. Clearly, after some time they all reach a saturation point, and from there onwards the depth remains constant or even decreases. This non-linearity can be explained by the fact that laser radiation is attenuated exponentially within medium and the rebounced bubbles traverse in opposite direction to incoming bubbles, hence giving rise to such chaotic behaviour.

As is seen in Fig. 11.20, the transported depth of DRN due to cavitation bubbles ranges between 1–4 mm for 8–15.3 kW cm^{-2}, respectively. Of course, macroscopic flow of material from one phase to another is possible at equilibrium. Hence, to maintain a strong evaporation, a certain overheating of the

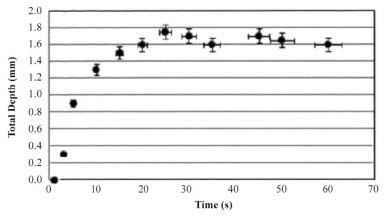

Figure 11.18. Total depth of cavity measured as a function of time at 3 W and 5 Hz.

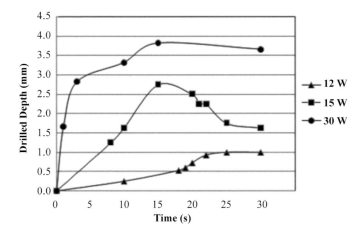

Figure 11.19. Drilled depth of cavity measured as a function of time at different powers.

condensed phase is necessary. Therefore, the knowledge of drilling or thermal evaporation velocity, Z_T, can be helpful to determine the dependence of temperature (T) on intensity (I) and the pressure at condensed phase (P_c) using the relation:

$$P_c = P_g + \left[\rho_c . Z_T . V_g \right] \tag{11.11}$$

where P_g is the pressure at gaseous phase, ρ_c is the density of gelatin at condensed phase, V_g the velocity of molecules, and

$$Z_T = I/\rho_c . L \tag{11.12}$$

Using Eq. (11.12) gives a value of ≈ 1.1 cm/s at threshold power of 3.1 kWcm^{-2} and 5.6 cm/s at 15 kW cm^{-2}, respectively. The major part of the energy needed to evaporate organic materials such as biological soft tissues with a considerable water content is consumed by the phase change of the contained water. Thus for gelatin and most soft tissues, the ratio I/Z_T will be essentially determined by the water content in (gcm^{-3}). During the drilling process, a liquid layer is present between the gaseous and the condensed phase. By the action of the existing pressure gradient, the liquid is pushed towards the origin of low pressure. Therefore, liquid material will be driven in radial direction towards the wall of the cavity and then escape along this wall from the evaporation wave front.

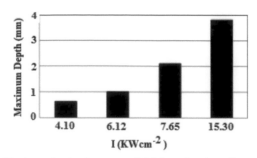

Figure 11.20. Maximum depth of transported DRN as a function of laser power density.

11.4 Early experimental results of thrombolysis using controlled release of tissue plasminogen activator (tPA) encapsulated by PLGA/CS nanoparticles delivered by pulse 532 nm laser (Mahmoodi et al. 2011)

The purpose of this study is to prepare cationic nanoparticles (NPs) by coating chitosan (CS) on the surface of PLGA NPs and evaluate the possibility of laser thrombolysis and photomechanical drug delivery in a blood clot using pulse 532 nm laser. *In vitro* tPA release showed a sustained release profile for three days. The mean particle size and encapsulation efficiency of tPA NPs were in the range of 280–360 nm and 46.7% ± 1.56, 50.8% ± 1.09, respectively. The encapsulation efficiency and the particles size were increased as a result of coating with CS. The release kinetic was evaluated by fitting the experimental data to two standard release equations. The results showed that the PLGA/CS NPs maintain the highest weight percentages of dissolved clot. Also, the thrombolysis process can be enhanced by delivering tPA into clot during laser ablation based on the photomechanical effect due to optical cavitation bubbles. Therefore, our studies could offer an alternative for currently existing method for acute myocardial infarction.

Introduction

Drug delivery systems are an area of study in which researchers from almost every scientific discipline can make a significant contribution (Buteica et al. 2010). Understanding the fate of drugs inside the human body is a high standard classical endeavor, where basic and mathematical analysis can be used to achieve an important practical end. No doubt the effectiveness of drug therapy is closely related to biophysics and physiology of drug movement through tissue. Therefore, drug delivery system requires an understanding of the characteristics of the system, the molecular mechanisms of drug transport and elimination, particularly at the site of delivery. In the last decade DDS have received much attention since they can significantly improve the therapeutic effects of the drug while minimizing its side effects. In chemical methods, cationic lipids, polymers, and liposomes can be used as a drug carrier (Konan et al. 2002) while physical methods such as high voltage electric pulse (Riviere and Heit 1997), CW ultrasound (Tachibana and Tachibana 1999), extra corporeal shock wave (Gambihler et al. 1992, Kodama and Tomita 2000), laser induced shock wave (Ogura et al. 2003), have been used as a driving force for drug delivery.

Laser thrombolysis is an interventional procedure to remove clot in occluded arteries using laser energy. It offers cost, recovery time, and safety advantages over bypass surgery, in which surgeons must replace arteries but laser thrombolysis are limited because they cannot completely clear thrombotic occlusions in arteries, typically leaving residual thrombus on the walls of the artery. A laser system capable of selectively targeting the clot is therefore desirable. This capability is offered by lasers emitting in the ultraviolet and visible regions, where the absorption by clot is much higher than that by artery. The principal chromophore of clot in the visible waveband is hemoglobin present in the red blood cells. Since higher absorption coefficients require less energy per unit area to achieve ablation, threshold for artery is higher than that for clot. Pulsed lasers operating in this waveband at radiant exposures between the thresholds for artery and clot can therefore selectively remove clot (Leach et al. 2004). Photomechanical drug delivery is a technique for localized drug delivery using laser-induced hydrodynamic pressure following cavitation bubble expansion and collapse.

Therefore, photomechanical drug delivery is used to enhance laser thrombolysis by delivering tPA into clot (Shangguan et al. 1998). CS is an amino polysaccharide (poly 1,4-D-glucoamine) coated NPs have been fabricated with muco-adhesion and enhanced permeability properties for nasal epithelium application (Yamamoto et al. 2005). CS is biocompatible, biodegradable, and non-toxic polymer. Furthermore, CS promotes the enhancement of drug transport across the cell membrane (Mao et al. 2001) and has been extensively applied in drug delivery systems and tissue engineering (Xu and Du 2003, Lanza et al. 2000). Since these NPs exhibit a positive potential in PBS solution due to protonization of its amine groups, and have been applied to deliver proteins or DNA (Xu and Du 2003, Lanza et al. 2000), therefore, they may be preferentially chosen as potentially safe and useful cations carriers for gene delivery (Tahara et al. 2008). CS is a weak base and is insoluble in water and organic solvents, however, it is soluble in dilute aqueous acidic solution with pH < 6.5. Particle size, density, viscosity, degree of deacetylation, and molecular weight are important characteristics of CS which influence the properties of pharmaceutical formulations based on CS. Pharmacology reperfusion therapy for acute myocardial infarction (AMI) and ischemic stroke characterized by ST-elevation in the electrocardiogram was incorporated into the armamentarium of clinicians over 18 years ago and has had an extraordinarily beneficial impact on outcome. A new tactic is to employ encapsulated fibrinolytic agents, whereby the lytic compound is sequestered in polymer microcapsules. Encapsulation has important effects, including acting as a shield to protect the drug from inactivation and increasing its half-life. Also, higher drug circulation in time allows the administration of a lower dosage, with decreased probability of side-effects. In addition, encapsulation may help to avoid bleeding complication by maintaining fibrinogen levels (Leach et al. 2004, Xie et al. 2007). Plasminogen activators (PAs) such as streptokinase (SK), urokinase, tPA, and genetically engineered one- and two-chain versions of tPA and urokinase have been administered effectively by intravenous infusion over a wide range of dosages. All of these agents show similar incidences and rates of reperfusion and problem with bleeding complications (Nguyen et al. 1990, Heslinga et al. 2009). tPA is a protein involved in the breakdown of blood clots. Specifically, it is a serine protease found on endothelial cells, the cells that line the blood vessels. As an enzyme, it catalyzes the conversion of plasminogen to plasmin, the major enzyme responsible for clot breakdown. Because it works on the clotting system, tPA is used in clinical medicine to treat only embolic or thrombolytic stroke. Its use is contraindicated in hemorrhagic stroke and head trauma. It may be manufactured by using recombinant biotechnology techniques. tPA created in this way may be referred to as recombinant tissue plasimogen activator or rtPA. It is used in diseases where blood clot is the prime issue, such as pulmonary embolism, myocardial infarction, and stroke. The clinical benefits of administering PAs for thrombolytic therapy may be markedly improved by developing new methods to promote clot lysis with reduced side effects. In this regard, a drug delivery strategy, such as encapsulating PAs (SK) into liposomes or polymeric microspheres as drug carriers to increase the therapeutic efficacy of conventional thrombolytic therapy has been demonstrated *in vitro* and *in vivo* animal models (Chung et al. 2008). Many groups have developed methods for producing PLGA microspheres by dissolving polymers in a solvent and precipitating it into a sphere, e.g., using solvent evaporation, solvent removal, spray-drying, or coacervation processes (Leach et al. 2003, Heslinga et al. 2009). The double-emulsion (water-in-oil-in-water), solvent evaporation/extraction method is one typical method widely used for the preparation of PLGA microspheres loaded with hydrophilic drug, such as therapeutic proteins. Many parameters determine the drug release behaviour from CS microspheres. These include concentration and molecular weight of the CS, the type and concentration of crosslinking agent, variables like stirring speed, type of oil, additives, crosslinking process used, drug CS ratio, etc. Drug release study from CS microspheres has generally shown that the release of the drug decreases with an increase in molecular weight and concentration of CS (Sinha et al. 2004). Typically, these microspheres will give out a very large burst of drug release upon immersion into the release medium. This initial burst release, referred to as the percentage/amount of drug release after 24 h, depends on the immediate diffusion of hydrophilic drug from polymer matrix, and complicated its correlation with the effective drug loading (Higuchi 1963, Hino et al. 2000, Zheng 2009). In this study, tPA-encapsulated PLGA and PLGA/CS were fabricated and drug delivery has been characterized in terms of particle size, thermal analysis, encapsulation efficiency, drug release profiles, weight of digested clot (%), and laser thrombolysis and photomechanical drug delivery. The release kinetics was evaluated by fitting the experimental data to Higuchie and Riger-Peppas equations.

Experimental

PLGA-encapsulated tPA NPs

Nanoparticles were fabricated via the W/O/W double emulsion solvent evaporation surface coating method, as previously described (Chung et al. 2008). Briefly, 3 ml of de-ionized aqueous recombinant human tissue-type plasminogen activator solution (rtPA) (Actilyse, Boehringer Ingelheim Pharma KG, Germany) with albumin as an emulsifier were poured into dichloromethane solution (DCM) (Merck, Germany) containing PLGA (50:50, Resomer RG 504H, Mw 48000, Bohringer Ingelheim, Germany), and then emulsified using a probe ultrasonicator (UP400S, hielscher, Germany) at 4 C to form an W/O emulsion. The W/O suspension at 4 C was added to 1 wt% of polyvinyl alcohol (PVA; Mw 22000, Merck), and emulsified using the same sonicator in a pulse mode several times to produce W/O/W emulsion. 0.5 wt% of PVA was added to the emulsion which was mechanically stirred. The suspension was evaporated at an ambient pressure to remove the solvent from the emulsified suspensions. The suspension that contained PLGA-encapsulated tPA NPs was centrifuged (Sigma, 3K30, RCF 25568, speed 16500 with rotor 12150H, Germany) at 4 C to separate the NPs from the suspension. Then, the NPS dried at a freeze dryer (Chaist, Alpha 1–2 LD plus, Germany) for storage.

CS-coated PLGA-encapsulated tPA NPs

To prepare the CS solution (low molecular, 80–85% deacetylation, Merck) for this work, CS was dissolved in 1% acetic acid solution, and similarly PLGA NPs was followed, except that 0.1 wt% CS solution and 0.5 wt% PVA solution were added, instead of PVA 0.5% solution, to the aforementioned W/O/W emulsion with continuously stirring.

Characterization and morphology of NPs

The size of NPs in aqueous solution was determined at 25 C using laser light scattering with zeta potential measurement (Zetasizer ZS, Malvern, UK). The zeta potential of various NPs in de-ionized water was determined using the same analyzer. The samples were prepared by suspending the freeze dried NPs in 5 ml deionized water. Transmission electron microscopy (TEM, Philips CM 10, HT 100 k) was used to determine the shape and study surface morphology of the NPs. This was done by placing the solution of NPs on a 200 mesh size copper grid that had been coated with carbon. Then, 2 wt% phosphotangstic acide was used to stain the NPs on the copper grid. After the NPs were air-dried at room temperature, the morphology of the stained NPs was observed. The experiment were repeated three times and results were presented as means and standard deviations from the triplicate (n = 3). Significance in data between different process variables was assessed using all data points obtained over multiple batches via student's t-test and one way ANOVA with post-test. P value < 0.05 was considered significant.

FTIR spectroscopy

The Fourier transform infrared spectroscopy (FTIR) absorption spectra of the PLGA and PLGA/CS NPs were obtained using an FTIR spectrum analyzer at 4 cm^{-1} resolution (Nicolet, Magna-IR Spec. 550, USA). To identify CS in PLGA/CS NPs, 5 mg of the NPs was mixed with KBr and then their spectra were obtained using the analyzer. The absorption spectra were recorded in the range 1000–4000 cm^{-1}.

AFM topographical analysis

The typical scanning probe microscopy (SPM) forces are mechanical contact force, Van der Waals force, capillary forces, electrostatic forces, magnetic force, etc. AFM relies on the interaction between the specimen and a nanometric tip attached to a cantilever, which scans the sample surface. Individual particles, size information (length, width, and height) and other physical properties (such as morphology and surface texture) are measured by AFM. A Dualscope/Rasterscope system (C26, DME, Denmark) was used for all imaging by AFM. The microscope was equipped with a scanner that had a maximum XY scan range of 50 by 50 μm and a Z range of 2.7 μm, and was operated by means of a Scan Master (95–50E), a real-time closed-loop scanning control system that allows for the accurate measurement, repositioning, and zooming in on selected features. The images were acquired by using silicon nitride cantilevers with high-aspect ratio conical silicon tips; the force constants were 0.1 N/m for contact-mode imaging. AFM was used to study the morphology of the PLGA and PLGA/CS NPs.

DSC analysis

The differential scanning calorimetry (DSC) (Mettler Toledo, DSC 823e, Switzerland) was used to analyze the effects of the coating and drug on the thermal properties of the PLGA and PLGA/CS NPs. The NPs were weighted in standard aluminum pans. DSC curves were obtained at heating rate of 5°C/min and temperature range of 0–550°C. The heating chamber was continuously purged with nitrogen gas at a rate of 30 ml/min.

Measuring tPA concentration

Measuring tPA aqueous solution was analyzed using HPLC (BIO-TEK Kontorn Inst., Detector 535, Italy) equipped with a C18 column at 37 C. The quantity of tPA was determined from the absorption intensity at the wavelength 254 nm. The same method was employed to determine the encapsulation efficiency (EE*) and release profiles of PLGA and PLGA/CS encapsulated tPA NPs.

In vitro release studies

Encapsulation efficiency for tPA loaded NPs were determined by HPLC method. The unencapsulated tPA concentration in the emulsion suspension was determined using the HPLC method after the NPs had been centrifuged and collected. 7.5 mg of NPs was dissolved in dichloromethane (DCM) and then 2.5 ml of isotonic phosphate buffer solution (PBS, pH 7.4) was added to the solution to extract the tPA. The quantity of the collected tPA was determined using HPLC. 30 mg dried tPA loaded NPs was suspended in 25 ml PBS with 1 wt% sodium azide which were shaken at 70 rpm at 37 C; 1 ml of the dissolution was periodically drawn out to analyze tPA by the HPLC. The PBS with sodium azide was replaced with equal volumes of fresh medium. The experiment was performed for a week.

Mathematical analysis of the drug release

In order to study tPA release mechanism from the PLGA NPs and PLGA/CS NPs, 2 models can be considered to fit the experimental data. Model 1 is based on the Higuchi equation which describes the Fickian diffusion of drug (Higuchi 1963). Higuchi is the first to derive an equation to describe the release of a drug from a polymer as the square root of a time-dependent process based on Fickian diffusion (Eq. 11.13)

$$\frac{M_t}{M_0} = Q_t = \sqrt{2DS\varepsilon(A - 0.5S\varepsilon)} \times \sqrt{t} = K_H \sqrt{t} \tag{11.13}$$

$$K_H = \frac{X}{\sqrt{t_x}} \tag{11.14}$$

where, Q_t is the amount of drug released in time (t), D is the diffusion coefficient, S is the solubility of drug in the dissolution medium, ε is the porosity, A is the drug content per cubic centimeter of polymer, and k_H is the release rate constant for the Higuchi model. Percentage drug released at the t_x is X% (Eq. 11.14). For example, for an ideal t_{100} hour release profile (where t_{100} is the time required for 100% drug release), k_H is equal to $100/(t_{100})^{1/2}$ (Gohel 2000). Model 2 is described by the Riger-Peppas equation (Eq. 11.15) (Riger and Peppas 1987):

$$\frac{M_t}{M_0} = Kt^n \qquad\qquad (11.15)$$

where, M_t/M_∞ is the fractional drug release, t is the release time, and n is the diffusional exponent that can be related to the drug transport mechanism. When $n = 0.5$, the drug release mechanism is Fickian diffusion, when $n = 1$, zero-order release occurs. When the value of n is between 0.5 and 1, anomalous (non-Fickian) is observed. These mathematical models are valid only for the first 60% drug release.

Clot preparation

Venous blood was repeatedly collected from a healthy volunteer and anticoagulated into 5 ml glass tubes (inner diameter 13 mm) containing 0.5 ml of 105 mmol l^{-1} sodium citrate. Aliquots of 1 ml of anticoagulated blood were recalcified with 100 μl of 100 mmol l^{-1} calcium chloride in a glass tube. The tubes were incubated for 2 hr at 37°C in a water bath and then clots were removed from the tube and being washed with 154 mmol l^{-1} sodium chloride. This method described by Cintas et al. allowed us to prepare whole blood clots with a good reproducibility in size and weight (Cintas et al. 2004). Clots were weighted before and after experiment. The mean weight of clots was measured prior to experiment as follows: 459.3 mg in the case of tPA only, 259.3 mg with PLGA NPs, and 228.4 mg with PLGA/CS. In the next step, NPs and tPA solution were added to clots separately and were placed in the occlusive tubes filled with PBS buffer. The tubes were then sealed and shaken at 70 rpm and 37°C. The thrombus dissolution was monitored using a fast digital CCD camera (Panasonic Super Dynamic WV-CP450) connected to an optical microscope (Prior-UK). Thrombolysis was expressed as the relative reduction in clot weight (%) and the weight percentage of dissolved clot defined by equation.

Weight of digested clot % = (Weight of clot at the start) – (Weight of residual clot)/
(Weight of clot at the start)   (11.16)

Optical set up

Drug delivery experiments were performed by using a frequency-doubled Nd:YAG laser (532 nm) with 10 ns pulse duration. As it can be seen in Fig. 11.21, the output of the laser was focused by a 500 μm spot size at the surface of clot. Clot removal measurements were made by exposing the sample to a predetermined number of pulses, n, at pulse repetition frequency of 2 Hz and the weight of clot loss was measured before and after each experiment. The laser beam scanned the entire clot surface at 2.33 mms^{-1} and number of scans of 2 (Ns = 2), as seen in Fig. 11.22.

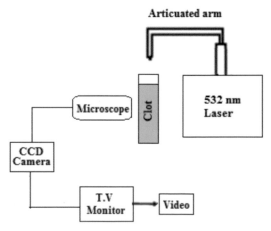

Figure 11.21. The experimental setup.

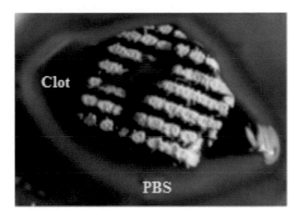

Figure 11.22. The scanned clot surface with laser at Ns = 2.

Results

Characterizations of PLGA and PLGA/CS NPs

The spherical shape and the shell layer of the PLGA/CS NPs are shown by TEM micrographs (Fig. 11.23). TEM micrographs of tPA encapsulated PLGA and PLGA/CS NPs show that they were spherical with solid cores. The main component of the shell layer of NPs in Fig. 11.23b is CS. The micrographs shown in Fig. 11.23 indicate that the tPA-PLGA-CS nanoparticles are larger than tPA-PLGA nanoparticles without CS layer as the corresponding sizes are given in Table 11.3. The hydrodynamic diameter of CS coated PLGA NPs increases gradually with initial CS concentration. Figure 11.24 shows 2-D and 3-D images of tPA encapsulated PLGA and PLGA/CS NPs. AFM images show their spherical shape and acceptable dispersion.

The positive zeta potential (Table 11.3) and FTIR spectroscopy of CS coated PLGA NPs confirmed the presence of CS on PLGA NPs. Figure 11.25 illustrates a comparison between the FTIR spectra of CS, PLGA, and PLGA/CS NPs. FTIR measurements results confirmed the presence of the CS on the surface PLGA/CS NPs. The characteristic absorption bands of amine group (NH) and OH, NH3+, CH, CN at CS at 3431, 2923, 2853, and 1629 cm^{-1}, respectively were observed. The peaks at 1095, 1184, and 1759 cm^{-1} and peaks around 3000 cm^{-1} are attributed to PLGA. The strong peak at 1759 cm^{-1} is due to the C = O stretch. The peaks at 3431 cm^{-1} corresponds to stretching and libational modes of hydroxyl.

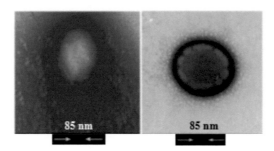

Figure 11.23. TEM micrographs (a) tPA-PLGA NPs, and (b) tPA-PLGA/CS NPs.

Table 11.3. The particle size, zeta potential, and encapsulation efficiency of the nanoparticles (The data presented mean ± SD with n = 3).

Sample	Size (nm)	Zeta Potential (mV)	PDI	EE*
tPA-PLGA NPs	282 ± 4.96	−8.92 ± 0.51	0.192	46.7 ± 1.56
tPA-PLGA/CS NPs	366 ± 2.94	+5.95 ± 0.17	0.334	50.8 ± 1.09

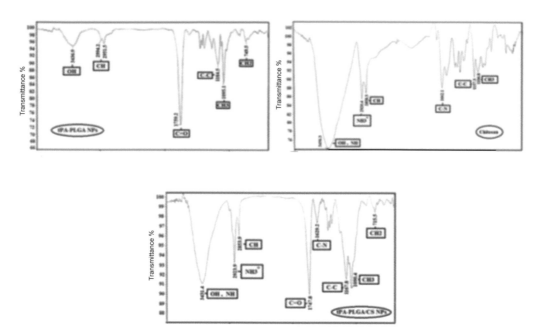

Figure 11.24. 2D and 3D AFM images of (a) tPA-PLGA NPs, and (b) tPA-PLGA/CS NPs.

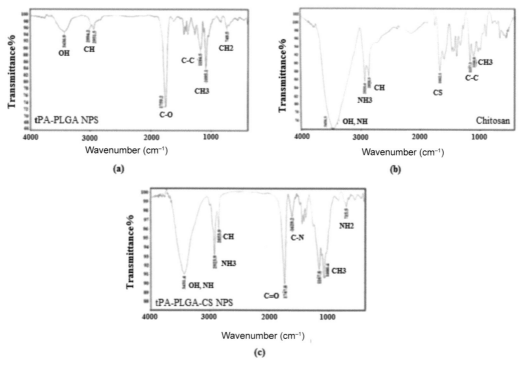

Figure 11.25. FTIR spectroscopy for (a) tPA-PLGA NPs, (b) CS, and (c) tPA-PLGA/CS NPs.

Thermal analysis

Figure 11.26 illustrates the comparison between the DSC curve for PLGA and PLGA/CS NPs and provides a qualitative and quantitative information about the physical state of drug in NPs and in the control samples, i.e., the pure PLGA, the pure CS, the mixture of PLGA and CS and tPA. The pure tPA (Fig. 11.26a) shows

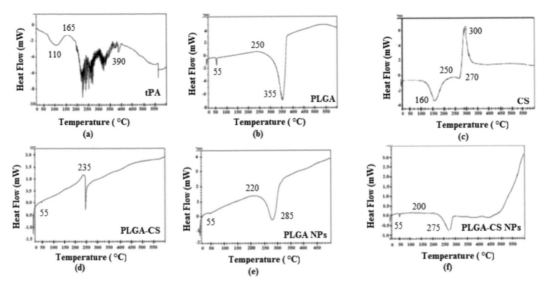

Figure 11.26. DSC curves for (a) tPA, (b) PLGA, (c) CS, (d) the mixture of PLGA and CS, (e) tPA-PLGA NPs, and (f) tPA-PLGA/CS NPs.

an endothermic peak that corresponds to the glass transition (Tg) at 110°C. After Tg, two peaks are observed due to the thermal decomposition of the drug, with maximum temperatures around 165 and 390°C. The pure PLGA exhibit an endothermic event (55°C) referring to the relaxation peak that follow Tg (Fig. 11.26b). No melting point was observed, because PLGA appears amorphous in nature. The thermal stability of PLGA is until 250°C and the thermal decomposition has begun at approximately 355°C. The DSC curve of CS (Fig. 11.26c) shows an endothermic peak (160°C) referring to Tg. The onset of thermal degradation of the CS is observed at 270°C. The thermal degradation in nitrogen is exothermic, and corresponding result is observed at 300°C. The curve of CS shows that the polymer presents thermal stability until 250°C. Figure 11.26 illustrates the mixture of PLGA and CS curve. The curve shows two endothermic peak that referring to Tg of the PLGA and CS. The thermal degradation of the mixture of PLGA and CS is observed at 250°C. This thermal decomposition begins approximately at the same temperature as the pure PLGA and CS. The DSC curve of PLGA NPs (Fig. 11.26e) corresponds to the relaxation enthalpy of PLGA (55°C). It can be observed that the nanoencapsulation process did not affect the polymer structure because the pure PLGA presented the same value for relaxation enthalpy. The thermal decomposition of PLGA NPs begins approximately at 285°C. Figure 11.26 shows two endothermic peaks of PLGA/CS NPs that correspond to Tg of PLGA (55°C) and thermal degradation of the CS (275°C).

tPA release from NPs

The EE* of tPA encapsulated PLGA and PLGA/CS NPs are found to be 46.7% ± 1.56, 50.8% ± 1.09, respectively (Fig. 11.27). Effect of coating with CS on loading efficiency might be caused by an ionic interaction between tPA and CS and prevented leakage of tPA from emulsion droplet during evaporation process. Drug release from NPs involves three different stages: the first stage is an initial burst followed by drug diffusion, the second stage is governed by swelling of the polymer by inward diffusion of water during which the drug is dissolved and can diffuse out. The third stage is characterized by the erosion phase, in which polymer degradation occurs (Xu and Czernuszka 2008). Initially, high release rate was observed due to the dissolution of surface adhered drug. The drug release of PLGA and PLGA/CS NPs were monitored during the first hour which accounted for 11% and 7.8%, respectively. After the initial release, it continued significantly for 2 days where 55% and 65% of tPA for PLGA and PLGA/CS was released respectively (Fig. 11.28).

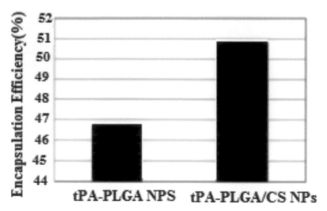

Figure 11.27. The EE* of tPA-PLGA and tPA-PLGA/CS NPs.

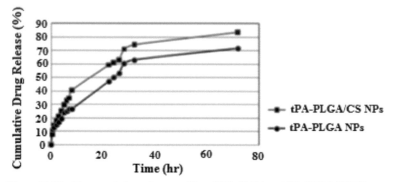

Figure 11.28. The cumulative release profiles of tPA-PLGA and tPA-PLGA/CS NPs.

Evaluation of release kinetic

The release kinetic was evaluated by fitting the experimental data to standard release equations (Riger-Peppas and Higuchi equation) (Eq. 11.13 and Eq. 11.15). From the analysis of the first phase (< 10% of drug released) and the last phase (> 65% of drug released), can be deduced that Higuchi square-root of time model ($R2 > 0.99$) (Fig. 11.29) and Riger-Peppas equations ($R2 > 0.99$) (Fig. 11.30) for PLGA/CS NPs (Table 11.4). The drug release mechanism is non-Fickian diffusion ($n > 0.5$). The best fit was obtained for both models.

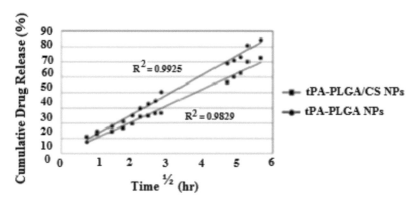

Figure 11.29. Drug release profiles from tPA-PLGA NPs and tPA-PLGA/CS NPs in PBS at pH 7.4 predicted by Higuchi equation.

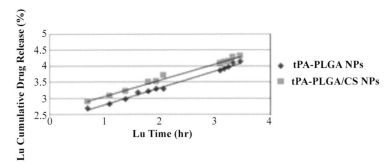

Figure 11.30. Drug release profiles from tPA-PLGA NPs and tPA-PLGA/CS NPs predicted by Riger-Peppas equation.

Table 11.4. The release parameters calculated by Higuchi and Riger-Peppas equations.

Sample	Riger-Peppas equation			Higuchi equation		
	R1	n	K	R2	K_H	K_H theory
tPA-PLGA NPs	0.9911	0.5286	12.80	0.9829	10.627	11.16
tPA-PLGA/CS NPs	0.9917	0.5038	9.63	0.9925	12.868	13.20

Thrombolysis of tPA-NPs

The thrombolysis of clots in an occlusive tube was examined by adding tPA only, PLGA NPs and PLGA/CS NPs into PBS solution. Thrombus weight reduction in each group is summarized in Table 11.5. The highest digested clot was obtained with PLGA/CS NPs (21.6%), while with tPA only the lowest (8.05%), suggesting the effect and important of the interaction between the CS and blood clot (Fig. 11.31). Therefore, PLGA/CS NPs could serve as an effective vehicle for local delivery of tPA in an attempt to alleviate the systemic side effects of the drug and to enhance its efficacy in thrombolytic therapy.

Laser thrombolysis and photomechanical drug delivery

Laser induced thrombolysis by photomechanically driven NPs was investigated at room temperature. Mean weight of clots before laser exposure was 100 mg in group I: tPA only, 299.3 mg in group II: PLGA NPs,

Table 11.5. The weight of digested clots percent after exposure to NPs (after 1 hr).

Sample	Initial weight (mg)	Final weight (mg) after exposure to NPs	Weight of digested clot (%)
tPA only	459.3	422.3	8.05
tPA-PLGA NPs	259.3	219	15.54
tPA-PLGA/CS NPs	228.4	179	21.62

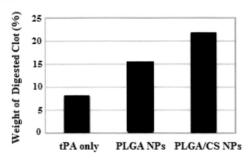

Figure 11.31. Plot of thrombolysis and weight of digested clots percent after exposure to NPs (after 1 hr).

and 316.2 mg in group III: PLGA/CS NPs. As it can be seen from the Fig. 11.32, the total weight loss (Eq. 11.17) increases with increasing the fluence. However, it behaves linearly up to 70 Jcm^{-2} there onwards the curve shows a nonlinear behaviour. A maximum weight loss of 69 mg is achieved at 135 Jcm^{-2}.

Total weight loss = (Weight of clot at the start) − (Weight of residual clot)   (11.17)

Weight reduction of clots in each group after laser exposure is summarized in Table 11.6. The next step was to study the percent of clot dissolution under the influence of tPA release at different times. The rate of thrombolysis obtained for PLGA/CS NPs was highest at different times (Fig. 11.33). Results presented in this study demonstrated the possibility of using photomechanical drug delivery to enhance the thrombolysis process by delivering nanoparticles into clot during the laser thrombolysis procedure or possibly to remove the clot residual after laser-clot ablation. It must also be noticed that even at higher values the produced temperature should be less than the material (PLGA or CS) melting temperature, which was so in our case. For example, the weight of digested clot percent after laser exposure is 33.27% for photomechanical drug delivery, compared to 21.6% for drug delivery in group PLGA/CS NPs, 31.13% for photomechanical drug delivery compared to 15.54% for drug delivery in group PLGA NPs, and 17% for photomechanical drug delivery compared to 8.05% for drug delivery in group tPA only. The results show that the PLGA/CS NPs maintain the highest weight percentages of dissolved clot.

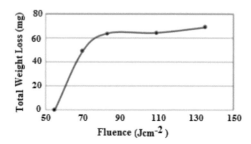

Figure 11.32. The total weight loss of clot versus fluence.

Table 11.6. Laser thrombolysis of clot after exposure to NPs (after 1 hr).

Sample	Initial weight (mg)	Final weight (mg) after laser exposure	Weight of digested clot (%)
tPA only	100	83	17
tPA-PLGA NPs	299.3	206.1	31.13
tPA-PLGA/CS NPs	316.2	211	33.27

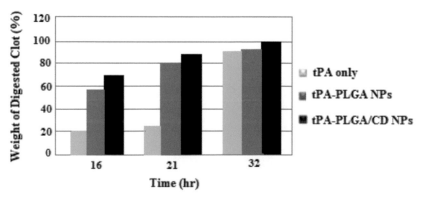

Figure 11.33. The weight of digest clot percent after laser exposure with F = 109 J cm^{-2} at different times.

Discussion

PLGA particulate drug delivery systems have been widely used for biomacromolecules such as peptides, proteins or nucleic acids (Cohen-Sela et al. 2009, Takeuchi et al. 2001). In this study, the tPA encapsulated PLGA and PLGA/CS were fabricated by double emulsion solvent evaporation (W/O/W). Sustained and localized release, as well as *in vivo* stabilization can be achieved using PLGA particles. However, during preparation, organic solvents and shear stress can denature or deactivate the biopolymers incorporated. The EE* of biopolymers in the particles is essentially low and results in the consumption of a large quantity of biopolymers in the preparation (Guo and Gemeinhart 2008). Hence surface coating of PLGA particles seems to be useful in reducing their effect. In this report, CS was used to coat PLGA NPs due to their cationic charge, biodegradability, and mucoadhesive properties. In addition, CS coated PLGA NPs have been proposed for delivery of protein drugs. CS has been shown to possess mucoadhesive properties due to molecular attractive force formed by electrostatic interaction between positively charged CS and negatively charged surfaces. These properties may be attributed to: (1) strong hydrogen bonding groups like –OH, -COOH, (2) strong charges, (3) high molecular weight, (4) sufficient chain flexibility, and (5) surface energy properties. The electrostatic attraction is likely the predominant driving force, especially in the formation of the first monomolecular adsorption layer (Park et al. 2001). The adsorption of CS continues even though a positively charged surface has been achieved, in which hydrogen bond (N-H) or van der waals force can be involved. At high concentration of CS, it is possible that the subsequent layer of CS could be adsorbed on the first layer and has no direct contact with the surface. With more layers added, CS chains would repel each other due to the same charge but be attracted and interact through hydrophobic interactions, van der waals forces, and hydrogen bonds (Sinha et al. 2004, Guo and Gemeinhart 2008). The reasons for encapsulating tPA as the thrombolytic drug are due to: (i) the extremely short half life (< 5 min) renders the need for administering a high dose (1.25 mg/kg) of tPA. However, the effective therapeutic dose range of tPA at the thrombuse site is only around 0.45–1 µg/ml (Park et al. 2001), (ii) due to administration of this high dose, clinical use of tPA is often associated with a high incidence of bleeding complication, and (iii) in order to prevent restenosis for up to several months, prolonged attenuation of thrombus by utilizing a delivery carrier for thrombolytic drug has been suggested. CS was chosen as coating on the surface PLGA for encapsulation of tPA, mainly because zeta potential of fibrinogen solution is –38.5 at pH of 7.4 (Chung et al. 2008). Hence, it would be reasonable to postulate that the zeta potentials of fibrins in blood clots have negative charge and that may facilitate the penetration of the NPs into clots. Morphology and spherical shape of NPs is shown by TEM micrographs and AFM images and is shown size of the tPA encapsulated PLGA/CS NPs is larger than PLGA NPs. The hydrodynamic diameter of CS coated PLGA NPs increases gradually with initial CS concentration. The increased particle size can be attributed to the increased viscosity of CS and the increased amount of adsorbed CS on the surface of PLGA NPs. The positive zeta potential and FTIR spectroscopy (Fig. 11.25) of CS coated PLGA NPs confirmed the presence of CS on PLGA NPs. Guo and Geimenhart (2008) reported that continuous adsorption of CS on PLGA NPs do not affect the apparent zeta potential at high concentration (greater than 0.4–0.6 g/l). The zeta potential with increased initial CS can be indicative of saturated adsorption of CS on PLGA NPs. However, the amount of adsorbed CS on PLGA NPs increases with the initial CS concentration and saturation of adsorption. The small size and the high surface energy of PLGA NPs play an important role for multilayer adsorption of CS. The increase of NPs size and the spectra of NPs with peaks at 1629, 2923, 2853, and 3431 cm^{-1} confirm the formation of the CS (Fig. 11.2b) on the PLGA NPs surface. The DSC curves of PLGA NPs (Fig. 11.26) and PLGA/CS NPs (Fig. 11.26f) correspond to relaxation enthalpy of pure PLGA (55°C). It can be observed that the nanoencapsulation process did not affect the polymer structure because the pure PLGA presented the same value for relaxation enthalpy. The DSC study did not detect any drug material in the NPs, i.e., the endothermic peak of tPA was not observed. Thus, it can be concluded that the drug incorporated into the NPs was in an amorphous polymer. The thermal decomposition of PLGA NPs and PLGA/CS NPs has begun in a lower temperature than that of the pure PLGA and CS. The nanoparticles are more exposed to the thermal degradation because their sub-micrometric size makes the superficial area larger. In relation to polymer, since NPs show wider superficial area they degrade easier. They were not observed peaks in approximately 355°C and 300°C, that seem to be characteristic of pure PLGA and CS (curves b and c, Fig. 11.26), confirming the previous data that show PLGA NPs and PLGA/CS NPS to have lower thermal stability than pure PLGA and CS. The thermal decomposition of PLGA/CS NPs is lower than thermal decomposition of PLGA NPs. The coating of NPs with CS makes the superficial area larger and shows wider superficial area they degrade easier. The PLGA/CS is more reactive than the pure polymers due to their wider superficial area and, consequently, they suffer thermal decomposition more quickly. EE* of PLGA/CS NPs was higher compared to PLGA NPs. Effect of coating with CS on loading efficiency might be caused by an ionic interaction between tPA and CS and prevented leakage of tPA from emulsion droplet during evaporation process. The drug release of PLGA and PLGA/CS NPs were monitored during the first hour of release which accounted for 11% and 7.8%, respectively. This difference is explained by the fact that it takes some times for CS to degrade and let tPA to diffuse out, as well as the fact that higher hydrodynamic pressure is experienced in the opposite direction (i.e., acting as resistance). However, after this short time some degradation and PBS uptake has taken place, as a result of which the release trend gradually increases. Longer drug release time due to the diffusion process is much slower compared with the initial release. Several concurrent processes, such as interactions between tPA and CS and between CS and PLGA, most probably influence the release of tPA. Therefore, depending on the ratios of the different components in each particle type, the influence of the increased CS solubility in acidic media (pH = 5) on the release of the drug, is not directly proportional to the CS content of each NPs. Faster release from the PLGA/CS NPs in media is attributed to the higher solubility of CS at lower pH (Manca et al. 2008). The final stage was the release of drug for few days where the process was completed. The complete release of the drug from the NPs occurred only after complete erosion or degradation of the NPs. Sustained release of tPA is sufficient to prevent the formation of new thrombus. In order to prevent restenosis for up to several months, the tPA should be release in controlled manner for a longer period of time. Indeed, several researches have indicated a lower rate of restenosis using a local infusion of tPA (Gellman et al. 1991). Therefore, our studies could offer and alternative for currently existing antithrombotic therapies.

Efficient thrombolysis appears to be dependent upon transport of the tPA into clot, which is a function of both diffusion and convection. The tPA incorporated in the NPs retained its activity, as confirmed by the fibrin clot lysis assay (Fig. 11.31). The weight percentage of dissolved clots is shown in the following order, PLGA/CS NPs (21.6%) > PLGA NPs (15.54%) > tPA (8.05%). The highest dissolved clot rate was obtained with PLGA/CS NPs, suggesting the effect and importance of the interaction between the CS and blood clot. Therefore, PLGA/CS NPs could serve as an effective vehicle for local delivery of tPA in an attempt to alleviate the systemic side effects of the drug and to enhance its efficacy in thrombolytic therapy. Laser thrombolysis is another method of optomechanical removal of clot that is currently under investigation. The goal of laser thrombolysis is to safely obliterate the embolus into microscopic fragments small enough to pass through the capillary circulation. Laser thrombolysis for acute stroke uses a low laser energy pulse of laser tuned to the hemoglobin absorption peak or facilitated by an exogenous administered chromophore. The absorbed energy vaporizes the hemoglobin molecule and adjacent water molecules to create a vapor bubble that expands and contracts to create shock waves that focally shatter the embolus (Nesbit et al. 2004). We demonstrate the possibility of using photomechanical drug delivery (compared to drug delivery) to enhance the thrombolysis process by delivering nanoparticles into clot during the laser irradiation and possibly to remove the clot residual after initial laser-clot ablation. Since 532 nm laser pulse is absorbed more efficiently by blood clot than by the surrounding arterial wall, thus, the clot can be heated and vaporized without damaging adjacent structures and reducing the chance of a new clot forming. Avoiding damage to the arterial wall is also important in the prevention of re-stenosis, or renewed narrowing. This demonstrates that a 532 laser pulse can enhance delivering of tPA into clot. The main operating mechanism with this laser in an absorbing liquid media such as blood is due to rapid generation of acoustic waves via thermoelastic mechanism and vaporization (photothermal). Further, the rapid breakdown and plasma formation cause heating of a small volume of liquid around the focus of a converging lens leads to the formation of a body of high-temperature vapour called a cavitation bubble (photomechanical). Most explanations have focused on cavitation-related processes such as microstreaming around the bubbles in stable cavitation, or microjetting in unstable cavitation, both of which can alter the structure of clots. In all cases, microbubbles may also increase the number of available binding sites for fibrinolytic enzyme molecules by stretching or damaging clot fibers. Therefore, nanoparticles are likely driven into the clot by thermomechanical waves (ultrasonics) at low fluencies and also by hydrodynamic flow due to the cavitation microbubble formation at higher values. These results suggest that PLGA/CS NPs could serve as an effective vehicle for local delivery of tPA in cardiological applications.

11.5 Fabrication and characterization of magnetoplasmonic liposome carriers
(Hassannejad and Khosroshahi 2013)

Phospholipid liposome encapsulating gold-coated superparamagnetic iron oxide nanostructures is developed. Gold nanoshells were fabricated by a multistep procedure through electroless plating of Au on the surface of the gold decorated superparamagnetic iron oxide nanoparticles (SPIONs). They were then stabilized using polyvinyl pyrolidone (PVP) with the molecular weight of 25 kDa, followed by their encapsulation within hydrophilic core of liposomes, composed of egg yolk phosphatidylcholine (EPC): cholesterol (CHOL) with a molar ratio of 2:1 and an efficiency of 94%. Surface chemistry, hydrodynamic size and electrokinetic potential, morphology and optical properties of magnetoplasmonic liposomes (MPLs) were studied by FT-IR, DLS, TEM, and UV-Vis spectroscopy, respectively. FT-IR results showed the presence of amine functional groups on the surface of SPIONs as well as coordination of the nitrogen and oxygen atoms of PVP to the Au atoms at the surface of gold nanoshells. The effect of surface coating on the stability of nanostructures was discussed. The obtained results show that the fabricated hybrid nanostructures are potentially useful for delivery of plasmonic nanoparticles to cells and can be used as exogenous absorber in laser thermal therapy.

Introduction

Liposomes are spherical, concentric bilayered vesicles surrounded by a phospholipid membrane. Due to their structure, chemical composition and colloidal size, all of which can be controlled by preparation methods, exhibit several properties which are useful in number of applications. Liposomes can be made entirely from naturally occurring substances and are therefore nontoxic, biodegradable and non immunogenic. The most important properties are colloidal size, i.e., a uniform distributions in the range of 20 nm to 10 μm. Due to their amphilic character, liposomes are powerful solubilizing system for a wide range of compounds. Also, the ease of surface modification and a good biocompatibility profile make them an appealing approach for increasing the circulating half-life of proteins and peptides. They may contain hydrophilic compounds, which remain encapsulated in the aqueous interior, or hydrophobic compounds, which may escape encapsulation through diffusion out of the phospholipid membrane. Liposomes can be engineered to adhere to cellular membranes to deliver a drug payload or transfer drugs via endocytosis process. Since the description of unique optical properties of noble metal nanoparticles, which deviate from the bulk materials, by Gustav Mie who solved Maxwell's electrodynamic equations for a homogeneous sphere in 1908 (Bohren and Huffman 1983) a vast majority of researches have been carried out for the development of noble metal nanoparticles with different structures as well as their applications in biomedicine. Noble metal nanoparticles can be used as a biosensor (Khlebtsov and Khlebtsov 2007), an exogenous absorber for laser-induced thermal therapy (Kumar and Abraham 2012, Melancon et al. 2011) or laser soldering (Khosroshahi and Nourbakhsh 2011). Wavelength of plasmon resonance (λ_{SPR}), the extinction cross-sections, and the ratio of scattering to absorption efficiency at λ_{SPR} are critical optical properties of noble metal nanoparticles which can be tuned by size, shape, and the dielectric properties of the surrounding medium.

Recently, the influence of assembly of nanoparticles, number of the nanoparticles in the nanocluster as well as the distance of the particles from one another on optical properties of plasmonic nanoparticles has been assessed based on experimental results and theoretical calculations (Liu et al. 2008, Melancon et al. 2011, Hassannejad and Khosroshahi 2013). The influence of the number of assembled nanoparticles and the structure of the nanoclusters on the absorption efficiency has been theoretically investigated (Khlebtsov et al. 2006). Also, Liu et al. (2009) studied the dependence of the optical characteristics of gold nanoshells on the inter-particle distance. Recently we reported a time dependent post synthesis Doppler shift by gold/SPION nanostructures due to self-assembly (Hassannejad and Khosroshahi 2013). The assembly of plasmonic nanoparticles within the live cells is important in diagnostic and therapeutic applications. Zharov et al. (2006)

used antibody-conjugated gold nanoparticles to accumulate them within cells. Also, nanoparticles can be embedded within polymeric matrices, microspheres, as well as liposomes. Hydrophilic and hydrophobic nanoparticles can be incorporated into the lipid bilayer or the core of the liposome, respectively. Park et al. prepared gold nanoparticles of 3–4 nm loaded into the bilayer of liposomes and evaluated the fluidity changes of bilayer due to nanoparticle loading (Park et al. 2006). Also, Paasonen et al. (2010) fabricated multilamellar liposomes with embedded gold nanoparticles of 2–4 nm. In addition, there are some reports about the deposition of gold nanoparticles onto the surface of liposomes (Paasonen et al. 2010, Saua et al. 2009, Leung et al. 2011). Here, we developed unilamellar liposomal carriers encapsulating PVP-stabilized gold nanoshells. The variation in the λ_{SPR} of gold nanoparticles is too limited. Gold nanoshells are found to have optical cross-sections comparable to and even higher than the nanoparticles. Additionally, it has been reported that the λSPR can be rapidly increased by either increasing the total nanoshell size or increasing the ratio of the core to shell radius (Jain et al. 2006). Encapsulation efficiency is the most important properties of liposomes in drug delivery applications. Here, we applied thin film hydration method to encapsulate stabilized hydrophilic gold nanoshells within the core of liposomes. In addition, the large number of nanoshells per liposome offer the advantage of developed hybrid nanostructures for delivery of magnetoplasmonic nanoparticles within a live cell with higher efficiency.

Materials and methods

Chemical and reagents

All analytical reagents were used without further purification. Ferric chloride hexahydrate (FeCl3.6H2O, 99%), ferrous chloride tetrahydrate (FeCl2.4H2O, 99%), hydrochloric acid (HCl, 37%), sodium hydroxide, chloroform, formaldehyde solution (H2CO, 37%), absolute ethanol and polyvidone 25 were purchased from Merck. Gold (iii) chloride trihydrate (HAuCl4.3H2O, ≥ 49% Au basis), 3-aminopropyltriethoxysilane (APTES), egg yolk phosphatidylcholine (EPC), and cholesterol (CHOL) were purchased from Sigma. Tetrakis (hydroxymethyl) phosphonim chloride (THPC) was an 80% aqueous solution from Aldrich. Deionized water (18 MΩ) was provided by a Milli-Q system and deoxygenated by vacuum for 1 hour prior to the use.

Synthesis of SPIONs: As described in the preceding sections

Synthesis of gold coated SPIONs

Gold coated SPIONs were fabricated by a multistep procedure through electroless plating of Au onto precursor nanoparticles (Brinson et al. 2008, Hassannejad and Khosroshahi 2013). The surface of SPIONs was functionalized with APTES to generate an amine terminated surface (Khosroshahi and Ghazanfari 2012). Amine functionalization was performed by adding APTES (35 µl) to the suspension of SPIONs in ethanol. H$_2$O (1 ml) was introduced into the reaction medium to initiate the hydrolysis. The reaction was allowed to proceed for 7 hours at room temperature and then rinsed by applying an external magnetic field and redispersing with ethanol to remove excess unreacted chemicals. A colloidal gold solution containing ~ 2 nm Au particles was prepared using THPC as the reductant according to Duff and Baker (1993) method and was refrigerated for 2–3 weeks before use. Precursor nanoparticles were prepared by adding amine terminated SPIONs in ethanol (1 ml of 0.0128 M) into THPC gold solution (40 ml) and NaCl (4 ml of 1 M) and refrigerated for 12 hours. Subsequently, precursor nanoparticles were isolated and redispersed in deoxygenated deionized water with the final concentration of 1.28 mM. A plating solution was prepared by mixing HAuCl4 solution (3 ml of 1%) with aqueous solution of K$_2$CO$_3$ (200 ml of 1.8 mM) and aged for 24–48 h in the dark. Subsequently, a continuous gold shell was grown around the SPIONs through reduction of AuCl$_4$-ions in the plating solution by formaldehyde onto the precursor nanoparticles. Complete shell growth took about 7 min, which was monitored by absorbance measurements.

PVP-stabilized gold nanoshells

PVP solution was prepared by dissolving PVP (27.1 mg /ml) in water and ultrasonication of the solution for 30 min at room temperature (Graf et al. 2006). In order to prepare PVP-coated gold nanoshells, in a typical procedure, obtained nanoshell dispersion in water (2 ml) was centrifuged at 4000 g for 25 min. Subsequently, supernatant (1 ml) was replaced by PVP solution (1 ml) and the obtained mixture stirred for 24 hours at room temperature. Next, it was centrifuged twice under 4000 g for 25 min and washed with Milli-Q water in order to remove free PVP from solution.

Fabrication of liposomal vesicles

Liposomes were composed of EPC:CHOL at a molar ratio of 2:1. A lipid mixture of chloroform stocks was prepared and dried at 42°C under nitrogen stream and further placed in a vacuum overnight. The lipid films were hydrated at a concentration of 20 mM EPL in HEPES buffered saline (HBS, 25 mM HEPES, 140 mM NaCl, pH 7.4) at 65°C for 2 h (vortexed for 30 s every 5 min). After hydration, 15 min of sonication (Tecna 20, 190 W) was applied to break down any larger vesicles. Subsequently, the samples underwent 5 cycles of freeze-thaw including 10 min at −196°C, 10 min at 65°C, and 30 s vortexing between cycles.

Preparation of magnetoplasmonic liposomes

Liposomal vesicles encapsulating hydrophilic gold nanoshells were prepared according to the procedure described above. In this case, the lipid film was hydrated with the PVP-coated gold nanoshell solution instead of HBS. Unencapsulated nanoparticles were removed by centrifuging at 400 g for 5 min, after which the supernatant liposomal dispersion was centrifuged at 20000 g for 30 min to precipitate the liposomes encapsulating gold nanoshells.

Characterization

Transmission electron microscopy (TEM) was performed using a CM 200 FEG STEM Philips-M.E.R.C. operating at the voltage of 200 kV. Liposomes were observed by TEM following negative staining with uranyl acetate. Liposomes were diluted with distilled water and dropped on a PDL-coated copper grid. The excessive sample was removed with filter paper and air-dried for 1 min at room temperature. Subsequently, uranyl acetate solution (10 µl of 1%) was dropped onto the grid. After 1 min, the excess staining solution was removed with filter paper and was allowed to dry in the air before introduction into the microscope. Fourier Transform Infrared Spectroscopy (FT-IR) spectra were recorded by TENSOR27 FT-IR spectrometer. The obtained nanoparticles were dried, mixed with KBr, and compressed into a pellet. UV-Vis spectroscopy of nanoparticle suspensions was taken on a CARY100 UV-Vis spectrophotometer with a 10 mm optical path length quartz cuvette. The mean particle size and polydispersity of the liposomal vesicles were determined using Dynamic Laser Light Scattering (DLS) method. The scattered light intensity at 90° was measured by light scattering photometer (Brookhaven instrument). The zeta potential was measured as the particle electrophoretic mobility by means of laser microelectrophoresis in a thermostated cell at room temperature. Every sample measurement was repeated 5 times. Encapsulation efficiency of gold nanoshells within the liposomes was determined by inductively coupled plasma mass spectrometry (ICP-MS). Samples for ICP-MS (VARIAN 735-ES) analysis were frozen, lyophilized, and dissolved in nitric acid hydrochloride, prepared by adding nitric acid (100 µL) and hydrochloric acid (300 µL of 37%) for 72 h to dissolve particles. Then, samples were diluted to 2 mL with HNO3 (1.6 mL of 2%) and analyzed via ICP-MS against standards (Maltzahn et al. 2009).

Theory of parameter affecting optical properties of gold nanostructures

It is known that the optical resonance is a function of size and shape of the nanoparticles. In addition, the surface plasmon peak is greatly influenced by the local dielectric environment. The change of the size of nanoparticles relative to the wavelength of light can produce different order of polarization ranging from the lowest dipolar to higher order multipoles. In the case of particles much smaller than the wavelength of light, the electron oscillation can be considered to be predominantly dipolar in nature. In the dipolar mode, the polarizability of a sphere of volume V is given by the Clasius-Mossotti relation (Kelly et al. 2002):

$$\alpha_p(\omega) = 3\varepsilon V \frac{\varepsilon_p(\omega) - \varepsilon_m}{\varepsilon_p(\omega) + 2\varepsilon_m} \tag{11.18}$$

where, ε_0 is permittivity of vacuum, ε_m is the dielectric constant of the surrounding medium, and ε_p is dielectric function of metal particle. Equation (11.18) incorporates the dependence of polarizability on the dielectric function of the metal and polarizability has a strong maximum when $\varepsilon = -2\varepsilon_m$. Then, an increase of the dielectric constant of the medium results in an increase of negative value of ε required satisfying the plasmon resonance condition, resulting in a red shift of the plasmon resonance wavelength. Furthermore, an increase in the medium dielectric constant results in the weakening of the Coulombic restoring force on the displaced electron cloud and hence lowering the plasmon oscillation frequency. Thus, surface plasmon frequency is sensitive to any changes in the refractive index of the local medium around the particle, including adsorption of molecules or change of the solvent. Additionally, plasmon shifts have been observed due to the perturbation of the conduction electron density of the nanoparticles caused by adsorbate-metal interactions (Mulvaney et al. 2006). Chemical interaction of the electrons with adsorbates can also results in a broadening of the plasmon resonance band, which is known as chemical interface damping (Hovel et al. 1993). Moreover, formation of three-dimensional clusters changes the absorption and scattering properties of plasmonic nanoparticles because of the delocalization of the SPR. Correspondingly, the color of a system varies. Cluster formation of plasmon particles, the number of particles in the cluster, as well as the distance between the particles in close approximation changes the intensity and position of λ_{SPR}.

Statistical analysis

Number of particle size based on TEM micrographs is the average of at least 50 measurements and reported as mean ± standard deviation. The SPSS 15.0 was used to perform the calculations.

Results and discussions

FTIR

FT-IR measurements were carried out to delineate the surface characteristics of nanoparticles. Figure 11.34 shows the FT-IR spectra of bare SPION (a), amine-functionalized SPION (b), PVP (c) and PVP-covered gold nanoshell (d). The broad band at region of 3550–3200 cm^{-1} with moderate intensity is assigned to the presence of –OH groups at the surface of nanoparticles. In Fig. 11.34a, the peaks at 444 and 579 cm^{-1} are assigned to the vibration of Fe-O bond, which are characteristic bands of magnetite. The broad band at 1623 cm^{-1} and the splitted band at 3414 cm^{-1} can be attributed to the N-H stretching vibration and NH$_2$ bending mode of free NH$_2$ groups, respectively. Also, it can be seen that the characteristic bands of the Fe-O bond of amine-functionalized SPIONs shift to higher frequencies of 620 and 477 cm^{-1} compared with that of bare SPIONs (at 579 and 444 cm^{-1}). These shifts have been attributed to the replacement of –H at the Fe-O-H groups on the surface of SPION by the more electronegative group of –Si(O$^-$)$^{2-}$ which leads to the enhancement of bond force constant for Fe-O bonds (Ma et al. 2003). The FT-IR spectrum of PVP (Fig. 11.34c) mainly consists of two bands at 1282 and 1664 cm^{-1} corresponding to the vibration of C-N and carbonyl group in pyrrolidone ring (Murat and Nazan 2005). Similar bands are also seen in the FT-IR spectrum of PVP-coated gold nanoshells. However, compared to the spectrum of PVP, the resonance peak of C-N, at 1282 cm^{-1}, was shifted to 1475 cm^{-1} and the band of C = O, at 1664 cm^{-1}, red shifted to 1647 cm^{-1}. The change of the spectrum indicates that the absorption of PVP on the gold shell is not on the basis of electrostatic attraction, but Au atoms on the surface of nanoparticles would coordinate with N and O atoms of PVP, which is consistent with previously reported results (Liu et al. 2010).

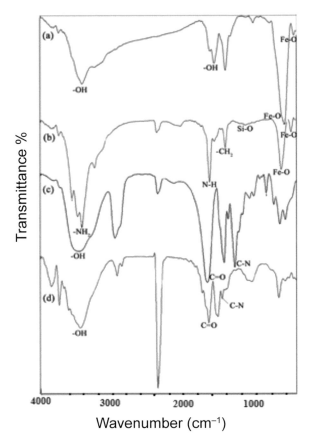

Figure 11.34. FT-IR spectra of bare SPION (a), amine-functionalized SPION (b), PVP (c), and PVP-covered gold-coated SPION (d).

DLS

According to the Derjarguin–Landau–Verwey–Overbeck (DLVO) theory, the stability of colloidal suspension results from the equilibrium between attractive (i.e., van der Waals) and repulsive (i.e., electrostatic) forces. For magnetic suspensions, magnetic dipolar forces between two particles must be added in order to promote the attraction force between the particles. Thus, electrical double layer is not enough to prevail against to coagulation in many conditions such as changing the pH value and ionic strength or in physiological medium. Coating of nanoparticles by polymers develops steric repulsion force which depends on molecular weight of the polymer and its density. Controlling the strength of these forces is a key parameter to elaborate nanoparticle suspensions with good stability. In aqueous solutions, the Fe atoms coordinate with water molecules, which dissociate readily to leave a hydroxylated surface. The hydroxyl groups on the surface of iron oxide are amphoteric and may react with acids or bases. Dependent on the pH of the solution, the relative abundance of pro-tonated or deprotonatoned hydroxyl groups governs the electrokinetic potential of iron oxide particles in the absence of absorbing ions other than H+. The corresponding surface reactions may be expressed as:

$\equiv FeOH + H+ \leftrightarrow \equiv FeOH2+$

$\equiv FeOH \leftrightarrow FeO- + H+$

In our case, an electrokinetic potential of -29.7 ± 0.68 mV at neutral pH was obtained for bare SPIONs which is consistent with previously reported values (Sun et al. 1998). Subsequently, surface hydroxyl groups exchanged by amine groups through silanization reaction using APTES. The zeta potential of amine-functionalized SPIONs increased to $+16.6 \pm 1.62$ mV. The pKa value of amine groups is about 10 and at neutral pH they are protonated. Therefore, the increase of the zeta potential to positive value indicates the successful grafting of APTES on the surface of SPIONs. The zeta potential value of gold colloids with an average size of ~ 2 nm formed using THPC reducing agent was –40.91 ± 1.14 mV. Therefore, by mixing of gold colloids with amine-functionalized SPIONs in a mixture of water and ethanol with a pH value of 9, the negatively charged gold colloids readily attached to the SPIONs led to the decrease of the zeta potential value of amine-functionalized SPION to –19.17 ± 0.27. The zeta potential of gold nanoshells and the surface potential of PVP-coated gold nanoshells were measured –21.63 ± 0.9 and –22.77 ± 0.73, respectively. The measured properties of synthesized nanoparticles are summarized in Table 11.7. The effect of surface coating on the stability of SPIONs is observable from DLS data. The volume-weighted hydrodynamic size measured by DLS for SPIONs, amine-functionalized SPIONs, gold nanoshells and PVP-coated nanoshells was 201.4, 95.4, 57.7 and 102.5 nm, respectively. The reduced hydrodynamic size of amine-functionalized SPIONs shows more stability of nanoparticle suspension after silanization reaction. This fact confirms that, apart from the electrostatic repulsion due to a zeta potential of +16.6 ± 1.62, steric repulsion arising from grafting of the APTES to the nanoparticles increased the stability of amine-functionalized SPIONs. Coating of the amine-functionalized SPIONs with a continuous thin layer of gold reduced the hydrodynamic size of gold nanoshells to 57.7 nm. At temperatures below the blocking SPIONs have a zero magnetic moment. However, it has been shown that residual forces, of magnetic dipolar origin, acting between SPIONs lead them to clump (Dobson and Gray 2009). The reduced size of gold-coated SPIONs could be due to the reduction of this residual forces. After PVP coating of gold nanoshells, the hydrodynamic size increased to 102.5 nm, which is because the immobilization of long chain molecules of PVP at the surface of the nanoparticles. This result agrees well with the previously reported thickness in the case of PVP adsorbed on palladium nanoparticles (Hirai and Yakura 2001). Fluctuation in the measured hydrodynamic size of synthesized nanoparticles is illustrated in Fig. 11.35.

Table 11.7. Properties of synthesized nanoparticles in different steps of fabrication.

Samples	TEM size (nm) ± SE	DLS volume-weighted size (nm) (PDI)	Electrophoretic potential (mV) ± SE
SPION	9.5 ± 1.4	201.4 (0.224)	–29.79 ± 0.68
SPION-NH₂	---	95.4 (0.283)	+16.60 ± 1.62
Gold colloid	2.34 ± 0.62	---	–40.91 ± 1.14
Precursor NP	---	---	–19.17 ± 0.27
SPION/gold nanoshell	15.8 ± 3.5	57.7 (0.25)	–21.63 ± 0.9
PVP-coated nanoshell	---	102.5 (0.288)	–22.77 ± 0.73
Nanoshell-encapsulated liposome	179.73 ± 69.93	290.5 (0.311)	–40.91 ± 1.14

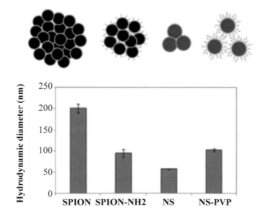

Figure 11.35. Schematic representation of the fluctuation in the measured hydrodynamic size of SPIONs, amine-functionalized SPIONs (SPION-NH2), gold nanoshells (NS) and PVP-coated gold nanoshells (NS-PVP) is shown in the upper part of the figure, and the histogram of hydrodynamic diameter of mentioned nanoparticles is shown in the lower part of the figure.

TEM

The bright field TEM micrographs of particles at different steps of nanoshell fabrication are presented in Fig. 11.36. Based on TEM micrographs, the average diameter of SPIONs and gold nanoshells was 9.5 ± 1.4 and 15.8 ± 3.5 nm, respectively. The larger size of SPIONs and gold nanoshells measured by DLS compared with TEM results indicates the slight agglomeration (Figs. 11.36a and 11.36c, respectively).

The TEM micrograph of MPLs is shown in Fig. 11.37. Encapsulation of a large number of nanoparticles into the hydrophilic inner site of liposome indicates high encapsulation efficiency of the prepared magnetoplasmonic liposmes. Also, the clear margin of magnetoplasmonic liposomes in TEM micrographs indicates a collection of PVP-coated gold nanoshells surrounded by a lipid bilayer. An average diameter of 179.73 ± 69.93 nm was obtained for magnetoplasmonic liposomes. The thickness of the lipid bilayer membrane surrounding the collection of nanoshells was 6.5 ± 1.6 nm measured by NIH ImageJ software

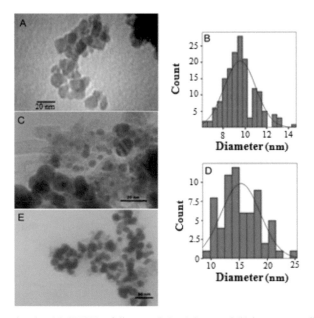

Figure 11.36. TEM images showing (a) SPIONs of diameter 9.5 ± 1.4 nm and (b) its corresponding size distribution, (c) gold nanoshells of diameter 15.3 ± 3.5 nm and (d) its corresponding size distribution and (e) PVP-coated gold nanoshells.

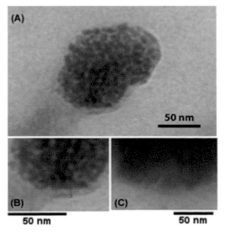

Figure 11.37. (a) TEM image of gold nanoshell-encapsulated liposome showing the phospholipid bilayer (visualized by negative staining using 1% uranylacetate) surrounding a collection of PVP-coated gold nanoshells. In (b) and (c) the bilayer thickness is indicated by red lines.

(http://rsb.info.nih.gov/ij/). Similarly, a value of 7–8 nm was also reported for lipid bilayer membrane (Floris et al. 2011). These data suggest that the formed vehicles have unilamellar liposomal structure.

Encapsulation efficiency

Encapsulation efficiency of gold MPLs was calculated using ICP-MS results through the formula (W1/W) × 100%, where W is initial concentration of Fe (mg/ml) in hydration solution and W1 is encapsulated concentration of Fe (mg/ml) in liposomes. An encapsulation efficiency of 94% was obtained. In order to evaluate the effect of PVP coating on encapsulation efficiency, we also fabricated magnetoplasmonic liposomes using as-synthesized gold nanoshells (without PVP coating). An encapsulation efficiency of 24% was obtained. These results indicate that stability of hydration suspension has a great effect on encapsulation efficiency of liposomes. In some reports, the encapsulation efficacy of prepared nanoparticle-loaded liposomes has not been reported (Paasonen et al. 2010) and this makes the comparison difficult. However, the encapsulation efficiency of our prepared nanoparticle-loaded liposomes is more than those reported by (Sabaté et al. 2008) for similar nanoparticle concentration used to prepare magnetic nanoparticle-loaded liposomes. Furthermore, as mentioned above, TEM micrograph of magnetoplasmonic liposomes show that the obtained liposome has a unilamellar structure. In previous reports, it has been shown that sonication can break down the large liposomes. Sonication can also produce unilamellar liposomes (Kim et al. 2007). Therefore, our hypothesis is that stabilization of gold nanoshells through PVP coating and application of sonication during the fabrication procedure resulted in the formation of unilamellar liposomes with a high gold nanoshell encapsulation efficiency.

Optical properties of fabricated MPLs

As shown in Fig. 11.38, the surface plasmon resonance wavelength of synthesized gold nanoshells was 540 nm, which red shifted to 554 nm after coating with PVP. As mentioned in the theory, this red shift

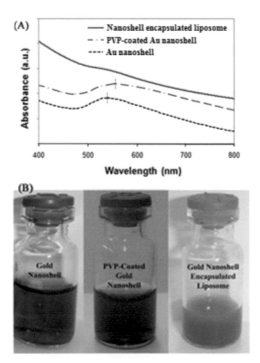

Figure 11.38. (a) Absorption measurements of gold nanoshell, PVP-coated gold nanoshell and nanoshell-encapsulated liposome. Optical images of aqueous dispersion of gold nanoshells, PVP-coated gold nanoshells and gold nanoshell-encapsulated liposomes are shown in (b).

can be due to the increased dielectric constant of the medium after coating with PVP. Also, encapsulation of PVP-coated nanoshells within liposomal structure caused to damping and broadening of absorption band. This broadband can be attributed to the size distribution of prepared MPLs and contribution from different number of gold nanoshells collected within liposomes.

Furthermore, visual observation of MPL solution (Fig. 11.38) confirms the high encapsulation efficiency. The difference between colors of aqueous dispersion of PVP-coated gold nanoshells compared to gold nanoshell-encapsulated liposomes can be due to the encapsulation of a collection of gold nanoshells within the inner part of the liposomes. Physical nature of these optical effects is related to strong electromagnetic interaction between plasmon nanoparticles due to assembly. In addition, the change of the medium refractive index caused by phospholipids encapsulating nanoshells can result in the shift of the λSPR. Although the complexes of gold nanoparticles with liposomes are known (Kojima et al. 2008) to the best of our knowledge, the present study is the first report on the gold nanoshell-loaded liposomes. Delivery of gold nanostructures to desirable cells using targeting moiety or carries (e.g., liposomes or polyelectrolyte hollow capsules) can be used to accumulate nanoparticles directly within live cells. It has been observed that the closed packing of the nanoparticles resulted in non-linear or synergistically amplified photothermal effects, strongly enhancing their diagnostic and therapeutic ability (Zharov et al. 2005). Recently, the influence of nanoparticle aggregation on the efficiency of electromagnetic absorption has been studied in order to lower the threshold fluence level for biomedical applications, such as laser-induced photothermal therapy. Optical amplification photothermal therapy with plasmonic nanoclusters has been reported by Khlebtsov et al. (2006). In order to evaluate the maximal absorption of single particle and cluster structures, they introduced the parameter of absorption amplification, which defines the enhancement of cluster absorption cross section C_{abs} in comparison to the simple sum of absorption cross section for isolated nanoparticles NC_{abs}. They found that when the number of cluster nanoparticles N is small, the electromagnetic coupling results in an increase in the absorption efficiency, and reaches a saturated value at $N > 20$. Then, the obtained hybrid structure in the present study could be a good candidate for laser-induced thermal therapy application.

Keywords: PLGA, PVA, Surfactant, Emulsifier, Nanosphere, Drug release, Betamethasone, Size distribution, Encapsulation efficiency, Superlong CO_2 laser, Chitosan, Fast photography, Photothermal deflection, Laser drug delivery, Laser thrombolysis, Frequency doubled Nd:YAG, PLGA/CS nanoparticles, Tissue plasminogen activator, Drug delivery, Superparamagnetic iron oxide nanoparticle, Gold nanoshell, PVP, Magnetoplasmonic Liposome, Stability.

References

Adams, M., A. Lavasanifar and G. Kwon. 2003. Amphiphilic block copolymers for drug delivery. J. Pharm. Sci. 92: 1343–1355.

Andersson-Engels, S. and H. Stepp. 2010. Therapeutic laser application and tissue interactions: bringing light into clinical practice. J. Biophoton 3: 259–260.

Asshauer, T. and G. Delacretz. 1994. Acoustic transient generation in pulsed holmium laser ablation under water. SPIE. Laser Tissue Interact. 2134A: 423–433.

Birbrair, A., T. Zhang, Z. Wang, M. Messi and J. Olson. Mintz. 2014. Type-2 pericytes participate in normal and tumoral angiogenesis. Am. J. Physiol. Cell Physiol. 307: C25–38.

Bodmeier, R. and J. McGinity. 1988. Solvent selection in the preparation of poly(D,L-lactide) microspheres prepared by the solvent evaporation method. Intl. J. Pharmaceutics 43: 179–186.

Bohren, C.F. and D. Huffman. 1983. Absorption and scattering of light by small particles. John Wiley & Sons, Inc.

Brinson, B., J. Lassiter, C. Levin, R. Bardhan, N. Mirin and N. Halas. 2008. Nanoshells made easy: improving Au layer growth on nanoparticle surfaces. Langmuir. 24: 14166–14171.

Buteica, A., D.I. Mihaiescu, A. Grumazescu and B. Vasile. 2010. The antibacterial activity of magnetic nanofluid: Fe_3O_4/oleic acid/cephallosporins core/shell/adsorption shell proved on *S. aureus* and *E. coli* and possible applications as drug delivery systems. Digest J. of Nanomat. and Biostructure 5: 927–932.

Brannon-Peppas, L. 1995. Recent advances on the use of biodegradable microparticles and nanoparticles in controlled drug delivery. Int. J. Pharm. 116: 1–9.

Bremond, N., M. Arora, M.D. Stephan and D. Lohse. 2006. Interaction of cavitation bubbles on a wall. Phys. Fluids 18: 121505.

Chawla, S. and M. Amiji. 2002. Biodegradable poly(e-caprolectone) nanoparticles for tumor-targeted delivery of tamifoxen. Intl. J. Pharma. 249: 127–138.

Chung, S. and E. Mazur. 2009. Surgical applications of femtosecond lasers. J. Biophoton. 2: 557–572.

Chung, T., S. Wang and W. Sai. 2008. Accelerating thrombolysis with chitosan-coated plasminogen activators encapsulated in poly-(lactide-co-glycolide) (PLGA) nanoparticles. Biomaterials 29: 228–237.

Cintas, P., F. Nguyen, B. Bonen and V. Larrue. 2004. Enhancement of enzymatic fibrinolysis with 2-MHz ultrasound and microbubbles. J. Thrombosis and Haemostasis 2: 1163–1166.

Cohen-Sela, E., M. Chorny, N. Koroukhov, H.D. Danenberg and G. Golomb. 2009. A new double emulsion solvent diffusion technique for encapsulating hydrophilic molecules in PLGA nanoparticles. J. Cont. Release 133: 90–95.

Coussios, C. and R. Roy. 2008. Applications of acoustics and cavitation to noninvasive therapy and drug delivery. Ann. Rev. Fluid Mechan. 40: 395–420.

Diaci, J. and J. Mozina. 1992. A study of blast waveforms detected simultaneously by a microphone and a laser probe during laser ablation. J. App. Phys. A 55: 352–358.

Dobson, J. and E. Gray. 2009. Residual attractive force between superparamagnetic nanoparticles. 1–21. doi:arXiv:0902.3684v1.

Duff, D., G. Baiker and A. Edwards. 1993. A new hydrosol of gold clusters. J. Chem. Soc. Chem. Commun. 115: 96–98.

Dyer, P.E., M.E. Khosroshahi and S. Tufft. 1993. Studies of laser-induced cavitation and tissue ablation in saline using a fibre-delivered pulsed HF laser. Appl. Phys. B: 56: 84–93.

Floris, A., A. Ardu, A. Musinu, G. Piccaluga, A. Fadda, C. Sinico and C. Cannas. 2011. SPION@liposomes hybrid nanoarchitectures with high density SPION association. Soft Matter 7: 6239–6247.

Frenz, M., F. Konz, H. Pratisto, P.W. Heinz, S. Alexander and I. Vitaly. 1998. Starting mechanisms and dynamics of bubble formation induced by a Ho:Yttrium aluminum garnet laser in water. Appl. Phys. 84: 5905.

Graf, C., S. Dembski, A. Hofmann and E. Rühl. 2006. A general method for the controlled embedding of nanoparticles in silica colloids. Langmuir 22: 5604–5610.

Galanzha, I., J. Kim and V. Zharov. 2009. Nanotechnology-based molecular photoacoustic and photothermal flow cytometry platform for *in vivo* detection and killing of circulating cancer stem cells. J. Biophoton 2: 25–735.

Gambihler, S., M. Delius and J.W. Ellwart. 1992. Transient increase in membrane permeability of L1210 cells upon exposure to lithotripter shock waves *in vitro*. Naturwissenschaften 79: 328–329.

Garinol, M., V. Fievez and V. Pourcelle. 2007. PEGylated PLGA-based nanoparticles targeting M cells for oral vaccination. J. Cont. Rel. 120: 195–204.

Gellman, J., S. Ligal and Q. Chen. 1991. Effect of lovastatin on intimal hyperplasia after balloon angioplasty: a study in an atherosclerotic hypercholesterolemic rabbit. J. Am. Coll. Cardiol. 17: 251–259.

Gohel, M., M. Panchal and V. Jogani. 2000. Novel mathematical method for quantitative expression of deviation from the Higuchi model. AAPS Pharm. Sci. Tech. 1(4) article 31.

Gregorcic, P., R. Petkovsek and J. Mozina. 2008. Measurements of cavitation bubble dynamic based on a beam-deflection probe. J. Appl. Phys. 93: 901–905.

Guan, X., D. Quan, K. Liao and T. Wang. 2008. Preparation and characterization of cationic chitosan-modified poly(D,L-lactide-co-glycolide) copolymer nanospheres as DNA carriers. J. Biomater. Appl. 22: 353–371.

Guo, C. and R. Gemeinhart. 2008. Understanding the adsorption mechanism of chitosan onto poly(lactide-co-glycolide) particles. Eur. J. Pharm. Biopharm. 70: 597–604.

Hassannejad, Z. and M.E. Khosroshahi. 2013. Synthesis and evaluation of time dependent optical properties of plasmonic-magnetic nanoparticles. Opt. Mater. 35: 644–651.

Hellman, A., K. Rau, H. Yoon and V. Venugopalan. 2008. Biophysical response to pulsed laser microbeam-induced cell lysis and molecular delivery. J. Biophoton. 1: 24–35.

Heslinga, M., E. Mastria and O.E. Adefeso. 2009. Fabrication of biodegradable spheroidal microparticles for drug delivery applications. J. Contr. Release 38: 235–242.

Hickey, T., D. Kreutzer, D. Burgess and F. Moussy. 2005. Dexamethasone/PLGA microspheres for continuous delivery of on anti-inflammatory drug for implantable medical devices. Biomaterials 23: 1649–1656.

Higuchi, T. 1963. Mechanism of sustained-action medication. Theoretical analysis of rate of release of solid drugs dispersed in solid matrices. J. Pharmaceut. Sci. 52: 1145–1149.

Hino, T., Y. Kawashima and S. Shimabayashi. 2000. Basic study for stabilization of w/o/w emulsion and its application to transcatheter arterial embolization therapy. Adv. Drug Deliv. Rev. 45: 27–45.

Hirai, H. and N. Yakura. 2001. Protecting polymers in suspension of metal nanoparticles. Polym. Adv. Tech. 12: 724–733.

Hobbs, S., W. Monsky, F. Yuan and W. Roberts. 1998. Regulation of transport pathways in tumor vessels: role of tumor type and microenvironment. Proc. Natl. Acad. Sci. 95: 4607–4612.

Hovel, H., S. Fritz, A. Hilger and U. Kreibig. 1993. Width of cluster plasmon resonances: bulk dielectric functions and chemical interface damping. Phys. Rev. B 48: 18178–18188.

Jain, P., K. Lee, I. El-Sayed and M. El-Sayed. 2006. Calculated absorption and scattering properties of gold nanoparticles of different size, shape, and composition: applications in biological imaging and biomedicine. J. Phys. Chem. B 110: 7238–7248.

Kakimoto, S., T. Moriyama and T. Tanabe. 2007. Dual-ligand effect of trasferrin and transforming growth factor alpha on polyethyleneimine-mediated gene delivery. J. Cont. Rel. 120: 242–249.

Kataoka, K., A. Harada and Y. Nagasaki. 2001. Block copolymer micelles for drug delivery: design, characterization and biological significance. Adv. Drug. Del. Rev. 47: 113–131.

Kelly, K., E. Coronado, L. Zhao and G. Schatz. 2002. The optical properties of metal nanoparticles: the influence of size, shape, and dielectric environment. J. Phys. Chem. B 107: 668–677.

Kim, S., L. Haimovich-Caspi, L. Omer, Y. Talmon and E. Franses. 2007. Effect of sonication and freezing–thawing on the aggregate size and dynamic surface tension of aqueous DPPC dispersions. J. Colloid Interf. Sci. 311: 217–227.

Khlebtsov, B., V. Zharov, A. Melnikov, V. Tuchin and N. Khlebtsov. 2006. Optical amplification of photothermal therapy with gold nanoparticles and nanoclusters. Nanotechnology 17: 5167–5179.

Khlebtsov, B. and N. Khlebtsov. 2007. Biosensing potential of silica/gold nanoshells: sensitivity of plasmon resonance to the local dielectric environment. J. Quant. Spectrosc. Radiat. Transfer. 106: 154–169.

Khosroshahi, M.E., S. Mansoori and A. Jafari. 2006. A preliminary analysis of drug delivery using a super long chopped pulse Co2 laser. The fourth IASTED Int. Conf. on Biomed. Eng. Austria. 519: 101–104.

Khosroshahi, M.E., M. Enyati, S. Shafiei and J. Tavakoli. 2007. Evaluation of drug release from PLGA nanospheres containing betamethasone. SPIE Proc. 6633: 66331E-1-E11.

Khosroshahi, M. and M. Nourbakhsh. 2011. *In vitro* skin wound soldering using SiO2/Au nanoshells and a diode laser. Medical Laser Application 26: 35–42.

Khosroshahi, M.E. and L. Ghazanfari. 2012. Synthesis and functionalization of SiO_2 coated Fe_3O_4 nanoparticles with amine groups based on self-assembly. Mat. Sci. and Engineering C 32(5): 1043–1049.

Kodama, T. and Y. Tomita. 2000. Cavitation bubble behavior and bubble–shock wave interaction near a gelatin surface as a study of *in vivo* bubble dynamics. Appl. Phys. B 70: 139–149.

Kodama, T., M. Hamblin and A. Doukas. 2000. Cytoplasmic molecular delivery with shock waves: importance of impulse. Physical J. 79: 1821–1832.

Kojima, C., Y. Hirano, E. Yuba, A. Harada and K. Kono. 2008. Preparation and characterization of complexes of liposomes with gold nanoparticles. Colloid Surf. B 66: 246–252.

Konan, Y., R. Gruny and E. Allemann. 2002. State of the art in the delivery of photosensitizers for photodynamic therapy. J. Photochem. Photobiol. B 66: 89–106.

Kost, J. and R. Langer. 2001. Responsive polymeric delivery systems. Adv. Drug Del. Rev. 46: 125–148.

Kumar, C. and J. Abraham. 2012. Laser immunotherapy with gold nanorods causes selective killing of tumor cells. Pharmacol. Res. 65: 261–269.

Lanza, R., R. Langer and J. Vancanti. 2000. Principles of Tissue Engineering. 2nd. (ed.). Academic Press, San Diego.

LaVan, D., T. McGuire and R. Langer. 2003. Small scale systems for *in vivo* drug delivery. 2003. Nature Biotech. 21: 1184–1191.

Leach, J., E. Orear, E. Patterson, Y. Miao and A. Johnson. 2003. Accelerated thrombolysis in a rabbit model of carotid artery thrombosis with liposome-encapsulated and microencapsulated streptokinase. Throm. Haemost. 90: 64–70.

Leach, J., E. Patterson and E.A. Orear. 2004. Distributed intraclot thrombolysis: mechanism of accelerated thrombolysis with encapsulated plasminogen activators. J. of Thrombosis and Haemostasis 2: 1548–1555.

Leroux, J., E. Allemann and Da. Jaeghere. 1996. Biodegradable nanoparticles-from sustained release formulations to improved site specific drug delivery. J. Cont. Rel. 39: 339–350.

Liu, C., C. Mi and B. Li. 2008. Energy absorption of gold nanoshells in hyperthermia therapy. IEEE Trans. Nanobiosci. 7: 206–214.

Liu, X., J. He, J. Lu and X. Ni. 2009. Effect of surface tension on a liquid-jet produced by the collapse of a laser-induced bubble against a rigid boundary. Opt. Laser Technol. 41: 21–24.

Liu, H., P. Hou, W. Zhang and J. Wu. 2010. Synthesis of monosized core–shell Fe3O4/Au multifunctional nanoparticles by PVP-assisted nanoemulsion process. Colloid Surf. A 356: 21–27.

Leung, S., X. Kachur, M. Bobnick and M. Romanowski. 2011. Wavelength- selective light-induced release from plasmon resonant liposomes. Adv. Funct. Mater. 21: 1113–1121.

Loo, S., C. Ooi and Y. Boey. 2004. Polymer degradation and stabili. 83: 259–265.

Maltzahn, G., J. Park, A. Agrawal, N. Bandaru and S. Das. 2009. Computationally guided photothermal tumor therapy using long-circulating gold nanorod antennas. Cancer Res. 69: 3892–3900.

Ma, M., Y. Zhang, W. Yu, H. Shen, H. Zhang and N. Gu. 2003. Preparation and characterization of magnetite nanoparticles coated by amino silane. Colloid Surf. A 212: 219–226.

Mao, K. Roy, V.L. Troung-Le and K.A. Janes. 2001. Chitosan-DNA nanoparticles as gene carriers: synthesis, characterization and transfection efficiency. J. Contrl. Release 70: 399–421.

Manca, M., G. Loy, M. Zaru and S. Antimisiaris. 2008. Release of rifampicin from chitosan, PLGA and chitosan-coated PLGA microparticles. Colloids and Surfaces B: Biointerfaces 67: 166–170.

Mahmoodi, M., M.E. Khosroshahi and F. Atyabi. 2011. Dynamic study of PLGA/CS nanoparticles delivery containing drug model into phantom tissue using CO_2 laser for clinical applications. J. Biophot. 4: 403–414.

Mahmoodi, M., M.E. Khosroshahi and F. Atyabi. 2011. Early experimental results of thrombolysis using controlled release of tissue plasminogen activator encapsulated by PLGA/CA nanoparticles delivered by pulse 532 nm laser. Digest J. Nanomat. Biostr. 6: 889–905.

Mastsumoto, A., Y. Matsukawa and T. Suzuki. 2005. Drug release characteristics of multi-reservoir type microspheres with poly (dl-lactide-co-glycolide) and poly (dl-lactide). J. Cont. Rel. 106: 172–180.

Mastsumoto, A., Y. Mastsukawa, T. Suzuki and H. Yoshino. 2007. Drug release characteristics of multi-reservoir type microspheres with PLGA and PLA. J. Cont. Rel. 106: 172–180.

Matsumoto, J., Y. Nakada, K. Sakurai, T. Nakamura and Y. Takahashi. 1999. Preparation of nanoparticles consisted of poly(L-lactide)-poly(ethylene glycol)-poly(L-lactide) and their evaluation *in vitro*. Intl. J. Pharmaceutics 185: 93–101.

Melancon, M., W. Lu, M. Zhong, M. Zhou and G. Liang. 2011. Targeted multifunctional gold-based nanoshells for magnetic resonance-guided laser ablation of head and neck cancer. Biomaterials 32: 7600–7608.

Moghimi, S., A. Hunter and J. Murray. 2001. Long circulating and specific nanoparticles: Theory to practice. Pharm. Rev. 53: 283–218.

Monsky, W., D. Fukumura, T. Gohongi and M. Ancukiewcz. 1999. Augmentation of transvascular transport of macromolecules and nanoparticles in tumors using vascular endothelial growth factor. Cancer Res. 59: 4129–4135.

Moore, A., J. Basilion, E. Chiocca and H. Weissleder. 1998. Measuring transferrin receptor gene expression by NMR imaging. Biochem. Biophys. Acta. 1402: 239–249.

Mulvaney, P., J. Pérez-Juste, M. Giersig, L. Liz-Marzán and C. Pecharromán. 2006. Drastic surface plasmon mode shifts in gold nanorods due to electron charging. Plasmonics 1: 61–66.

Murat, S. and A. Nazan. 2005. Radiation synthesis of poly(N-vinyl-2-pyrrolidone)-κ-carrageenan hydrogels and their use in wound dressing applications. I. Preliminary laboratory tests. J. Biomed. Mater. Res. A 74: 187–196.

Murray, J. and J. Carmichael. 1995. Targeting solid tumors: challenges, disappointments and opportunities. Adv. Drug Del. Rev. 17: 117–127.

Nguyen, P., E. Orear, A. Johnson and E. Patterson. 1990. Accelerated Thrombolysis and reperfusion in a canine model of myocardial infarction by liposomal encapsulation of streptokinase circulation research 66: 875–875.

Nesbit, G., G. Luh, R. Tien and S. Barnwell. 2004. New and future endovascular treatment strategies for acute ischemic stroke. J. Vasc. Interv. Radiol. 15: S103–S110.

Ogura, M., S. Sato, M. Terakawa, H. Wakisaka and M. Uenoyama. 2003. Delivery of photosensitizer to cells by the stress wave induced by a single nanosecond laser pulse. Jpn J. Appl. Phys. 42: L977.

Olesen, S. 1986. Rapid increase in blood brain barrier permeability during sever hypoxia and metabolic inhabitation. Brain Res. 368: 24–29.

Palanker, D., I. Turovets and A. Lewis. 1997. Dynamics of ArF excimer laser-induced cavitation bubbles in gel surrounded by a liquid medium. Laser Surg. Med. 21: 294–300.

Panyam, J., W. Zhou, S. Prabha and S. Sahoo. 2002. Rapid Endothelial Escape of Poly(DL-lactide-co-glycolide) Nanoparticles: Implications for Drug and Gene Delivery 16: 1217–1226.

Park, Y., J. Liang, Z. Yang and V. Yang. 2001. Controlled release of clot-dissolving tissue-type plasminogen activator from a poly(l-glutamic acid) semi-interpenetrating polymer network hydrogel. J. of Cont. Release 75: 37–44.

Park, S., J. Mun and S. Han. 2006. Loading of gold nanoparticles inside the DPPC bilayers of liposome and their effects on membrane fluidities. Colloid Surf. B 48: 112–118.

Paasonen, L., T. Sipilä, A. Subrizi, P. Laurinmäki and S. Butcher. 2010. Gold-embedded photosensitive liposomes for drug delivery: triggering mechanism and intracellular release. J. Controlled Release 147: 136–143.

Pjanovic, R., N. Vragolovic, J. Giga and R. Grulovic. 2010. Diffusion of drugs from hydrogels and liposomes as drug carriers. J. Chem. Technol. Biotech. 85: 693–698.

Riger, P. and N. Peppas. 1987. A simple equation for description of solute release II. Fickian and anomalous release from swellable devices. J. Contr. Release 5: 37–42.

Riviere, J. and M. Heit. 1997. Electrically-assisted transdermal drug delivery. Pharm. Res. 14: 687–697.

Sabaté, R., R. Barnadas-Rodríguez, J. Callejas-Fernández, R. Álvarez and J. Estelrich. 2008. Preparation and characterization of extruded magnetoliposomes. Inter. J. Pharmaceutics 347: 156–162.

Saltzman, W. and W. Olbricht. 2002. Building drug delivery into tissue engineering. Drug Discovery 1: 177–186.

Saua, T., A. Urban, S. Dondapati, M. Fedoruk, M. Horton and A. Rogach. 2009. Controlling loading and optical properties of gold nanoparticles on liposome membranes. Colloid Surf. A 342: 92–96.

Shangguan, H., L. Casperson, A. Shearin and S. Prahl. 1996. Investigation of cavitation bubble dynamics using particle image velocimetry: implications for photoacoustic drug delivery SPIE. Lasers in Surg. 2671: 104–115.

Shangguan, H., K. Gregory, L. Casperson and S. Prahl. 1998. Enhanced laser thrombolysis with photomechanical drug delivery: an *in vitro* study. Laser Surg. Med. 23: 151–160.

Shuai, X. and A. Nasongkla. 2004. Micellar carriers based on block copolymers of poly(e-caprolactone), and poly(ethylene glycole) for doxorubicine delivery. J. Cont. Rel. 98: 415–426.

Sinha, V., A.K. Singla, S. Wadhawan, R. Kaushik and R. Kumria. 2004. Chitosan microspheres as a potential carrier for drugs. Int. J. Pharm. 274: 1–33.

Soppimath, K., T. Aminabhavi and A. Kulkarni. 2001. Biodegradable polymeric nanoparticles as drug delivery devices. J. Cont. Rel. 249: 1–20.

Sun, Z., F. Su, W. Forsling and P. Samskog. 1998. Surface characteristics of magnetite in aqueous suspension. J. Colloid Interf. Sci. 197: 151–159.

Tachibana, K. and S. Tachibana. 1999. Application of ultrasound energy as a new drug delivery system. Jpn. J. Phys. 38: 3014–3019.

Tahara, K., T. Sakai, H. Yamamoto, H. Takeuch and Y. Kawashima. 2008. Establishing chitosan coated PLGA nanosphere platform loaded with wide variety of nucleic acid by complexation with cationic compound for gene delivery. Int. J. of Pharma. 354: 210–216.

Takeuchi, H., H. Yamamoto and Y. Kawashima. 2001. Mucoadhesive nanoparticulate systems for peptide drug delivery. Adv. Drug Del. Rev. 47: 39–54.

Weindel, K., J. Moringlane, D. Marm and H. Weich. 1994. Detection of quantification of vascular endothelial growth factor/ vascular permeability factor in brain tumor tissue and cyst fluid: the key to angiogenesis? Neurosurgery 35: 439–448.

Weissleder, H., C. Cheng and A. Bogdanova. 1997. Magnetically labelled cells can be detected by MRI imaging. J. Magn. Reson. Imag. 7: 258–263.

Wieland, A., T. Houchin-Ray and L. Shea. 2007. Non-vitral vector delivery from PEG-hyaluronic acid hydrogels. J. Cont. Rel. 120: 233–241.

Willams, J., R. Lansdown, R. Sweitzer and M. Romanoski. 2003. Nanoparticle drug delivery for intravenous delivery of topoisomerase inhibitors. J. Cont. Rel. 91: 167–172.

Xie, Y., M. Kaminski and M.D. Torno. 2007. Physicochemical characteristics of magnetic microspheres containing tissue plasminogen activator. J. Magnetism and Magnetic Material. 311: 376–378.

Xu, Y. and Y. Du. 2003. Effect of molecular structure of chitosan on protein delivery properties of chitosan nanoparticles. Int. J. Pharma. 250: 215–226.

Xu, Q. and J. Czernuszka. 2008. Controlled release of amoxicillin from hydroxyapatite-coated poly(lactic-co-glycolic acid) microspheres. J. Cont. Release 127: 146–153.

Yamamoto, H., Y. Juno, S. Sugimoto, H. Takeuchi and Y. Kawashima. 2005. Surface-modified PLGA nanosphere with chitosan improved pulmonary delivery of calcitonin by mucoadhesion and opening of the intercellular tight junctions. J. Contrl. Release. 102: 373–381.

Yeh, T., W. Zhang and S. Ildastad. 1993. Intracellular labelling of T-cells with superparamagnetic contrast agents. Mag. Res. Med. 30: 617–627.

Yuan, F., M. Dellian, D. Fukumura and M. Leunig. 1995. Vascular permeability in human tumor xenograft: molecular size dependence and cut-off size. Cancer Res. 55: 3752–3756.

Zhao, R., R. Xu, Z. Shen, J. Lu and X. Ni. 2007. Experimental investigation of the collapse of laser-generated cavitation bubbles near a solid boundary. Opt. Laser Technol. 39: 68–972.

Zheng, W. 2009. A water-in-oil-in-oil-in-water (W/O/O/W) method for producing drug-releasing, double-walled microspheres. Int. J. of Pharma. 374: 90–95.

Zharov, V., K. Mercer, E. Galitovskaya and M. Smeltzer. 2006. Photothermal nanotherapeutics and nanodiagnostics for selective killing of bacteria targeted with gold nanoparticles. Biophys. J. 90: 619–627.

Zharov, V., E. Galitovskaya, C. Johnson and T. Kelly. 2005. Synergistic enhancement of selective nanophotothermolysis with gold nanoclusters: Potential for cancer therapy. Lasers Surg. Med. 37: 219–226.

Zharov, V., J. Kim, D. Curiel and M. Everts. 2005. Self-assembling nanoclusters in living systems: application for integrated photothermal nanodiagnostics and nanotherapy. Nanomedicine 1: 326–345.

12

Theranostic: Cancer Diagnosis and Therapy

12.1 Introduction

Cancer is a complicated disease caused by genetic instability and accumulation of multiple molecular alterations causing the cells to introduce uncontrolled proliferation, genomic, and chromosomal instability, and is the leading cause of death worldwide. In 2007, it was estimated that about 10 million cases of cancer occurred globally, with nearly 1.43 million new cases and 560,000 deaths projected to occur in the US in the year 2008 (American Cancer Society 2008). According to Cancer Research Society of Canada, about 196,900 new cases of cancer were expected in 2015 in Canada, i.e., 1 person every 3 minutes, every day. Similarly, Cancer Statistics Center of American Cancer Society predicted that in 2016, there will be an estimated 1,685,210 new cancer cases diagnosed, and 595,690 cancer deaths in the US. The projected numbers of new cancer cases and deaths in 2016 should not be compared with previous years to track cancer trends because they are model-based and vary from year to year for reasons other than changes in cancer occurrence. Age-standardized incidence and death rates should be used to measure cancer trends. Metastasis of cancerous cells from the primary site (i.e., tumor) to other organs in the body is governed by their ability to leave the tumor and invade through membranes and tissues, survive in circulation by avoiding immune attack and residing in surrounding tissues. To maintain growth, cancer cells need to initiate the formation of new blood vessels, hence providing a constant supply of nutrients. After a cancer is metastasized in the body, it becomes almost impossible to treat and often leads to patient mortality.

Therefore, the major concern of current cancer research is to develop clinically useful technologies for improved diagnosis and treatment of the disease in patients. However, the current cancer treatment consists of doses of compounds that are non-specific and highly toxic. The inability of conventional diagnosis techniques to detect cancer early and at a curable stage further hinders effective treatment options. The cancer treatment strategy has remained essentially unchanged: surgical resection of the tumor followed by either chemotherapy, radiotherapy, or a combination of both, which normally cause unselective damage to healthy tissue (Hull et al. 2014). Also, treatment failure can be due to a number of reasons, such as the presence of residual cells left after surgical removal of the tumor, resistance to chemotherapies, and physiological obstructions to treatments such as blood brain barrier (Alexis et al. 2010). The main obstacles in effective prevention of cancer are: early detection, poor drug availability, nonspecific systemic drug distribution, inadequate drug delivery to tumor, and inability to monitor therapeutic responses in real time (Gindy and Prud'homme 2009). Fortunately, during the last decade significant scientific research and progress have been made in understanding of cancer at the genetic, molecular, and cellular levels, hence providing valuable opportunities for cancer diagnosis and treatment. Parallel to this, nanotechnology, which is one of the most popular research areas particularly in biomedical applications, could offer potential solutions to many of the aforementioned problems. One key branch of nanotechnology in nanomedicine is nanomaterials, as discussed in Chapter 9. Engineered nanoparticles open the door to new noninvasive strategies for cancer therapy: (a) Nanoparticle-enhanced photothermal therapy (PTT) where nanostructures such as nanoshells, nanorods, and carbon nanotubes are used due to their strong absorption in NIR region, (b) Nanoparticle-enhanced radiotherapy (RT) where AuNPs can enhance the effect of radiotherapy on tumors thus, reduced toxicity to surrounding normal tissues, (c) Nanoparticle-enhanced radiofrequency therapy (RF) where by using AuNPs-induced heating helps to achieve tumor cell destruction without inserting probes into tissue as in traditional RF ablation, and (d) Nanoparticle-enhanced theranostic. The term theranostic was coined by Funkhouser (2002) to define a combined modality of therapeutic and diagnostic. Such a combination acting as a single system is capable of providing more specific and efficient system for detecting and treating diseases in a single clinical procedure. Utilizing NPs as theranostic agent is a promising approach where it is possible to selectively localize them in a tumor without additional undesirable side effects, such as damaging the surrounding healthy tissues. It was discussed in the previous chapter that tumor blood vessels tend to be diluted and leaky, hence NPs can easily be extravasated from the blood pool into tumor and be retained due to poor lymphatic drainage leading to EPR effect. Also, nanomaterials are effectively used for drug delivery, cancer cell targeting via protein, and small molecule binding, intracellular drug release, *ex vivo* diagnostic applications, and bioimaging. An ideal multifunctional theranostic system must meet the following conditions for safe use: (a) rapidly and selectively accumulate inside target, (b) efficiently deliver a required amount of drug without complications, (c) be cleared from body within hours or biodegraded into nontoxic products.

12.2 Theranostic nanomaterials

By definition, theranostic nanomaterials are those materials which satisfy the requirements of imaging and therapy with no side effects or cytotoxicity. Electromagnetic radiation from visible to longer wavelengths are attractive sources for transferring energy to living tissues. However, as it is explained in Chapter 6, the depth of the penetration of photons within the tissue depends strongly on the wavelength of source and the target-specific chromophore. The therapeutic part of theranostic is known as hyperthermia. The examples of such sources are radio frequency (RF), microwaves (MW), ultrasound (US), and laser radiation. The application of suitable nanomaterials can greatly enhance both imaging and PPT due to EPR effect. Now, let us quickly remind ourselves that in the case of metallic nanoparticles, SPR (see 9.3.3) is a localized surface plasmons (LSP). When a photon interacts with a NP, LSP is produced, due to which two processes can occur: (a) either the photons decay radiatively by emission of photons, which can be used for imaging purpose based on the scattering process, or (b) they decay non-radiatively based on the electron-hole excitation, i.e., absorption. As a result of thermalization via phonon scattering with the ion lattice, the NPs are heated and it is this generated heat which is used for therapeutic purpose. Also, it is noteworthy that the position of LSP strongly depends on both the material type and the size of NP. For example, for aluminium (UV) (Knight et al. 2012), silver (blue) (Scholl et al. 2012), gold (green), and copper (red) (Chan et al. 2007).

Magnetic nanoparticles (MNPs): A special kind of MNPs, i.e., SPIONs (see §9.2) exhibit interesting properties, such as superparamagnetism, high saturation field, and extra anisotropy. Their small size facilitates them with an effective surface area, low sedimentation rate, tissular diffusion, and reduced dipole-dipole moment. In addition, the capabilities such as attachment to a functional molecule, giving target magnetic properties, permitting manipulation and transportation to a particular location through the control of an external magnetic field produced by, for example, a permanent magnet-all make SPIONs potential candidate for theranostic. Prior to their clinical applications, a full consideration must be given to biocompatibility, biodegradability, nanotoxicity (see §9.6), stability, shape, and size of MNPs. The stability in turn is controlled by NP dimension and surface chemistry. They must be coated with a biocompatible polymer after synthesis in order to prevent agglomeration, thus providing monodispersivity as much as possible. Once MNPs are heated up by alternating magnetic field gradient, they can be used as hyperthermia agents to destroy tumoric cells. The *in vivo* applications are grouped into (a) Therapeutic: hyperthermia and drug targeting, and (b) Diagnosis: NMR, MRI, and *in vitro* applications are mainly diagnostics.

Gold nanoparticle (GNPs): It is well established that GNPs provide a versatile platform for theranostic applications due to their biocompatibility and surface modification capability. The surface of gold has a significant affinity for thiol groups or amines, enabling these NPs to be easily PEGylated, i.e., modifying their surface with PEG for improved biocompatibility. Additionally, the scattering properties (extrinsic) of GNPs make them suitable candidates for optical and spectroscopic tags, imaging, and biological sensing. However due to lack of intrinsic fluorescent properties, they cannot be used for optical imaging. Spherical GNPs in the range of 20–30 nm strongly absorb light between 520–530 nm, i.e., the position of resonance peak, and some interesting results have been achieved using pulsed and cw lasers (Afifi et al. 2013, Mendoza-Nova et al. 2013, Li et al. 2009). However, the main problem of using the spherical GNPs for PTT is that the position resonance peak lies between 520 and 580 nm, where hemoglobin and oxyhemoglobin also strongly absorb light in this range. Therefore, healthy tissue can be thermally damaged due to unwanted radiation exposure, making them less ideal for PTT. Another advantage of GNPs is that they have a higher atomic number and X-ray absorption coefficient than iodine, which makes them potential contrast agents for computed tomography (CT) and radiotherapy sensitizers (Kim et al. 2009).

Gold Nanoshells (GNSs): These structures are composed of a dielectric core (e.g., SiO_2 or Fe_3O_4) surrounded by a thin gold layer. Depending on the core-shell ratio, the SPR is easily tunable throughout the NIR region (700–1200 nm). Also, they are easily modified for simultaneous imaging and PTT. The number of GNSs delivered to a tumor is determined by the radius of the NS, i.e., larger the size, the less NSs can be delivered. In a study, Bardhan et al. (2010) used multimodal GNS with iron oxide for MRI and ICG on the surface as NIR fluorophore, PEG for a better biocompatibility, and antibodies for higher and more specific biodistribution and uptake into the tumor (Bardhan et al. 2009).

Nanorods (NRs): As it was mentioned, the SPR of AuNPs varies between 520 and 580 nm, which is a serious limitation for their application as an *in vivo* contrast agent due to high scattering by stratum corneum of skin tissue and high absorption by hemoglobin. On the other hand, the therapeutic window covers a range between 650–1100 nm, where the optical absorption by tissues is minimum due to low absorption and scattering of hemoglobin and water. Thus, an alternative approach is to use NRs which are basically ellipsoidal structures, with shorter axis being about 10–45 nm, and the longer axis about 50 nm to several hundred nanometers with two distinct modes of (i) transverse and (ii) longitudinal. The resonance position is tunable throughout NIR region by changing the aspect ratio, i.e., as it is increased, the longitudinal plasmon mode red-shifted significantly and the transverse mode blue-shifted slightly.

Carbon nanoparticles (CNPs): The three naturally occurring allotropes of carbon are graphite, diamond, and amorphous carbon. Carbon nanotubes are allotropes of carbon and fullerene with a significant thermal conductivity, mechanical stability, and electrical properties. Their structure is comprised of a graphene sheet rolled at defined angles. The properties of these materials are strongly influenced by combination of angles and radii, and whether the nanotube has metallic or semiconductor properties. A multi-walled nanotubes (MWCNTs) consists of number of concentric layers of single-wall nanotubes (SWCNTs). Carbon nanoparticles are being explored widely for use in cancer treatment. Studies reveal that cancer treatment using radio waves can heat and destroy a tumor, lymphoma, or metastasized cancer. In an experiment Burke et al. (2009) used a cw Nd:YAG laser to irradiate MWCNTs and showed that kidney tumor could be treated in this way. He used one single short 30-sec treatment with low laser intensity (3 Wcm^{-2}), which was sufficient to achieve a complete ablation of the tumor.

Liposomes: These are spherical phospholipid bilayers with sizes varying between 50 and 1000 nm, that can spontaneously form in aqueous media to form either water-soluble or water-insoluble anti-cancer drugs and proteins within hydrophilic core or inside their phospholipid bilayer. Liposomes are increasingly being used as nanocarriers for pharmaceuticals. Depending on their phospholipid composition, the properties of the liposomes are tunable. When cholesterol is added into the liposomes, the melting temperature of liposome can be set to a defined temperature.

Dendrimers: Dendrimers are a class of well-defined nanostructured macromolecules with a three dimensional structure composed of three architectural components: a core, an interior of shells (generations) consisting of repeating branch-cell units, and terminal functional groups (the outer shell or periphery)

(Tomalia 2005). They are synthesized from a polyfunctional core by adding branched monomers that react with the functional groups of the core, in turn leaving end groups that can react again (Menjoge et al. 2010). One such example is poly (amidoamine) (PAMAM), which acts as a template or stabilizer for preparation of inorganic nanocomposites. Some important properties of these structures include a large number of end groups, the functionable cores, the nanoporous nature of the interior at higher generations (Peng et al. 2008). Also, their chemical structures, molecular weight, and molecular size can provide special type of functionality, which play a role in developing fields of materials science.

12.3 Hyperthermia

12.3.1 Background

Using heat to treat cancer is by no means a modern concept, and in fact traces back to 3000 BC, where cautery was used until the mid-19th century, when the heating effect of electric current was noticed and developed. 'Diathermy' is a term given to the process of using currents with frequencies of several hundred kilohertz to produce heat at depth in tissues. Hyperthermia is classed into two categories: (i) Mild hyperthermia, where a temperature rise is high enough to cause partial cell killing and to damage and sensitize cancer cells to chemotherapy and radiotherapy (Svaanad et al. 1990), (ii) thermos-ablation, where the temperature rise exceeds 46°C and causes cell necrosis (Lopez-Molina et al. 2008). The early recorded microwaves in cancer therapy was at 375 MHz, then developed to 3000 MHz using a power magnetron after World War II.

1) Basically, the mechanism of MW or RF (500 kHz–10 MHz) diathermy is based on induced dipole moments during the field and tissue interaction, where the charges are displaced, producing permanent dipole moments. Once they are aligned, the heat produced as a result of work done is then absorbed by the tissue. It was not until late 1960s that the interaction of electromagnetic field with biological tissues for deep tumor treatment and the related questions, regarding solution to the problem of heating tissues, uniform thermal distribution, preventing healthy tissues from undesirable damage, applicator design, etc. were considered seriously. For frequencies in the range of 10–2450 MHz the penetration depth of high water content tissues (e.g., skin and muscle) is of the order of 200–20 mm. In low water content tissues (e.g., fat and bone) the values are more varied since the electrical properties of these are more sensitive to small variations in water content. Typically, penetration depths are an order of magnitude greater and wavelengths are about three times greater than those for high content tissues. In the case of superficial tumors, the applicator can be placed in contact with skin so that the treatment field is quite well defined and power requirements are modest and stray electromagnetic radiation can be made minimum. However, in the case of deep tumors, it is more challenging and the main goal is to produce therapeutic temperatures throughout tumors deep in the body in a predictable way. This involves careful and confined deposition of energy inside whole tumor, which itself is placed inside a healthy tissue environment. Thus, possible differences in blood perfusion within tumor and normal tissues are then relied upon to achieve differences in temperature, and hence to avoid unnecessary thermal damage.

2) Ultrasound hyperthermia. This extends from 300 kHz to 3 MHz and the diffraction spreading of the beam from transducers of, say 40–100 mm diameter is small because of the small wavelengths involved (the wavelength at 1 MHz is $\approx$ 1.5 mm in soft tissue). Ultrasonic penetration into soft tissue at these frequencies is such that the intensity is halved over a distance of roughly 25 wavelengths and is greater than that associated with MW techniques. However, the major disadvantages are (a) the significant differences in acoustic impedance between soft and hard tissues (bone) or gas, thus causing considerable reflection and little transmission across these interfaces, and (b) the high absorption coefficient for US in bone. Another technique which was developed in 1970s is to implant 'seeds' of ferromagnetic material into tumor and subsequently heat them in an RF magnetic field. The ferromagnetic material is heated to a much greater extent than the surrounding tissues and a local region of therapeutic temperatures can be achieved due to heat transport from seeds. Curie temperature of these seed materials has been chosen between 45–50°C to obtain automatic

temperature regulation within the implant. In hyperthermia, the resolution and accuracy should be at least 0.25°C because of the strong dependence of biological responses on temperature. An acceptable spatial resolution of 5–10 mm and a temporal resolution of a few seconds is desirable to monitor the time-varying temperatures observed during treatments.

3) Laser hyperthermia-Problems with RF technique include: indifferent energy localization to the target organ with excessive heating of the superficial tissues and non-uniform heating patterns which result in variable temperature profiles. Microwave applications suffer from significant loss of tissue penetration for frequencies greater than 1000 MHz and unacceptable temperature gradients associated with coaxial applicators. The main drawback of ultrasound is the loss of penetration due to interaction with gas or bone, thus restricting its applications for most thoracic and abdominal use. Lasers, as fully explained in Chapter 3, have distinct optical properties which make them unique in many ways. With regard to hyperthermia, one such property is monochromacity, which governs the wavelength selectivity by an organ and predictable induction of tissue is expected. Also, light can be delivered by an optical fibre to target area with minimal loss of power, and for larger target areas, bundles of fibre can be utilized.

12.3.2 Physical principle of SPION-enhanced hyperthermia

There are four different mechanisms by which magnetic materials can generate heat in an alternating magnetic field (AMF) (Van der Zee 2002):

(a) generation of eddy currents in magnetic particles with size > 1 μm, (b) hysteresis losses in magnetic particles > 1 μm and multidomain magnetic particles, (c) relaxation losses in superparamagnetic single domain particles (SPIONs), and (d) frictional losses in viscous suspensions. When MNPs are subject to AMF, energy is produced in the form of heat, which then dissipates into surrounding medium, and if the temperature is sufficiently high, can destroy the cancer cells. A major advantage of employing MNPs (or GNPs in their own case) is that AMF can be localized in a certain region of body where MNPs are collected. By varying the frequency, current of AMF, size, and composition of the MNPs, the temperature generated from the MNPs can be controlled. It is thought that the heat is generated through Neel relaxation and Brownian motion. The Neel mechanism is explained through the motion of magnetic moments inside the particle in the magnetic field of the coil, the AMF causes the magnetic moments within MNPs to rotate, producing internal friction. When the field is turned off, the moments return to equilibrium position. At this stage, the energy is released in the form of thermal energy. The Neel time constant is defined as

$$\tau_N = \tau_0 e^{\Delta E/k_B T} \tag{12.1}$$

where ΔE is the activation energy and $k_B T$ is the thermal energy.

Brownian motion requires the rotation of the MNPs as a whole, therefore, the heat is generated through frictional movement in its surroundings. MNPs can be trapped inside biological tissues, which in turn block free rotation of the particles, hence preventing the generation of frictional heat. The Brownian constant of time is defined as

$$\tau_B = \frac{3\eta V_B}{k_B T} \tag{12.2}$$

where V_B is the hydrodynamic volume, i.e., the total volume of a particle coated with surfactant, η is the viscosity of the suspension medium.

12.3.3 Physical principle of GNP-enhanced radiotherapy and imaging

Cancer therapy largely relies on chemotherapy and radiotherapy in which most anti-cancer drugs are taken up by cells with high proliferation rate, such as cancer cells. However, it is an accepted fact that normal tissue also suffer from chemotherapeutic drugs resulting in significant side effects. Despite the long journey since the advent of X-ray in nineteenth century and significant improvements in machines, imaging and therapy techniques and services, some major issues still remain unresolved including: local control of the primary tumor, normal tissue toxicity, requirement of high doses of radiation, and insufficient contrast resolution. Indeed from a therapeutic point of view, radiosensitizing can enhance the dose specifically absorbed by tumor tissue leading to a better tumor killing. Radiation therapy has mainly focused on: (a) increasing the dose radiation delivered to the tumor, (b) sensitizing the radioresistant part of tumor cells to conventional doses of radiation, and (c) targeting cancer cells while applying radiation therapy. Similarly, from imaging point of view, short imaging times of traditional iodine-based contrast agents, low sensitivity and resolution can be improved by using agents with enhanced X-ray attenuation capabilities. It at this stage where the history of radiation oncology shows us how valuable multidisciplinary approaches and ideas succeeded to bridge between life science and physical science. One such loud and clear example which has recently been highlighted is the use of nanomaterials such as GNPs. In addition to all the advantages of GNPs which were discussed, one more property should be mentioned which plays a key role with respect to radiosensitization, i.e., gold has high atomic number (Z_{Au} = 79, that is number of protons). It is known that high Z materials produce X-rays more efficiently, thus allowing high absorption and enhancement of ionizing radiation as well as superior X-ray attenuation for imaging applications.

While the energy of most of the electrons striking the target is dissipated in the form of heat, the remaining few electrons produce useful X-rays. Every now and then, one of these electrons gets close enough to the nucleus of a target atom to be deviated from its path and emits an X-ray photon (i.e., Bremsstrahlung or braking radiation) that has some of its energy. The amount of Bremsstrahlung produced for a given number of striking electrons depends on two factors: (i) the Z of the target—the more the protons, the greater the acceleration of the electrons (ii) the kilovolt (kV) peak-the faster the electrons, the more likely it is that they will penetrate into the region of the nucleus. Sometimes a fast electron strikes a K-shell electron in a target atom and knocks it out of its orbit (i.e., Auger/Coster-Kronig electrons). The vacancy in the K shell is filled immediately when an electron from an outer shell of the atom falls into it. In either of above cases, the ejected particles form tracks of ionization in the tissue. In the case of high Z NPs, the secondary particles locally enhance the physical dose delivered around the metallic NPs (Butterworth et al. 2012). Photoelectric phenomena are dominant at kV energies and directly proportional to Z-number of the material. Therefore, photoelectric cross-sections of gold are much higher than materials such as tissue, containing carbon (Z = 6), hydrogen (Z = 1), nitrogen (Z = 7), and oxygen (Z = 8). Cho (2005) has demonstrated that the yield of electrons is increased up to 10 times when 0.1% w/w of GNPs are incorporated into biological tissue irradiated with kV radiation beam with energy of < 200 keV, and approximately double when the same tissue is irradiated with megavoltage clinical beam ($\approx$ 6 MeV). Leehtman et al. (2011, 2013) have shown that the effectiveness of GNP-mediated radiosensitization depends on the size of GNPs, the rate of photoelectric absorption, the characteristics of the Auger electrons, and the position of GNPs inside the cell. Berbeco et al. (2011) suggested that GNPs can enhance the tumor-killing efficacy of 6 MV X-ray by increasing radiation dose to the tumor microvasculature and endothelial cells.

12.4 Applications

12.4.1 Experimental validation and simulation of Fourier and non-Fourier heat transfer equation during laser nano-phototherapy of lung cancer cells: An in vitro assay (Khosroshahi et al. 2014)

This paper investigates the numerical scheme extended to solve the non-Fourier form of bioheat transfer equation and the experimental trials which were conducted to validate the numerical simulation. MNPs were prepared via co-precipitation and modified with a silica layer. The amino modified Fe_3O_4/SiO_2 nanoshells were covered with gold colloids producing nanoshells of $Fe_3O_4/SiO_2/Au$ (MNSs). *In vitro* assays were performed to determine the effect of apoptosis of QU-DB lung cancer cells based on the cells morphology changes. Cell damage was reduced by decreasing the power density of laser. Also, a larger area of damage on cell culture plates was observed at longer intervals of laser irradiation. The effect of nanoshell concentration and irradiation rate has been evaluated. The experiment confirmed a hyperbolic behaviour of thermal propagation. The results revealed that three dimensional implementation of bioheat equation is likely to be more accurate than two dimensional study.

Introduction

The latest statistics show that cancer remains one of the leading causes of death worldwide, accounting for 7.6 million deaths (around 13% of all deaths) in 2008 (WHO). However, advances in nanotechnology have changed the very foundations of cancer diagnosis, treatment, and prevention, and hence offer some exciting possibilities to keep pace with today's advances in cancer treatment (Srinivas et al. 2002, Choi et al. 2010). In recent years, conventional surgical treatments of cancer have been rendered ineffective, because these techniques are extremely invasive and usually associated with high morbidity. Among recent technologies for cancer treatment, thermal therapies employing a variety of heat sources, including ultrasound (Jolesz and Hynynen 2002), microwaves (Seki et al. 1999, Gazelle et al. 2000), radiofrequency (Mirza et al. 2001), lasers (Amin et al. 1993, Nolsøe et al. 1993) can provide a minimally invasive alternative to conventional surgical treatment of solid tumors. Technological advancements, such as small, compact, high-power laser systems with actively cooled applicators, have introduced highly promising modalities for cancer therapy, most commonly the photothermal and the photodynamic therapy (McKenzie and Carruth 1984, Wang et al. 2010, Simon et al. 2013, Nicolodelli et al. 2013). On the other hand, emergence of noble metal nanostructures with remarkable set of optical, chemical and physical properties, has regulated thermal energy into target regions delivered by optical fibres to provide a lethal dose of heat with as little damage to surrounding healthy tissue as possible (Huang et al. 2007, Skrabalak et al. 2007). Gold nanoshells are spherical particles with diameters typically ranging in size from 10 to 200 nm and are composed of a dielectric core covered by a thin gold shell. Unique to nanoshells, is their localized surface plasmon resonance (LSPR) which greatly intensifies their interaction with the electromagnetic field. The light interaction with metal induces resonance effect, which arises from collective oscillations of conductive metal electrons at the nanoshell surface. This subsequently couples with the surface plasmons to create self-sustaining, propagating electromagnetic waves known as surface plasmon polaritons (SPPs).

Relative thickness of the core and shell layers of the nanoparticle has a key role in the plasmon resonance characteristic and the resultant optical absorption of nanoshells (Loo et al. 2005, Khosroshahi et al. 2011, Khanadeev et al. 2011, Avetisyan et al. 2012, Hasannejad and Khosroshahi 2013). The absorption band of core-shell particles can be tuned by adjusting the ratio of the thickness of the gold shell to the diameter of the dielectric core to enable photothermal therapy in appropriate regions (Oldenburg et al. 1998). From a photothermal therapy perspective, the wave length of maximal absorption and the absorption cross-section are key features to consider when selecting a particle for hyperthermia. Meanwhile, size and surface characteristics of the nanoparticle are of prime importance in the biodistribution and rapid clearance of nanoparticle from the blood which affects nanoparticle delivery to target sites (Huang et al. 2007, Skrabalak et al. 2007). In order to optimize the delivery of gold nanoparticles and enhance ablative therapy, functionalization of nanoparticles and their surface modification with cargoes such as peptides, antibodies, and small molecule ligands have been reported in the literature (Oldenburg et al. 1998, Loo et al. 2005, Kumar et al. 2008, Khosroshahi and Ghazanfari 2012). Other advantages of gold nanoparticles, including biocompatibility and non-cytotoxicity, have opened several additional promising research avenues for further optimization of the gold nanoparticle-mediated photothermal therapy (Pankhurst et al. 2003, Lewinski et al. 2008, Murphy et al. 2008).

Recent developments in computational modelling of thermal therapy have attempted to model the heating profile of irradiated tissue, which could be essential for effective clinical translation (Elliott et al. 2007, Vera and Bayazitoglu 2009). Accurate modeling and simulation of thermal distribution and temperature elevation of nanoparticle-laden tissue is of importance for describing heat transfer in a tissue and would lead to optimized thermal ablation in solid tumors. Numerous mathematical models have been proposed to gain further information on the thermal behaviour and heat affected zone of nanoparticle-laden tissue. In most of them, the temperature distributions in the tissue were obtained using the heat transfer equation proposed by Pennes (1948). Previous studies have employed both parabolic heat transfer equation (PHTE) and hyperbolic heat transfer equation (HHTE) to model heating of biological tissues, however, many of them considered laser heating source as a generation term without dealing with plasmonic heating source. The principle goal of this report is to compare the experimental and numerical results in order to achieve a qualitative understanding of the nanoshell-assisted laser hyperthermia, where for the simulation, the PHTE and HHTE were solved numerically using a finite element analysis.

Materials and methods

Synthesis and coating Fe$_3$O$_4$/SiO$_2$ nanoshells with gold

Fe$_3$O$_4$ NPs and SiO$_2$ coated Fe$_3$O$_4$ NPs were synthesized via chemical coprecipitation and Stober methods, respectively as described before (Khosroshahi and Ghazanfari 2012). Finally, the Fe$_3$O$_4$/SiO$_2$ nanoparticles were coated with 2–3 nm gold nanoparticles to get a dark pink solution, which is characteristic of nanoshell formation, as suggested (Pham et al. 2002, Ji et al. 2007).

Preparation of cells and gold coated Fe$_3$O$_4$/SiO$_2$ nanoshells compound

QU-DB lung cancer cells (purchased from the Pasteur Institute, National Cell Bank of Iran) were seeded in 96-well tissue culture plates and incubated at 37°C and 5% CO$_2$. Dulbecco's Modified Eagle Medium (DMEM-GIBCO) supplemented with 10% fetal bovine serum (FBS-GIBCO) was used as cell culture medium (C.C.M.). Serum-free cell culture medium containing nanoparticles maintained under UV for 4 hours before adding to cell cultures. After 24 hours incubation period, cell culture medium was replaced with two different concentrations of gold nanoshell suspension including 0.01 and 0.1 mg/ml. The nanoshells used in our experiments had a diameter of ~85 nm (75–100 nm) with an average shell thickness of ~35 nm which was measured with transmission electron microscopy (TEM). TEM micrograph (Fig. 12.1a) shows clustering of small gold NPs assembled on the surface of larger silica NPs. The AFM image in Fig. 12.1b indicates some possible agglomeration causing surface rough morphology.

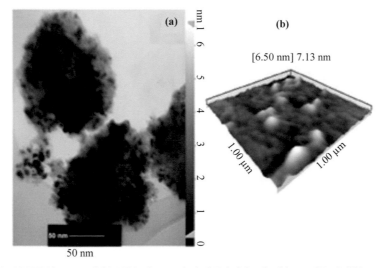

Figure 12.1. (a) TEM image and (b) AFM micrographs in 3-D-height of gold coated Fe$_3$O$_4$/SiO$_2$ nanoshells.

In vitro assay

The lung cancer cells were first incubated with serum free cell culture medium containing synthesized gold coated Fe$_3$O$_4$/SiO$_2$ nanoshells for 24 hours. The cell-NP medium was then irradiated by a NIR diode laser at 800 nm ± 10 nm with focal spot of 7 mm^2 to evaluate the heat induced apoptosis. Cells were divided into two treatment groups. Severe hyperthermic treatment with 184, 157, and 71 W/cm^2 for a minute and mild hyperthermic treatment with 42 and 14 W/cm^2 for 3 minutes. The temperature was monitored by a digital thermometer with 0.1°C precision (CHY502A1, MULTI LOGGER), connected to a laptop for further processing. The effects of hyperthermic treatment and heat-induced apoptosis were evaluated according to alteration of cell morphology. Living QU-DB lung cancer cells have fibroblast-like morphology, while damaged cells shrink and have rounded shape (Joanitti et al. 2010). Cell membrane, cytoskeleton (Kong et al. 2000) intracellular proteins (Lee et al. 2009), nucleic acid, and mitochondrial function are molecular effectors during hyperthermia, and it has been shown that actin filaments become insoluble during hyperthermia (Nikfarjam et al. 2005). Studies have shown the shrinkage or morphological alterations of endothelial cells in response to heat stress which have been attributed to disaggregation of the cytoskeleton after hyperthermia (Kong et al. 2000). This phenomenon has been supported independently in electron microscopic studies (Clark et al. 1983). Changes in cell membrane function are generally considered to be the main cause of cell death. Observation of altered membrane fluidity and permeability with increase in temperature, support this concept (Nikfarjam et al. 2005). These phenomena may become evident during the recovery phase of the cell to the base-line temperature, but not immediately after heating (Clark et al. 1983). Therefore, cells undergoing apoptosis shrink and exhibit cytoplasmic and chromatin condensation and in the final stages they fragment into small apoptotic bodies (Soto-Cerrato et al. 2005). Figure 12.2a illustrates normal morphology of cancer cells, i.e., before treatment. To determine the effect of laser radiation on cultured cells without nanoparticles, they were irradiated at 157 W/cm², and as is seen in Fig. 12.2b, no significant change was observed in cell morphology.

By increasing the exposure time to 180 seconds at lower power densities, the damaged area was extended, and more cells at the region far from the laser beam were affected because of heat transfer. Figure 12.3 demonstrates the cellular morphology changes at 157 W/cm² for one minute. As shown in Fig. 12.3, cells in the irradiated region have a circular shape, which is the characteristic of apoptotic cells (Joanitti et al. 2010). The percentage of apoptosis was calculated by dividing the total number of rounded cells by the total number of cells at the focal point of the laser, as well as the immediate surrounding area (6 × 104 μm²). At 184 and 157 W/cm² and irradiation time of 60s all the cells suffered apoptosis. But, the

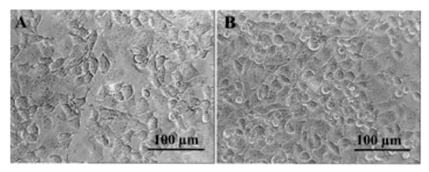

Figure 12.2. Optical microscopy of (a) control cells (untreated tumoric cells) 24 hours after subculture and (b) the cells after laser treatment without nanoshells.

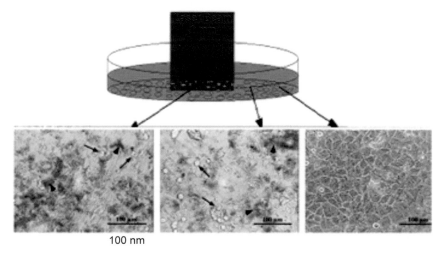

100 nm

Figure 12.3. Illustration of QU-DB lung cancer cells after laser irradiation at different powers of 157 W/cm² for 60 s at 0.1 mg/ml. Three different parts were photographed and depicted in a row: the focal point of the laser beam at the center (left), the adjacent region (middle) and far region (right). Arrow head: nanoshells colonies; arrow: dead cells.

heat-inducted death was reduced to 92.78% at 71 W/cm² during the same period of time. The percentage of damaged cells and gold nanoshells decreases with the increase of distance from the center of the beam. In this situation, the percentage of damaged cells was reduced to 57% and 47.15% at 42 and 14 W/cm², respectively. This experiment was repeated three times in order to prove the observed reproducibility of the data. Furthermore, the effect of NPs concentration on cell apoptosis is shown in Fig. 12.4, where the amount of damaged cells is reduced by decreasing the concentration to 0.01 mg/ml at 157 W/cm² during a one minute exposure.

The results indicate that the concentration of nanoshells had significant effects on the amount of heat generated at a given power density. For core–shell, the NP efficiency parameter has the form (Pustovalov et al. 2009)

$$\frac{\Delta T_0}{I_0} = \frac{K_{abs} r_1}{4k_\infty} \times \left[1 - \exp\left(-\frac{3k_\infty t_p}{r_1^2 (c_0 \rho_0 r_0^3 + c_1 \rho_1 (1 - r_0^3/r_1^3))} \right) \right] \tag{12.3}$$

where I_0 is the intensity of the laser radiation during pulse duration, tp and K_{abs} is the efficiency factor of absorption, k_∞ is the coefficient of thermal conduction of the ambient medium, c_0, ρ_0 and c_1, ρ_1 are the heat capacity and density of the material of the core (Magnetite-Silica) and shell (Gold) accordingly, r_0 and r_1 are the radii of the core and shell and the thickness of the shell $r_0 = r_1 - r_0$. The maximum value of the parameter $\Delta T_0/I_0$ represents the efficiency of transformation of absorbed optical energy by NPs into thermal energy. In our case this corresponds to about 12% and 7% for C.C.M. + MNSs at 0.1 mg/ml and 0.01 mg/ml + QU-DB lung cancer cells, respectively. By increasing the power density, the temperature increased faster and higher. One important aspect of this finding was that the maximum temperature of 56 and 59°C of C.C.M. decreased to ≈ 46 and 50°C for 0.01 mg/ml and 0.1 mg/ml, respectively, which likely is attributed to the protein adsorption in the presence of cells. Optical microscopy showed that the majority of cells have become circular due to induced thermal stress. Clearly most of the gold-coated Fe_3O_4/SiO_2 nanoshells are accumulated at the center of the wells, where the laser beam was focused. This may be due to the movement of nanoshells in the direction of the force gradient towards the center of the beam (Missirlis and Spiliotis 2002).

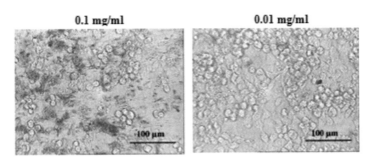

Figure 12.4. Illustration of QU-DB lung cancer cells after hyperthermia treatment at 157 W/cm² and two different concentrations of gold coated Fe_3O_4/SiO_2 nanoshells: 0.1 mg/ml (left) and 0.01 mg/ml (right) at 60s. More colonies and apoptotic cells can be seen in the sample with concentration of 0.1 mg/ml.

Mathematical framework

The well-known Fourier's law of heat conduction presents a linear relationship between the heat flux through a material and the gradient of temperature (T), whose differential form is:

$$\bar{q}(\bar{r},t) = -K\nabla T(\bar{r},t) \tag{12.4}$$

where K and ∇ are thermal conductivity of material in W/mK and gradient operator, respectively. The Fourier's law is simple in mathematics and has been widely used, even though it is only an empirical relationship. In principle, however, the Fourier's law leads to an unphysical infinite heat propagation speed within a continuum field for transient heat conduction processes because of its parabolic characteristics, which is in contradiction to the theory of relativity (Joseph and Preziosi 1989, Cahill et al. 2003). To overcome this spatio-temporal challenge, especially in ultra-small scales, the CV model proposed by Cattaneo and Vernotte (Cattaneo 1958, Vernotte 1961):

$$\tau\frac{\partial\bar{q}(\bar{r},t)}{\partial t} + \bar{q}(\bar{r},t) = -K\nabla T(\bar{r},t) \tag{12.5}$$

where τ denotes the relaxation time that tissue responds to the heat perturbation. The CV model gives rise to a wave-type of heat conduction equation, namely, hyperbolic heat conduction equation. The introduced time-derivative term in the CV model describes a wave nature of heat propagation at a finite speed, which has been proved in both theory and experiments (Vernotte 1961). The natural extension of this model yields a constitutive relation called the single-phase-lagging heat conduction model, which is written as follows:

$$\bar{q}(\bar{r},t+\tau) = -K\nabla T(\bar{r},t) \tag{12.6}$$

It has been further extended to the dual-phase-lagging (DPL) model by Tzou (1996) which is given as:

$$\bar{q}(\bar{r},t+\tau_q) = -K\nabla T(\bar{r},t+\tau_T) \tag{12.7}$$

where τ_T and τ_q are the phase lags of the temperature gradient and the heat flux vector in second, respectively. The first order Taylor expansion of Eq. (12.7) gives:

$$\bar{q}(\bar{r},t) + \tau_q\frac{\partial\bar{q}(\bar{r},t)}{\partial t} \cong -K\left\{\nabla T(\bar{r},t) + \tau_T\frac{\partial}{\partial t}[\nabla T(\bar{r},t)]\right\} \tag{12.8}$$

Taking the divergence of (12.8) and substituting $\nabla\cdot\bar{q}$ to the energy equation established at a general time t:

$$-\nabla\cdot\bar{q}(\bar{r},t) + Q(\bar{r},t) = C_p\frac{\partial T(\bar{r},t)}{\partial t} \tag{12.9}$$

which leads to the *T* representation of the DPL model:

$$\nabla^2 T(\bar{r},t) + \tau_T\frac{\partial}{\partial t}\nabla^2 T(\bar{r},t) + \frac{1}{K}[Q(\bar{r},t) + \tau_q\frac{\partial Q(\bar{r},t)}{\partial t}] = \frac{1}{\alpha}\frac{\partial T(\bar{r},t)}{\partial t} + \frac{\tau_q}{\alpha}\frac{\partial^2 T(\bar{r},t)}{\partial t^2} \tag{12.10}$$

where k and Q(r,t) are thermal diffusivity (m²/s) and volumetric heating source (W/m³). It should be noted that when $\tau_q = \tau_T$ and, (12.4) reduces to Fourier's law, and DPL model in (12.10) becomes the classical diffusion equation. If $\tau_T = 0$, Eq. (12.10) becomes the CV wave model originated by Cattaneo (1958), Vernotte (1961). The propagation speed is defined as:

$$C = \sqrt{k/\tau} \tag{12.11}$$

which is also called "thermal wave speed". For $\tau = 0$, C is infinitely high in accordance with the instantaneous heat propagation predicted by the Fourier model. Equation (12.10) is of considerable importance in the investigation of a variety of heat transfer problems. The most commonly used form of Eq. (12.10) to solve heat transfer problems for either a biological fluid or tissue is Pennes bioheat equation, because of its conciseness and validity. The bioheat transfer equation was first introduced by Pennes (1948) to model heat transfer in perfused tissue such that:

$$\rho C\frac{\partial T}{\partial t} = \nabla\cdot(K\nabla T) + C_b\dot{V}(T_a-T) + \dot{Q}_s + \dot{Q}_m \tag{12.12}$$

where ρ, C, $\dot{V}$, $\dot{Q}_s$, $\dot{Q}_m$, C_b, and T_a are density of tissue (kg/m³), specific heat of tissue (J/Kg K), blood perfusion rate (Kg/m³s), heat generation due to external heat source (W/m³), tissue metabolic heat generation (W/m³), specific heat of blood (J/Kg K), and artery temperature (K), respectively. Comparing the results of numerical modeling with the experimental measurements have demonstrated that the traditional Pennes' equations has yielded incorrect results as the thermal relaxation time of tissue is eliminated in this parabolic heat conduction equation. Therefore, in this study thermal wave model of bio-heat transfer (TWMBT) based on finite speed of heat propagation is compared to the well-known Pennes' equation based on infinite heat propagation in biological tissues. Liu et al. introduced that the thermal wave model of bio-heat transfer in the basic equation to describe TWMBT can be written as follows (Liu et al. 1997):

$$\nabla.[K\nabla T(\bar{r},t)] + C_b \dot{V}(T_a - T) + \dot{Q}_s + \dot{Q}_m + \tau[-C_b \dot{V}\frac{\partial T}{\partial t} + \frac{\partial \dot{Q}_m}{\partial t} + \frac{\partial \dot{Q}_s}{\partial t}]$$

$$= \rho C[\tau(\frac{\partial^2 T(\bar{r},t)}{\partial t^2}) + \frac{\partial T(\bar{r},t)}{\partial t}$$

(12.13)

The blood perfusion $\dot{V}$ and $\dot{Q}_m$ metabolic term are neglected in the *in vitro* model. Volumetric heat generation Q_s due to spatial electromagnetic heat source is expressed as follows (Welch and van Gemert 1995):

$$\dot{Q}_s = \alpha I$$

(12.14)

where α and I are absorption coefficient of tissue (m^{-1}) and the irradiance (W/m^2) of an isotropic point source emitting P_{Laser} (W) within an infinite homogeneous medium, which can be formulated as follows (Duderstadt and Hamilton 1976):

$$I = \frac{P_{Laser}}{4\pi d_0 r}\exp(-\gamma_{eff}.r)$$

(12.15)

where P_{Laser} (W) is power of the light source, γ_{eff} (m^{-1}) is the effective attenuation coefficient, r(m) is the radial distance from the source, and d_0 (m) is the optical diffusion distance, so γ_{eff} is (Wyman et al. 1989):

$$\gamma_{eff} = \sqrt{3\alpha(\alpha+\beta_r)}$$

(12.16)

where β_r is reduced scattering coefficient (m^{-1}) which is a lumped property incorporating the scattering coefficient β (m^{-1}), and g = <cos (θ)> is the first moment of the scattering phase function, called scattering anisotropy.

$$\beta_r = \beta(1-g)$$

(12.17)

Also,

$$d_0 = \frac{1}{3(\alpha+\beta_r)} = \frac{\alpha}{\gamma_{eff}^2}$$

(12.18)

Moreover, an additional term accounts for thermal energy release by the gold nanoshells should be added to the Eq. (12.14):

$$\dot{Q}_s = \alpha.I.[1-10^{-\varepsilon Lc}]$$

(12.19)

where the term in the bracket is plasmonic heating induced by exposure to laser irradiation with ε, L, and c being the wavelength-dependent molar absorptivity (extinction coefficient), the distance the light travels through the material (i.e., the path length), and the concentration of absorbing species according to the Beer-Lambert's law.

Thermophysical properties of nanoparticles

In order to analyze the modeled conditions, thermophysical properties of materials used in our experiments were taken from literature or calculated by the formulas summarized by Buongiorno (2006):

$$\rho_{nf} = (1-f)\rho_f + f\rho_p$$

(12.20)

where n_f, f, ρ, and φ denote the nanofluid, base fluid, nanoparticles, and particle volume concentration. It should be noted that for calculating the specific heat of nanofluid some of prior researchers have used the following correlation (Pak and Cho 1998):

$$C_{nf} = (1-f)C_f + f\,C_p \tag{12.21}$$

It is modified and presented by Buongiorno (2006) as follows:

$$C_{nf} = \frac{(1-f)\rho_f C_f + f\rho_p C_p}{\rho_{nf}} \tag{12.22}$$

The most commonly used thermal conductivity equation was proposed by Avsec and Oblak (2007) for the mixtures containing micrometer size particles; it is assumed that this equation is applicable for the nanofluids:

$$\frac{K_{nf}}{K_f} = \frac{K_p + (n-1)K_f + (n-1)(1+\beta)^3 f\,(K_p - K_f)}{K_p + (n-1)K_f - (1+\beta)^3 f\,(K_p - K_f)} \tag{12.23}$$

In the above equation, n is the empirical shape factor and is equal to 3 for spherical nanoparticles, and β is ratio of nanolayer thickness to particle radius. The thermal conductivity increases by decreasing the diameter of the nanoparticles. As there is a large uncertainty in the thermophysical properties of biological tissues and due to the temperature dependency of these properties, we have chosen a set of values based on comparing the parameters from different sources. In the present study, the average diameter of the observed three layer core/shell $Fe_3O_4/SiO_2/Au$ nanoparticles was 85 nm (with respective thickness of 35/15/35 nm). Density, heat capacity, and thermal conductivity of the prepared nanofluid were calculated using the above relations. Properties of the base fluid (C.C.M.), nanofluid (suspension containing spherical nanoparticles), gold nanoshells, QU-DB lung cancer cells, the laser, and culture dish parameters are shown in Table 12.1 (Duck 1990).

Table 12.1. Biological and thermophysical parameters used in simulation.

Cell culture medium (DMEM)	
Specific heat capacity (C_f)	4.18 ($Jg^{-1}K^{-1}$)
Density (ρ_f)	0.99 (gcm^{-3})
Thermal conductivity (K_f)	0.6 ($Wm^{-1}K^{-1}$)
Absorption coefficient (α_f)	1 (cm^{-1})
Three layer core-shell nanoparticles ($Fe_3O_4/SiO_2/Au$)	
Specific heat capacity C_p	111.65 ($Jkg^{-1}K^{-1}$)
Density (ρ_p)	19.3 (gcm^{-3})
Thermal conductivity (K_p)	318 ($Wm^{-1}K^{-1}$)
Particle volume concentration (φ)	0.1&0.01 ($mgcm^{-3}$)
Size (d_p)	85 (nm)
Thermal diffusivity of gold (k = $K/\rho C$)	$127 \times 10^{-6}\,(m^2s^{-1})$
Absorption coefficient (α_p)	$7.66 \times 10^9\,(cm^{-1})$
Characteristic length (x)	$x = d_p = 85$ (nm)
QU-DB lung cancer cells	
Specific heat capacity (C_c)	3.5 ($Jg^{-1}K^{-1}$)
Density (ρ_c)	1 (gcm^{-3})
Thermal conductivity (K_c)	0.0028 ($Wcm^{-1}K^{-1}$)
Absorption coefficient (α_c)	0.25 (cm^{-1})
Size (d_c)	10 (μm)
Thermal relaxation time (τ_c)	1.7×10^{-4} (s)
Laser and culture dish parameters	
Laser irradiance rate (I)	14, 42, 71, 157, 184 (Wcm^{-2})
Diameter of culture dish (d_d)	10 (mm)

Boundary and initial conditions

The geometry used to simulate the temperature distribution was based on a 3-D model consisting of cylindrical cell culture dish, in which a volume of material with three different layers: a single cell layer (thickness: diameter of a cancer cell of 10 μm and confluency of 99%), a plasmonic gold nanoparticle layer incubated on the cultured lung cancer cell layer (thickness: diameter of one three layer nanoparticle of 85 nm) with cell culture media above these two layers (height: 7 mm). The gold nanoparticles were first internalized by cancer cells and then the volume was irradiated by a 810 nm diode laser with a rectangular output beam at different power densities ranging from 14 to 184 W/cm² to study the photothermal process. It should be noted that the Eq. 12.13 is analyzed in the polar coordinates as the experimental domain is cylindrical. It is assumed that the tissue is initially at the physiological temperature of 37°C:

$$T_i = T(0,r,z) = 37°C \tag{12.24a}$$

Another initial condition is

$$\frac{\partial T}{\partial t}(0,r,z) = 0 \tag{12.24b}$$

Due to the cylindrical symmetry of the geometry in which the heat equation should be analyzed, temperature elevation was solved in the radial direction only. Three types of boundary conditions are commonly used during the solving of the heat transfer model:

$$\frac{\partial T}{\partial r}(0,z,t) = 0, \frac{\partial T}{\partial r}(R,z,t) = 0 \tag{12.25a}$$

$$T(r,0,t) = T_\infty, T(R,z,t) = T_\infty, k\frac{\partial T}{\partial z}(r,L,t) = \begin{cases} q & r \prec r_i \\ 0 & r \succ r_i \end{cases} \tag{12.25b}$$

Because of the complexity of the model the following assumptions are considered.

(1) Radiation emission from the tissue phantom is neglected because the tissue blackbody intensity is much smaller than the incident laser intensity; (2) tissue optical and thermal properties are thermally stable during the heat transfer process; (3) blood perfusion and thermal evaporation and/or phase change of tissue during the heat transfer process are not considered; (4) fluid phase and nanoparticles are in thermal equilibrium with zero relative velocity.

Solution scheme

The heat transfer behaviour of the system is modeled by using finite element modeling (FEM) using a commercial FEM package (Comsol Multiphysics 3.2a) for solver execution. The software implemented a 2-D and 3-D cylindrical modeling of the phantom and laser in a cylindrical coordinate system. Figure 12.5 shows a typical setup of the problem by the software. To ensure mesh quality and validity of solution, the mesh was refined until there was less than a 0.5% difference in solution between refinements.

Results and discussion

In this paper, temperature distributions in a GNP-containing cell layer during a continuous wave laser irradiation has been obtained both experimentally and numerically. The experimental trials were conducted in three cases: direct focusing of continuous wave diode laser with different intensities on the (i) the cell culture media containing cancer cells only, (ii) the cell culture media containing gold nanoparticles only, and (iii) the cell culture media containing both cancer cells and gold nanoparticles. The experimental results are compared to the numerical results obtained using solution of thermal wave model of bio-heat transfer equation. The results of numerical modeling obtained from both hyperbolic non-Fourier and parabolic Fourier equation are compared with all three experimental cases. Two common pathways of cell death underlying laser-enabled cell damages to specific cellular structures (e.g., plasmatic membranes, nuclei,

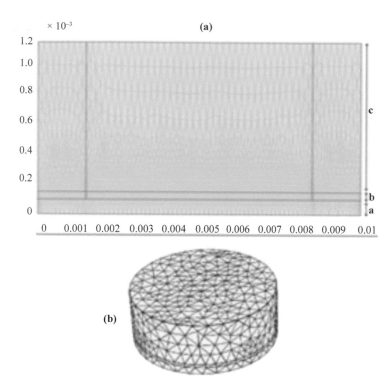

Figure 12.5. The meshed structure of computational domain for (a) 2-D and (b) 3-D simulation. In the 2-D simulation, a, b, c represent the cultured cancer cells, GNPs layer and culture medium, respectively.

cytoskeletons or organelles) are apoptosis and necrosis pathways, depending on the properties of gold nanoparticles (composition, shape and size), their concentration and location in subcellular regions and laser parameters (irradiance, type, and irradiation time) (Tong et al. 2007).

Effect of continuous irradiation on temperature profile

Figure 12.6(a,b) shows the experimental and simulation results obtained from hyperbolic non-Fourier indicating the effect of laser irradiance on the temperature variation of the GNP-containing cancer cell layer at 0.01 mg/ml. As it is observed, at lower irradiances the temperature rise is very similar, whereas at higher values the experimental results tend to deviate slightly at later time intervals where they become more significant, i.e., faster deviation at shorter times. The reason for mismatch in their growth pattern can be attributed to isolated boundaries in the model which led to a sharp increase in the temperature of thin cell layer at the bottom of the dish.

Effect of concentration of gold nanoparticles on temperature profile

Based on the SPR absorption in GNPs, an energy relaxation is followed through non-radiative decay channels which results in an increase in kinetic energy, leading to overheating of the local environment around the light-absorbing species. Since, the photothermal effect on tissue is a function of temperature, two different concentrations of GNPs (0.01 mg/ml and 0.1 mg/ml) were used to investigate the local temperature distribution and thermolysis in *in vitro* culture medium. By using an appropriate value of GNPs concentration, c for the plasmonic heating term in Eq. 12.19, we analyzed the influence of nanoparticles on the thermal history at 184 W/cm². It is clear from Fig. 12.7 that the maximum temperature at 140 s using 0.1 mg/ml is higher than 0.01 mg/ml. The increase in temperature by increasing the concentration

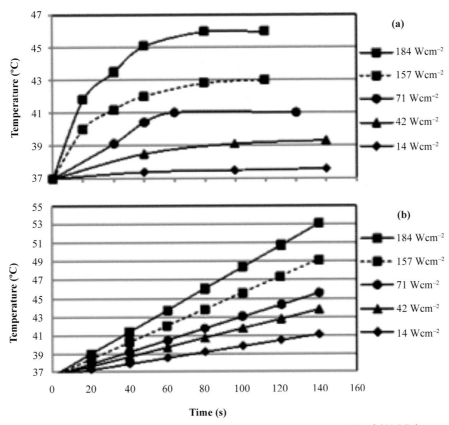

Figure 12.6. (a) Experimentally and (b) numerically-obtained data for temperature rise (ΔT) of QU-DB lung cancer cells incubated with culture medium containing 0.01 mg/ml of MNPS over a period of 3 minutes at various laser irradiance.

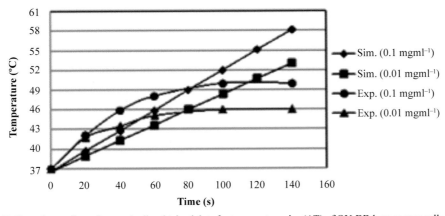

Figure 12.7. Experimentally and numerically-obtained data for temperature rise (ΔT) of QU-DB lung cancer cells incubated with culture medium containing various concentrations of MNPs (0.01 and 0.1 mg/ml) over a period of 3 minutes at 184 W/cm².

of nanoparticles can be due to the density of the nanoparticles arrangement on the cell membrane and the possibility of Au NPs aggregation, hence resulting in a stronger LSPR and thus, more efficient photothermal effects.

Figure 12.8(a,b) illustrates the temperature contours of irradiated culture medium with and without MNSs. As is normally expected, the distribution of laser irradiance follows a Gaussian mode, however, the straight path of temperature gradient in our case is due to the rectangular laser beam used for irradiation.

Time = 140   Contour: T-273.15   Contour Color: T

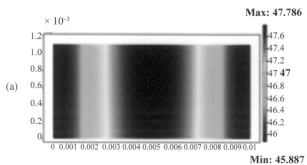

(a)

Time = 140   Contour: T-273.15   Contour Color: T

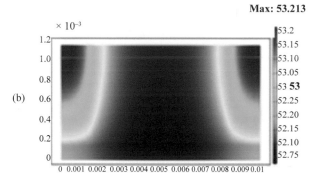

(b)

Time = 140   Contour: T-273.15   Contour Color: T

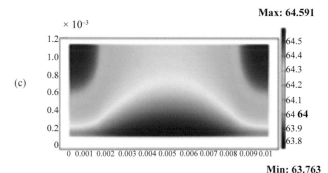

(c)

Figure 12.8. Temperature contour of (a) irradiated cancer cells incubated with MNPs-free medium (MNPs concentration = 0), (b) irradiated cancer cells incubated with MNPs-containing medium (MNPs concentration = 0.01 mg/ml) and (c) irradiated MNPs suspended in culture medium (MNPs concentration = 0.01 mg/ml) without cancer cells. Laser power density in all cases is 184 W/cm².

Effect of fourier and non-fourier model on temperature profile

The experimental and the numerical results are compared using thermal wave model of bio-heat transfer equation. It is observed that experimentally measured temperature distribution is in good agreement with

Time = 140   Contour: T-273.15   Contour Color: T

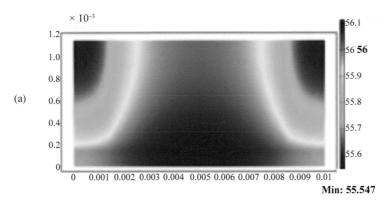

Time = 140   Contour: T-273.15   Contour Color: T

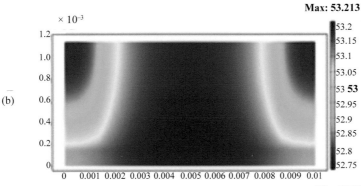

Figure 12.9. Temperature contours of irradiated cancer cells incubated with MNPs-containing medium (MNPs concentration = 0.01 mg/ml) at power density of 184 W/cm^2. (a) Numerically-obtained heat gradient based on Fourier and (b) non-Fourier conduction model.

that predicted by simulation of non-Fourier hyperbolic heat conduction model. Temperature contours of irradiated cancer cells incubated with 0.01 mg/ml of MNSs based on Fourier and non-Fourier conduction model are shown in Fig. 12.9.

Comparison of results of 2-D and 3-D modeling

The geometry used to simulate TWMBT equation was based on a 2-D and 3-D model consisting of a cylindrical cell culture dish including a cancer cell layer situated at the bottom of the dish surrounded by GNPs and culture media. Temperature changes of irradiated cancer cells at 184 W/cm^2 using 0.01 mg/ml of MNSs for experimental, 2-D and 3-D simulation are shown in Fig. 12.10. The boundary and slice representation of 3-D temperature gradients are presented in Fig. 12.11, where the spatio-temporal temperature distribution of irradiated MNSs-laden cancer cells is clearly distinguished with its maximum at the center shown by red.

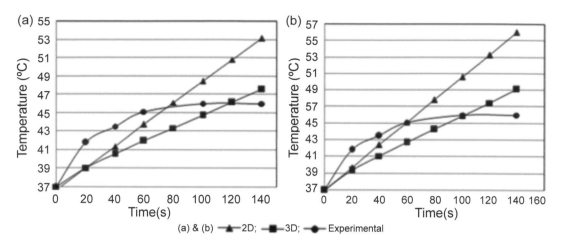

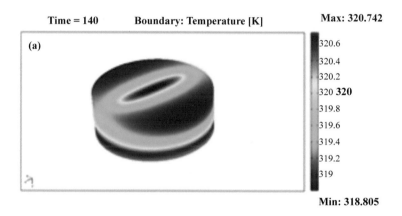

Figure 12.10. Dimensionality effects on the profile of irradiated QU-DB lung cancer cells incubated with MNPs-containing culture medium (MNPs concentration = 0.01 mg/ml) over a period of 150 seconds at the power density of 184 W/cm². Simulation trials conducted based on both (a) non-Fourier and (b) Fourier conduction model.

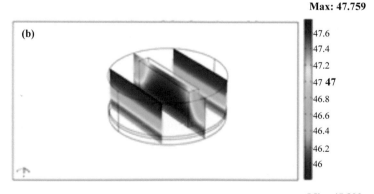

Figure 12.11. (a) Boundary and (b) slice representation of 3-D temperature contours of irradiated cancer cells incubated with MNPs-containing medium (MNPs concentration = 0.01 mg/ml) at power density of 184 W/cm². Black edges in (b) indicates the computational domain.

12.4.2 Synthesis and characterization of SPION functionalized third generation dendrimers conjugated by gold nanoparticles and folic acid for targeted breast cancer laser hyperthermia: An in vitro assay (Khosroshahi et al. 2015)

Superparamagnetic iron oxide nanoparticles (SPION) were synthesized and functionalized by polyamidoamine (PAMAM) dendrimer. Magnetodendrimer samples were conjugated by gold nanoparticles (Au-NPs) using two reducing agents of sodium borohydride and hydrazine sulfate. Pre-synthesized 10-nm Au-NP were used to evaluate the efficiency of conjugation method. Laser Induced Fluorescence Spectroscopy (LIFS) of these materials showed that the nanocomposite and magnetodendrimers have the fluorescence properties covering the whole range of visible spectrum. For targeting and the biocompatibility purpose, the synthesized materials were conjugated by folic acid molecules. Laser-induced hyperthermia was performed using Au-NPs. The samples were characterized using X-ray diffractometry (XRD), transmission electron microscopy (TEM), Fourier transform infrared (FTIR) spectroscopy, UV-Visible spectroscopy, and fluorescent spectroscopy. Two cell lines of breast cancer, i.e., MCF 7 and MDA MB 231, were chosen for cytotoxicity evaluation of the synthesized nanostructures. The MDA MB 231-IDAF Hydr. combination exhibited the highest viability% (50 µg/mL) before laser irradiation, and highest cell apoptosis and crystallization after irradiation, compared to other combinations and MCF7 cell lines. The preliminary results confirmed the possibility of employing the above system as a nanoprobe theranostic platform for bioimaging and therapy of breast cancer cells.

Introduction

Synthesis and application of magnetic nanoparticles have found a great attention in many scientific fields including optic, electronic or medicine, and biomedical engineering as contrast agent, magnetic targeting drug delivery, cell labeling, and cancer treatment (Sun et al. 2005). Among different methods of synthesis, coprecipitation is relatively an easy and simple procedure which is used in this research. To overcome the aggregation and improvement in stability of nanoparticles, modification in different steps may be performed including synthesis condition, surfactant addition, or coating fabrication. Dendrimers as nanostructured macromolecules are assembled from a polyfunctional core by adding branched monomers that react with the functional groups of the core, in turn leaving end groups with the ability to react again (Menjoge et al. 2010). Dendrimers provide many opportunities for the functionalization of the NP surfaces with tunable surface chemistry (Tajabadi et al. 2013), where different fluorophores can be also be attached for generating luminescent dendrimers (Larson and Tucker 2001, Rezvani Alanagh et al. 2014). One of the most widely used cancer-targeting ligands is folic acid (FA), which targets FA receptors that are overexpressed in several human carcinomas, including breast, ovary, lung (Grabchev et al. 2003, Li et al. 2010). In this study, the optimal magnetite nanoparticles were chosen, coated with third generation PAMAM dendrimer, and finally functionalized with Au-NP via different preparation methods. We report the results of (i) Synthesis and characterization of SPION (iron-oxide)-PAMAM-AuNP-FA nanocomposites (IDAF) using sodium borohydrate (IDAF-NaBH$_4$) and hydrazine sulfate (IDAF-Hydr.) as reducing agents and pre-synthesized Au-NP (IDAF-10 nm), (ii) Evaluation of cytotoxicity and uptake of IDAF nanocomposites by MDA MB 231 and MCF 7 breast cancer cell lines, and (iii) Evaluation of laser-induced thermal response and viability after cellular uptake and irradiation.

Materials and methods

Iron chlorides (III) (FeCl$_3$.6H$_2$O), Iron Sulfate (FeSO$_4$.7H$_2$O), and Ethanol (C$_2$H$_5$OH) were purchased from Merck Company. Ammonium Hydroxide (NH$_4$OH), Methyl Acrylate (CH$_2$= C(CH$_3$) COOCH$_3$), Ethylenediamine (C$_2$H$_4$(NH$_2$)$_2$), Sodium Borohydrate (NaBH$_4$), Hydrazine sulfate (H$_6$N$_2$O$_4$S), Gold colloid solution (10 nm), Folic Acid, Fetal Bovine Serum (FBS) were obtained from Sigma (USA).

Magneto-dendrimer synthesis

Magneto-dendrimers were synthesized via three different procedures.

i)   Sodium borohydrate as a reducing agent (IDA-NaBH$_4$ (Iron oxide-Dendrimer-Au)
     A solution of tetracholoroauric acid (HAuCl$_4$) solution (5 mM) was prepared and added to the suspension of third generation magnetodendrimer (1% w/v) with the same volume under N$_2$ atmosphere. In order to produce complex between Au (III) and amide or amine group of dendrimer, the resulting mixture was vigorously stirred for one hour at darkness. After that, the amount of 5 mL of aqueous sodium borohydrate solution (0.1 M) was added drop-wise to the reaction mixture.

ii) Hydrazine sulfate as a reducing agent (IDA Hydr)
     Here, stable Au-NPs were produced by adding hydrazine sulfate aqueous solution (25 mM) to the solution of magneto-dendrime-HAuCl$_4$ complex and stirring it for 2 hours. The particles were rinsed with ethanol five times using magnetic separation, and resulted in sample IDA Hydr.

iii) Gold nanoparticles (pre-synthesized Au NP-10 nm)
     Au-NPs were directly added to magneto-dendrimer suspension under N$_2$ atmosphere. The mixture was stirred for an hour to complete the reaction, and resulted in sample IDA NP.

Synthesis of folic acid functionalized magnetodendrimer-gold complex (IDAF)

Magnetodendrimer-gold complex was functionalized via carbodiimide reaction. Folic acid (0.085 mmol) and EDC (1.2 mmol) with the molar ratio of 1/14 (Fa/EDC) were reacted in the solution of DMF (27 mL) and DMSO (9 mL) under N$_2$ atmosphere for an hour. This organic mixture was added drop-wise to aqueous mixture of magnetodendrimer-gold complex and stirring continued for 3 days. The final nanoparticles were purified using magnetic separation and centrifugation. These nanoparticles were named as IDAF-NaBH$_4$, IDAF 10 ($\times$ 10 concentration of NaBH$_4$), DAF Hydr (IDAF-Hydr.), and IDAF NP.

Characterization

The presence of PAMAM, gold, and folic acid typical bonds on the surface of magnetite nanoparticles were proved by Fourier transform infrared (FTIR) spectroscopy (BOMEM, Canada). Particle size and morphology of magnetite nanoparticles were determined by transmission electron microscopy (TEM, Philips CM-200-FEG microscope, 120 kV). The amount of gold nanoparticles attached to the magnetodendrimer was estimated using wavelength-dispersive X-ray spectroscopy (SEM–WDX, XL30, Philips, USA). The fluorescent properties of nanoparticles were determined using fluorescence Spectro Fluorophotometer (RF-1510, Shimadzu, Japan). The fluorescence microscopy of cells were performed by Axioscope (Zeiss, Germany). The MDA MB231 cells were cultured on coverslips placed in a 12 well plate. After 24 h, ID (third generation dendrimers-G3), IDAF-NaBH$_4$, IDAF 10, IDAF Hydr, and IDAF NP nanoparticles with the concentration of 100 µg/mL were added to each well and incubated for a further 24 hours. The cells were fixed at 4% glutaraldehyde (Sigma, UK) solution in PBS for 1 h. The cellular uptake of nanoparticles were observed by SEM (XL30, Philips, USA). Furthermore, wavelength dispersive X-Ray analysis (WDX, Philips, USA) based on Fe element was performed to observe map distribution of nanoparticles attached to the cells. The cells with concentration of 1×10^4 were then seeded on coverslips following the addition of nanoparticles. After 24 h, the medium was removed, the cells rinsed with PBS and the fluorescent emission of cells containing nanoparticles was detected by a fluorescence microscope (Axioscop, Zeiss, Germany). For the purpose of hyperthermia, the MDA MB231 cells were cultured in a plate for 24 hours prior to addition of optimal nanoparticles (with the concentration of 50 µg/mL). After addition and incubation for further 24 hours, non-reacted nanoparticles were washed with PBS twice and fresh culture medium was added. Each well was irradiated by 534 nm laser for 10 minutes and the efficiency of hyperthermia was evaluated using MTT assay.

In vitro tests

Evaluation of cytotoxicity

Human breast cancer cell lines MDA MB 231 and MCF 7 were obtained from the National Cell Bank (NCBI, Pasture Institute of Iran). The cells were cultured in RPMI 1640 (GIBCO, USA) supplemented with 10% fetal bovine serum (FBS, GIBCO, USA) and seeded onto a 96 well-plate at a density of 15×10^3 cells per well. Serial dilutions of nanoparticles (5 μg/mL–250 μg/mL) were added following incubation at 37°C, 5% CO_2. The same medium without any particle was considered as control. After 24 h, the culture medium was removed and replaced by 100 μl of MTT (3-(4,5-dimethylthiazol-2-yl)-2,5-diphenyltetrazolium bromide, Sigma, USA). The formation of formazan crystals was checked by optical microscope and the supernatant removed after 4 h. In order to dissolve formazan crystals, 100 μl of isopropanol was added to each well. Subsequently, the plate was placed in incubator for 15 minutes. The absorbance of each well was read using microplate reader (stat fax-2100, AWARENESS, Palm City, USA) at 545 nm. The results were reported in the form of relative cell viability compared to control sample (which could be calculated by the following equation):

$$\% \text{ Viability} = \frac{A_{545(\text{magnetic sample})}}{A_{545(\text{Control})}} \tag{12.26}$$

Evaluation of IDAF uptake

Cell uptake of ID (G3), IDAF-NaBH₄, IDAF-10, IDAF-Hydr and IDAF-NPs were evaluated at the same condition. Prior to addition of nanoparticles, cells were seeded for 24 hours and then three different concentrations of 50, 100, and 250 μg/mL of each group of nanoparticles were added to MDA MB 231 and MCF 7 cells media. The plate was incubated for 24 hours and then the supernatant solution extracted and placed in the fresh 96-well plate at the same position. The cells were washed with 100 μL fresh PBS and the resultant solution was placed into another fresh 96-well plate (the absorption of these wells were reported as a loosely attached particles). Finally, cell membrane was dissolved and the resultant absorption reported as uptaken nanoparticles. The modified iron oxide nanoparticles have characteristic maximum absorption in the range of 350–400 nm. Therefore, the particle absorptions were reported at three maximum wavelengths of 350, 360, and 370 nm.

Results and discussions

TEM analysis

Figure 12.12 shows that nanocomposites synthesized by NaBH₄ reducing agents are larger than those obtained by hydrazine sulfate and gold colloids, which is mainly due to ions interaction with surface amine group of magnetodendrimer (Shi et al. 2006, Divsar et al. 2009, Hoffman et al. 2011). However, the observed homogeneous distribution when hydrazine sulfate was used as a reducing agent could be

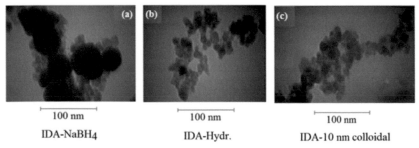

Figure 12.12.   TEM image of (a) IDA-NaBH₄, (b) IDA-Hydr and (c) IDA-NP (colloidal 10 nm).

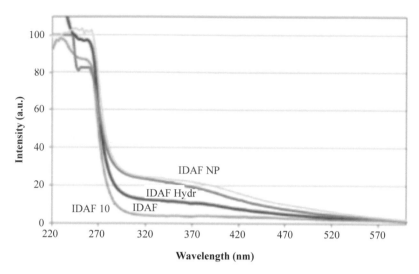

Figure 12.13. UV-vis spectra of IDA-NaBH$_4$, IDA-Hydr., IDA-Np, IDA (*10).

explained by entrapment and formation of gold nanoparticles on the cavity of magnetodendrimer due to their smaller size (Torigoe et al. 2001).

UV-Vis spectroscopy of IDAF nanocomplex

UV-vis spectroscopy was used to prove the presence of targeting moiety (i.e., folic acid molecule) in the final nanostructures conjugated with folic acid molecules. As it is seen in Fig. 12.13, all the samples revealed a maximum absorption peak around 270 nm, which is the characteristics of folic acid moieties (Majoros et al. 2006, Shi et al. 2009). In order to prove the effect of folic acid on cell uptake, G3 was used as control.

FTIR of IDAF nanocomplex

In the magnetodendrimer FTIR spectrum, the peaks at 581 and 629 cm^{-1} depict the existence of iron oxide phase at all of synthesized structures, amide band at 1570 and 1630 cm^{-1} represent the characteristics of PAMAM dendrimer, and the gold nanoparticles interact with amine terminated dendrimers stronger than carboxyl terminated dendrimers (Esumi et al. 2000). Furthermore, according to Satoh et al. (2002), the FTIR and UV-vis evaluations depend on the size of dendrimer and their generations. For this reason, at lower generations external type and in higher generations mixed type could be observed (Satoh et al. 2005). Type I amide band (wavenumber of 1630 cm^{-1}) is generally related to C=O stretching vibration (70–85%), and directly appertains to combination and structure of polymer backbone. Type II amide band (wavenumber 1570 cm^{-1}) represents N-H bending vibration (20%) (Grabchev et al. 2003, Li et al. 2010, Baykal et al. 2012). The band at 1630 cm^{-1} shows that the gold nanoparticles interact with N-H groups in magnetodendrimer structure, whereas the polymer backbone relatively remains as its pure structure. IDAF nanoparticles indicates two new peaks at 1155 and 1227 cm^{-1} as an evidence for C=C and C-H bond of aromatic segment in folic acid molecules (Chandrasekar et al. 2007, Singh et al. 2008). This proves the proper attachment of folic acid molecules to the IDA nanoparticles synthesized by different methods.

In vitro cytotoxicity: MTT

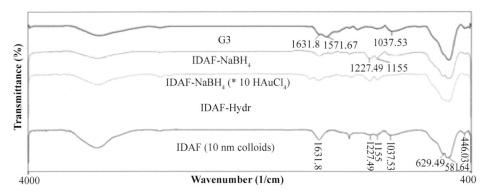

Figure 12.14. FTIR spectra of IDAF-NaBH₄, IDAF-* 10, DAF-Hydr. and DAF-NP nanoparticles.

MTT results shown in Fig. 12.15 verify that all formulations of synthesized nanoparticles are biocompatible up to the concentration of 50 μg/mL for the MDA MB231 (Fig. 12.15a) and 25 μg/mL for MCF7 cell lines (Fig. 12.15b). For IDAF-10 and IDAF-Hydr, the biocompatibility is at higher concentrations. Generally, a higher range of viability obtained for MDA MB231 than MCF7 cell lines in contact with the samples can be explained by the key role played by folate receptor on the surface of MDA MB231 cells. Folic acid is considered as a vital vitamin for cell growth and the presence of this moiety in the structure of nanoparticles enhances the cell viability. NH₂ groups on the surface of ID specimen electrostatically interact with cell surface and form clusters of nanoparticles which may be harmful to cells (Biswal et al. 2009). It has been reported that surface modification of dendrimers may improve their biocompatibility (Nam et al. 2009).

Cellular uptake of IDAF nanocomplex

The optical microscope pictures shown in Fig. 12.16 demonstrates the results of IDAF nanocomplex uptake by MDA MB231and MCF7 cells where a superior uptake of gold and folic acid functionalized nanoparticles by MDA MB231 cells is observed. Since MDA MB231 cells are overexpressed by folate receptors at the surface than the MCF cells, this leads to more uptake of nanoparticles. The selective reaction between folic acid molecules and the folate receptors on the surface act as lock and key, which results in the formation of vesicle around the nanoparticles. Therefore, they can enter the cells via endocytosis mechanism. On the other hand, the interaction between the charges of magnetodendrimer surface and cells membrane is nonspecific, which results in lower degree of endocytosis. As seen in Fig. 12.17, IDAF-Hydr. are uptaken more than any other nanoparticles at all concentrations by MDA MB231 cells than MCF 7 cells. Higher interaction of IDAF Hydr with these cell lines could be explained by entrapped gold nanoparticles, which effectively modify the structure of magnetodendrimer reducing the nonspecific interaction with cell surfaces. It should be noted that the uptake of ID (G3) sample is explained by fluid phase endocytosis, whereas for folic acid functionalized nanoparticles interpreted by receptor mediated endocytosis (Pradhan et al. 2007). The results confirm the efficiency and specificity of the second route.

Fluorescence imaging of nanoparticles uptake

It has been shown that after addition of HAuCl₄, the fluorescence intensity is red shifted towards the longer wavelength (Hong et al. 2007, Khosroshahi and Nourbakhsh 2010). After adding the reducing agent, the peaks are changed considerably, which shows the close attachment of Au-NPs to the dendrimers. The shift of fluorescence spectra is explained by strong interaction between gold crystals and amine groups of dendrimer (Torigoe et al. 2001). Optical properties of Au-NPs are highly sensitive to their particle size and have an effective influence on the fluorescence spectra of dendrimer (Wu et al. 2011). This is because of

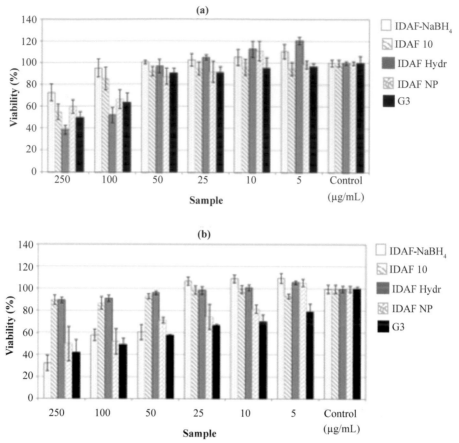

Figure 12.15. MTT analysis of (a) MDA MB 231 and (b) MCF7 cell lines in close contact with ID (G3), IDAF-NaBH$_4$, IDAF-* 10, IDAF-Hydr, and IDAF-NP.

the internal interaction between flexible structure of dendrimer and rigid structure of entrapped Au-NPs, whereas the larger particles damp the fluorescence of dendrimers. These phenomena could be explained in terms of fluorescence resonance energy transfer (FRET) (Arias et al. 2001).

In this study, IDA-Hydr nanocomposites strongly changed the initial fluorescent spectra of ID, i.e., the shape and location of peaks were sharply changed. In most cases, the fluorescence spectra of IDA-Hydr are stronger than other nanoparticles with highest signals at about 525 nm and 550 nm, respectively. One reason for this is more likely due to their smaller size which helps them to be entrapped easily by dendrimers and hence intensify the fluorescence signals. Figure 12.18 shows the fluorescence microscopy images of the MDA MB231 cell lines containing different nanoparticles excited at different wavelengths using blue, green, and red filters. All nanomagnetodendrimer formulations showed high cell staining capability, which indicates the nanoparticles are well uptaken by the cells, either by endocytosis or by attachment to the membrane surface. The cells structure did not exhibit any spherical shape, confirming the nanoparticles' high biocompatibility, except at higher concentration where some changes occurred due to rearrangement of cytoskeleton combination, such as actin and tubulin (Gupta et al. 2004, Gupta and Gupta 2005). Overall, these results are in good agreement with other researches on the dendrimer/folic acid nanoparticles (Quintana et al. 2002, Majoros et al. 2006, Shi et al. 2009, Biswal et al. 2009), and indicate that all formulations are highly efficient in fluorescent labeling of breast cancer cells.

MDA MB 231

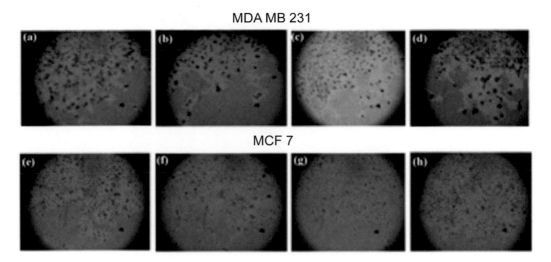

MCF 7

Figure 12.16. Optical microscope images of IDAF-NaNH$_4$, IDAF-* 10, IDAF-Hydr, and IDAF-NP nanoparticles endocytosed by (a–d) MDA MB 231 and (e–h) MCF 7 cell lines.

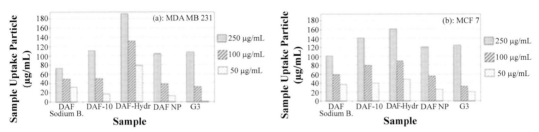

Figure 12.17. Uptake of nanoparticles by (a) MDA MB231, and (b) MCF7 cell lines at different concentrations.

Thermal response of IDAF nanocomplex

The temperature distribution around optically-stimulated plasmonic nanoparticles can be described by the following equation:

$$\rho c \frac{\partial T}{\partial t} = \nabla . (k \nabla T) + \langle p \rangle \tag{12.27}$$

where T is the local temperature, ρ, c, and k represent density, specific heat capacity, and thermal conductivity of material, respectively. Here $< p >$ is the average heat power dissipated inside the NP and the heat power is given by $P = < p > . V_{NP}$. As the TEM results show, the use of NaBH$_4$ as a reducing agent produced clusters of Au-NPs which consists of a greater particle size than the other formulation. Therefore, it is expected to produce higher temperature, as seen in Fig. 12.19. If we assume that all the energy absorbed by nanoparticles is expended for heating up the surrounding medium, then Q$_s$ or absorbed laser power per unit volume of nanoparticles is

$$Q_s = Q (1-10^{-A}) \tag{12.28}$$

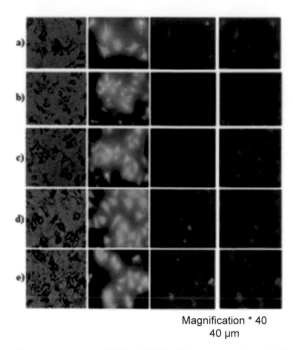

Magnification * 40
40 µm

Figure 12.18. Fluorescence microscope images of MDA MB231cell lines containing (a) ID (G3) (b) IDAF-NaBH$_4$, (c) IDAF-* 10, (d) IDAF-Hydr, and (e) IDAF-NP nanoparticles.

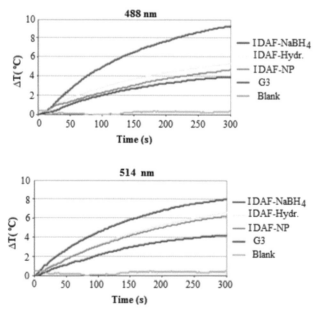

Figure 12.19. The effect of laser irradiation at two different wavelengths of (a) 488 nm and (b) 514 nm on thermal behaviour of different synthesized nanoparticles.

where A is the optical density of absorbed nanoparticles and Q is the laser power per unit volume of nanoparticles. The direct absorption of laser power by cells is ignored due to negligible absorption cross-section compared to structures containing nanoparticles. The optical density for IDAF-Hydr and IDAF-10 nanoparticles uptaken by MDA MB231 cells were calculated 0.3466 and 0.2681, respectively. As a result, it can be deduced that $\approx 55\%$ of initial laser power is used to produce local heat for IDAF-Hydr nanoparticles

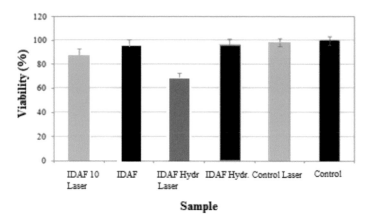

Figure 12.20. Viability evaluation of MDA MB231 cells containing nanoparticles after irradiation by tunable argon laser at 200 mW.

in contrast to the IDAF-10 with ≈ 46%. Therefore, DAF-Hydr nanoparticles could cause a higher degree of cell death after laser irradiation (Fig. 12.20). It is conclusive that the presence of nanoparticles within the cells have a key influence in laser-induced heating in comparison to using laser only where the viability is almost the same as control.

12.4.3 Nanoshell-mediated targeted photothermal therapy of HER2 human breast cancer cells using pulsed and continuous wave lasers: an in vitro study (Khosroshahi et al. 2014)

In this study we report the apoptosis induction in HER2 overexpressed breast cancer cells using pulsed, continuous wave lasers and PVP-stabilized magneto-plasmonic nanoshells (PVP-MPNS) delivered by immunoliposomes. The Immunoliposomes containing PVP-MPNS were fabricated and characterized. Heating efficiency of the synthesized nanostructures was calculated. The effect of functionalization on cellular uptake of nanoparticles was assessed using two cell lines of BT-474 and Calu-6. The best uptake result was achieved by functionalized liposome (MPNS-LAb) and BT-474. Also, the interaction of 514 nm argon (Ar) and Nd:YAG second harmonic 532 nm lasers with nanoparticles was investigated based on the temperature rise of the nanoshells suspension and the release value of 5(6)-carboxyfluorescein (CF) from CF/MPNS-loaded liposomes. The temperature increase of the suspensions after 10 consecutive pulses of 532 nm and 5 minutes of irradiation by Ar laser were measured approximately 2°C and 12°C, respectively. The irradiation of CF/MPNS-loaded liposomes by Ar laser for 3 minutes resulted in 24.3% release of CF and in the case of 532 nm laser the release was laser energy dependent. Furthermore, the comparison of CF release showed a higher efficiency for the Ar laser than by direct heating of nanoshell suspension using circulating water. The percentage of cell apoptosis after irradiation by Ar and 532 nm lasers were 44.6% and 42.6%, respectively. The obtained results suggest that controlling the NP-laser interaction using optical properties of nanoshells and the laser parameters can be used to develop a new cancer therapy modality via targeted nanoshell and drug delivery.

Introduction

Magneto-plasmonic nanoshells (MPNS), a class of nanoparticles (NPs) composed of magnetic core covered by plasmonic shell, are promising structures in the field of bioimaging and therapy (Cho et al. 2006, Pham et al. 2008, Khosroshahi et al. 2011, Ghazanfari and Khosroshahi 2014, Khosroshahi and Ghazanfari 2012). Plasmonic NP (PNP)-mediated laser hyperthermia is currently emerging as a novel approach of cancer therapy, where the cancer cells are destroyed through laser-induced heating of PNPs on the surface or within the cells (Sun et al. 2013, Huang et al. 2007). The unique optical properties of PNPs are derived from localized surface plasmon resonance (LSPR), a collective and coherent oscillation of conduction electrons with respect to all the ions, which results in strong scattering and absorption of incident radiation at a specific wavelength depending on the size and shape of the nanostructure (Nourbakhsh and Khosroshahi 2011). Laser irradiation at the LSPR increases the temperature of the NPs as well as their surrounding environment depending on the optical properties of the NPs and parameters of the laser. Two mechanisms are thought to lead to cell death: (i) irradiation of NPs using continuous wave (cw) laser causing heating of NPs and subsequently, the heat conduction to the surrounding medium leads to the plasmonic photothermal therapy (Cheng et al. 2009), (ii) when NPs are irradiated by a short pulsed laser (i.e., femto to nano-second pulse duration). Provided the pulse duration is smaller than the relaxation time of surrounding medium, the heat is confined during the pulse and no heat is transferred from NP to its ambient. This results in a thermoelastic expansion of medium, which leads to photoacoustic waves or temperature gradients around the NPs which generates transient vapor microbubbles. In the latter case, the violent collapse of microbubbles produces some mechanical effects which can cause cell death. It has been reported that the laser fluence threshold significantly decreases with the increase of the size of NP cluster (Lapotko et al. 2006, Kitz et al. 2011). The plasmonic response of metallic nanostructures to either continuous or pulsed laser irradiation and the resulting thermal effects are of particular interest for cell destruction or triggered release. Cebrián et al. (2013) have used continuous wave laser for heating the nanostructures. They showed the illumination of silica-gold nanoshells or hollow gold nanoparticles with 808 nm laser resulted in temperature increase of 10 and 30°C, respectively. Li et al. (2013) and Fernandez et al. (2012) have reported photothermal therapy results from absorption of 808 nm cw laser by gold nanostructures. Also, Khosroshahi et al. (2012) have reported a temperature rise of 9°C resulting from irradiation of a three-layered nanostructure of Fe_3O_4/SiO_2/Au using 800 nm cw diode laser. Lapotko et al. (2006a,b) have used 532 nm pulsed-laser to irradiate gold NPs to generate nanobubbles for diagnostic and therapeutic applications at the cellular level. They showed that generated nanobubbles can lead to cell death through rupturing the target cells membranes.

Improvement of cell internalization and aggregation of NPs within cells using liposome carriers can significantly enhance the efficacy of NP-mediated laser hyperthermia. Liposomes are the most recognized of the advanced delivery systems and consist of a lipid bilayer encapsulating an internal aqueous compartment. In our previous work, we developed liposome carriers containing a large number of gold nanoshells (Hassannejad et al. 2014). Therefore, the uptake of a liposome carrier can produce a NP cluster within a live cell, and subsequently results in a significant enhancement of the efficacy of photothermal therapy. Also, the selectivity of the photothermal therapy can be achieved by conjugating the targeting moieties, such as monoclonal antibodies or aptamers (Steinhauser et al. 2006, Barrajón-Catalán et al. 2010, Zhang et al. 2011, Melancon et al. 2014), which can accelerate the accumulation of NPs within the desired cells. In the current study, we experimentally evaluated the efficiency of two different light sources (i.e., pulsed 532 nm and continuous wave 514 nm Ar lasers) for nanoshell-mediated targeted laser hyperthermia and drug delivery. Although the laser-NP interaction using these lasers have been reported previously, the comparison of different mechanisms using the same nanostructure has not been reported. For this purpose, the MPNS-loaded liposomes (MPNS-L) were first successfully synthesized and then the cells internalization was achieved through functionalization of MPNS-L by Herceptin (MPNS-LAb), a monoclonal antibody against HER2 receptors with overexpression of 18–28% of human breast cancers (Huang et al. 2006). The two aforementioned lasers were used to investigate the following objectives: (i) Laser-nanoshell interaction based on temperature change of the nanoshell suspension, (ii) The cumulative release of CF in each case, and (iii) Finally to evaluate the nanoshell-mediated laser thermal therapy using TUNEL assays.

Materials and methods

Chemicals

All analytical reagents were used without further purification. Ferric chloride hexahydrate ($FeCl_3.6H_2O$, 99%), ferrous chloride tetrahydrate ($FeCl_2.4H_2O$, 99%), chloroform, hydrochloric acid (HCl, 37%), absolute ethanol, sodium hydroxide, formaldehyde solution (H_2CO, 37%), ammonium thiocyanate (NH_4SCN), and polyvinylpyrrolidone (polyvidone25, PVP) were purchased from Merck. Tetrakis (hydroxymethyl) phosphonim chloride (THPC) was an 80% aqueous solution from Aldrich. Gold (iii) chloride trihydrate (HAuCl$_4$.3H$_2$O, ≥ 49% Au basis), 3-aminopropyltriethoxysilane (APTES), egg yolk phosphatidylcholine (EPC), cholesterol (CHOL), and 5(6)-carboxyfluorescein (CF) were purchased from Sigma.1,2-distearoyl-*sn*-glycero-3-phosphoethanolamine-N-[maleimide(polyethyleneglycol)-2000] (ammonium salt) (DSPE-PEG(2000)-Mal) was purchased from Avanti® Polar Lipids. Ultra centrifugal filter was purchased from Amicon® Millipore Company. The TdT-mediated dUTP nick end labelling (TUNEL) kit was purchased from Roche. HERCEPTIN®(Roche) was provided by Cancer Research Center, Shahid Beheshti University of Medical Sciences. The BT-474 and Calu-6 cell lines were supplied by Avicenna Research Institute, Shahid Beheshti University of Medical Sciences. Deionized water (18 MΩ) was provided by a Milli-Q system and deoxygenated by vacuum for 1 hour prior to the use.

Cell lines

BT-474 human breast carcinoma cell lines, as HER2-positive cells, and Calu-6 human lung carcinoma cell lines, as HER2-negative cells, were grown in 75-cm^2 plastic tissue culture flasks in RPMI-1640 supplemented with 10% fetal bovine serum (FBS) and 1% penicillin/streptomycin at 37°C in a humidified 5% CO$_2$ atmosphere. For TUNEL assay, the cells were seeded on cover slips (1cm^2) and imaged using a Ziess (Axioskop 2 plus) upright microscope.

Fabrication of magnetoplasmonic nanoshell-loaded liposome (MPNS-L)

Superparamagnetic iron oxide nanoparticles (SPION) were synthesized using a well-known coprecipitation method (Khosroshahi and Ghazanfari 2012, Hassannejad and Khosroshahi 2013). MPNS were synthesized and the surface of SPIONs were covered by a thin layer of gold through an electroless plating of Au onto the SPIONs and subsequently stabilized by PVP. In order to fabricate MPNS-loaded liposomes, a lipid mixture of chloroform stocks composed of EPC:CHOL at a molar ratio of 2:1 was dried at 42°C under N$_2$ stream, and further placed in a vacuum overnight. The lipid films were hydrated at a concentration of 20 mM EPC in the PVP-MPNS solution at 65°C for 2 h (vortexed for 30 s every 5 min). After hydration, 15 min of sonication (Tecna 20, 190 W) was applied, and finally the samples underwent 5 cycles of freeze-thaw, including 10 min at −196°C, 10 min at 65°C, and 30 s vortexing between cycles. Unencapsulated MPNSs were removed by centrifuging at 400 g for 5 min, after which the supernatant liposomal dispersion was centrifuged at 20000 g for 30 min to precipitate the liposomes encapsulating nanoparticles.

Preparation of Herceptin functionalized MPNS-loaded liposomes (MPNS-LAb)

Functionalization procedure of synthesized MPNS-L has been adopted from the previously reported post-insertion technique (Iden and Allen 2001). This technique consists of the following steps: (1) thiolation of antibody, (2) preparation of micelle composed of DSPE-PEG (2000)-Mal, (3) covalent link of antibody to the terminus of polyethylene glycol (PEG) chains on the surface of micelle through the reaction of thiol with maleimide, and (4) transfer of antibody conjugated phospholipids from micelles to synthesized MPNS-L. In our case, Herceptin was thiolated using the reaction of 12 mg/ml antibody with 2-iminothiolane (Traut's reagent) at 1:4 molar ratio in degassed 0.1 M phosphate buffer, 1 mM EDTA, pH 8, for 1 h at room temperature, in an inert N$_2$ atmosphere, and in a silicon-coated glass vial. Unreacted 2-iminothiolane was removed by centrifugation (4000 g, 10°C, 15 minutes) three times using 30 kDa cutoff centrifugal ultrafilters. The quantification of immobilized thiol groups was carried out using Ellman's test (Ellman 1959). In order to prepare micelles, dried lipid films containing DSPE-PEG(2000)-Mal were hydrated at a concentration of 1 mM in degassed 0.1 M phosphate buffer, 1 mM EDTA, pH 7.4 at 65°C for 1 h (vortexed for 30 s every 15 min). Finally, 20 min of sonication (Tecna 20, 190 W) at 60°C was applied and the covalent attachment of the thiolated antibody to the PEG terminus of Mal-PEG-DSPE micelles took place inside siliconized coated glassware in an inert N_2 atmosphere during an overnight incubation at room temperature. For transferring antibody conjugated phospholipids from micelles to MPNS-L, the functionalized micelles were incubated with the MPNS-L suspension for 1 h at 60°C, at EPC:DSPE molar ratio of 1:0.05. Free antibodies were removed by centrifugation (15000 g, 4°C, 25 minutes). The obtained immunoliposomes were dispersed in PBS or cell culture medium according to the next experiment.

Preparation of 5(6)-carboxyfluorescein (CF)/MPNS-loaded liposome

CF/MPNS-loaded liposomes were prepared similar to MPNS-L, except that in this case, the lipid layer was hydrated by MPNSs dispersed within 100 mM solution of CF with the same concentration of nanoparticles. The free CF was removed by centrifuging 5 times at 15000 g for 30 min (Hollmann et al. 2007).

Characterization methods

Scanning electron microscopy (SEM) was performed using a Hitachi S4160 field emission machine with an accelerating voltage of 15 KV. Transmission electron microscopy (TEM) was performed using a CM 200 FEG STEM Philips-M.E.R.C. operating at 200 kV. TEM imaging of MPNS-L was perfomed following negative staining with uranyl acetate. Liposomes were diluted with distilled water and dropped on a PDL-coated copper grid, the excess sample was then removed with a filter paper and air-dried for 1 min at room temperature. Subsequently, uranyl acetate solution (10 µl of 1%) was added onto the grid. The excess staining solution was removed after 1 min with a filter paper and was allowed to dry in the air before introducing into the microscope. NIH Image J software (http://rsb.info.nih.gov/ij/) was used to measure the sizes of particles based on TEM micrographs. The magnetization measurements were carried out at 300 K and in a magnetic field (H) up to 9 kOe with a vibrating sample magnetometer (VSM-PAR 155) that can measure magnetic moments as low as 10^{-3} emu. UV-Vis spectroscopy of nanoparticle suspensions was taken on a CARY100 UV-Vis spectrophotometer with a 10 mm optical path length quartz cuvette. Encapsulation efficiency of gold nanoshells within the liposomes was determined by inductively coupled plasma mass spectrometry (ICP-MS). Samples were frozen, lyophilized, and dissolved in nitric acid hydrochloride (composed of 100 µL of nitric acid and 300 µL of 37% hydrochloric acid) for 72 h. The samples were later diluted with HNO_3 (2% V/V) to produce a final volume of 2 mL, which was analyzed with ICP-MS and compared against standards (Kim and Nie 2005).

Theoretical background of laser-induced heating of plasmonic nanoparticles

The processes of laser-induced heating and heat transfer between spherical plasmonic particles and surrounding medium with no mass transfer are well described and established by some research groups, e.g., Pustovalov et al. (2008, 2009). Accordingly, heating of a spherical nanoparticle by laser pulses can be calculated using the following equation

$$\rho_0 c_0 V_0 \frac{dT_0}{dt} = \frac{1}{4} I_0(t) Q_{abs} S_0 - J_c S_0 \qquad (12.29)$$

with the initial condition of $T_0\,(t=0) = T_i$ where $\int_0^{r_0} q_0(t) 4\pi r^2 dr = \frac{1}{4} I_0(t) Q_{abs} S_0$, ρ_0 (g/cm³) and c_0 (J/g.K) are the density and the specific heat capacity of the nanoparticle material, V_0 (cm³) and S_0 (cm²) are the volume and the surface area of the nanoparticle respectively, T_0(K) is the temperature of the particle volume, t (s) is the time, I_0 (W/cm²) is the intensity of laser radiation, T_i(s) is the initial temperature of the particle and the surrounding tissue, J_c (W/cm²) is the energy flux density removed from nanoparticles by heat conduction under quasi-stationary heat exchange with ambient tissue, and Q_{abs} is the absorption efficiency factor. The maximal value of spherical nanoparticle temperature T_{max} at the end of laser pulse with duration, t_p under constant radiation intensity I_0 is

$$T_{max} = T_i + \frac{I_0 Q_{abs} r_0}{4k_i}\left[1 - \exp\left(-\frac{3k_i t_p}{c_0 \rho_0 r_0^2}\right)\right] \tag{12.30}$$

where K_m is the thermal conductivity of the ambient medium. Accordingly, the efficiency parameter of nanoparticle heating $\Delta T_0 / I_0$ can be defined using the following equation

$$\frac{\Delta T_0}{I_0} = \frac{T_{max} - T_i}{I_0} = \frac{Q_{abs} r_0}{4K_m}\left[1 - \exp\left(-\frac{3K_m t_p}{c_0 \rho_0 r_0^2}\right)\right] \tag{12.31}$$

For a nanoshell structure with the core and shell radii of r_c and r_s, respectively, the efficiency parameter of heating can be defined as follows:

$$\frac{\Delta T_0}{I_0} = \frac{Q_{abs} r_s}{4K_m} \times \left[1 - \exp\left(-\frac{3K_m t_p}{\tau_T}\right)\right] \tag{12.32}$$

where $\tau_T = r_s^2 \left(c_c \rho_c r_c^3 / r_s^3 + c_s \rho_s \left(1 - r_c^3 / r_s^3\right)\right) / 3K_m$ is characteristic time, c_c, ρ_c and c_s, ρ_s are the heat capacity and density of the material of the core and shell, respectively. The details of the mathematical approach to obtain the above mentioned equations have been provided in the references of Pustovalov et al. (2008, 2009). According to the Eq. (12.32) for laser pulse duration shorter than the thermal relaxation time, τ_T, the laser energy can be confined within the particle and the loss of heat from NPs by heat conduction during the time t_p can be ignored. For $t_p > \tau_T$ heating of both the particle and the surrounding medium is possible and the heat conduction occurs during the time t_p which will determine the maximal value of temperature. The required parameters for calculating the characteristic time and heating efficiency of our synthesized nanoshells are: $r_c = 4.75$ nm and $r_s = 7.65$ nm, heat capacity of magnetite and gold $c_c = 0.651$ J/g.K, $c_s = 0.13$ J/g.K, as well as density of magnetite and gold $\rho_c = 5.21$ g/cm³, $\rho_s = 19.3$ g/cm³, respectively. The embedding medium was considered to be water with a thermal conductivity of $K_m = 0.609$ W/m.K.

Laser-induced heating of MPNS

Suspension of PVP-MPNS in PBS was irradiated using a cw Ar laser (Melles Griot/43 Series Ion Laser-USA: 350 mW at 514 nm) and with 532 nm second harmonic pulsed Nd:YAG laser (S-504L, Songic International Limited, 8–10 ns pulse duration, 1–6 Hz), where the wavelength overlaps with the absorption band of synthesized MPNSs. For this purpose, 100 µl of the suspension of PVP-MPNS with concentrations of 25, 50, 100, and 300 µg/ml was added to each well of a 96-well cell culture plate and divided in two groups (n = 3 per group). First group was irradiated with 350 mW and 2 mm spot diameter Ar laser for 5 minutes, and the second group was irradiated with 532 nm laser with 859 mJ pulse energy (10 pulses at 1 Hz) and spot diameter of 500 µm. In a separate experiment, the suspension of MPNS-L with the nanoparticle concentration of 100 µg/ml was exposed to Ar laser for 5 min. In all samples the suspension temperature rise was measured using a digital K-type thermocouple thermometer (CHY502A1, CHY Firemate Co., Taiwan) with a probe diameter of 0.5 mm and a response time of 0.1 s, which was placed parallel and 2 mm away from the laser beam.

Release study

The controlled release of CF from MPNS-loaded liposomes was studied based on the fluorescence increase due to the release and subsequent dilution of the encapsulated self-quenching CF (Hossann et al. 2007). Briefly, for quantification of entrapped CF, liposome suspension (1 mM) was diluted 10 times by the solution of 2% Triton X-100 in water. After heating at 45°C for 15 min and vigorous mixing, 20 µl of this solution was adjusted to a total volume of 1 ml using phosphate buffer (0.1 M, pH 8) and the fluorescence (Ex. 493 nm/Em. 513 nm) was measured using fluorescence spectrophotometer (Varian, Carry eclipse). The obtained value was taken as 100% release (I_∞). Temperature dependent CF release was measured after 5 min incubation of 10 times-diluted sample at desired temperature (I_t), after which 20 µl of this solution was adjusted to a total volume of 1 ml using phosphate buffer (0.1 M, pH 8). For quantification of laser-induced release, suspension of liposomes was exposed to Ar laser ($\lambda = 514$ nm) for 3 min and 10 pulses of Nd:YAG laser second harmonic ($\lambda = 532$ nm, 1 Hz). Subsequently, fluorescence intensity was measured using fluorescence spectrophotometer and release value of CF was calculated as:

$$\text{CF release (\%)} = [(I_t - I_0)/(I_\infty - I_0)] \times 100 \tag{12.33}$$

where I_0 is the fluorescence baseline. In our conditions, the laser irradiation had no effect on the CF fluorescence intensity, which is confirmed by measurement of the fluorescence intensity of CF solutions with different concentrations before and after laser irradiation.

Cellular uptake study

In order to quantify the cellular uptake of nanoparticles, BT-474 and Calu-6 cell lines were cultured in separate wells of a 24-well cell culture plate, at a density of 3×10^4 cells/well and incubated at 37°C and 5% CO_2 for 48 h. Subsequently, cell culture medium was replaced by 500 μl of the suspension of MPNS, MPNS-L and MPNS-LAb in complete cell culture medium (100 μg/ml concentration of nanoparticle) and incubated at the same condition for additional 2 h (Davda and Labhasetwar 2002). After the incubation period, the cells were washed three times with ice cold PBS. Then, the cells were solubilized by 50 μl ice cold lysis buffer and the cell lysates were diluted to 100 μl with PBS. From each well, 10 μl of the cell lysate were used to determine the total protein content using spectrophotometer (Nanodrop) and the remains of the cell lysate was lyophilized and used to measure Fe content by ICP-MS. Measurement of the protein content was performed to normalize the Fe content in the ICP-MS experiment to the number of cells analyzed.

TUNEL analysis for detection of nanoshell-mediated laser hyperthermia

BT-474 cells were seeded at a density of 5×10^3 cells on 1 cm^2 cover slips. After 48 h of incubation at 37°C and 5% CO_2, the cell culture medium was replaced by MPNS-LAb suspended in complete cell culture medium (100 μg/ml concentration of NP). After 2 h of incubation at 37°C and 5% CO_2, the cells were washed with complete cell culture medium and divided in two groups, one irradiated by Ar laser for 5 min and the other irradiated by 10 consecutive pulses of 532 nm laser. After irradiation, they were incubated for another 1 h and then the apoptosis was measured using TUNEL assay kit according to the manufacturer's instruction. Briefly, the cells were fixed with paraformaldehyde (4% in PBS, pH 7.4) for 30 min at room temperature, washed 3 times with PBS, permeabilized with ice cold 0.1% Triton X-100 in 0.1% sodium citrate for 2 min, washed twice with PBS and finally incubated with 50 μl TUNEL reaction mixture in a humidified atmosphere for 60 min at 37°C in the dark. Subsequently, the cells were washed with PBS twice. Cells nuclei were counterstained for 5 min in 5 mg/ml Hoechst 33342 and mounted on a slide in aqueous no-fade solution. The samples were analyzed under a Ziess Axioskop 2 plus fluorescent microscope. For TUNEL and Hoechst 33342 the excitation wavelengths were 470 nm and 361 nm, respectively with the corresponding emission wavelengths of 520 nm and 486 nm. One hundred cells were analyzed per irradiation condition, and the experiment was performed twice.

Results

Electron microscopy

The micrographs of electron microscopy of superparamagnetic iron oxide nanoparticles (SPIONs), MPNS, and MPNS-L are presented in Fig. 12.21. Based on TEM micrographs, the average diameter of SPION and MPNS are found to be 9.5 ± 1.4 and 15.8 ± 3.5 nm, respectively (Fig. 12.21 A–F). Figure 12.21 G indicates the TEM micrograph of MPNS-L with a diameter of 179.73 ± 69.93 nm which have encapsulated MPNSs cluster inside unilamellar liposomes. The thickness of the lipid bilayer membrane was 6.5 ± 1.6 nm (Fig. 12.21h).

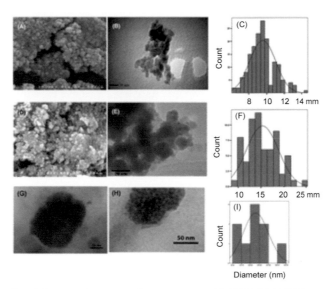

Figure 12.21. Micrographs of electron microscopy of nanostructures: (a) SEM, (b) TEM images of SPIONs and (c) its corresponding size distribution based on TEM, (d) SEM, (e) TEM image of MPNSs and (f) its corresponding size distribution based on TEM, (g) TEM image of MPNS-loaded liposomes showing the phospholipid bilayer (visualized by negative staining using 1% uranyl acetate) surrounding a collection of PVP-MPNS and (I) its corresponding size distribution. The bilayer thickness is indicated by a red line in (h).

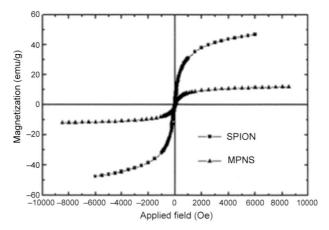

Figure 12.22. The magnetization as function of applied magnetic field of SPION (-■-) and MPNS (-▲-) at 300 K.

VSM

The magnetization as a function of applied magnetic field of SPION and MPNS at 300 K is shown in Fig. 12.22. No hysteresis loop is observed for these nanoparticles, which implies their superparamagnetic behaviour. The saturation magnetization Ms of SPION was determined to be 47.62 emu g^{-1} at 6 kOe which decreases to the 12 emu g^{-1} for MPNS, respectively.

Encapsulation efficiency

Encapsulation efficiency of MPNSs was calculated using ICP-MS results using the formula $(W_1/W) \times 100\%$, where W is initial concentration of Fe (mg/ml) in hydration solution and W_1 is encapsulated concentration of Fe (mg/ml) in liposomes. An encapsulation efficiency of 94% was obtained.

Laser-induced heating of MPNS

Suspension of PVP-MPNS in PBS was irradiated with a Ar laser and 532 nm second harmonic pulsed Nd:YAG laser, where the wavelength overlaps with the absorption band of synthesized nanoparticles (Fig. 12.23a). The temperature increase of the PVP-MPNS suspension with the concentration of 300 µg/ml was recorded after 10 consecutive pulses, which was about 2°C above the ambient temperature. When PVP-MPNS suspension was irradiated by Ar laser, the temperature raised substantially, and as it is shown in Fig. 12.23b, the temperature increase is dependent on the concentration and the maximum temperature rise of 12°C was obtained at concentration of 300 µg/ml. Also, the encapsulation of PVP-MPNS within liposome carriers had no significant effect on the temperature change of the suspension during irradiation by Ar laser (Fig. 12.23b).

Using the Eq. (12.32), a characteristic time of $\tau_T = 8.74 \times 10^{-11}$ s was calculated for synthesized nanoshells, which is smaller than pulse duration of 532 nm laser ($\tau_p = 8 \times 10^{-9}$ s). Therefore, no thermal confinement takes place and some heat exchange is expected. In addition, according to Eq. (12.31), the heating efficiency of nanoshells was determined to be 2.06×10^{-5} cm^2 K/W, which is in the order of magnitude reported for spherical silica-gold core shell NPs with the same dimension (Pustovalov et al. 2009).

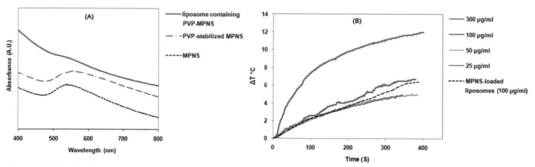

Figure 12.23. (A) Absorption measurements of MPNS, PVP-stabilized MPNS and liposome containing PVP-MPNS, (B) temperature increase of MPNS suspension with different concentrations of 25, 50, 100, 300 µg/ml and MPNS-loaded liposomes with the NP concentration of 100 µg/ml during irradiation by a continuous wave Ar laser.

Release study

The cumulative release (%) of CF from the CF/MPNS-encapsulated liposomes after irradiation by both lasers is summarized in Table 12.2. Irradiation by Ar laser for 3 min resulted in 24.3% release, whereas 532 nm induced release was laser energy dependent, and a maximum value of 28.52% was obtained using the energy of 1 J. Therefore, to understand the mechanism of CF release from liposomes, the cumulative release (%) of CF was measured at different temperatures, ranging from 37°C to 90°C. The results are summarized in Table 12.3. A maximum release value of 24.57% was obtained after 5 min incubation of the liposomes at 90°C.

Table 12.2. Laser-induced release of CF from CF/NP-encapsulated liposomes after irradiation by Ar ion laser and the Nd/YAG laser second harmonic.

Type of Laser	%R
Argon	
λ = 514 nm, irradiation period: 3 min (P = 350 mW)	24.3
Nd:YAG laser second harmonic E = 551 mJ	23.2
λ = 532 nm f = 1 Hz, E = 859 mJ	27.3
n = 10 pulses, E = 1000 mJ	28.52

Table 12.3. Cumulative release of CF (%R) from liposomes after 5 min incubation of the CF/NP encapsulated liposomes at desired temperature.

Temperature (°C)	%R after 5 min incubation
37	16.87
42	16.9
50	18.04
–6	18.21
80	18.90
90	24.57

Cellular uptake study

Effects of the targeting moiety on the cellular uptake of the MPNS by HER2 overexpressing cell line of BT-474 was measured by quantification of the iron/cell protein ratio in cells incubated with MPNS, MPNS-L, or MPNS-LAb. The results are shown in Fig. 12.24. The uptake of MPNS-LAb (4.84 ± 0.8 mg/mg) was about 9.7 and 2.4-fold higher than that of MPNS (0.5 ± 0.4 mg/mg) and MPNS-L (2.01 ± 0.38 mg/mg), respectively. Additionally, in order to evaluate the effect of HER2 expression on the cellular uptake of MPNS, Calu-6 cell line as a HER-2 negative control sample was exposed to the aforementioned three different formulations. It was observed that the magnitude of iron/cell protein ratio was approximately 5 folds lower than that of HER2-overexpressing BT-474 cell lines, and functionalization of liposomes showed no significant effect on cellular uptake of MPNS by Calu-6 cells, in comparison to MPNS-L.

Detection of laser-induced apoptosis by TUNEL assay

Before performing the TUNEL assay, the cytotoxicity of synthesized nanoshells had to be evaluated through a well-known test, MTT. Based on the MTT assay, we showed that the used MPNS concentration and the laser energy had no significant effect on cell viability. In addition, the results of cellular uptake assay answered our question about the feasibility of targeted delivery of MPNS-LAb to HER2 overexpressing cells. Therefore, in order to evaluate the laser-induced apoptosis, the effect of laser irradiation was evaluated

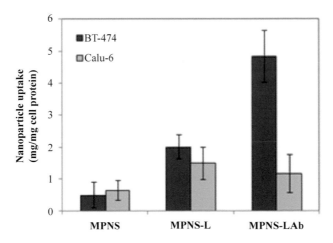

Figure 12.24. Cellular uptake of NPs normalized to cell protein content: BT-474 and Calu-6 cell lines were exposed to suspension of MPNSs, MPNS-L or MPNS-LAb in complete cell culture medium (100 µg/ml concentration of nanoparticle) for 2 h. Internalization was measured by ICP-MS. A significant increase of iron content per protein in BT-474 cell line was obtained after functionalization of MPNS-loaded liposomes with Herceptin. Functionalization of liposomes had no significant effect on cellular uptake of NPs by Calu-6 cells.

in BT-474 cell lines. As shown in Fig. 12.25, irradiation of BT-474 cells after antibody-mediated endocytosis of MPNP-LAb using both cw laser and pulsed laser resulted in the apoptosis, which is indicated by circles around TUNEL positive cells. The percentage of cell apoptosis after irradiation by Ar and pulsed 532 lasers was 44.6% and 42.6%, respectively.

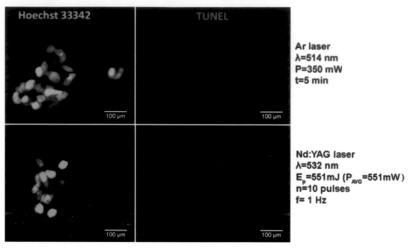

Figure 12.25. TUNEL staining following laser irradiation of BT-474 cells containing MPNS-LAb: Blue indicates the nucleus stained by Hoechst 33342. Green indicates TUNEL-positive cells, corresponding to apoptotic cells. The TUNEL positive cells are indicated by dashed circles.

Discussion

We designed and applied a novel nanostructure for targeted laser-induced apoptosis in HER2 overexpressing human breast cancer carcinoma. The high encapsulation efficiency of PVP-MPNS was obtained which confirms a successful transport of gold nanoshells towards the desired cells. Based on the LSPR peak of the synthesized gold nanoshells, we used two light sources of Ar laser and second harmonic Nd:YAG pulsed laser. Nanoparticle-mediated heat generation using Ar laser was sufficient to induce thermal damage to BT-474 cells exposed to fabricated MPNS-AbL. Also, laser-triggered release of the CF (as a model of hydrophilic drug) from MPNS-L was evaluated using both aforementioned lasers. The payload release from liposome carriers can be strongly affected by the lipid composition of the bilayer. At temperatures above the gel phase transition temperature (T_m) of lipids, the incorporation of CHOL into the bilayer has a stabilizing effect. The interaction between the cholesterol and phospholipids results in an increase in membrane unity, as has been shown by an increase in the mechanical stiffness of the membranes (Skirtach et al. 2005). In addition, the previous studies have shown that enhanced CF release at high temperature could be attributed to the change of the permeability and not to disruption of the liposome membrane (Yoshimoto et al. 2011). Therefore, the low percentage release of CF from fabricated liposomes due to direct heating of liposomes by circulating constant-temperature water could be explained by the vesicle rigidity as well as short evaluation time of the release in our experiment. Gold nanostructures can serve as energy absorption centers supplied by a laser beam. Following the laser irradiation of gold nanostructures, local heating produced due to temperature rise is transferred to the vicinity of absorbing nanostructures and the lipid bilayer causes the release of the vesicle contents. The comparison between the results obtained from laser-induced heating using cw laser and the cumulative release of CF shows the higher efficiency of release triggered by cw laser irradiation than direct heating of liposomes by circulating water. It can be concluded that the use of gold nanoshells as localized heating source within liposome carriers has more effect on permeability of bilayers in comparison to heating by circulating constant-temperature water. As it was reported by Khosroshahi et al. (2014), the irradiation of MPNSs by cw diode laser generated a significant heating effect with a hyperbolic distribution function. Also, TEM micrographs of fabricated MPNS-L indicate the cluster of a large number of the MPNSs in the immediate vicinity of the bilayer, which allow an efficient heat transfer directly to the bilayer upon cw Ar laser irradiation, leading to release of encapsulated dye.

The physical processes associated with the photothermal interaction at λ_{SPR} depend on the nanoparticle characteristics (e.g., shape, size, and the absorption cross section), as well as laser parameters. Using the pulsed laser with fluence lower than NP damage threshold can result in the temperature rise of the suspension of NPs, as reported previously (Pustovalov et al. 2008). But, at fluences above NP damage threshold melting or even evaporation of gold and subsequently generation of the vapor bubble may result around superheated NPs due to vaporization of the surrounding medium. This has been named photothermal bubble generation, which implies that the thermal energy results in phase transition around the NP (Lapotko 2009). In our case, CF/MPNS-encapsulated liposomes were irradiated at three different pulsed laser energy levels of 551, 859, and 1 J, which resulted in release values of 23.2%, 27.3%, and 28.52%, respectively. Based on the temperature increase of about 2°C above the ambient temperature measured during the laser irradiation, it is tentatively assumed that we have a photothermal bubble generation with possible cellular thermal damage. In summary, our results demonstrated that nanoshell-mediated targeted photothermal therapy is feasible, provided the light source is chosen carefully based on the main objective of the therapy. For example, in the case of controlled release of therapeutic proteins, which may be sensitive to heat, using a pulsed laser can be appropriate. However, if the controlled hyperthermia and increasing the cellular uptake of small drug molecules, such as chemotherapy drugs, is the main objective, using a cw laser seems to be a more appropriate choice.

12.4.4 *In vitro application of doxorubicin loaded magnetoplasmonic thermosensitive liposomes for laser hyperthermia and chemotherapy of breast cancer* (Khosroshahi et al. 2015)

We describe doxorubicin loaded magnetoplasmonic thermosensitive liposomes (MPTL-DOX), which are designed to combine features of magnetic drug targeting and laser hyperthermia-triggered drug release. The synthesized magnetite/gold nanoshells are stabilized using polyvinyl pyrolidone (PVP) with mean crystallite size of 15.8 ± 3.5 nm. The liposome formulation DPPC:cholesterol:DSPE-PEG2000 at 80:20:5 molar ratio shows DOX release of less than 5% at 37°C following 24 h incubation. MPTL-DOX shows encapsulation efficiencies of about 95% and 74% for DOX and magnetoplasmonic nanoshells (MPNS), respectively. The MPTL-DOX formulation displays a desired temperature sensitivity with 65% and 100% DOX release following laser irradiation and then 24 h incubation at 37°C, respectively. The rate of DOX release from liposome using this formulation is 0.09 which was obtained by heating to 43°C, and agrees well with the first kinetic model. A temperature rise between 4–12°C was achieved for MNS using 25 µg/ml and 300 µg/ml after 400 s, respectively. For cytotoxicity measurement, one untreated (control) and two treatment groups are studied. The first treatment groups are: with MPNS only, with MPTL only, and laser irradiation only. The second treatment groups are: laser hyperthermia using MPTL, MPTL with magnetic field (MF), MPTL-DOX, and MPTL-DOX with MF. MPTL-DOX is targeted to breast cancer cell lines (MCF-7 cells) under a permanent magnetic field and exhibits a substantial increase in cytotoxicity and apoptotic effects. The results suggest that externally guided drug targeting can trigger drug release using an exogenous absorber in laser hyperthermia which can be used advantageously for thermo-chemotherapy of cancers.

Introduction

Engineered nanomaterials hold great promise in drug delivery systems (Puvvada 2011, Yiv and Uckun 2012, Gowda et al. 2013). Novel magnetic nano-formulations such as liposomes, metallic/nonmetallic, and polymeric nanoparticles have increased the ability to deliver drugs for which conventional therapies have shown limited efficacy. When magnetoliposomes containing iron oxide nanoparticles are exposed to a magnetic field, the liposomal temperature exceeds transition temperature and the contents are released (Babincova et al. 2002). Heating techniques may be improved by using a magnetic field localized to therapeutic site, for instance a tumor (Landon et al. 2011, Tsalach et al. 2014, Candido et al. 2014). Hassannejad et al. (2014) have recently demonstrated that gold-coated superparamagnetic iron oxide nanoparticles (SPIONs) encapsulated by phospholipid liposomes can be used as exogenous absorbers in laser thermal therapy. Moreover, gold nanoparticles were conjugated with the anticancer drug Doxorubicin, for drug delivery to liver cancer recently (Syed et al. 2013). When gold nanostructures are irradiated by laser, the absorbed optical energy raises their temperature, hence acting as a localized heat source that is quickly equalized within the nanoparticles. The heat is then transferred to the surrounding environment determined by their thermal relaxation time and laser pulse duration. Therefore, light-triggered thermal properties of liposomal Au nanostructures are different from the classical thermosensitive liposomes (Paasonen et al. 2010). Au nanostructures absorb energy at a characteristic wavelength and exhibit surface plasmon resonance (SPR) (Lukianova-Hleb et al. 2011, Hassannejad and Khosroshahi 2013). Only part of the absorbed energy is emitted as photoluminescence while most of it is converted to heat (Fenske and Cullis 2008). Therefore, light-induced heating of liposomal Au nanostructures by UV, visible, and near-infrared to release liposome-entrapped drugs has developed (Yavlovich et al. 2010). In addition to the required elements for triggered drug release, an optimized delivery system for cytotoxic drugs should have biophysical properties (e.g., stealth properties) to favour passive accumulation in tumors upon intravenous administration. This study is a novel approach towards implementing a PEG-shielded thermosensitive liposome encapsulating the DOX as a drug together with PVP-stabilized magneto-plasmonic nanoshells (MPNS), enabling magnetic drug targeting by static gradient magnetic fields and laser hyperthermia as a trigger for drug release, producing a synergistic cytotoxic effect. To the best of our knowledge, this combination of magnetic targeting/laser hyperthermia/drug release is novel and has not been addressed previously.

Materials and methods

Chemicals and reagents

All analytical reagents are used without further purification. Ferric chloride hexahydrate ($FeCl_3.6H_2O$, 99%), ferrous chloride tetrahydrate ($FeCl_2.4H_2O$, 99%), hydrochloric acid (HCl, 37%), sodium hydroxide, chloroform, formaldehyde solution (H_2CO, 37%), absolute ethanol, Triton X-100, and polyvidone25 are purchased from Merck (USA). Tetrakis (hydroxymethyl) phosphonim chloride (THPC) aqueous solution, Gold (III) chloride trihydrate ($HAuCl_4.3H_2O$, ≥ 49% Au basis), 3-aminopropyltriethoxysilane (APTES), and Doxorubicin hydrochloride (DOX) are purchased from Sigma-Aldrich (USA). Dipalmitoylphosphatidylcholine (DPPC), cholesterol (Chol), and 1,2-distearoyl-sn-glycero-3-phosphoethanolamine-N-[amino(polyethylene glycol)-2000] (ammonium salt) (DSPE-PEG2000) are purchased from Avanti Polar Lipids (USA). MCF-7 cell line is purchased from the Pasteur Institute (Iran). RPMI 1640 medium and fetal bovine serum (FBS) are purchased from GIBCO (USA). Annexin-V-FLUOS staining kit is purchased from Roche (Switzerland). Deionized water (18 MΩ.cm) is provided by a Milli-Q system and deoxygenated by vacuum for 1 hour prior to the use.

Synthesis of PVP-stabilized gold nanoshells

Gold coated superparamagnetic iron oxide nanoparticles (SPIONs) are fabricated by a multistep procedure, as described earlier (Khosroshahi and Ghazanfari 2012, Ghazanfari and Khosroshahi 2014). Briefly, SPIONs are synthesized by the coprecipitation method (Kou et al. 2008, Khosroshahi and Ghazanfari 2010, Khosroshahi and Ghazanfari 2012). Then the surface of SPIONs is functionalized with APTES to generate an amine terminated surface (Khosroshahi and Ghazanfari 2012). A colloidal gold solution containing ~ 2 nm Au particles is prepared according to the Duff et al. (1993) method. After that, a continuous gold shell is grown around the SPIONs. In order to prepare PVP-coated gold nanoshells in a typical procedure (Hassannejad et al. 2014), the obtained nanoshell dispersion in water (2 ml) is centrifuged at 4000 g for 25 min. Then 1 ml supernatant is replaced by 1 ml PVP solution and the obtained mixture is stirred for 24 hours at room temperature. After that, it is centrifuged twice under 4000 g for 25 min and washed with water in order to remove free PVP. As the hydrophilic head group (N-C = O) of PVP is attached to the surface of the particles, particle repulsion will occur due to steric interactions between polymers adsorbed on the particle's surface.

Preparation of magnetoplasmonic liposomes

Liposomes are composed of DPPC:Chol:DSPE-PEG2000 at a molar ratio of 80:20:5, as suggested by Pradhan et al. (2010). A lipid mixture of chloroform stocks is prepared and dried at 42°C under nitrogen stream and further placed in a vacuum overnight. The lipid film is hydrated with a buffer consisting of PVP-coated gold nanoshell dispersed in 300 mM Citrate (pH 4.0) at 60°C. After hydration, 15 min of sonication (Tecna 20, 190 W) is applied to break down any larger vesicles. Subsequently, the samples undergo 5 cycles of freeze-thaw, including 10 min at -196°C, 10 min at 65°C, and 30 s vortexing between cycles. Unencapsulated nanoparticles are removed by centrifuging at 400 g for 5 min, after which the supernatant liposomal dispersion is centrifuged at 20000 g for 30 min to precipitate the liposomes encapsulating gold nanoshells. Liposomes are obtained by extruding the mixture 15 times with an extruder (Avanti Polar Lipids) at 55°C through polycarbonate membrane filters (Whatman PLC, Maidstone, Kent) with a pore size of 100 nm. Encapsulation efficiency of MPTL is calculated using ICP-MS results through the formula (W1/W) $\times$ 100%, where W is initial concentration of Fe (mg/ml) in hydration solution and W1 is encapsulated concentration of Fe (mg/ml) in the liposomes.

Doxorubicin loading into the magnetoplasmonic liposomes (MPTL-DOX)

Doxorubicin, a weak base cation with a pKa of 8.3, is encapsulated into the extruded liposomes using a pH-gradient loading protocol as described by Mayer et al. (1986) with a slight modification: the exterior pH of the extruded liposomes is adjusted to 8 with sodium carbonate solution (500 mM) creating a pH gradient. The preheated liposomes are incubated with doxorubicin hydrochloride (DOX:lipid weight ratio of 1:10); with respect to the amount of original total lipid used for the liposome preparation at 60°C for 1 h. Unencapsulated DOX is removed by passing the liposome through a Sephadex-G50 (fine) column at a flow rate of 0.5 ml/min with HEPES buffered saline (10 mM HEPES pH 7.4 and 140 mM NaCl) as the eluent. The resulting liposomes (MPTL-DOX) are stored at 4°C until further use. The DOX concentration of the liposomes is determined by a Cary Eclipse spectro-fluorimeter equipped with ThermoScan Software (Varian, Palo Alto, CA) at 485 nm excitation and 590 nm emission wavelength. 20 μl DOX loaded liposomes are incubated in 1 ml HEPES buffered saline for up to 60 min and the fluorescence intensity is measured after various incubation times. Before measurement, the samples are allowed to cool down to room temperature. For quantification, a calibration curve is obtained with a dilution series of free doxorubicin in 1% Triton X-100 in HEPES buffered saline is used. Using the following formula, entrapment efficiency (%) = (encapsulated drug in liposomes/amount of total drug) $\times$ 100% (Nie et al. 2012).

Cells and cell culture

The MCF-7 breast cancer cells are cultivated in RPMI 1640 medium supplemented with 10% FBS and maintained at 37°C in a 5% CO_2 incubator.

Cytotoxicity study

Cytotoxicity studies are done using MTT (3-(4,5-dimethylthiazol-2-yl)-2,5-diphenyltetrazolium bromide) tetrazolium reduction assay. As suggested by Kulshrestha et al. (2012) 1×104 cells per well are cultivated in 96-well plates overnight. The control group is untreated cells and the first MCF-7 treatment groups are: with magnetoplasmonic nanoshells only, with MPTL (at a lipid concentration of 10 mM) only, and with laser irradiation only. For the control (untreated) group, the cells are washed with PBS, and after that the fresh cell culture media is placed in an incubator for the next 24 h. For the MPNS and MPTL treatments, the cells are cultured in 200 μl medium containing nanoshells and MPTL (at lipid concentration of 10 mM), respectively. In order to study the effect of magnetic fields on nanoliposomes, during the first hour of incubation, the culture plates are positioned on the 96-well format magnetic plate (Chemicell-Germany) with a field gradient of 50–130 T/m. After 75 min, the cells are washed with PBS and incubated for another 24 h with fresh medium. The second treatment groups are: laser hyperthermia mediated by MPTL only,

MPTL with magnetic field (MF), MPTL-DOX only, and MPTL-DOX with MF all at lipid concentration of 10 mM. *In vitro* hyperthermia of MCF-7 cells consisting of liposomes containing magneto-plasmonic nanoshells is done using Argon laser (Melles Griot/43 Series Ion Laser-USA) at 350 mW for 5 minutes with or without DOX. The thermometer is connected at the other end to a Windows-based laptop where the results are displayed on the screen. During the experiment the temperature is maintained at $37 \pm 0.4°C$ recorded by a digital thermometer (Model No. HP-34420A).

In vitro evaluation of thermo-chemotherapy

In vitro evaluation of cellular uptake is based on 15 min incubation of cells in a solution containing Ca_2+ ions and annexin V-FITC (at a final concentration of 1 μg/ml). The annexin V-binding buffer consists of 10 mM HEPES-NaOH, pH 7.4, 150 mM NaCl, 5 mM KCl, 1 mM MgCl2, and 1.8 mM $CaCl_2$. The stained cells are mounted on slides and immediately visualized under the fluorescence microscope. Procedure of preparation of the multihybrid nanoliposomes is illustrated in Fig. 12.26.

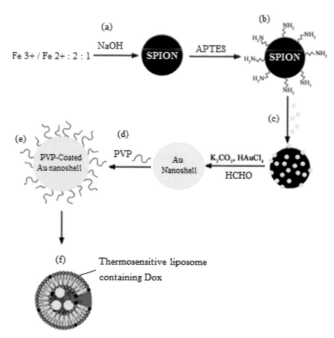

Figure 12.26. Preparation procedure of the nanoliposomes. (a) synthesis of SPION, (b) functionalization of SPION with APTES, (c) colloidal gold attachment to the amine groups, (d) gold nanoshell growth, (e) PVP coating on the surface of gold nanoshell, (f) magnetoplasmonic nanoshells and Dox co-loaded liposome.

Characterization

Transmission electron microscopy (TEM) as performed using a CM 200 FEG STEM Philips-M.E.R.C. operating at the voltage of 200 kV. Liposomes are observed by TEM following negative staining with uranyl acetate. Liposomes are diluted with distilled water and dropped on a PDL-coated copper grid. The excessive sample is removed with filter paper and air-dried for 1 min at room temperature. Subsequently, uranyl acetate solution (10 μl of 1%) is dropped onto the grid. After 1 min the excess staining solution is removed with filter paper and is allowed to dry in the air before introduction into the microscope. Fourier Transform Infrared Spectroscopy (FT-IR) spectra are recorded by TENSOR27 FT-IR spectrometer. The obtained nanoparticles are dried, mixed with KBr and compressed into a pellet. UV-VIS spectroscopy of nanoparticle suspensions is taken on a CARY100 UV-VIS spectrophotometer with a 10 mm optical path length quartz cuvette. The mean hydrodynamic radius and polydispersity of the liposomal vesicles are determined using Dynamic Laser Light Scattering (DLS). The scattered laser light intensity at 90° is measured by light scattering photometer using a wavelength of 488 nm (Brookhaven instrument Corporation, USA). Stability of magnetoliposomes formulation is evaluated by measuring the zeta potential. The zeta potential is measured as the particle electrophoretic mobility of charged, colloidal suspensions by means of laser microelectrophoresis in a thermostatted cell at room temperature (Brookhaven Instruments Corporation, USA). Every sample measurement is repeated 5 times. Encapsulation efficiency of gold nanoshells within the liposomes is determined by inductively coupled plasma mass spectrometry (ICP-MS). Samples for ICP-MS (VARIAN 735-ES) analysis are frozen, lyophilized, and dissolved in nitric acid hydrochloride, prepared by adding nitric acid (100 μL) and hydrochloric acid (300 μL of 37%) for 72 h to dissolve particles. Then, samples are diluted to 2 mL with $HNO3$ (1.6 mL of 2%) and analyzed via ICP-MS against standards. Magnetization measurements are carried at 300 K in a magnetic field (H) of up to 20 kOe with a vibrating sample magnetometer (Meghnatis Daghigh Kavir Co. VSM/AGFM) that can measure magnetic moments as low as 10^{-3} emu. For the magnetization measurements, NPs are in dry powder form obtained by evaporating the water from the solution. The samples are dried by freeze dryer (Pishtaz Engineering Co. Model: FD-4).

Statistical analysis

All experiments are performed at least in triplicate. The value of particle size determined by TEM micrographs is the average of at least 50 measurements and reported as mean ± standard deviation. The SPSS 15.0 is used to perform the calculations. Paired-sample t-test is used to compare the difference between the control and treated groups. P values of < 0.05 are considered statistically significant.

Results and Discussion

FTIR

Figure 12.27 shows the FT-IR spectra of bare SPION (a), amine-functionalized SPION (b), PVP (c), and PVP-covered gold nanoshell (d). The broad band at region of 3550–3200 cm^{-1} with moderate intensity is assigned to the presence of –OH groups at the surface of nanoparticles. The peaks at 444 and 579 cm^{-1} in Fig. 12.27a are assigned to the vibration of Fe-O bond, which are characteristic bands of magnetite. The broad band at 1623 cm^{-1} and the split band at 3414 cm^{-1} can be attributed to the N-H stretching vibration and NH_2 bending mode of free NH_2 groups, respectively. Also, it can be seen that the characteristic bands of the Fe-O bond of amine-functionalized SPIONs shift to higher frequencies of 620 and 477 cm^{-1} compared to that of bare SPIONs (at 579 and 444 cm^{-1}). These shifts have been attributed to the replacement of –H at the Fe-O-H groups on the surface of SPION by the more electronegative group of $-Si(O-)2-$ which results in the enhancement of bond force constant for Fe-O bonds. The FTIR spectrum of PVP (Fig. 12.27c) mainly consists of two bands at 1282 and 1664 cm^{-1} corresponding to the vibration of C-N and carbonyl group in pyrrolidone ring. Similar bands are also seen in the FT-IR spectrum of PVP-coated gold nanoshells. However, comparing with the spectrum of PVP, the resonance peak of C-N, at 1282 cm^{-1}, was shifted to 1475 cm^{-1} and the band of C = O, at 1664 cm^{-1}, red shifted to 1647 cm^{-1}. The change of the spectrum indicates that the absorption of PVP on the gold shell is not on the basis of electrostatic attraction, but gold atoms on the surface of nanoparticles would coordinate with N and O atoms of PVP which is consistent with previously reported results (Liu et al. 2010). FTIR confirms the presence of a PVP coating on the nanoshells.

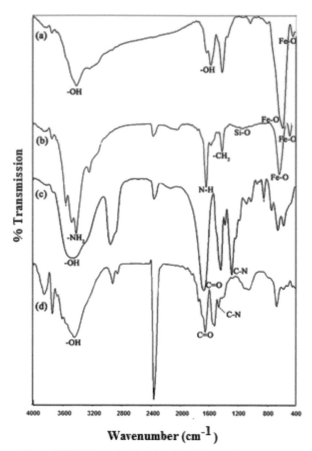

Figure 12.27. FTIR spectra of bare SPION (a), amine-functionalized SPION (b), PVP (c) and PVP-covered SPION/gold nanoshells (d).

DLS

The effect of surface coating on the stability of SPIONs is observable from DLS data. The volume-weighted hydrodynamic size measured by DLS for nanostructures are summarized in Table 12.4. The reduced hydrodynamic size of amine-functionalized SPIONs shows more stability of nanoparticle suspension after silanization reaction. This effect can be also seen after coating of the amine-functionalized SPIONs with a continuous thin layer of gold, which reduced the hydrodynamic size of gold nanoshells to 57 nm. After PVP coating of gold nanoshells, the hydrodynamic size increased to 102 nm, which is because of the nanoshell's surface functionalization with long chain PVP molecules. This result agrees well with the previously reported thickness in the case of PVP adsorbed on palladium nanoparticles (Hirai and Yakura 2001). The hydrodynamic diameter of the MPTL-DOX is 240 nm. The size distribution of this formulation is quite homogenous as polydispersity index is around 0.19.

Table 12.4. Properties of synthesized nanoparticles in different steps of fabrication.

	TEM size ± SE (nm)	DLS volume-weighted size (PDI) (nm)	Electrophoretic potential ± SE (mV)
SPION	9.5 ± 1.4	201 (0.22)	−29 ±
SPION/Au nanoshell	–	57 (0.21)	−21 ± 0.9
PVP-coated nanoshell (MPNS)	15.8 ± 3.5	102 (0.22)	−3.0 ± 0.7
MPTL MPTL-DOX	97.5 ± 5.7 –	142 (0.20) 240 (0.19)	−40 ± 0.8 −39 ± 0.6

VSM

Figure 12.28 shows the magnetization curve for magnetite core and gold nanoshells at ambient temperature. It indicates the superparamagnetic behaviour of nanostructures. It can be deduced that the magnetite NPs have magnetization saturation (Ms) of about 46.94 emu/g. Absence of hysteresis loss with zero coercivity in the magnetization curve suggests the superparamagnetic nature of the particles. The Ms value of the resultant gold nanoshells decreases to 11.98 emu/g, when the gold is added. With the same magnetite core size and gold shell thickness of 3.5 nm, the Ms value for the synthesized nanoshells in this paper is larger than that reported by Xu et al. (2007).

TEM

The physical size of particles at different steps of nanoshell fabrication is determined by bright field TEM. Based on TEM micrographs (Fig. 12.29), the average diameter of SPIONs and SPION/gold nanoshells are 9.5 ± 1.4 and 15.8 ± 3.5 nm, respectively. TEM image confirms the formation of magnetoplasmonic liposome (Fig. 12.30). The clear margin of each encapsulated nanoparticle indicates the steric hindrance of PVP-covered nanoshells. Based on TEM micrographs, the average diameter of SPION/gold nanoshells are 15.8 ± 3.5 nm. It is observed that MPNS are packed within the liposomes. The thickness of the lipid bilayer membrane surrounding the collection of nanoshells is 6.5 ± 1.6 nm measured by NIH Image J software (http://rsb.info.nih.gov/ij/), suggesting the formation of unilamellar liposomal structure. A value of 7–8 nm is also reported for lipid bilayer membrane (Floris et al. 2011).

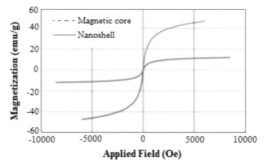

Figure 12.28. (a) Variation of magnetization with applied magnetic field for bare magnetite core and (b) magnetoplasmonic nanoshells.

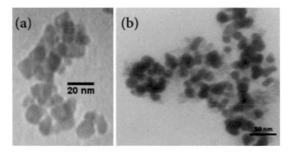

Figure 12.29. TEM images showing (a) SPIONs of diameter 9.5 ± 1.4 nm and (b) SPION/gold nanoshells.

Encapsulation efficiency of nanoshells

A magnetoplasmonic nanoshells (MPNS) encapsulation efficiency of 54% is obtained. Higher encapsulation of MPNS results in higher heating ability, therefore it increases the toxicity of the liposomes. In this aspect, this magnetoplasmonic liposomes is superior to the others reported in literature (Pradhan et al. 2010).

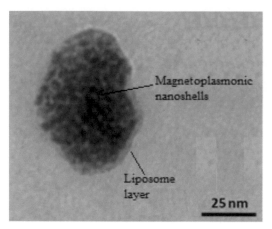

Figure 12.30. TEM image of gold nanoshell-encapsulated liposome.

The concentration of nanoshells has a significant effect on the amount of heat generated at a given power density. This effectively indicates that not only do the MPNSs play an important role in generating thermal effect, but also that an enhanced absorption cross section for spherical metal nanoshells can be achieved at optimized value of concentration for a better laser-hyperthermia (Ghazanfari and Khosroshahi 2014). The absorption efficiency of our synthesized MPNS corresponds to 0.656 at λ_{SPR} of 531 nm. Maximum value of the parameter $\Delta T/I$ shows the efficiency of transformation of absorbed optical energy by MPNS into the thermal energy, where T is the temperature and I is constant intensity of laser radiation during pulse duration. In our case, the nanoshell efficiency parameter equals $2 \times 10^{-5}°C \; cm^2/W$.

Furthermore, an experiment was set up to measure the temperature of the aqueous medium containing dispersed gold nanoshells and magnetoplasmonic liposomes, where the cuvette containing the sample was irradiated by laser at 17 W/cm² for 400 s. A thermistor probe (Redfish Sensors Inc., Model QTGB-14 D3) with an accuracy of 0.15% was placed in the solution to monitor the temperature change where it was recorded by a thermometer (Model No. HP-34420A). The output of the thermometer was connected to a Windows-based laptop where the results were displayed. As it is shown in Fig. 12.31, at low concentrations, the temperature of MPNS increases steadily and linearly up to 4°C in about 300 s where it reaches the turning point and saturates after 400 s. At 100 μg/ml the temperature reaches its maximum of 6.5°C, but when the concentration was increased to 300 μg/ml, the temperatures increases linearly up to 8°C in about 120 s where it shows a turning point and at this stage the temperature rise gradually until it is maximized at 12°C after 400 s. Such a phenomenon can be due to the arrangement, density, and potential for aggregation of Au nanoshells. Therefore, it results in a stronger surface plasmon absorption of light and more efficient photothermal effects. All the experiments demonstrate that the temperature increases with increasing MPNs concentration and the exposure time. However, in the case of MPNS encapsulated liposomes, as seen in Fig. 12.32, the maximum temperature obtained was about 6°C after 400 s which as expected is less than the case of those without liposome. These results clearly confirm that the fabricated

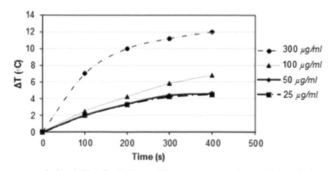

Figure 12.31. Temperature variation (ΔT) of MPNSs at different concentrations with irradiation time at 17 W/cm⁻².

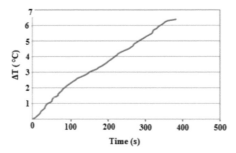

Figure 12.32. Temperature variation (ΔT) of MPNS encapsulated liposomes at 100 μg/ml with irradiation time.

MNSs are not only suitable candidates for hyperthermia tumor therapy, but even with liposome carriers the temperature increase is sufficient to cause the hyperthermic effect about 42–45°C. The question of how fast and what temperature is generally achievable entirely depends on the MPNS concentration, the laser power, and the irradiation time.

Laser induced fluorescence spectroscopy (LIF)

The fluorescence response of Dox was studied at room temperature using 488 nm wavelength of argon laser, which is close to its excitation wavelength. The emission spectrum was recorded and processed by Spectrasuit software. The results of LIF experiment for Dox, TL, TL-Dox, and MPTL-Dox are shown in Fig. 12.33, where a peak at 590 nm corresponding to Dox emission is observed. A small bump at 550 nm is thought to be due to Au nanoshell response.

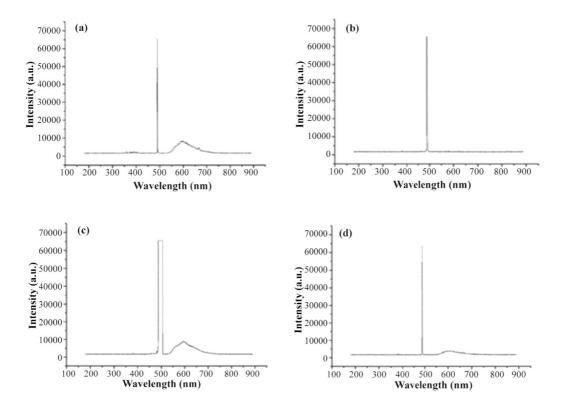

Figure 12.33. LIF spectra (a) free Dox, (b) liposomes, (c) Dox loaded liposomes, (d) Dox and gold nanoshells co-loaded liposomes.

Recent studies have indicated that AuNPs act as good quenchers of many fluorescence donors, due to the nanosurface energy transfer (NSET) effect (Wang et al. 2011). Addition of gold nanoshells to TL-Dox result in a significant quenching of doxorubicin fluorescence (Fig. 12.33d), demonstrating the presence of NSET between the doxorubicinyl groups and Au nanoshells.

Encapsulation efficiency of DOX and drug release study under laser irradiation

The drug encapsulation efficiency of 95% for DOX-loaded magnetoplasmonic liposome is calculated. The liposome formulation DPPC:cholesterol:DSPE-PEG2000 shows DOX release of less than 5% at 37°C following 24 h incubation. This particular lipid composition has Tm at around 41.3°C (Pradhan et al. 2010), as a thermosensitive formulation, so minimal leakage at 37°C and triggered DOX release at 43°C is expected. DOX release from magnetoplasmonic liposomes are 65% and 100% in 50% FBS following 5 min Argon ion laser (350 mW, $\lambda = 514$ nm) irradiation and 24 h incubation at 37°C, respectively. Laser induced hyperthermia raises the temperature from 37°C to 43°C, which leads to the phase transition of the lipid combination causing massive release of the encapsulated drug. Most of the magnetic liposomes reported in earlier studies (Viroonchatapan et al. 1998) have been composed of DPPC alone, which shows a high burst of drug release even at 37°C. By adding saturated lipids, the compressibility moduli of the liposome could be increased.

Furthermore, it has been established that drug release from low temperature sensitive liposomes occurs via grain boundary permeabilization when it is heated into the region of its phase transition temperature (Landon et al. 2011). However, the grain boundary structures of the bilayer could bind proteins that are responsible for opsonization. Therefore, in order to reduce the toxicity (by avoiding the opsonization) a few mol% of DSPE-PEG2000 is added to cover the bilayer (Landon et al. 2011).

Drug release from thermosensitive liposomes

As reported by Pradhan et al. (2010), phase transition temperature of the liposome prepared with formulation of DPPC:CHOL:DSPE-PEG2000 at the molar ratio of 80:20:5 is ~ 42°C. In this report, the drug release rate from similar lipid composition is measured as a function of time at 43°C. The release rate of thermosensitive liposome varies according to the composition of liposome, its preparation procedure, and heating temperature (Yatvin et al. 1981). The relation between percentage release and exposure time is found to follow the first-order kinetics expressed as (Woo et al. 2008)

$$\%R(t) = R_c(1 - e^{-k_{rel}t})$$
(12.33)

where % R(t) is the percentage of drug released at exposure time t, krel is liposome release rate, and Rc is the total percentage of drug released at a given heating temperature. It is assumed that at t = 0 the temperature is 37°C. This equation is used to fit the experimental data obtained at 43°C (Yatvin et al. 1981). From the best fitting curve (shown in Fig. 12.34) obtained by using nonlinear least squares method, the release rate is found to be 0.07 for TL-Dox and 0.09 for MPTL-Dox. In addition, doxorubicin release from both of the formulations are assessed (Table 12.5).

Cytotoxicity study

Figure 12.35 shows the cytotoxic effect of laser, MPNS, and MPTL on MCF-7 cells. The untreated (control) and first treated (i.e., exposure of untreated cells to laser, MPNS, or MPTL) groups are non-toxic. After being heated, the cells develop resistance to heat, which reduces the likelihood of being destroyed by direct thermal cytotoxic effects. Because hyperthermia alters the cell walls by means of so-called heat shock proteins, cancer cells then react much more effectively to the radiation (Burke et al. 2012). So before the laser hyperthermia experiment, the cells are normally preheated, which in our case was done using a water bath (Lab Companion, USA). The heating effect of surrounding liquid medium on viability of MCF-7 and L-929 cells was assessed after being heated for 5 min at the temperature of 43°C. The cell viability is significantly (~ %50) decreasing in L-929 cells, but as for MCF-7 cells, there is no significant difference

Table 12.5. Doxorubicin release from thermosensitive liposomes irradiated with Ar ion laser (350 mW).

Sample	24 hr–37°C	5 min Ar Laser Irradiation	24 hr–37°C
TL-DOX	5%	12%	69%
MPTL-DOX	15%	65%	100%

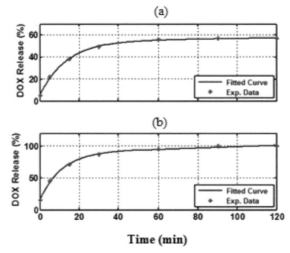

Figure 12.34. Rate of nanoliposomes drug release (a) TL-Dox, (b) MPTL-Dox with drug concentration of 0.13 μg/ml at 43°C.

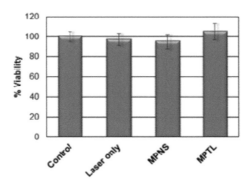

Figure 12.35. Cytotoxicity profile of control (untreated) and first treated (exposure of untreated cells to laser, MPNS, and MPTL) groups (mean ± SD; n = 3, P > 0.05).

between control and treated cells. The cytotoxic effects of laser hyperthermia and chemotherapy using the prepared formulation as single and combined modalities are illustrated in Fig. 12.36. Data are presented as a percentage of the cell viability, where viability of control group is taken as 100%.

Magnetic guidance is one of the strategies for the accumulation of nanoparticles. Therefore, when the magnetic field is applied, most of the MNS are accumulated at the bottom of the wells, where the cells are present. After that, based on the SPR absorption in gold nanoshells, an energy relaxation is followed through a non-radiative decay channel, which results in an increase in kinetic energy, leading to overheating of the local environment around the light-absorbing species. Clearly, the hyperthermia effects are expected to be higher, where the applied magnetic field have accumulated for most of the nanoparticles around the cells. Because it increases the possibility of Au NPs aggregation, it results in a stronger localized SPR, and thus more efficient photothermal effects. Moreover, the combined laser hyperthermia treatment and magnetically targeting MPTL-DOX, at doxorubicin concentration of 0.5 μg/ml (IC-50 of MCF-7 cells) (Osman et al. 2012) and 0.1 μg/ml result in less than 1% and less than 15% cell viability (Fig. 12.36), respectively. An

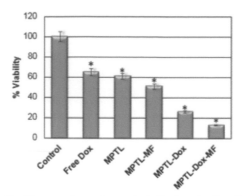

Figure 12.36. Cytotoxicity profile of the second treated group including laser irradiated MPTL and MPTL-DOX formulations on MCF-7 cells (mean ± SD; n = 3, *P < 0.05), where permanent magnetic field (MF) is applied during the incubation of some samples, as indicated.

analysis of these combined treatments using Valeriote's formula (Valeriote and Lin 1975) shows that the magnetically targeted MPTL-DOX and laser hyperthermia treatments are synergistic in nature.

Fluorescence microscopy

Figure 12.37 shows that the internalized nanoliposomes release doxorubicin in the acidic organelles of MCF-7 cells, which would activate the fluorescence of doxorubicin quenched by Au nanoshells due to NSET. The fluorescence microscopy images of MPTL-DOX in MCF-7 cells are obtained by a fluorescence microscope Eclipse 80i (Nikon, Japan). DOX-MPNS loaded liposomes are incubated with MCF-7 cells for about 75 min (with and w/o MF) and irradiated with Ar laser at 37°C. The image (a) shows the red fluorescence in the area or the nucleus of the MF applied to MPTL-DOX in MCF-7 cells. The nucleus of the cells in MPTL-DOX-w/o MF (d) does not show this fluorescence. This confirms that under magnetic field, the drug loaded NPs are internalized by the cells. It has been reported that chemosensitivity to DOX in MCF7 is due to the decreased level of DNA double-strand break repair proteins (Henning et al. 2007). Aroui et al. (2010) have shown that the major mechanism of DOX activity is the inhibition of topoisomerase II and stabilization of a ternary drug-topoisomerase II (TOPO II)-DNA complex, causing DNA damage and induction of apoptosis. Furthermore, Prasad et al. (2007) have shown that hyperthermia causes apoptosis

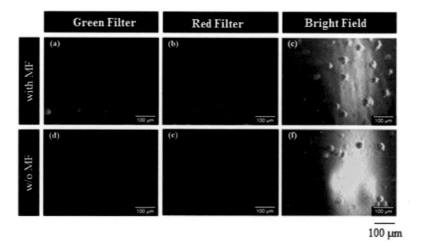

100 μm

Figure 12.37. Uptake of doxorubicin loaded MPTL by MCF-7 cells, the cells are incubated with drug loaded nanostructures for about 75 min, (a–c) with permanent magnetic field (MF), (d–f) without (MF) and irradiated with Ar laser at 37°C. The images are obtained by the fluorescence microscope equipped with green and red filters for, Annexin V-FITC and DOX, respectively (n = 3).

by irreversibly damaging the actin and tubulin structures of cells. Hyperthermia damages different cellular structures, such as enzyme complexes required for DNA synthesis and repair (George and Singh 1982). We believe that the presence of gold nanoshells enhances the laser hyperthermia effect in a controlled manner.

In addition, apoptosis is a mode of cell death that is accompanied by specific alterations to the plasma membrane. In Fig. 12.37c,f, membrane blebbing can be identified, which is characteristic of apoptotic cells (Massart et al. 2004). Redistribution of phosphatidylserine from the inner to the outer plasma membrane leaflet has become one of the most widely used markers for apoptotic cells in mammals. This is largely due to the availability of annexin V probe as a sensitive phosphatidylserine-binding protein. The FITC-conjugated annexin V-binding assay provides a very specific, rapid, and reliable technique to detect apoptosis. Analysis of fluorescence microscopy images is conducted to reveal the enhanced cell apoptosis caused by the magnetoplasmonic nanoshells and doxorubicin under combined chemotherapeutic and hyperthermia therapies. Therefore, this experiment indicates the doxorubicin loading into the liposomes in addition to indicating the potential application of this hybrid nanosystem in fluorescence imaging.

Keywords: Theranostic, Hyperthermia, Laser hyperthermia, Enhanced radiotherapy, Bioheat equation, Gold nanoshell, Lung cancer cells, Surface plasmon resonance, Third generation nanodendrimers, Folic acid, Breast cancer cells, Fluorescence microscopy, Magnetoplasmonic nanoshells, Doxorubicin, Thermosensitive liposomes, Cytotoxicity.

References

Afifi, M., S. El-Sheikh and M. Abdelsalam. 2013. Therapeutic efficacy of plasmonic photothermal nanoparticles in hamstrer buccal pouch carcinoma. Oral Surg. Med. Pathol. Radiol. 115: 743–751.

Alexis, F., E. Pridgen and R. Langer. 2010. Nanoparticle technologies for cancer therapy. Handb Exp. Pharmacol. 197: 55–86.

American Cancer Society. Cancer facts and figures 2008. http://www.cancer.org/downloads/STT/2008CAFFfinalseculred.pdf.

Amin, Z., J. Donald, A. Masters, R. Kant, A.C. Steger and S.G. Bown. 1993. Hepatic metastases:interstitial laser photocoagulation with real time US monitoring and dynamic CT evaluation treatment. Radiology 187: 339–347.

Arias, J., V. Gallardo and S. Gomez-Lopera. 2001. Synthesis and characterization of poly(ethyl-2-cyanoacrylate) nanoparticles with a magnetic core. J. of Cont. Rel. 77: 309–321.

Aroui, S., S. Brahim, M. Waa and A. Kenani. 2010. Cytotoxicity, intracellular distribution and uptake of doxorubicin and doxorubicin coupled to cell-penetrating peptides in different cell lines: a comparative study. Biochem. Biophys. Res. Commun. 391: 419–425.

Avsec, J. and M. Oblak. 2007. The calculation of thermal conductivity, viscosity and thermodynamic properties for nanofluids on the basis of statistical nanomechanics. Int. J. Heat Mass Tran. 50: 4331–4341.

Avetisyan, Y., A. Yakunin and V. Tuchin. 2012. Novel thermal effect at nanoshell heating by pulsed laser irradiation: hoop-shaped hot zone formation. J. Biophotonics 5: 734–744.

Babincova, M., P. Cicmanec, V. Altanerova, C. Altaner and P. Babinec. 2002. AC-magnetic field controlled drug release from magnetoliposomes: design of a method for site-specific chemotherapy. Bioelectrochemistry 55: 17–9.

Bardhan, R., W. Chen and C. Perez-Torres. 2009. Nanoshells with targeted simultaneous enhancement of magnetic field and optical imaging and photothermal therapeutic response. Adv. Funct. Matter. 19: 3901–3909.

Bardhan, R., W. Chen and M. Bartels. 2010. Tracking of multimodal therapeutic nanocomposites targeting breast cancer *in vivo*. Nano Lett. 10: 4920–4928.

Barrajón-Catalán, E., M. Menéndez-Gutiérrez, A. Falco, A. Carrato, M. Saceda and V. Micol. 2010. Selective death of human breast cancer cells by lytic immunoliposomes: correlation with their HER2 expression level. Cancer Lett. 290: 192–203.

Baykal, A., M. Toprak, Z. Durmus and M. Senel. 2012. Synthesis and characterization of dendrimer-encapsulated iron and iron-oxide nanoparticles. J. Supercond. Nov. Mag. 25: 1541–1549.

Berbeco, R., W. Ngwa and G. Makrigiorgos. 2011. Localized dose enhancement to tumour blood vessel endothelial cells via megavoltage x-rays and targeted gold nanoparticles. Int. J. Radiat. Oncol. Biol. Phys. 81: 270–276.

Biswal, B., M. Kavitha, R. Verma and E. Prasad. 2009. Tumor cell imaging using the intrinsic emission from PAMAM dendrimer: a case study with HeLa cells. Cytotechnology 61: 17–24.

Burke, A., X. Ding and R. Singh. 2009. Long term survival following a single treatment of kidney tumours with multiwalled carbon nanotubes and NIR radiation. Proc. Natl. Acad. Sci. USA. 106: 12897–12902.

Buongiorno, J. 2006. Convective transport in nanofluids. J. Heat Transfer. 128: 240–250.

Burke, A., R. Singh, D. Carroll, J. Wood and R. D'Agostino. 2012. The resistance of breast cancer stem cells to conventional hyperthermia and their sensitivity to nanoparticle-mediated photothermal therapy. Biomaterials 33: 2961–2970.

Butterworth, K., S. McMahon and F. Currel. 2012. Physical basis and biological mechanisms of gold nanoparticle radiosensitization. Nanoscale 4: 4830–4838.

Cahill, D., W. Ford, K. Goodson, G. Mahan, A. Majumdar and H.J. Maris. 2003. Nanoscale thermal transport. J. Appl. Phys. 93: 793–818.

Candido, N., M. Calmon, S. Taboga, J. Bonilha and M. dos Santos. 2014. High efficacy in hyperthermia-associated with polyphosphate magnetic nanoparticles for oral cancer treatment. J. Nanomed. Nanotechol. 3: 1–11.

Cattaneo, C. 1958. Heat conduction. Compt. Rend. 247: 431–433.

Cebrián, V., F. Martín-Saavedra, L. Gómez, M. Arruebo, J. Santamaria and N. Vilaboa. 2013. Enhancing of plasmonic photothermal therapy through heat-inducible transgene activity. Nanomedicine 9: 646–656.

Chan, G., J. Zhao and E. Hicks. 2007. Plasmonic properties of copper nanoparticles fabricated by nanosphere lithography. Nano Lett. 7: 1947–1952.

Chandrasekar, D., R. Sistla, F. Ahmad and R. Khar. 2007. The development of folate-PAMAM dendrimer conjugates for targeted delivery of anti-arthritic drugs and their pharmacokinetics and biodistribution in arthritic rats. Biomaterials 28: 504–512.

Cheng, F., C. Chen and C. Yeh. 2009. Comparative efficiencies of photothermal destruction of malignant cells using antibody-coated silica@Au nanoshells, hollow Au/Ag nanospheres and Au nanorods. Nanotechnology 20: 425104–425113.

Cho, S. 2005. Estimation of tumour dose enhancement due to gold nanoparticles during typical radiation treatments: a preliminary Monte Carlo study. Phys. Med. Biol. 50: N163–73.

Cho, S., B. Jarrett, A. Louie and S. Kauzlarich. 2006. Gold-coated iron nanoparticles: a novel magnetic resonance agent for T1 and T2 weighted imaging. Nanotechnology 17: 640–644.

Choi, Y., J. Kwak and J. Park. 2010. Nanotechnology for early cancer detection. Sensors 10: 428–455.

Clark, A., H. Robins, J. Vorpahl and M. Yatvin. 1983. Structural changes in murine cancer associated with hyperthermia and lidocaine. Cancer Res. 43: 1716–1723.

Davda, J. and V. Labhasetwar. 2002. Characterization of nanoparticle uptake by endothelial cells. Inter. J. Pharm. 233: 51–59.

Divsar, F., A. Nomani, M. Chaloosi and I. Haririan. 2009. Synthesis and characterization of gold nanocomposites with modified and intact polyamidoamine dendrimers. Microchim. Acta. 165: 421–426.

Duck, F. 1990. Physical Properties of Tissue: A Comprehensive Reference Book. Academic Press, London.

Duderstadt, J. and L. Hamilton. 1976. Nuclear Reactor Analysis. Wiley, New York.

Duff, D.G., A. Baiker and P. Edwards. 1993. A new hydrogel of gold clusters. 1. formation and particle size variation. Langmuir 9: 2301–2309.

Ellman, G. 1959. Tissue sulfhydryl groups. Arch. Biochem. Biophys. 82: 70–77.

Elliott, A., J. Schwartz, J. Wang, A. Shetty, J. Hazle and J.R. Stafford. 2007. Analytical solution to heat equation with magnetic resonance experimental verification for nanoshell enhanced thermal therapy. Lasers Surg. Med. 40: 660–5.

Esumi, K., A. Suzuki, A. Yamahira and K. Torigoe. 2000. Role of poly(amidoamine) dendrimers for preparing nanoparticles of gold, platinum, and silver. Langmuir. 16: 2604–2608.

Eyer, P., F. Worek, D. Kiderlen, G. Sinko, A. Stuglin, V. Simeon-Rudolf and E. Reiner. 2003. Molar absorption coefficients for the reduced Ellman reagent: reassessment. Analyt. Biochem. 312: 224–227.

Fernandez Cabada, T., C. de Pablo, A. Serrano and P. Guerrero Fdel. 2012. Induction of cell death in a glioblastoma line by hyperthermic therapy based on gold nanorods. Int. J. Nanomedicine 7: 1511–1523.

Fenske, D. and P. Cullis. 2008. Liposomal nanomedicines. Expert Opin. Drug Deliv. 5: 25–44.

Floris, A., A. Ardu, A. Musinu, G. Piccaluga and A. Fadda. 2011. SPION@liposomes hybrid nanoarchitectures with high density SPION association. Soft Matter 7: 6239–6247.

Funkhouser, J. 2002. Reinventing pharma: the theranostic revolution. Curr. Drug Disc. 2: 17–19.

Gazelle, G., S. Goldberg, L. Solbiati and T. Livraghi. 2000. Tumor ablation with radio-frequency energy. Radiology 217: 633–646.

George, K. and B. Singh. 1982. Synergism of chlorpromazine and hyperthermia in two mouse solid tumours. Br. J. Cancer 45: 309–313.

Ghazanfari, L. and M.E. Khosroshahi. 2014. Simulation and experimental results of optical and thermal modeling of gold nanoshells. Mater. Sci. Eng.: C 42: 185–191.

Gindy, M. and R. Prud'homme. 2009. Multifunctional nanoparticles for imaging, delivery and targeting in cancer therapy. Export Opinion. 6: 865–878.

Gowda, R., N. Jones, S. Banerjee and G. Robertson. 2013. Use of nanotechnology to develop multi-drug inhibitors for cancer therapy. J. Nanomed. Nanotechnol. 4: 1–16.

Grabchev, I., V. Bojinov and J.M. Chovelon. 2003. Synthesis, photophysical and photochemical properties of fluorescent poly(amidoamine) dendrimers. Polymer. 44: 4421–4428.

Gupta, A., M. Gupta, S. Yarwood and A. Curtis. 2004. Effect of cellular uptake of gelatin nanoparticles on adhesion, morphology and cytoskeleton organisation of human fibroblasts. J. Cont. Rel. 95: 197–207.

Gupta, A. and M. Gupta. 2005. Cytotoxicity suppression and cellular uptake enhancement of surface modified magnetic nanoparticles. Biomaterials 26: 1565–1573.

Hasannejad, Z. and M.E. Khosroshahi. 2013. Synthesis and evaluation of time dependent optical properties of plasmonic–magnetic nanoparticles. Opt. Mat. 35: 644–65.

Hassannejad, Z., M.E. Khosroshahi and M. Firouzi. 2014. Fabrication and characterization of magnetoplasmonic liposome carriers. Nanosci. & Tech. 1: 1–9.

He, J. 1999. Electrostatic multilayer deposition of gold–dendrimer nanocomposite. Chem. of Mat. 11: 3268–3274.

Henning, K., M. Natisha, J. Richard and K. Stowell. 2007. Differential regulation of DNA repair protein Rad51 in human tumour cell lines exposed to doxorubicin. Anticancer Drug 18: 419–425.

Hirai, H. and N. Yakura. 2001. Protecting polymers in suspension of metal nanoparticles. Polym. Adv. Technol. 12: 724–733.

Hoffman, L., G. Andersson, A. Sharma and S. Clarke. 2011. New Insights into the structure of PAMAM dendrimer/gold nanoparticle nanocomposites. Langmuir. 27: 6759–6767.

Hollmann, A., L. Delfederico, G. Glikmann, G. De Antoni, L. Semorile and E. Disalvo. 2007. Characterization of liposomes coated with S-layer proteins from lactobacilli. BBA - Biomembranes 1768: 393–400.

Hong, R., J. Li, J. Wang and H. Li. 2007. Comparison of schemes for preparing magnetic Fe_3O_4 nanoparticles. China Part. 5: 186–191.

Hossann, M., M. Wiggenhorn, A. Schwerdt, K. Wachholz, N. Teichert and H. Eibl. 2007. *In vitro* stability and content release properties of phosphatidylglyceroglycerol containing thermosensitive liposomes. Biochim. Biophy. Acta 1768: 2491–2499.

Huang, X., P. Jain, I. El-Sayed and M. El-Sayed. 2006. Determination of the minimum temperature required for selective photothermal destruction of cancer cells with the use of immunotargeted gold nanoparticles. Photochem. Photobiol. 82: 412–417.

Huang, X., P.K. Jain, I. El-Sayed and M. El-Sayed. 2007. Gold nanoparticles: interesting optical properties and recent applications in cancer diagnostics and therapy. Nanomed. 2: 681–693.

Huang, X., W. Qian, I. El-Sayed and M. El-sayed. 2007. The potential use of the enhanced nonlinear properties of gold nanospheres in photothermal cancer therapy. Lasers Surg. Med. 39: 747–753.

Hull, L., D. Farrel and P. Grodzinski. 2014. Highlights of recent developments and trends in cancer nanotechnology research. Biotechnol. Adv. 32: 666–678.

Iden, D. and T. Allen. 2001. *In vitro* and *in vivo* comparison of immunoliposomes made by conventional coupling techniques with those made by a new post-insertion approach. BBA - Biomembranes 1513: 207–216.

Ji, X., Sh. Ruping, A. Elliott, R. Stafford, E. Esparza-Coss and J. Bankson. 2007. Bifunctional gold nanoshells with a superparamagnetic iron oxide-silica core suitable for both MR imaging and photothermal therapy. J. Phys. Chem. C 111: 6245–6251.

Joanitti, G., R. Azevedo and S. Freitas. 2010. Apoptosis and lysosome membrane permeabilization induction on breast cancer cells by an anticarcinogenic Bowman-Birk protease inhibitor from Vigna unguiculata seeds. Cancer Lett. 293: 73–81.

Jolesz, F. and K. Hynynen. 2002. Magnetic resonance image-guided focused ultrasound surgery. Cancer J. 1: S100–12.

Joseph, D. and L. Preziosi. 1989. Heat waves. Rev. Modern Phys. 61: 41–73.

Khanadeev, V., B. Khlebtsov, S. Staroverov, I. Vidyasheva and A. Skaptsov. 2011. Quantitative cell bioimaging using gold-nanoshell conjugates and phage antibodies. J. Biophotonics 4: 74–83.

Khosroshahi, M.E. and L. Ghazanfari. 2010. Preparation and characterization of silica-coated iron-oxide bionanoparticles under N2 gas. Physica E 42: 1824–1829.

Khosroshahi, M.E. and M. Nourbakhsh. 2010. Preparation and characterization of selfassembled gold nanoparticles on amino functionalized SiO_2 dielectric core. World Academy of Science. Eng. and Tech. 64: 353–356.

Khosroshahi, M.E., M. Nourbakhsh and L. Ghazanfari. 2011. Synthesis and biomedical application of SiO_2/Au nanofluid based on laser-induced surface plasmon resonance thermal effect. J. Mod. Phys. 2: 944–953.

Khosroshahi, M.E. and L. Ghazanfari. 2012. Synthesis and functionalization of SiO_2 coated Fe_3O_4 nanoparticles with amine groups based on self-assembly. Mat. Eng. C. 32: 1043–1049.

Khosroshahi, M.E. and L. Ghazanfari. 2012. Physicochemical characterization of Fe_3O_4/SiO_2/Au multilayer nanostructure. Mater. Chem. Phys. 133: 55–62.

Khosroshahi, M.E. and L. Ghazanfari. 2012. Comparison of magnetic and rheological behaviour of uncoated and PVA-coated Fe_3O_4 nanoparticles synthesized under N_2 gas. J. Mag. Mag. Mater. 324: 4143–4146.

Khosroshahi, M.E., L. Ghazanfari and Z. Hassannejad. 2012. Preliminary results of treating cancerous cells of lung (QU-DB) by hyperthermia using diode laser and gold coated Fe_3O_4/SiO_2 nanoshells: an *in vitro* assay. Iran J. Med. Phys. 9: 253–263.

Khosroshahi, M.E., L. Ghazanfari and P. Khoshkenar. 2014. Experimental validation and simulation of Fourier and non-Fourier heat transfer equation during laser nano-phototherapy of lung cancer cells: An *in vitro* assay. J. Mod. Phys. 5: 2125–2141.

Khosroshahi, M.E., M. Tajabadi, Sh. Bonakdar and V. Asgari. 2015. Synthesis and characterization of SPION functionalized third generation dendrimer conjugated by gold nanoparticles and folic acid for targeted breast cancer laser hyperthermia: an *in vitro* assay. World Cong. Med. Phys. & Biomed. Eng. 823–826.

Khosroshahi, M.E., Z. Hassannejad, M. Firouzi and A. Arshi. 2015. Nanoshell-mediated targeted photothermal therapy of HER2 human breast cancer cells using pulsed and continuous wave lasers: an *in vitro* study. Lasers Med. Sci. 30: 1913–1922.

Khosroshahi, M.E., L. Ghazanfari, M. Firouzi and V. Sandoghdar. 2015. Application of doxorubicin loaded magnetoplasmonic thermosensitive liposomes for laser hyperthermia and chemotherapy of breast cancer. J. Nanomed. Nanotech. 6: 1–9.

Kim, G. and S. Nie. 2005. Targeted cancer nanotherapy. Mat. Today 8: 28–33.

Kim, S., I. Haimovich-Caspi, I. Omer, Y. Talmon and E. Franses. 2007. Effect of sonication and freezing-thawing on the aggregate size and dynamic surface tension of aqueous DPPC dispersions. .J Colloid Interface Sci. 311: 217–227.

Kim, D., J. Kim and Y. Jeong. 2009. Antibiofouling polymer coated gold@iron oxide nanoparticle as a usual contrast agent for CT and MRI. Bull. Korean Chem. Soc. 30: 1855–1857.

Kitz, M., S. Preisser, A. Wetterwald, M. Jaeger, G. Thalmann and M. Frenz. 2011. Vapor bubble generation around gold nanoparticles and its application to damaging of cells. Biomed. Opt. Express 2: 291–304.

Knight, M., L. Liu and Y. Wang. 2012. Aluminium plasmonic nanoantennas. Nano Lett. 12: 6000–6004.

Kong, G., R. Braun and M. Dewhirst. 2000. Hyperthermia enables tumor-specific nanoparticle delivery: effect of particle size. Cancer Res. 60: 4440–4445.

Kou, G., S. Wang, C. Cheng, J. Gao and B. Li. 2008. Development of SM5-1-conjugated ultrasmall superparamagnetic iron oxide nanoparticles for hepatoma detection. Biochem. Biophys. Res. Comm. 374: 192–197.

Kulshrestha, P., M. Gogoi, D. Bahadur and R. Banerjee. 2012. *In vitro* application of paclitaxel loaded magnetoliposomes for combined chemotherapy and hyperthermia. Colloids and Surfaces B: Biointerfaces 96: 1–7.

Kumar, S., J. Aaron and K. Sokolov. 2008. Directional conjugation of antibodies to nanoparticles for synthesis of multiplexed optical contrast agents with both delivery and targeting moieties. Nature Protocols 3: 314–320.

Landon, C., J. Park, D. Needham and M. Dewhirst. 2011. Nanoscale drug delivery and hyperthermia: the materials design and preclinical and clinical testing of low temperature-sensitive liposomes used in combination with mild hyperthermia in the treatment of local cancer. The Open Nanomed. J. 3: 38–64.

Lao, L. and R. Ramanujan. 2004. Magnetic and hydrogel composite materials for hyperthermia on human mammary carcinoma cells *in vitro*. J. Mag. Mag. Mater. Med. 15: 1061–1064.

Lapotko, D., E. Lukianova and A. Oraevsky. 2006. Selective laser nano-thermolysis of human leukemia cells with microbubbles generated around clusters of gold nanoparticles. Lasers Surg. Med. 38: 631–642.

Lapotko, D., E. Lukianova, M. Potapnev, O. Aleinikova and A. Oraevsky. 2006. Method of laser activated nano-thermolysis for elimination of tumor cells. Cancer Lett. 239: 36–45.

Lapotko, D. 2006. Laser-induced bubbles in living cells. Lasers Surg. Med. 38: 240–248.

Lapotko, D. 2009. Pulsed photothermal heating of the media during bubble generation around gold nanoparticles. Inter. J. Heat Mass Transfer. 52: 1540–1543.

Larson, C. and S. Tucker. 2001. Intrinsic fluorescence of carboxylate-terminated polyamido amine dendrimers. Appl. Spect. 55: 679–683.

Lee, Y., K. Wong, J. Tan, P. Toh, Y. Mao and V. Brusic. 2009. Overexpression of heat shock proteins (HSPs) in CHO cells for extended culture viability and improved recombinant protein production. J. Biotechnol. 143: 34–43.

Leehtman, E., N. Chattopadhyay and Z. Cai. 2011. Implications on clinical scenario of gold nanoparticles radiosensitization in regards to photon energy, nanoparticle size, concentration and location. Phys. Med. Biol. 56: 4631–4637.

Leehtman, E., S. Mashouf and N. Chattopadhyay. 2013. A Mont Carlo model of gold nanoparticle radiosinsitization accounting for increased radiobiological effectiveness. Phys. Med. Biol. 58: 3075–3087.

Lewinski, N., V. Colvin and R. Drezek. 2008. Cytotoxicity of nanoparticles. Small 4: 26–49.

Li, J., L. Wang and X. Liu. 2009. *In vitro* cancer cell imaging and therapy using transferrin-conjugated gold nanoparticles. Cancer. Lett. 274: 319–326.

Li, J., Q. Chen and L. Yang. 2010. The synthesis of dendrimer based on the dielectric barrier discharge plasma grafting amino group film. Surf. Coat. Tech. 205: S257–S260.

Li, J., J. Han, T. Xu, C. Guo, X. Bu and H. Zhang. 2013. Coating urchinlike gold nanoparticles with polypyrrole thin shells to produce photothermal agents with high stability and photothermal transduction efficiency. Langmuir 29: 7102–7110.

Liu, J., X. Zhang, C. Wang, W. Lu and Z. Ren. 1997. Generalized time delay bioheat equation and preliminary analysis on its wave nature. Chin. Sci. Bull. 42: 289–292.

Liu, H., P. Hou, W. Zhang and J. Wu. 2010. Synthesis of monosized core–shell Fe_3O_4/Au multifunctional nanoparticles by PVP-assisted nanoemulsion process. Colloid Surf. A 356: 21–27.

Loo, C., A. Lowery, N.J. Halas, J. West and R. Drezek. 2005. Immunotargeted nanoshells for integrated cancer imaging and therapy. Nano Lett. 5: 709–711.

Loo, C., L. Hirsch, M. Lee, E. Chang, J. West, N.J. Halas and R. Drezek. 2005. Gold nanoshell bioconjugates for molecular imaging in living cells. Opt. Lett. 30: 1012–1014.

Lopez-Molina, J., M. Rivera, M. Trujillo et al. 2008. Asseeement of heat transfer equation in theoretical modeling for radiofrequency heating techniques. The Open Biomed. Eng. J. 2: 22–27.

Lukianova-Hleb, E., A. Oginsky, D. Shenefelt, R. Drezek and J. Hafner. 2011. Rainbow plasmonic nanobubbles: synergistic activation of gold nanoparticle clusters. J. Nanomed. Nanotechol. 2: 1–8.

Majoros, I., Myc, A., T. Thomas et al. 2006. PAMAM Dendrimer-based multifunctional conjugate for cancer therapy: synthesis, characterization, and functionality. Biomacromolecules. 7: 572–579.

Massart, C., R. Barbet, N. Genetet and Gibassier. 2004. Doxorubicin induces fas-mediated apoptosis in human thyroid carcinoma cells. Thyroid. 14: 1–11.

Mayer, L.D., M. Bally and P. Cullis. 1986. Uptake of adriamycin into large unilamellar vesicles in response to a pH gradient. Biochim. Biophys. Acta 857: 123–126.

McKenzie, A.L. and J.A. Carruth. 1984. Lasers in surgery and medicine. Phys. Med. Biol. 29: 619–641.

Melancon, M., M. Zhou, R. Zhang, C. Xiong, P. Allen, X. Wen and Q. Huang. 2014. Selective uptake and imaging of aptamer- and antibody-conjugated hollow nanospheres targeted to epidermal growth factor receptors overexpressed in head and neck cancer. ACS NANO 8: 4530–4538.

Mendoza-Nova, H., G. Ferro-Flores and B. Ocampo-Garcia. 2013. Laser heating of gold nanospheres functionalized with octreotide: *in vivo* effect on HeLa cell viability. Photomed. Laser Surg. 31: 17–22.

Menjoge, A., R. Kannan and D. Tomalia. 2010. Dendrimer-based drug and imaging conjugates: design considerations for nanomedical applications. Drug Discovery Today. 15: 171–185.

Mirza, A., B. Fornage, N. Sneige, H. Kuerer et al. 2001. Radiofrequency Ablation of Solid Tumors. Cancer J. 7: 95–102.

Missirlis, Y. and A. Spiliotis. 2002. Assessment of techniques used in calculating cell-material interactions. Biomol. Eng. 19: 287–294.

Murphy, C., A. Gole, J.W. Stone, P. Sisco, A.M. Alkilany, E. Goldsmith and S. Baxter. 2008. Gold nanoparticles in biology: beyond toxicity to cellular imaging. Acc. Chem. Res. 41: 1721–1730.

Nam, K., H. Hahn, B. Kim, H. Lim and H. Kim. 2009. Biodegradable PAMAM ester for enhanced transfection efficiency with low cytotoxicity. Biomaterials. 30: 665–673.

Nedelcu, G. 2008. Magnetic nanoparticles impact on tumoural cells in the treatment by magnetic fluid hyperthermia. Digest J. Nanomat. Biost. 3: 103–107.

Nie, Y., L. Ji, H. Ding, L. Xie and L. Li. 2012. Cholesterol derivatives based charged liposomes for doxorubicin delivery: preparation, *in vitro* and *in vivo* characterization. Theranostics 2: 1092–1103.

Nicolodelli, G., D. Angarita, N. Inada, L. Tirapelli and V. Bagnato. 2013. Effect of photodynamic therapy on the skin using the ultrashort laser ablation. J. Biophotonics. 8: 1–7.

Nikfarjam, M., V. Muralidharan and C. Christophi. 2005. Mechanisms of focal heat destruction of liver tumors. J. Surg. Res. 127: 208–223.

Nolsøe, C., S. Torp-Pedersen, F. Burcharth, T. Horn and S. Pedersen. 1993. Interstitial hyperthermia of colorectal liver metastases with US-guided Nd:YAG laser with a diffuser tip: a pilot clinical study. Radiology 187: 333–337.

Nourbakhsh, M. and M.E. Khosroshahi. 2011. An *in vitro* investigation of skin tissue soldering using gold nanoshells and diode laser. Lasers Med. Sci. 26: 49–55.

Oldenburg, S., R. Averitt, S. Westcott and N.J. Halas. 1998. Nanoengineering of resonances. Chem. Phys. Lett. 288: 243–247.

Osman, A., H. Bayoumi, S. Al-Harthi, Z. Damanhouri and M. ElShal. 2012. Modulation of doxorubicin cytotoxicity by resveratrol in a human breast cancer cell line. Cancer Cell International 12: 1–8.

Paasonen, L., T. Sipila, A. Subrizi, P. Laurinmaki and S. Butcher. 2010. Gold-embedded photosensitive liposomes for drug delivery: triggering mechanism and intracellular release. J. Cont. Rel. 147: 136–143.

Pak, B. and Y. Cho. 1998. Hydrodynamic and heat transfer study of dispersed fluids with submicron metallic oxide particles. Exp. Heat Transfer. 11: 151–170.

Pankhurst, Q., J. Connolly, S. Jones and J. Dobson. 2003. Applications of magnetic nanoparticles in biomedicine. J. Phys. D: Appl. Phys. 36: R167–181.

Peng, X., Q. Pan and G. Rempel. 2008. Bimetallic dendrimer-encapsulated nanoparticles as catalysts: a review of the research advances. Chem. Soc. Rev. 37: 1619–1628.

Pennes, H. 1948. Analysis of tissue and arterial blood temperatures in the resting human forearm. J. Appl. Physiol. 1: 93–122.

Pham, T., J. Jackson, N. Halas and T. Lee. 2002. Preparation and characterization of gold nanoshells coated with self-assembled monolayers. Langmuir 18: 4915–4920.

Pham, T., C. Cao and S. Sim. 2008. Application of citrate-stabilized gold-coated ferric oxide composite nanoparticles for biological separations. J. Mag. Mag. Mater. 320: 2049–2055.

Pradhan, P., J. Giri, R. Banerjee and J. Bellare. 2007. Cellular interactions of lauric acid and dextran-coated magnetite nanoparticles. Journal of Magnetism and Magnetic Materials 311: 282–287.

Pradhan, P., J. Giri, F. Rieken, C. Koch and O. Mykhaylyk. 2010. Targeted temperature sensitive magnetic liposomes for thermo-chemotherapy. J. Cont. Rel. 142: 108–121.

Prasad, N.K., K. Rathinasamy, D. Panda and Bahadur. 2007. Mechanism of cell death induced by magnetic hyperthermia with nanoparticles of γ-Mn$_x$Fe$_{2-x}$O$_3$ synthesized by a single step process. J. Mater. Chem. 17: 5042–5051.

Puvvada, N. 2011. Nanomedical platform for drug delivery. J. Nanomed. Nanotechnol. 2: 1–5.

Pustovalov, V., A. Smetannikov and V. Zharov. 2008. Photothermal and accompanied phenomena of selective nanophotothermolysis with gold nanoparticles and laser pulses. Laser Phys. Lett. 5: 775–792.

Pustovalov, V., L. Astafyeva and B. Jean. 2009. Computer modeling of the optical properties and heating of spherical gold and silica-gold nanoparticles for laser combined imaging and photothermal treatment. Nanotechnology 20: 225105.

Pustovalov, V., L. Astafyeva and B. Jean. 2009. Computer modeling of the optical properties and heating of spherical gold and silica-gold nanoparticles for laser combined imaging and photothermal treatment. Nanotech. 20: 1–11.

Quintana, A., E. Raczka, L. Piehler and I. Lee. 2002. Design and function of a dendrimer-based therapeutic nanodevice targeted to tumor cells through the folate receptor. Pharm. Res. 19: 1310–1316.

Rezvani Alanagh, H., M.E. Khosroshahi, M. Tajabadi and H. Keshvari. 2014. The effect of pH and magnetic field on the fluorescence spectra of fluorescein isothiocyanate conjugated SPION-dendrimer nanocomposites. J. Supercond. Nov. Mag. 27: 2337–2345.

Satoh, K., T. Yoshimura and K. Esumi. 2005. Effects of various thiol molecules added on morphology of dendrimer–gold nanocomposites. J. Colloid Interf. Sci. 2002. 255: 312–322.

Scholl, J., A. Koh and J. Dionne. 2012. Quntum plasmon resonances of individual metallic nanoparticles. Nature 483: 421–427.

Seki, T., M. Wakabayashi, T. Nakagawa, M. Imamura, T. Tamai and A. Okamura. 1999. Percutaneous microwave coagulation therapy for patients with small hepatocellular carcinoma: comparison with percutaneous ethanol injection therapy. Cancer. 85: 1694–1702.

Shi, X., T. Ganser, K. Sun, L. Balogh and J. Baker. 2006. Characterization of crystalline dendrimer-stabilized gold nanoparticles. Nanotechnology 17: 1072–1078.

Shi, X., S. Wang, M. Shen, M. Antwerp and X. Chen. 2009. Multifunctional dendrimer-modified multiwalled carbon nanotubes: synthesis, characterization, and *in vitro* cancer cell targeting and imaging. Biomacromolecules 10: 1744–1750.

Simon, T., S. Boca-Farcau, A.M. Gabudean, P. Baldeck and S. Astilean. 2013. LED-activated methylene blue-loaded Pluronic-nanogold hybrids for *in vitro* photodynamic therapy. J. Biophotonics 6: 950–959.

Singh, P., U. Gupta, A. Asthana and N. Jain. 2008. Folate and folate-PEG-PAMAM dendrimers: Synthesis, characterization, and targeted anticancer drug delivery potential in tumor bearing mice. Bioconjugate Chem. 19: 2239–2252.

Skirtach, A., C. Dejugnat, D. Braun, S. Susha, A. Rogach and W. Parak. 2005. The role of metal nanoparticles in remote release of encapsulated materials. Nano Lett. 5: 1371–1377.

Skrabalak, S., J. Chen, L. Au, X. Lu, X. Li and Y. Xia. 2007. Gold nanocages for biomedical applications. Adv. Mater. 19: 3177–3184.

Soto-Cerrato, V., B. Montaner, M. Martinell, M. Vilaseca, E. Giralt and R. Perez-Tomas. 2005. Cell cycle arrest and proapoptotic effects of the anticancer cyclodepsipeptide serratamolide (AT514) are independent of p53 status in breast cancer cells. Biochem. Pharmacol. 71: 32–41.

Srinivas, P., P. Barker and S. Srivastava. 2002. Nanotechnology in early detection of cancer. Lab. Invest. 82: 657–662.

Steinhauser, I., B. Spänkuch, K. Strebhardt and K. Langer. 2006. Trastuzumab-modified nanoparticles: optimisation of preparation and uptake in cancer cells. Biomaterials 27: 4975–4983.

Svaasand, L., C. Gomer and E. Morinelli. 1990. On the physical rationale laser-induced hyperthermia. Lasers Med. Sci. 5: 121–127.

Syed, A., R. Raja, G. Kundu, S. Gambhir and A. Ahmad. 2013. Extracellular biosynthesis of monodispersed gold nanoparticles, their characterization, cytotoxicity assay, biodistribution and conjugation with the anticancer drug doxorubicin. J. Nanomed. Nanotechol. 4: 1–6.

Sun, Y., L. Duan, Z. Guo and Y. DuanMu. 2005. An improved way to prepare superparamagnetic magnetite-silica core-shell nanoparticles for possible biological application. J. Mag. Mag. Mater. 285: 65–70.

Sun, X., G. Zhang, R. Keynton, M. O'Toole, D. Patel and A. Gobin. 2013. Enhanced drug delivery via hyperthermal membrane disruption using targeted gold nanoparticles with PEGylated Protein-G as a cofactor. Nanomedicine 9: 1214–1222.

Tajabadi, M., M.E. Khosroshahi and Sh. Bonakdar. 2013. An efficient method of SPION synthesis coated with third generation PAMAM dendrimer. Colloids and Surfaces A: Physicochem. Eng. Aspects 431: 18–26.

Tomalia, D. 2005. Birth of a new macromolecular architecture: dendrimers as quantized building blocks for nanoscale synthetic polymer chemistry. Prog. Polym. Sci. 30: 294–324.

Tong, L., Y. Zhao, T. Huff, M. Hansen, A. Wei and J. Cheng. 2007. Gold nanorods mediate tumor cell death by compromising membrane integrity. Adv. Mater. 19: 3136–3141.

Torigoe, K., A. Suzuki and K. Esumi. 2001. Au (III)–PAMAM interaction and formation of Au–PAMAM nanocomposites in ethyl acetate. J. Colloid Interf. Sci. 241: 346–356.

Tsalach, A., I. Steinberg and I. Gannot. 2014. Tumor localization using magnetic nanoparticle-induced acoustic signals. IEEE Trans. Biomed. Eng. 61: 2313–2323.

Tzou, D. 1996. Macro- to Microscale Heat Transfer: The Lagging Behaviour. Taylor & Francis, Washington DC.

Valeriote, F. and H. Lin. 1975. Synergistic interaction of anticancer agents: a cellular perspective. Cancer Chemother. Rep. 59: 895–900.

Van der Zee, J. 2002. Heating the patient: a promising approach. Ann. Oncol. 13: 1173–1184.

Vera, J. and Y. Bayazitoglu. 2009. A note on laser penetration in nanoshell deposited tissue. Int. J. Heat Mass Tran. 52: 3402–3406.

Vernotte, P. 1961. Exact and analytic-numerical solutions of lagging models of heat transfer in a semi-infinite medium. Compt. Rend. 252: 2190–2191.

Viroonchatapan, E., H. Sato, M. Ueno, I. Adachi and J. Murata. 1998. Microdialysis assessment of 5-fluorouracil release from thermosensitive magnetoliposomes induced by an electromagnetic field in tumor-bearing mice. J. Drug Target 5: 379–390.

Wang, K., J. Finlay, T. Busch, S. Hahn and T. Zhu. 2010. Explicit dosimetry for photodynamic therapy: macroscopic singlet oxygen modeling. J. Biophotonics 3: 304–318.

Wang, F., Y. Wang, S. Dou, M. Xiong and T. Sun. 2011. Doxorubicin-tethered responsive gold nanoparticles facilitate intracellular drug delivery for overcoming multidrug resistance in cancer cells. ACS Nano 5: 3679–3692.

Welch, A. and M. van Gemert. 1995. Optical-thermal response of laser-irradiated tissue. Plenum Press, New York.

World Health Organization: WHO

Woo, J., G. Chiu, G. Karlsson, E. Wasan and L. Ickenstein. 2008. Use of a passive equilibration methodology to encapsulate cisplatin into preformed thermosensitive liposomes. Int. J. Pharm. 349: 38–46.

Wu, C., C. Yu and M. Chu. 2011. A gold nanoshell with a silica inner shell synthesized using liposome templates for doxorubicin loading and near-infrared photothermal therapy. Int. J. of Nanomed. 6: 807–813.

Wyman, D., M. Patterson and B. Wilson. 1989. Similarity relations for the interaction parameters in radiation transport. Appl. Opt. 28: 5243–5249.

Xu, S., Y. Hou and S. Sun. 2007. Magnetic core/shell Fe_3O_4/Au and Fe_3O_4/Au/Ag nanoparticles with tunable plasmonic properties. J. Am. Chem. Soc. 129: 8698–8699.

Yatvin, M., J. Weinstein and W. Dennis. 1981. Selective delivery of liposome-associated cisdichlorodiammineplatinum (II) by heat and its influence on tumor drug uptake and growth. Cancer Res. 41: 1602–1607.

Yavlovich, A., B. Smith, K. Gupta, R. Blumenthal and A. Puri. 2010. Light-sensitive lipid-based nanoparticles for drug delivery: design principles and future considerations for biological applications. Mol. Memb. Biol. 27: 364–381.

Yiv, S. and F. Uckun. 2012. Lipid spheres as attractive nanoscale drug delivery platforms for cancer therapy. J. Nanomed. Nanotechnol. 3: 1–6.

Yoshimoto, M., T. Furuya and N. Kunihiro. 2011. Temperature-dependent permeability of liposome membrane incorporated with Mg-chlorophyll. Colloids Surf. A 387: 65–70.

Zhang, Y., H. Hong and W. Cai. 2011. Tumor-targeted drug delivery with aptamers. Curr. Med. Chem. 18: 4185–4194.

13

Biomedical Imaging

13.1 Introduction

Bioimaging, in general, is one of the major streamlines of comprehensive cancer care in both diagnosis and research, with significant advantages of real time monitoring, minimal or no invasive action, and operational over relatively wide ranges of time and size scales involved in biological and pathological processes. Bioimaging plays a great role in different stages of cancer management: Prediction, screening, biopsy for detecton, staging, prognosis, therapy planning, therapy guidance, and therapy response (Kent et al. 2004, Lee et al. 2004, Feme 2005, Lehman 2007, Brindle 2008). According to Kumar (2006), biomarkers identified from the genome and proteome can be selectively targeted and chemical binding can improve their imaging signal. Various pharmaceutical therapies that have been developed for cancer are classed as cytotoxic, antihormonal, immunotherapeutic, and molecular targeted. Imaging can help the molecular targeted therapies to control their effectiveness and include: signal transduction, angiogenesis, cell cycle inhibitors, apoptosis inducers, and epigenetic modulators (Brindle 2003). There are numerous medical imaging techniques each with advantages and limitations, see Table 13.1.

In contrast to above techniques, the molecular imaging is a combined functional and structural imaging modality, which effectively can be used to achieve the health benefit from understanding the spatial mapping at the whole body level and molecular processes within cells and tissues. Various targeted agents for cancer markers are, for example: epidermal growth factor receptor (EGFR), $\alpha_v \beta_3$ integrin, vascular endothelial growth factor (VEGF), carcinoembryonic antigene (CEA), and folate receptors (FR). Clearly, the development of minimally invasive targeted therapy and drug delivery should be based on the guided imaging system. Most clinical imaging systems are based on the interaction of electromagnetic radiation with body tissues and fluids, except ultrasound which is based on the reflection, scattering, and the frequency shifts of acoustic waves (i.e., Doppler effect). Ultrasound also has the capability of imaging tissue elasticity, and thus can be employed in differential diagnosis of breast cancer, prostate cancer, liver fibrosis, because cancer tissues are less elastic than normal tissue and ultrasound elastography (Lerner et al. 1990, Pallwein et al. 2007). High frequency electromagnetic radiation such as γ-rays, X-rays, or UV light is ionizing can cause mutation, hence leading to cancer. In contrast, non-ionizing radiation imaging systems including IR spectroscopy, microwave imaging spectroscopy, photoacoustic, and thermoacoustic imaging which are readily used for imaging pose no such danger. However, both groups of imaging systems have one point in common, they vary in physical properties including sensitivity, temporal, and spatial resolution. In addition, the imaging systems produce images that have differences in contrast. The differences in contrast can be due to changes in physical properties caused by the endogenous nature of the tissue, e.g., radiation absorption, reflection, transmission, magnetic relaxivity, magnetic susceptibility, oxygenation, spectral distribution, electrical impedance, mechanical elasticity, etc., or exogenous mechanisms, e.g., radiation absorption, reflection, emission, magnetic relaxivity, magnetic susceptibility, isotope spectra,

Table 13.1. Advantages and limitations of some of clinical cancer diagnostic and imaging systems.

Modality	Advantages	Disadvantages
CBE/BSE	• Inexpensive • Non-invasive	• Effectiveness depends highly on the individual and the examiner proficiency • Small size tumors cannot be detected by palpation • Unnecessary physician visits • Increased anxiety and false assurance
X-ray mammog	• Relatively fast • Widely available	• Involves X-ray radiation and can cause carcinogenesis • Regular checks of machine to prevent overdosing the patients • Ineffective for high breast density particularly for women between 20s–40s • Very limited tests per year • Pain & discomfort during a test • Risks of +ve and –ve false response • Possible anxiety and psychological stress
Ultrasound	• Can differentiate between cystic and solid mass • Can be used to guide biopsy procedure • High resolution	• False +ve results when detecting dense breast tissue • False –ve results with palpable mass • Low contrast
MRI	• High spatial resolution • Good soft tissue contrast • Excellent anatomical and functional information • Suitable for dense breast	• Injection of Gadolinium • Incapable of measuring molecular events, e.g., protease activity and gene expression • Relatively large acquisition time • Expensive equipment • Low sensitivity • Possible false +ve results followed by the its consequences • Cannot be used for patients with pacemaker or breast reconstruction involving metals
PET	• Provides biochemical information • High sensitivity • 3-D imaging • Capable of monitoring changes in tumor metabolism and drug biodistribution • Specificity • Sensitivity • Fast detection time	• Limited anatomical information • Requires specialized equipment • Requires radio-nucleotide facilities • Expensive equipment • Low spatial resolution
SPECT	• Simultaneous multiple probes Detection in contrast to PET • Specificity • Sensitivity • Fast detection time	• Lower sensitivity than PET • Low spatial resolution
CT	• High-sensitivity anatomical imaging • 3-D imaging	• Use of Iodine-based compounds • Limited functional information • Poor soft tissue contrast • Requires expensive equipment • Lower resolution
Optical	• Wide applicability • Covering a wide optical range (Vis-IR) for imaging • Comparatively inexpensive • Versatile • Sensitive • Fluorescence excitation possible	• Hard to differentiate between background noise and diagnostic signal • High scattering in tissue • Poor image quality due to close spacing between auto-fluorescence of normal tissue and fluorescence of contrast agents

CBE: Clinical breast examination, BSE: Breast self-examination, MRI: Magnetic resonance imaging, PET: Positron emission tomography, SPECT: Single-photon emission computed tomography, CT: Computerized tomography fluorescence, perfusion, hypoxia, etc. Finally, it is believed that the sensitivity and specificity of diagnostic systems can be improved by combining the systems as one system known as *multimodal system*, which will be discussed in the next section.

13.2 Single, multimodal imaging systems and contrast agents

The single modal imaging systems that are widely used today in the clinical practice are:

1. *Nuclear imaging*: This includes nuclear magnetic resonance (NMR), PET, and SPECT. PET and SPECT are both quantitative methods in the sense that they provide *in vivo* distribution images of injected radioisotopes. Both systems provide information about physiological activity such as glucose metabolism, blood flow, and perfusion but suffer from providing structural or anatomical information. The major differences, however, are that SPECT allows simultaneously, the labelling of various radioisotopes for number of compounds, which can influence the structure as well as function of biomolecules. PET on the other hand, shows higher sensitivity than SPECT, and is able to assess cellular activity at low levels (Park et al. 2006). A small animal study by Dolovich and Labiris (2004) reported that PET measures about 4 to 8 mm^2 and SPECT about 12 to 15 mm^3. The spatial resolution of PET is about 1 to 2 mm^3 and SPECT about 1 mm^3. Also, the radioactive contrast agents such as ^{99m}Tc and 111In used for SPECT require chelating moieties in the labelling of compounds. Most PET radioisotopes are short-lived, from a few minutes to 2 h, which implies on-site availability of cyclotron to produce them and hence increasing the cost of PET imaging. SPECT radioisotopes, however, last longer about 6 h allowing longer image acquisition time.

2. *CT*: This is a non-invasive method based on the use of computer-processed combinations of many X-ray images taken from different angles to produce cross-sectional (tomographic) images of specific areas of a scanned object, allowing the user to see inside the object without cutting. CT produces a volume of data that can be manipulated in order to demonstrate various bodily structures based on their ability to block the X-ray beam. Despite their high contrast resolution, they are limited by the variety of compatible agents thus cannot be used for labelling molecules. Kim et al. (2007) prepared long circulating PEG-coated gold nanoparticles as contrast agents for CT imaging and showed that these agents had two-fold high contrast in tumor than normal tissues on CT images.

3. *MRI*: It is the most versatile diagnostic imaging modality, capable of providing excellent structural, functional, and metabolic information. The system is based on the magnetism property of protons that align themselves in a very large magnetization field. These protons originate from water molecules (i.e., water proton ^1H) of our body. A radiofrequency is generated at a particular frequency called *resonance frequency*, and can flip the spin of a proton. When the electromagnetic field is switched off, the proton flips back to the original state, hence generating RF signal. This process is called *relaxation*. Therefore, the MRI signal originates from the differences between water content (T1) and magnetic relaxation times of the water protons (T2). The receiver coils measures this relaxation, which is turned into an image by a computer algorithm. MRI contrast agents are used to modify the relaxation rates at time T1 or T2. T1 contrast agents, such as gadolinium chelators enhance the positive signal on T1-weighted images, while T2 agents such as SPION-based decrease the signal intensity on T2-weighted images. There are some issues concerning the application of Gd-DTPA (diethyltriamine-pentaacetic acid) agents:
   (a) Its uptake in extravascular space as well as its unwanted enhancement of venous (and arterial) structures limits its potential, and (b) Gd is inherently toxic material in ionic form with a half-life of several weeks. Although, it is administered in the complex form, its stability is influenced by temperature, pH, concentration of surrounding ions and ligands (Weinmann et al. 1984).

4. *Optical imaging (OI)*: Broad optical imaging methods and microscopic techniques such as optical coherence tomography (OCT), diffuse optical tomography (DOT), multiphoton microscopy (MPM), confocal laser scanning microscopy (CLSM), fluorescence microscopy (FM), are used for bioimaging to visualize the structure of cells, tissues and to profile diseases at cellular and tissue level. These techniques are based on the ballistic photons for imaging, hence their imaging depth are limited due to strong backscattering that related to tissue tomography. OI technique operates in

the optical range of UV-Vis-IR and is divided into two groups of (a) bioluminescence imaging (BI) and (b) fluorescence imaging (FI). The former utilizes the emission generated by chemiluminescent reaction between an enzyme and its substrate, whereas the latter is based on the absorption of energy from an external exciting source, such as laser, halogen and xenon lamps, by a fluorophore, e.g., fluorescent proteins. FI is increasingly attractive in diseases detection but the optical penetration in biological tissue is significantly limited by different chromophores absorption and scattering. NIR light (650–950 nm) is minimally absorbed in biological tissues and physiological fluids such as blood, so it maximizes the efficient optical penetration depth up to centimeters. This increased photon transport improves the chance of identifying tissue targets below the surface. Since, tissue exhibits no autofluorescence in the NIR spectrum, the signal-to-noise (i.e., background contrast) can be maximized using fluorescence contrast agents responsive to NIR light. Without the knowledge (i.e., measurements) of the absorption, scattering, and anisotropy of the imaged tissue, only qualitative information is expected. NIR fluorescence imaging is available for laparoscopic, theracoscopic, and robot-assisted surgery. The main challenge in all these applications is optimized light source to enable sufficient fluorescence excitation and low-attenuation optics to detect low concentration of NIR fluorophores. In addition, limiting factors for laser-based light sources are skin, eye exposures, irreversible photochemical bleaching of the NIR fluorophores and tissue heating (Gioux et al. 2010).

The basic requirements for fluorophores to be used in bioimaging are: Solubility (or dispersibility), stability, specific target molecules association, high emission quantum efficiency, and no *bleaching* effect. Photobleaching is a term describing the chemical degradation of a fluorophore, resulting in diminishing and disappearing of fluorescence, which in turn can be because of photochemistry in the excited state, photooxidation in the presence of oxygen, or thermal degradation due to local heating by non-radiative processes. In any case, the important issue is the selection of an appropriate fluorophore, considering the above conditions, for an efficient excitation by a suitable laser wavelength available, for example, in microscope. The emission wavelength of the fluorophore must also be compatible with emission filters on the microscope. There are two categories of fluorophores used as fluorescence labeling in bioimaging:

(a) Those for targeting biological molecules without prior attachment to biomolecules which in this case, the hydrophilic or hydrophobic interaction of excitation wavelength with biomolecule or cell determines the labeling characteristic, (b) Those that need to be conjugated chemically to a biomolecule via oligonucleotides or protein ligands for selectivity at certain sites.

Intraoperative application of NIR imaging depends on the suitable contrast agents and intraoperative imaging system to visualize the other so called invisible contrast agent during surgery. Some contrast agents include diluted methylene blue with an excitation peak about 700 nm, indocyanine green (ICG) with fluorescence peak at 800 nm which is also approved by FDA, and 5-aminoievulinic acid (5-ALA) (Vahrmeijer et al. 2013). None of the above agents are ligand-targeted (i.e., covalently) although they show specificity in some clinical applications. More recently Khosroshahi et al. (2015, 2016) and Rezvani et al. (2014) used folate-conjugated fluorescine successfully to visualize the cancer cells. It may well be argued that fluorescine and other visible fluorophores are not optimal for cancer surgery because of light absorption and scattering result in interrogation of only the superficial layer and that high autofluorescence from surrounding tissue reduces contrast. However, the use of advance filters, signal processing, and contrast agents can indeed render hope or possibly obliterate the problems concerning the main fluorescence signal intensity and hence the imaging quality at a certain depths.

5. *Ultrasound (US)*: The US modality is well established and matured technology, it is relatively cheap and considerably patient friendly. It uses high frequency sound waves normally between 1–40 MHz to transmit the energy through skin tissue and reflect back from the internal organs at some distance within body, though higher frequency has also been used for tissue imaging (Yokosawa et al. 1996). USI is limited to hard and ossious structures such as bone or gas-containing organs such as lungs. To enhance the image quality some contrast agents can be utilized based on the different acoustic properties between them and scanned tissues. One such common agent is gas-containing micro (1–6 μm) or nanobubbles (10–100 nm) where the curvature in air-liquid interface can increase

the intensity of the backscattered signal and improve the echo effect. Xing et al. (2010) fabricated biocompatible nanobubbles by ultrasonication of monostearate and polyoxyethlene mixture then filled with perfluoropropane gas for tumor imaging. The micro and nanobubbles have also been used in photoacoustic imaging, which will be discussed in the next section.

Multimodal strategies

No mono-modality imaging system can provide all the required information in biomedical imaging technology. As mentioned above, each imaging modality has its own advantages and limitations in terms of sensitivity, resolution, accuracy, and quantitative capabilities. The major problem which is often faced with single-modality imaging is the inability to assure the conformance of diagnosis, which is very important factor in determining the treatment. The problem is solved by multimodal imaging system where a combination of techniques with complementary strengths offer unique benefits which are not met by individual methods. Therefore, utilizing such complementary imaging modes will greatly improve the diagnosis and treatment reliance and render extra comfort to both physicians and patients. Multimodal imaging techniques can be obtained in two different approaches: either to combine different imaging instruments into one unit, or to develop multimodal imaging agents.

Followings are some examples of first case:

- PET-CT (Cherry 2009)
- MRI-Optical (Josephson et al. 2002, Cha et al. 2011)
- MRI-CT (Kim et al. 2011)
- MRI-PET (Lee et al. 2008, Yang et al. 2011)
- MRI-PET-NIRF (Xie et al. 2010)
- MRI/SPECT (Madru et al. 2012)
- MRI-PA-Raman (Zerda et al. 2013)
- SPECT-CT-Agents (Jang et al. 2012)
- PA-US (Lashkari and Mandelis 2014, Khosroshahi et al. 2015)
- PA-OCT (Berer et al. 2015)
- PA-Fluorescence (Maeda et al. 2014)
- PA-US-Agents (Hannah et al. 2014, Wang et al. 2014)

Multimodal imaging agents

Although every individual imaging modality system has its particular contrast agents, multimodal imaging systems also require its customized multimodal contrast agents. Some examples are as follows:

1) *Gold-iron oxide nanoparticles (Au-SPION)*: has been used in MRI-PAI dual mode imaging by Jin et al. (2010), where they showed the defined structural characteristics and physical properties of this agent not only offer contrast for electron microscopy and MRI but also a new mode of magneto photoacoustic imaging. The (Au-SPION) provides a superior contrast compared to using only single conventional nanoparticles.

2) *Gold-iron oxide nanoclusters*: Small nanoclusters with optical, magnetic, and therapeutic functionality, designed by assembly of nanoparticle building blocks, offer broad opportunities for targeted cellular imaging, therapy, and combined imaging and therapy (Ma et al. 2009). Approximately 30 nm stable uniformly sized near-infrared (NIR) active, superparamagnetic nanoclusters formed by kinetically controlled self-assembly of gold-coated iron oxide nanoparticles. The nanoclusters of approximately 70 iron oxide primary particles with thin gold coatings display intense NIR (700–850 nm) absorbance.

3) *Single-walled carbon nanotubes (SWNTs)*: Kimura et al. (2012) fabricated new size-controlled and biocompatible (Gd2)3-DEG-gelatin nanoparticles for MRI and PAI. Single-walled carbon nanotubes (SWNTs) is another multimodal contrast agent which possess surface properties and biocompatibility similar to plasmonic nanoparticles with wide absorption that can produce strong photoacoustic signals.

4) *Perfluorocarbon (PFC) droplets*: Phase-change contrast agents transform liquid emulsions into microbubbles (MBs) contrast agents that can have both diagnostic and therapeutic functions. PFC droplets undergo a volumetric expansion when is subject to sufficient acoustic pressures delivered by an ultrasound transducer, called acoustic droplet vaporization (ADV) (Kripfgans et al. 2000). Similarly, when it is subject to optical irradiation, vaporization also occurs (ODV) (Strohm et al. 2010). Thus, when the laser fluence is below the vaporization threshold, the droplets remain in the liquid phase and can be used as a PA contrast agent. However, when the fluence exceeds the threshold, it induces droplet vaporization resulting in microbubbles which can be used for contrast enhanced ultrasound imaging. MBs can be composed of phospholipids, albumin, or polymer. These gas-filled can produce strong acoustic scattering relative to the surrounding tissue. In more advance form, AuMBs comprose albumin-shelled microbubbles with encapsulated gold nanorods. Wang et al. (2012) have investigated this system as PA/US dual modality contrast agent.

5) *Dye-doped PFC nanoparticles*: These contrast agents have been used as PAI-FI by (Akers et al. 2010). Spectroscopic characterization of the developed NIR dye-loaded perfluorocarbon-based nanoparticles for combined fluorescence and PA imaging revealed distinct dye-dependent photophysical behaviour. They demonstrated that the enhanced contrast allows detection of regional lymph nodes of rats *in vivo* with time-domain optical and photoacoustic imaging methods. Also, the use of fluorescence lifetime imaging provided a strategic approach to bridge the disparate contrast reporting mechanisms of fluorescence and PA imaging methods.

13.3 Imaging agents and multifunctionality

The progress and advances in nanobiotechnology during the last decade has resulted in significant achievements. On the hand, it seems, the everyday increasing clinical demands had a direct role in shaping, directing, and even accelerating part of this progress in specific directions. For example, the hetrogencity of cancers necessitates image-guided therapies, where personalized disease treatments are planned based on individual patients' pathological conditions and responses to the treatment. Consequently, as a result of such demands, the idea of *multifunctional* (i.e., multimoiety) nanoparticles was formed. Multifunctional nanoparticles are those that are capable of combining various functional features in one package acting as a single multifunctional nanoprobe for different purposes: detection, imaging, therapy, or drug delivery. Though the clinical demands provided the necessary motivation, it is however, important to acknowledge the fact that emergence of new advance nanoparticles itself is due to nanofabrication techniques advancement which render various possibilities for biomedical applications. Basically, a nanoparticle outer layer (normally with a suitable coating) can be linked to a specific targeting ligand that only recognizes the unique features of the surface of the target. In addition, other moieties can be attached simultaneously for other purposes, including imaging and drug delivery. Therefore, the function of such multifunctional structure depends on the application, which in turn governs the type of components that can be used. Let us remind ourselves that the high surface area-to-volume ratio facilitates surface loading capability with more cargoes such as targeting moieties, imaging and therapeutic agents, or other functional molecules. Once such a multifunctional structure is administrated to body, it can be triggered by light excitation (optically and thermally) or by magnetic field for diagnostic and therapeutic applications. However, prior to their use, a number of requirements ought to be satisfied: (a) biocompatibility, (b) non-toxicity, (c) dispersibility and stability in *in vivo* environment, (d) high selectivity, (e) long circulation time in the bloodstream, and (f) efficient clearance by the renal system. The next stage to consider is the synthesis process. The synthesis of nanoparticles has received a great deal of interest and attention because of their potential biomedical applications, which in turn are affected by the kind of surface modification. There are two types of modification methods: chemical and physical where the former offers a stronger and robust bonding and stable surface ligand. A proper surface modification determines how well biomolecules are conjugated on the nanoparticles. A wide variety of contrast agents and labels is required for different types of detection and imaging including MRI, PET, SPECT, and fluorescence-based imaging. While the last method is widely used for *in vivo* imaging, the others are more used for *in vivo* applications. An important class of nanoparticles comprises those made of inorganic materials such as metals, metal oxide, semiconductor, rare earth minerals, and silica. These materials possess unique electrical, optical, magnetic, and plasmonic properties due to quantum mechanical effects at nanoscale. Most nanocrystals can be fabricated with a great control on size, shape, composition, and physical properties. Potential single agents and functional nanoparticles that can be used for both therapy and bioimaging, as some described in Chapter 9, are: Dyes (for example, Indocyanine-green (ICG), Alexa Fluor 750, Evans blue, IRDye800CW, Methylene blue,…), gold nanoparticles, gold nanoshells, gold nanorods, nanocages, nanostars, nanobeacons, SPIONS, polymeric NPs (e.g., PLA, PEG, PEO, PPO and PLGA), dendrimers, Silica, QDs, and upconversion nanoparticles. Multimodal nanoparticles can often offer better spatial registration of different imaging modality and avoid excessive immune response caused by repeated challenge. A number of multimodal nanoparticles combine the use of a full body scan with an imaging modality that offers local images with higher resolution (Bao et al. 2013). This technique allows characterization of disease at multiple spatial scales. For example, SPIONs labeled with Cy5.5 can be used in both MRI and NIR imaging.

13.4 Fluorescence microscopy (FM)

A fluorescence microscope is an optical microscope that uses fluorescence and phosphorescence instead of (or in addition to) reflection and absorption to study properties of organic or inorganic material where it uses fluorescence to generate an image. The specimen is illuminated with light of a specific wavelength which is absorbed by the fluorophores, causing them to emit light of longer wavelengths (i.e., of a different color than the absorbed light). The illumination light is separated from the much weaker emitted fluorescence through the use of a spectral emission filter. Typical components of a fluorescence microscope are a light source (xenon arc lamp or mercury-vapor lamp or more advanced forms of high-power LEDs and lasers), the excitation filter, the dichroic mirror (or dichroic beam splitter), and the emission filter. The filters and the dichroic are chosen to match the spectral excitation and emission characteristics of the fluorophore used to label the specimen. In this manner, the distribution of a single fluorophore (i.e., color) is imaged at a time. Most fluorescence microscopes in use are epifluorescence microscopes, where excitation of the fluorophore and detection of the fluorescence are done through the same light path (i.e., through the objective). These microscopes are widely used in biology and are the basis for more advanced microscope designs, such as the confocal microscope and the total internal reflection fluorescence microscope.

13.4.1 *Imaging and therapeutic applications of optical and thermal response of SPION-based third generation plasmonic nanodendrimers* (Tajabadi et al. 2015)

In this study, 9 nm superparamagnetic iron oxide nanoparticles (SPION) were functionalized by polyamidoamine (PAMAM) dendrimer. Using tetracholoroauric acid (HAuCl$_4$), magnetodendrimer (MD) samples were conjugated by gold nanoparticles (Au-NPs). Two different reducing agents, i.e., sodium borohydride and hydrazine sulfate, and presynthesized 10-nm Au-NP were used to evaluate the efficiency of conjugation method. The samples were characterized using X-ray diffractometry (XRD), transmission electron microscopy (TEM), Fourier transform infrared (FTIR) spectroscopy, UV-visible spectroscopy, and fluorescence spectroscopy. The results confirmed that Au-NPs produced by sodium borohydrate and the pre-synthesized 10-nm Au-NPs were capped by MDs, whereas the Au-NP prepared by hydrazine sulfate as a reducing agent were entrapped by MDs. Optical properties of the MDs were studied by laser-induced fluorescence spectroscopy (LIF) within a wide range of visible spectrum. Also, based on the thermal analysis, all synthesized nanostructures exhibited a temperature increase using 488 nm and 514 nm wavelengths of a tunable argon laser. The new iron oxide-dendrimer-Au NPs synthesized by sodium borohydrate (IDA-NaBH$_4$) produced the highest temperature increase at 488 nm, whereas the other nanostructures particularly pure Au-NPs produced more heating effect at 514 nm. These findings suggest the potential application of these nanocomposites in the field of bioimaging, targeted drug delivery, and controlled hyperthermia.

Introduction

Recently, a variety of nanomaterials, including magnetite superparamagnetic iron oxide nanoparticles (SPION) and nobel metal nanoparticles such as gold, have been the focus of many research fields particularly in medicine and biomedical engineering, which has shown a promising advancement (Pankhurst et al. 2003, Berry and Curties 2003, Khosroshahi and Nourbakhsh 2011). Plasmonic nanoparticles exhibit unique optical properties with major advantages due to the photophysical properties: strong localized surface plasmon resonance (LSPR), surface-enhanced scattering, non-linear optical properties, tunable resonance across the Vis-NIR due to adjustable nanoparticle size and shape, biocompatibility due to their inert surface, nontoxicity, surface conjugation chemistry, i.e., they can be linked to specific ligands for tumor targeting, imaging and therapies, lack of photobleaching or blinking as with quantum dots, and very low oxidation (Wang et al. 2005, Shi et al. 2009, Thompson et al. 2012, Hassannejad and Khosroshahi 2013). Not only can gold nanoparticles (Au-NPs) operate as an optical signal transfer in plasmonic devices, but they can also be used as an useful platform for analytic-receptor interaction (Esumi et al. 2004). Au-NPs need surface treatment with different molecules to precisely perform desirable applications. There are some evidence of Au-NPs modification with silica, liposome, and linear polymers (Wang et al. 2009, Khosroshahi and Ghazanfari 2012). Researchers explicitly assert that poly(amidoamine) (PAMAM) dendrimers can act as a template or stabilizer for preparation of inorganic nanocomposites. The resultant nanocomposites have much applicable potential, such as gen vector, catalysis, resonance imaging agents, and nanocapsules (Shi et al. 2009, Shen and Shi 2010, Thompson et al. 2012). Since dendrimers have unique chemical structures, molecular weight, and molecular size which can provide special type of functionality, they received privileged attention in developing fields of materials science (Majoros et al. 2006, Syahir et al. 2009, Choi et al. 2012). Considering large number of terminal groups on the exterior of the molecule and interior voids, dendrimers introduce an attractive platform for metal ion chelates (Venditto et al. 2005). Indeed, dendrimer-entrapped inorganic nanoparticles (DENP) include a nanostructure where one or more inorganic nanoparticles with the diameter of less than 5 nm are entrapped within an individual dendrimer molecule. In the case of dendrimer-stabilized inorganic nanoparticles (DSNP), one inorganic nanoparticle which usually has the diameter larger than 5 nm is stabilized by multiple dendrimer molecules (Bronstein and Shifrina 2011). Evaluation of formation of both DENP and DSNP in the presence of amine-terminated PAMAM dendrimers with and without addition of reducing agents has been the subject of several studies over the past few years (Garcia and Baker 1998, Esumi et al. 2005, Hoffman et al. 2011). Most of chemical methods of Au-NP preparation include nucleation and then growth of gold clusters by reduction of a gold salt (Bronstein and Shifrina 2011). The bond is formed between gold nanoparticles and dendrimers as a result of interaction between coordinating groups such as –OH, –NH$_2$, or –COOH and gold ions (Sardar et al. 2009). The contemporary issues in cancer treatment are production of effective nanoprobes for tumor targeting and selective therapy (Li et al. 2009). Fine magnetite nanoparticles with simple production method, nearly uniform size distribution and high magnetization saturation were prepared in our previous study (Khosroshahi and Nourbakhsh 2010, Khosroshahi and Nourbakhsh 2011, Khosroshahi and Ghazanfari 2012, Tajabadi and Khosroshahi 2012, Tajabadi et al. 2013), the optimal magnetite nanoparticles were chosen, coated with third generation PAMAM dendrimer, and finally functionalized with Au-NP via different preparation methods. The main intention of the paper was to synthesize third generation dendrimers conjugated with Au-NPs using three methods of sodium borohydrate, hydrazine sulfate as the reducing agents and pre-synthesized Au-NP, and compare their fluorescent and optothermal properties with dendrimers for the purpose of biomedical application.

Materials and methods

Materials

Iron chlorides (III) (FeCl$_3$.6H$_2$O), Iron Sulfate (FeSO$_4$.7H$_2$O), and Ethanol (C$_2$H$_5$OH) were purchased from Merck Company. Ammonium Hydroxide (NH$_4$OH), Methyl Acrylate (CH$_2$ = C(CH$_3$)COOCH$_3$), Ethylenediamine (C$_2$H$_4$(NH$_2$)$_2$), Soduiom Borohydrate (NaBH$_4$), Hydrazine sulfate (H$_6$N$_2$O$_4$S), Gold colloid solution (10 nm), and tetracholoroauric acid (HAuCl$_4$) were obtained from Sigma Aldrich.

Formation of gold and magnetodendrimer

Dendrimer grafted magentite nanoparticles (magnetodendrimers-MDs) were synthesized based on our previous published report (Tajabadi et al. 2013). The gold coated MDs were synthesized using the three aforementioned procedures to achieve the following objectives: (i) to have efficient method of loading Au-NP, (ii) to improve the fluorescence properties of material, and (iii) to find the optimal optothermal properties.

a) *Using sodium borohydrate (IDA-NaBH$_4$):* A solution of tetracholoroauric acid (HAuCl$_4$) (5 mM) was prepared and added to the suspension of third generation magnetodendrimer (1% w/v) with the same volume under N$_2$ atmosphere. In order to produce the complex between Au (III) and amide or amine group of dendrimer, the resulting mixture was vigorously stirred for one hour in darkness. After that, 5 mL of aqueous sodium borohydrate solution (0.1 M) was added drop-wise to the reaction mixture. The following reactions lead to reducing Au (III) to zero charge Au (0) nanoparticles. The reaction was continued under a vigorous stirring for 2 hours at 25°C. The obtained nanoparticles are referred to as IDA-*NaBH$_4$*. These particles were rinsed with ethanol five times using magnetic separation. The same procedure was repeated with the tenfold concentration of HAuCl$_4$ and to evaluate the completion of the reactions, a UV-vis analysis was performed at 0, 15, 30, 45, 60, 90, and 120 minutes after addition of reducing agent. The product is referred as (IDA-10).

b) *Using hydrazine sulfate (IDA-Hydr):* The stable gold nanoparticles were produced by adding hydrazine sulfate (H$_6$N$_2$O$_4$S) aqueous solution (25 mM) to the solution of magnetodendrime-HAuCl$_4$ complex and stirring for 2 hours. The particles were rinsed with ethanol five times as before and the sample was named IDA-Hydr.

c) *Using gold nanoparticles (IDA-NP):* Au-NPs (purchased from sigma Aldrich) were directly added to magnetodendrimer suspension under N$_2$ atmosphere. The mixture was stirred for an hour to complete the reaction, and then particles rinsed five times with ethanol.

Characterization

Crystalline phase of nanoparticles was confirmed using X-ray diffraction with radiation of Cu Kα (XRD, λ = 0.15406 nm, FK60-40 X-ray diffractometer). The presence of PAMAM, gold formation on the surface of magnetite nanoparticles was proved by Fourier transform infrared (FTIR) spectroscopy (BOMEM, Canada). Particle size and morphology of nanocomposites were determined by transmission electron microscopy (TEM, Philips CM-200-FEG microscope, 120 kV). The amount of Au-NP attached to the magnetodendrimer was estimated using wavelength-dispersive X-ray spectroscopy (SEM–WDX, XL30, Philips, USA). The UV-vis spectra of nanoparticles were recorded using spectrophotometer (UV-2600, Shimadzu, Japan).

Experimental setup

The evaluation of fluorescence emission of ID (G3), IDA-10, IDA-Hydr, and IDA-NP nanoparticles at different excitation wavelengths was performed using an ion argon laser (Melles Griot-35MAP431) at 25°C. The fluorescence signals were detected by a 600 μm core diameter optical fiber (LIBS-600-6-SR, Ocean Optics) connected to spectrometer (UV-Vis USB 4000, Ocean Optics), as can be seen in Figure 13.1. In our case, the excitation wavelengths were 454, 457, 465, 472, 477, 488, 496, 502, and 514 nm. After obtaining the spectra of samples, they were smoothed by Gaussian model using Findgraph software. The next set up was to evaluate the efficiency of these nanoparticles in coloring the polymeric substrate, using two kinds of natural polymers, i.e., cotton and collagen. After the injection of nanoparticle solution to these substrates, fluorescence microscopy (Zeiss Axioshop-Germany) was used to study the materials' coloring.

Results and discussion

UV-vis evaluation

The concept of dendrimer nanocomposites is based on immobilization of preorganized metallic ions (Okugaichi et al. 2006). With respect to this concept, a dendrimer acts as a template or reactor to preorganization of ions and small molecules (Balogh et al. 1999). The full generation of dendrimeric nanoparticles are electron donors in aqueous medium and form a cation. In such cases, atoms and molecules could attach to internal space or external surface of dendrimer (He et al. 1999, Esumi et al. 2004). This preorganization can lead to attachment of precursor-dendrimer, which is a dynamic equilibrium between template and reactants. The dynamic equilibrium causes a homogeneous distribution of ions and molecules. At the second stage, a series of reactions lead to production of resultant hybrid materials. At this stage, mostly a reducing agent is added to precursor-dendrimer complex, and the complex loses HCl moieties, and Au-NPs are stabilized in the dendrimer structure (Balogh et al. 1999, Zhao et al. 1998). There are three different types of hybrid materials; i.e., internal, external, and mixed type.

In this work, in order to evaluate the formation of Au-NPs during the synthesis reaction, sampling was done at different reaction times and the UV-vis spectra of these samples were recorded. Figure 13.2 indicates that all samples have a unique absorption peak in the range of 520–540 nm, which reveal the

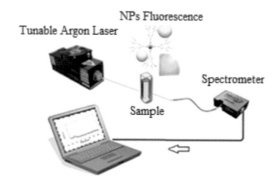

Figure 13.1. Experimental setup of laser-induced fluorescence spectroscopy for IDA nanocomposites.

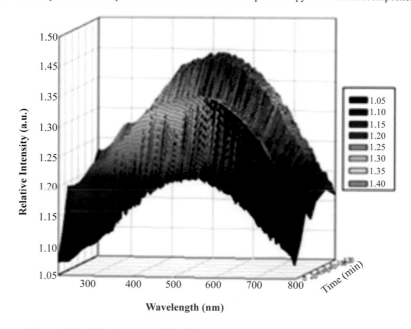

Figure 13.2. UV-vis spectra of dendrimer-gold complex during the synthesis.

formation of Au-NPs. Plasmonic peak around 520 nm corresponds to the collective oscillation of gold free electrons (Satoh et al. 2002, Shi et al. 2006). During the synthesis reaction, the intensity of plasmon resonance peak was increased over time and the peak shifted towards higher wavelengths with respect to increase in particle size.

At synthesis condition of dendrimer–gold nanocomposite and in the presence of $HAuCl_4$ molecules, amine group loses electrons and electrostatically interacts with $AuCl_4^-$ ions. In UV-vis spectrum of the condition prior to addition of reducing agent, an absorption peak was observed around 280 nm, which is the characteristic peak of bond formation between $AuCl_4^-$ and dendrimer (Kim et al. 2003). After addition of reducing agent, a broad peak around 520 nm was seen. This plasmonic peak is related to the collective oscillation of electrons. Other researches indicate that peaks at 280 and 320 nm represent the aggregation of Au-NPs (Mosseri et al. 1989, Divsar et al. 2009). It should be mentioned that location and shape of surface plasmon resonance is strongly dependent on the particle size of material and the particle aggregation results in reduction of gold plasmon band intensity (Jiang et al. 2010, Zhang et al. 2010). As it is seen in Figure 13.3, the peak ratio of 520 nm to 280 nm increases over the time, which indicates the formation of Au-NPs. However, this ratio shows a reducing trend after 90 minutes, which can be an indication of probability of aggregation and cluster formation of Au-NPs. No significant peak corresponding to Au NPs was observed in the UV-vis spectra shown in Figure 13.4 after purification of resultant material, which may suggest that the final structure contains discrete gold nanoparticles (i.e., trapped) in a dendrimer substrate. This phenomenon was previously reported by Westcott et al. (1998) and Zheng et al. (2003).

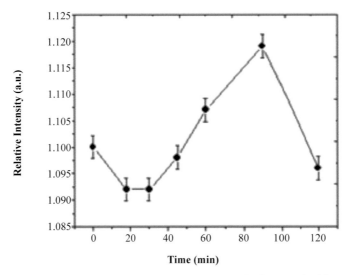

Figure 13.3. Change of intensity ratio of 520 nm to 280 nm peaks during synthesis of magnetodendrimer–gold nanocomposite.

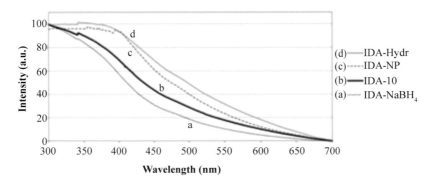

Figure 13.4. UV-vis spectra of magnetodendrimer–gold nanocomposite (a) IDA, (b) IDA 10, (c) IDA NP, (d) IDA Hydr.

TEM analysis

Figure 13.5 indicates that the nanocomposites synthesized using NaBH$_4$ are larger than those synthesized using hydrazine sulfate. Based on these results and other researchers' suggestions, on the presence of NaBH$_4$, the ions interact with surface amine group of magnetodendrimer (Torigoe et al. 2001, Zhang et al. 2010) and form larger particles at the expense of smaller particles. When hydrazine sulfate was used as a reducing agent, the homogeneous distribution and smaller particles were obtained, which could be explained as an entrapment and formation of Au-NPs on the cavity of magnetodendrimer (Torigoe et al. 2001).

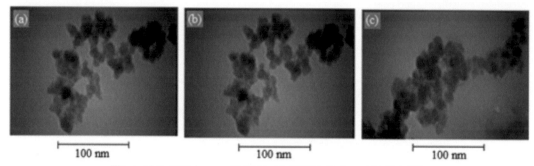

Figure 13.5. TEM image of (a) IDA-10, (b) IDA-Hydr, and (c) IDA-NP.

XRD analysis

In order to evaluate the presence of Au-NP in the final structure, XRD analysis was done (Fig. 13.6). The XRD patterns contain diffraction peaks at 2θ equal to 38, 44.3, 64.5, and 77.9 which represent (111), (200), (220), and (311) crystallographic plane, respectively which prove the FCC structure of gold (JCPDS No. 00-04-0784) (Arias et al. 2001, Wu et al. 2011, Streszewski et al. 2012). The broadening of the most intense peak of these nanoparticles demonstrates that the small size Au-NPs could be calculated by using the Scherrer equation (Eq. 13.1) (Faiyas et al. 2009). The calculation shows that the average particle size of Au-NPs obtained using NaBH$_4$ reducing agent is about 4 orders larger than those formed by hydrazine sulfate.

$$D = \frac{K \lambda}{\beta \cos \theta} \tag{13.1}$$

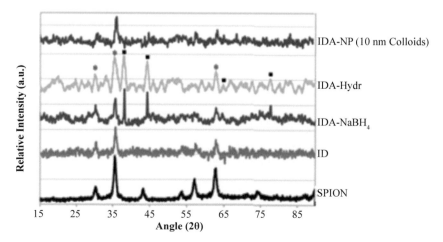

Figure 13.6. XRD pattern of (a) SPION, (b) ID, (c) IDA-NaBH$_4$, (d) IDA-Hydr, (e) IDA-NP (* represents magnetite phase and ■ indicates gold phase).

where, D, λ, and β represent the mean diameter of particles, the wavelength of incident X-ray, and the full width at half height (FWHM), respectively and constant K is equal to 0.9.

FTIR and WDX evaluation

FTIR analysis was used to prove the attachment of Au-NPs to magnetodendrimer shown in Figure 13.7. In the dendrimer-modified iron oxide nanoparticle (ID), the amide bands at 1570 and 1630 cm^{-1} represent the characteristics of PAMAM dendrimer. Esumi et al. believe that the interactions of Au-NPs with amine terminated dendrimers are stronger than carboxyl terminated dendrimers, as the FTIR bands of dendrimer are shifted while the half generations do not show any changes (Esumi et al. 2000). Furthermore, according to the FTIR and UV-vis evaluations of dendrimer depend on the size and their generations, at lower generations external type and at higher generations a mixed type could be observed (Satoh et al. 2002).

Type I amide band (wave number of 1630 cm^{-1}) is generally related to C=O stretching vibration (70–85%) and directly appertain to combination and structure of polymer backbone. Type II amide band (wave number 1570 cm^{-1}) represents the N-H bending vibration (20%) (Grabchev et al. 2003, Chou and Lien 2009, Li et al. 2010, Baykal et al. 2012). As shown in Figure 13.7, FTIR spectra regarding IDA complex samples do not contain the band at 1570 cm^{-1} and the band 1630 cm^{-1} remain without any changes. This shows that the Au-NPs interact with N-H groups of MD structure, whereas the polymer backbone relatively retains its original structure. In this figure, the peaks at 581 and 629 cm^{-1} represent the iron oxide phase at all synthesized structures. In order to quantitatively appraise attachment of Au-NPs to MD, WDX (Wavelength-dispersive X-ray spectroscopy) analysis was performed. The analysis confirms the presence of gold phase in the prepared nanoparticles (Fig. 13.8) (Streszewski et al. 2012), and Figure 13.9 shows the efficiency of synthesis in terms of relative counts of Fe:Au where hydrazine sulfate reducing agent has been shown to produce the best nanoparticles compared to other synthesis methods.

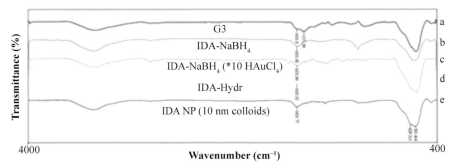

Figure 13.7. FTIR Spectra of (a) G 3, (b) IDA-NaBH$_4$, (c) IDA-10, (d) IDA-Hydr, (e) IDA-NP.

Laser-induced fluorescence spectroscopy

One of the early works regarding the fluorescence of PAMAM dendrimer was reported by Klajnart and Bryszewska (2002). It has been shown that after addition of HAuCL$_4$, the fluorescence intensity is red shifted towards the longer wavelength (Kim et al. 2003). After adding the reducing agent, the peaks are changed considerably, which shows the close attachment of Au-NPs to the dendrimers. The shift of fluorescence spectra could be explained by strong interaction between gold crystals and amine groups of dendrimer. Optical properties of Au-NPs are highly sensitive to their particle size and have an effective influence on the fluorescence spectra of dendrimer (Jiang et al. 2010, Zhang et al. 2010). This is because of the internal interaction between flexible structure of dendrimer and rigid structure of entrapped Au-NPs, whereas the larger particles damp the fluorescence of dendrimers. These phenomena could be explained in terms of fluorescence resonance energy transfer (FRET) (Zhang et al. 2010). In this study, IDA-Hydr nanocomposites strongly changed the initial fluorescent spectra of MD, i.e., the shape and location of peaks were sharply changed. In most cases, the fluorescence spectra of IDA-Hydr is stronger than others with

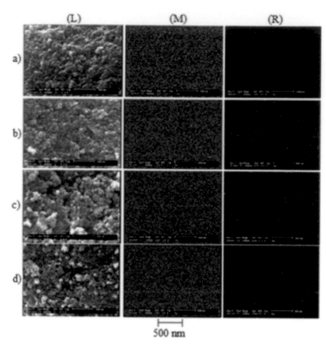

Figure 13.8. WDX images of (a) IDA-NaBH$_4$, (b) IDA-10, (c) IDA-Hydr, (d) IDA-NP nanoparticles at three different levels of synthesized nanoparticles (L), Fe element (M), and Au element (R), respectively.

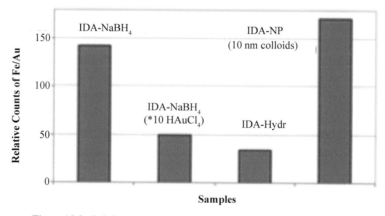

Figure 13.9. Relative counts of Fe/Au for different synthesized nanoparticles.

highest signals at about 525 nm and 550 nm, respectively. One reason for this is more likely due to their smaller size which helps them to be entrapped easily by dendrimers, and hence intensify the fluorescence signals, as we can see in Figure 13.10.

Considering the chemical structures of collagen and cotton, there is a possibility of hydrogen interaction between the hydroxyl group of the substrate and amine group of dendrimer nanocomposites, which produces a new fluorescent moieties with a time dependent behaviour. The longer the time, the more fluorescent moieties are produced hence, more intense fluorescence image could be obtained. Figures 13.11 and 13.12 represent the fluorescence image of nanoparticles with different formulation in close contact with collagen and cotton, respectively.

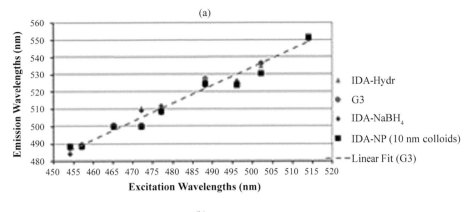

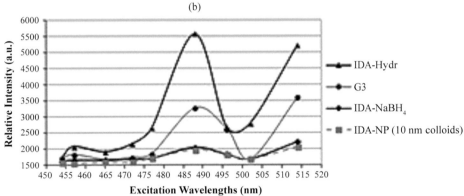

Figure 13.10. Fluorescence of emission wavelengths (a) and the relative intensities (b) of G3, IDA-NP, IDA-10, IDA-Hydr, IDA-NaBH$_4$ at different excitation wavelengths.

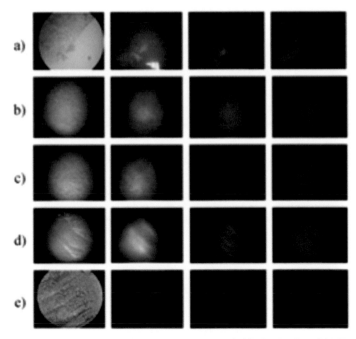

Figure 13.11. Fluorescence image of (a) G3, (b) IDA-NaBH4, (c) IDA-10, (d) IDA-Hydr, and (e) IDA-NP nanoparticles on the collagen substrate.

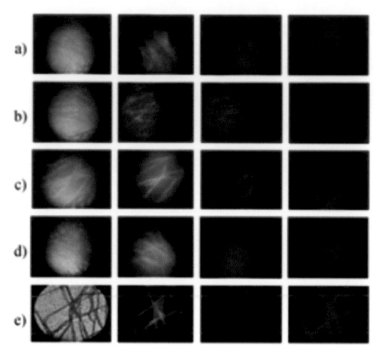

Figure 13.12. Fluorescence image of (a) G3, (b) IDA-NaBH$_4$, (c) IDA-10, (d) IDA-Hydr, and (e) IDA-NP nanoparticles on the cotton substrate.

Thermal response of synthesized nanoparticles

Figure 13.13 shows the thermal response of different synthesized nanocomposites at 488 nm (Fig. 13.13a) and 514 n (Fig. 13.13b) for 5 minutes. Clearly, the highest temperature rise was produced by IDA-NaBH$_4$ at 488 nm and pure Au-NPs at 514 nm due to its proximity to gold surface plasmon resonance (SPR) peak absorption at about 530 nm. It has been reported that photon excitation of metallic nanostructures leads to production of hot electron cloud which cools down in about 1 ps as a result of heat transfer within the nanoparticle lattice, which is then followed by phonon-phonon interactions in 100 ps where the metallic lattice transfers the heat to its surrounding medium and cools down (Lee and El-Sayed 2005, Jain et al. 2006, Govorov and Richardson 2007, Huang et al. 2008, Baffou et al. 2010, Ghazanfari and Khosroshahi 2014). The phenomena of energy absorption and increasing the temperature are well known in SPR frequencies, where these rapid changes of temperature lead to variety of applications of nanocomposites. The temperature distribution around optically-stimulated plasmonic nanoparticles can be described by the following equation (Sassaroli et al. 2009):

$$\rho c \frac{\partial T}{\partial t} = \nabla.\left(K\nabla T\right) + \langle p \rangle \tag{13.2}$$

where T is the local temperature, and ρ, c, and K represent density, specific heat capacity, and thermal conductivity of material, respectively. Here < p > is the average heat power dissipated inside the NP and the heat power is given by P = < p >. V_{NP} indicated using Eq. 13.3:

$$P = 4\pi R^3 K_{Au} \frac{c\varepsilon_w}{2} |E|^2 Im\left(\frac{\varepsilon_{Au} - \varepsilon_w}{\varepsilon_{Au} + 2\varepsilon_w}\right) = 4\pi R^3 K_{Au} \frac{c\varepsilon_w}{2} |E_0|^2 \left|\frac{3\varepsilon_w}{\varepsilon_{Au} + 2\varepsilon_w}\right|^2 Im\left(\frac{\varepsilon_{Au} - \varepsilon_w}{\varepsilon_{Au} + 2\varepsilon_w}\right) \tag{13.3}$$

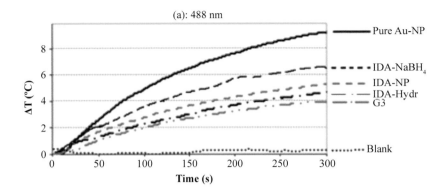

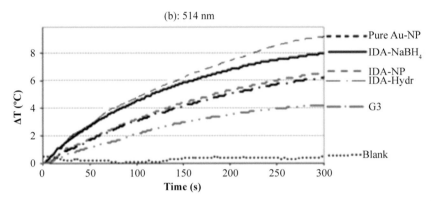

Figure 13.13. The effect of laser irradiation at two different wavelengths of (a) 488 nm and (b) 514 nm on thermal behaviour of different synthesized nanoparticles.

where c is the speed of light, ε_{Au} and ε_w are the permittivity of gold and water, respectively. This definition obtained from the original formula (Baffou and Rigneault 2011):

$$P = \sigma_{abs} I \qquad (13.4)$$

σ_{abs} is the optical absorption cross section of the gold nanoparticles, and I is the intensity of incoming light.

$$I = \frac{c\varepsilon_w}{2}|E|^2 \qquad (13.5)$$

and

$$E = E_0 \frac{3\varepsilon_w}{\varepsilon_{Au} + 2\varepsilon_w} \qquad (13.6)$$

After a transient evolution, materials reach steady state temperature profile under CW illumination. Dimensional analysis of the two diffusion equations demonstrates two time scale of the system:

$$\tau_d^w = \frac{\rho_w c_w}{K_w} R^2 = \frac{R^2}{k_w} \qquad (13.7)$$

$$\tau_d^{Au} = \frac{\rho_{Au} c_{Au}}{K_{Au}} R^2 = \frac{R^2}{k_{Au}} \qquad (13.8)$$

where k = K/ρc is thermal diffusivity (m² s⁻¹), τ_d^w and τ_d^{Au} represent the characteristic times associated with the evolution of the temperature profile in the surrounding water and inside Au-NP, respectively. Thermalization inside the nanoparticle happens much faster than the water, as k_{Au} is far greater than k_w. Hence, the best consideration of reaching comprehensive temperature profile of the total system is directed by the time scale τ_d^w (Baffou and Rigneault 2011). In the final steady state regime, Eq. 2 reduces to:

$$\nabla.(K\nabla T)(r) = -\langle p \rangle(r) \tag{13.9}$$

This equation is formally equivalent to Poisson's equation and produces a profile of temperature increase ΔT given by a Coulom potential outside the particle (Baffou et al. 2009).

$$T(r) = \frac{P}{4\pi K_w r} \qquad \text{for} \quad r \geq R \tag{13.10}$$

Substituting the Eq. 13.3 in Eq. 13.10, it gives the temperature increase at the surface of nanoparticle (i.e., r = R),

$$\Delta T(r) = \frac{I K_{Au} R^2}{K_w} \text{Im}\left(\frac{\varepsilon_{Au} - \varepsilon_w}{\varepsilon_{Au} + 2\varepsilon_w}\right) \approx 2.00 \times \frac{I K_{Au} R^2}{K_w} \tag{13.11}$$

Here, R represents the nanoparticle's radius and I is the intensity of incident beam. Equation (13.11) shows that temperature of the system containing plasmonic nanoparticles is proportional to the square of the nanoparticle radius, i.e., $\Delta T \propto R^2$. As the TEM results show, the use of sodium borohydrate as a reducing agent produced clusters of Au-NPs, which consists a greater particle size than the other formulation. Based on the above analysis, we expect to obtain a higher temperature in IDA-NaBH₄ shown in Figure 13.13. Also this figure indicates that IDA-Hydr formulation leads to the least significant changes in temperature, which could be described by its smaller particles size compared to other gold containing formulations. Furthermore, it was shown that temperature of NP changes with regard to their exciting wavelengths and hence the maximum spectral position of the plasmonic band, i.e., the temperature drastically decreases at both lower and higher wavelengths (Grabchev et al. 2003, Sassaroli et al. 2009, Baffou et al. 2010). As IDA nanoparticles contain clusters, their plasmonic peak may be obtained at 320 nm. The thermal analysis indicates that at shorter exciting wavelengths, these nanocomposites produce more heat than the longer wavelengths, and on the other hand longer wavelengths cause more temperature increase in the case of pure Au-NPs. This lies on the fact that the shorter exciting wavelength (488 nm) is closer to the plasmonic band of the Au-NPs than 514 nm.

13.4.2 Evaluation of cell viability and T2 relaxivity of fluorescein conjugated SPION-PAMAM third generation nanodendrimers for bioimaging (Khosroshahi et al. 2016)

This study has investigated the possibility of using fluorescent dendronized magnetic nanoparticles (FDMNPs) for potential applications in drug delivery and imaging. FDMNPs were first synthesized, characterized, and then the effect of Polyamidoamine (PAMAM) dendrimer functionalization and fluorescein isothiocyanate (FITC) conjugation on biocompatibility of superparamagnetic iron oxide nanoparticles (SPIONs) was evaluated. The nanostructures cytotoxicity tests were performed at different concentrations from 10 to 500 μg/mL using MCF-7 and L929 cell lines. The results showed that FITC conjugation diminishes the toxicity of dendronized magnetic nanoparticles (DMNP) mainly due to the reduction of surface charge. DMNP appears to be cytotoxic at the concentration levels being used for both cell lines. On the contrary, FDMNPs showed more biocompatibility and cell viability of MCF-7 and L929 cell lines at all concentrations. The fluorescence microscopy of FDMNPs incubated with MCF-7 cells showed a successful localization of cells, indicating their ability for applications such as a magnetic fluorescent probe in cell studies and imaging purposes. T2 relaxivity measurements demonstrated the applicability of the synthesized nanostructures as the contrast agents in tissue differential assessment by altering their relaxation times. In our case, the r2 relaxivity of FDMNPs was measured as 103.67 mM⁻¹ S⁻¹.

Introduction

The modification of superparamagnetic iron oxide nanoparticles (SPIONs) with other nanostructures has received much attention in recent years (Khosroshahi and Ghazanfari 2011, 2012, Unterweger et al. 2014). These nanoparticles (NPs) can be functionalized with biological molecules to make them interact with or even bind to a biological entity, thereby providing a controllable method of so-called targeting. In addition, due to their magnetic nature, they obey Coulomb's law, and hence can be manipulated by an external magnetic field (Pankhurst et al. 2003). It is this action at a distance and the penetration of magnetic field into tissue as well as other physiochemical advantages of magnetic nanoparticles MNPs such as biocompatibility that make them an ideal candidate for biomedical applications, for example anticancer drug delivery and imaging (Wolinsky and Grinstaff 2008, Mody et al. 2014). However, there are some major issues that should be considered in applications of NPs in cancer therapy without having a specific binding to cancerous cells. Number of investigations have shown the successful application of various protein ligands for conjugating the (MNPs) surface (Caminade et al. 2005, Khosroshahi and Ghazanfari 2012) but the specific ligand-receptor or antibody-antigen interaction occurs on the cell membrane, hence limiting their intercellular uptake of conjugated NPs. One approach to overcome such limitations is to employ dendrimers which are highly branched molecules and are mainly considered due to their unique spherical, symmetric structure, and properties.

Poly amidoamine (PAMAM) dendrimers are hydrophilic, biocompatible, monodisperse, cascade-branched macromolecules with highly flexible surface chemistry that facilitates functionalization which offers number of advantages (Falanga et al. 2013, Tajabadi et al. 2013, Alanagh et al. 2014). The hybrid nanostructure of PAMAM dendrimer with SPIONs is investigated as diagnosis and therapeutic agents to boost the clinical benefits of nanomedicine in several studies (Shen and Shi 2010, Khodadust et al. 2013). What makes them interesting in terms of imaging is their structural characteristics and internal spaces between their branches which are capable of encapsulating guest species (Jasmine et al. 2009, Tajabadi et al. 2015). The coupling of luminescent molecules to the periphery of dendrimers can make them a powerful sensing agent based on the photophysical properties of the dendrimer via energy transfer (Wang et al. 2007, Alanagh et al. 2014). Due to large number of terminal groups on PAMAM coating, higher quantity of fluorescein isothiocyanate (FITC) molecules or other similar molecules can be conjugated (Satija et al. 2007, Shi et al. 2008, Denora et al. 2013). To the best of our knowledge, the effect of FITC conjugated PAMAM biocompatibility of SPION, and hence is seldom analyzed on cells. However, the precise information about the biocompatibility of nanomaterials cannot be just evaluated by relying on the MTT tests, and other related evaluations are also required. The results of such investigations are expected to be very beneficial in terms of fabrications and modifications for biomedical applications. The extensive number of factors involved in the biocompatibility of nanomaterials both *in vitro* and *in vivo*, make a thorough and complete evaluation a difficult task to follow and understand independently the role of each influencers (Lee and MacKay 2005). Magnetic resonance (MR) is a dynamic and flexible technology that allows one to tailor the imaging study to the anatomic part of interest. With its dependence on the more biologically variable parameters of proton density, longitudinal relaxation time (T1), and transverse relaxation time (T2), variable image contrast can be achieved by using different pulse sequences and by changing the imaging parameters. Signal intensities of T1, T2, and proton density-weighted images relate to specific tissue characteristics. Certain contrast agents are predominantly used to shorten the T1 relaxation time, and these are mainly based on low-molecular weight chelates of the gadolinium ion (Gd (3^+)). The most widely used T2 shortening agents are based on iron oxide (FeO) particles, particularly SPIONs. Depending on their chemical composition, molecular structure and overall size, the *in vivo* distribution volume and pharmacokinetic properties vary widely between different contrast agents, and these largely determine their use in specific diagnostic tests (Li et al. 2013).

Magnetic resonance imaging (MRI) combined with contrast agents is believed to be the most effective and safest non-invasive technique for imaging of living bodies (Werner et al. 2008). Up to 50% of all MRI scans in the clinic, contrast agents are used to enhance image contrast (Paeng and Lee 2010). However, more attention has been paid to develop novel SPIONs with specific surface coating or functional moieties which facilitate their desired applications. The main advantage of SPIONs with respect to MRI are their ability to be easily visualized, change proton relaxation properties, hence providing a source of contrast for

MRI. Other advantages include their ability to be guided to target sites by means of an external magnetic field, and their ability to be heated in order to provide hyperthermia for cancer therapy. A basic need for an *in vivo* molecular probe imaging is sensitive detection probes and MRI images lack such sensitivity. While the optical imaging has the strengths of high sensitivity and direct detection of signals with optical devices, they have a poor penetration depth in soft tissues due to high scattering. Consequently, multimodal imaging systems are highly efficient approach for guided surgical therapy. Following our previous work regarding the synthesis, characterization of FDMNPs (Tajabadi et al. 2013), we intend to describe here, the results of cell viability and r2 relaxivity of MNPs and FDMNPs for possible application as bioimaging for tumors diagnosis in a multimodal probe.

Materials and methods

Nanocomposite synthesis

All the chemical reagents used in this research were analytical grade and used as received from Merck, except for FITC, which was purchased from Aldrich Chemical Co. without further purification. The detailed synthesis process of FDMNP is described in our previous work (Alanagh et al. 2014). Briefly, an aqueous solution of $FeCl_3.6H_2O$ (0.012 M) and $FeSO_4.7H_2O$ (0.006 M) was treated by ultrasonic wave, then added into ammonia aqueous solution (0.9 M) and stirred rigorously. To complete the co-precipitation reaction after 1 h of being stirred, it was continued for further 30 min at 70°C to modify the surface of nanoparticles. Then 149 mL of magnetite colloid ethanol solution and 1 mL H_2O was treated by ultrasonic wave for 30 minutes. 35 μL 3-aminopropyltriethoxysilane [$3NH_2 (CH2)_3Si (OC_2H5)$, APTS] was added into it with rapid stirring for 7 h. The final product of this process was used as base or zero generation (G0) for PAMAM dendrimer growth. The further dendrimer generation was initiated using 50 mL of 5 wt% G0 ethanol solution and adding 200-mL sample of 20% (v/v) methylacrylate ethanol solution to the suspension, then it was stirred by a magnetic pellet for 48 h. After rinsing, 40 mL of 50% (v/v) ethylenediamine ethanol solution was added and the suspension was immersed in an ultrasonicating water bath at room temperature for 3 h. The particles were rinsed five times with ethanol. Stepwise growth using methylacrylate and ethylenediamine was repeated until the desired number of generations (G1–G3) was achieved, as seen in Figure 13.14.

The product was then washed three times with ethanol and five times with deionized water (DIW). FDMNPs could be obtained by the reaction between the isosulfocyanic group of FITC and the amino groups of the DMNs. Here, 0.002 g/mL of ethanol solution of FITC (large excess of the amino groups) was added to 0.02 g/mL aqueous solution of magnetic particles grafted by third generation PAMAM. After 24 h of stirring in the dark at room temperature, the product was washed through four cycles of centrifugation/ethanol and centrifugation/DIW.

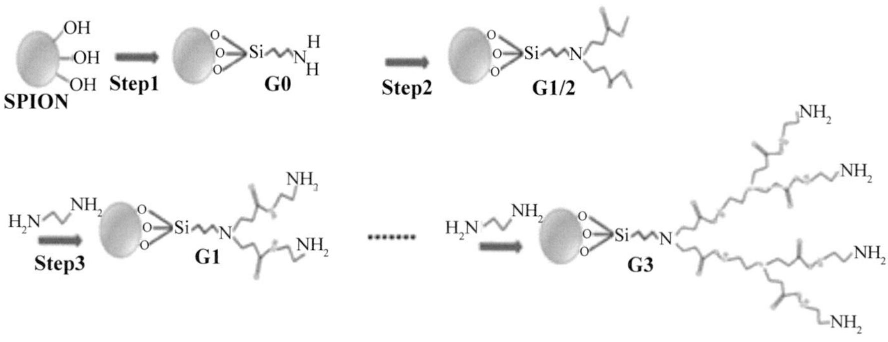

Figure 13.14. Schematic reaction of magnetite surface coating with PAMAM dendrimer.

Characterization instruments

The average size of nanocomposites was estimated using a transmission electron microscope (Model CM120, PHILIPS). Fluorescence spectroscopy (Perkin Elmer, Ls55) was used to evaluate the fluorescence at excitation wavelength of 495 nm for MNPs, DMNPs and FDMNPs. Zeta potential of DMNPs and FDMNPs were determined by zeta sizer (Malvern, Nano ZS). The samples were dried at 15°C in a vacuum for 6 hours before the measurements.

Culture of cell lines

Two cell line of MCF-7 (human breast cancer cells) and L929 (mouse fibroblasts) were obtained from National Cell Bank of Iran (NCBI) and Pasteur Institute of Iran. Cells were grown in DMEM at 37°C under 5% CO_2 in a humidified incubator. The cells were harvested, counted and transferred to 96-well plates (15000 cells per a well) and incubated for 24 h prior to the addition of nanoparticles. The NPs were processed and used in various concentrations, and the treated cells were then incubated for 24 h. 5 mg of MTT (3-[4,5-dimethylthiazol-2-yl]-2,5-diphenyltetrazolium bromide), the water soluble tetrazolium salt dissolved in 1 mL of phosphate-buffered saline (PBS), and 25 μL of the MTT solution were added to each of the 96 wells. The plates were wrapped in an aluminum foil and incubated at 37°C for 4 h. The solution in each well, containing media, unbound MTT, and dead cells, were removed by suction, and 200 μL of DMSO was added to each well. The plates were then shaken, and the optical density was measured using a microplate reader (Stat tax 2100, USA) at 575 nm. The relative cell viability (%) related to control wells containing cell culture medium without nanoparticles was calculated by [A1] test/[A2] control × 100, where [A1] test is the absorbance of the test sample and [A2] control is the absorbance of the control sample. Each MTT test was performed three times for each FDMNPs nanocomposite solution concentration and the average results were reported. The MCF-7 cells were then trypsinized, rinsed with DMEM, and washed twice with PBS to remove the excess nanoparticles which did not react with cells. The images of cancer cell line were acquired by an optical and fluorescence microscope using 400 × magnification.

MRI studies

T1 and T2 relaxivities of the samples were evaluated by 1.5 T GE Signa MRI Scanner at 0.01, 0.008, 0.004, and 0.002 mg (Fe)/mL concentrations at 25°C. T2 relaxation times axial spine echo (SE) sequences were obtained with TR = 1000 ms and echo time (E). The TE refers to time between the application of radiofrequency excitation pulse and the peak of the signal induced in the coil measured in milliseconds. The amount of T2 relaxation is controlled by TE, 10 ms. All pulse sequences were acquired with a 90 mm × 90 mm field of view (FOV), a matrix of 256 × 196 pixels, a slice thickness of 5 mm and one acquisition.

Results

Characterization

The transmission electron micrograph (Fig. 13.15a) shows that the freeze-dried FDMNPs are aggregated and form a cluster, which makes it hard to determine the nanoparticles' geometrical shape. The aggregation, results mainly from high surface-to-volume ratio, dipole-dipole interactions, the freeze-drying and sample treatment procedures. The particle size distribution from 5 to 14 nm with a normal distribution fit is shown in Figure 13.15b, where the mean particle size is about 10 nm with a standard deviation of about 2.1 nm.

The formation of FDMNPs in Figure 13.16 was confirmed by comparing the FT-IR spectra of MNPs-APTS, DMNPs and FITC. All the samples exhibited the characteristic peaks of Fe_3O_4 nanoparticles which are including: Fe_2^+-Fe_2^- band, observed at 590 cm^{-1} and Fe_3^+-Fe_2^- band observed at 445 cm^{-1} (Uzun 2010).

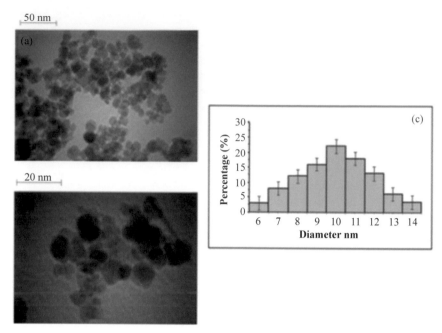

Figure 13.15. (a) TEM photograph of MNPs, (b) FDMNPs and (c) The particle size distribution from 5 to 14 nm with a normal distribution fit. The mean particle size is about 10 nm with a standard deviation of about 2.1 nm.

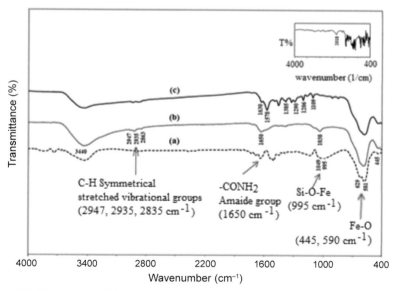

Figure 13.16. FTIR spectra of (a) MNPs-APTS, (b) DMNPs, (c) FDMNPs; inset: FTIR spectra of FITC.

The peaks at 995 cm^{-1} and 1049 cm^{-1} are due to presence of Si-O and C-N bonds, respectively (Lee and MacKay 2005). However, their frequencies are shifted to lower values, indicating strong Si bonding. These peaks apparently confirm the accuracy of the second stage of our synthesis, where the stretching vibration of Si–O at the surface of aminosilane–MNP is at 995 cm^{-1} which shifts to about 1038 cm^{-1} of the DMNPs due to the presence of highly electronegative –CO–NH groups (Pan et al. 2005), as shown in Figure 13.16a. This provides further evidence to confirm that the aminosilanization reaction was successfully achieved during the preparation.

The bending vibration of –NH$_2$ group is at 3440 cm^{-1} and for –CO–NH– group is at 1650 cm^{-1} which is in agreement with previous studies (Chou and Lien 2011, Karaoglu 2011). Also, it can be seen from Figure 13.16b, that compared to the G0 sample, the G3 DMNPs exhibits absorption bands at 2863, 2935, and 2947 cm^{-1} due to stretching vibration of the C–H bond. These observations reveal the presence of PAMAM dendrimer. The formation of the FITC-DMNP conjugate in Figure 13.16c is evident from the disappearance of the characteristic isothiocyanate stretching band of FITC at 2018 cm^{-1} (Neuberger 2005) (inset Fig. 13.16). This indicates that FDMNP does not have free FITC in its combination. The weakened absorbance band of NH$_2$ at 3400 ~ 3250 cm^{-1} compared with DMNPs spectrum and the disappearance of the absorbance band at 2000–2280 cm^{-1} of N = C = S may all indicate the formation of a thiourea bond that could be confirmed by the absorption peaks at 1150–1450 cm^{-1} (Zhang 2009). The 1150–1450 cm^{-1} bands are assigned to the reaction between the primary amine of the dendrimer surface and the isothiocyanate group of FITC. The absorption peaks of functional groups of FDMNPs are shown in Table 13.2.

The XRD pattern of FDMNP was shown in Figure 13.17. It has the same pattern as Fe$_3$O$_4$ nanoparticles (Chou and Lien 2011). The comparison of XRD patterns of unreacted FITC with FDMNP shows the absence of FITC peaks in the FDMNP. This confirms that the modification of MNPs by dendrimer and FITC did not alter the crystalline structure of MNPs. Based on the Scherrer equation (Liu et al. 2007) and using the width of most intense diffraction line, the average crystallite size for FDMNP was calculated as 14 ± 0.5 nm. The error for the grain size by Scherrer's equation can be up to 50% (Chou and Lien 2011).

Due to its extraordinary sensitivity and excellent specificity, fluorescence spectroscopy is considered as an appropriate analytical technique. In this study, fluorescence spectroscopy was performed to demonstrate the conjugation of FITC on DMNPs and also to evaluate the fluorescence at excitation wavelength of 495 nm. No emission due to MNPs and DMNPs was observed, whereas a strong fluorescence was recorded at 520 nm for FDMNPs (Fig. 13.18).

Zeta potential is believed to be a key parameter for evaluating the cellular reactions (Fontes et al. 2007). As is seen in Figure 13.19a, the numerical value of the zeta potential of DMNPs and FDMNPs were measured as +10.1 mV and –22.3 mV, respectively. The alteration of functional groups on the surface of

Table 13.2. Absorption peaks of functional groups of FDMNPs.

Peak (cm^{-1})	Functional group	Peak (cm^{-1})	Functional group
3400–3250	Primary amide	3000–2500	O-H
1630	C=O (stretching)	1578	C-N-H
1385, 1549	Secondary amide	1206	C=S
1290	C-N (stretching)	1109	C-O-C

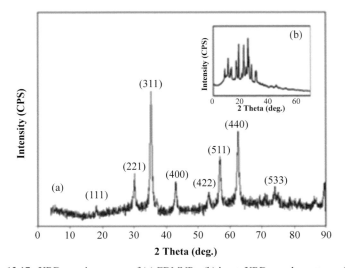

Figure 13.17. XRD powder pattern of (a) FDMNPs; (b) inset: XRD powder pattern of FITC.

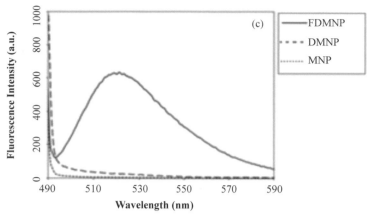

Figure 13.18. Fluorescence spectra of MNPs, DMNPs and FDMNPs at excitation wavelength of 495 nm.

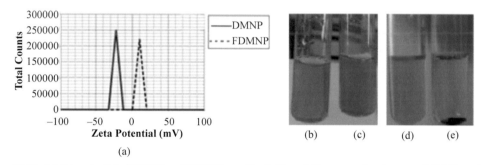

Figure 13.19. (a) Zeta potential of DMNPs and FDMNPs at pH = 7. The stability comparison between FDMNPs and MNPs after 15 minutes treatment with ultrasonic waves, (b) FDMNPs, (c) MNPs immediately after treatment with ultrasound, (d) and (e) NPs after 1 h of exposure.

nanocomposites due to the conjugation of the hydroxyl and carboxyl groups of FITC is the main reason for the decrease in zeta potential of the final product. Primary amine groups on PAMAM dendrimers surface are responsible for the positive surface charge of DMNPs and the negative charge of FDMNPs can be explained well due to hydroxyl and carboxyl groups of FITC. It is clear that the great amount of FDMNPs's zeta potential leads to their further stability. Figure 13.19(b,c,d,e) shows the stability comparison of FDMNPs and MNPs after 15 minutes treating them with ultrasonic waves.

Biocompatibility and cellular viability analysis

An ideal biomarker agent must be biocompatible and easily taken up by the cells. Therefore, the toxicity profile of the as-prepared ferrofluid was studied *in vitro*. To assess the biocompatibility, the interaction of SPIONs, SPION-D, and FDMNP with two cells of MCF-7 and L929 are analyzed with MTT assay. The MTT results of bare MNPs are not consistent with toxicity behaviour as expected due to oxidation effects of nanoparticles (Soenen et al. 2011). They exhibited low cell viability and did not follow a certain pattern of reduction or augmentation in toxicity by increasing the concentration. Some studies have shown that the increased concentration of NPs may trigger the cell viability (Huang et al. 2010). Since the unconjugated magnetite nanoparticles make higher DNA injuries due to further oxidation sites (Zhang et al. 2011), so these results are not reported. The results of MTT assay in both samples (DMNPs and FDMNPs incubated MCF-7 and L929 cell lines) after 24 hours and different concentrations from 10 to 500 µg/mL are shown in Figure 13.20. As it is seen, with the increase in the amount of concentration, the cellular compatibility of all samples is reduced.

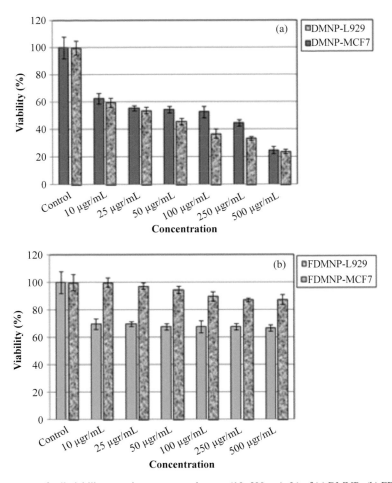

Figure 13.20. Percentage of cell viability at various exposure dosages (10–500 µg/mL) of (a) DMNPs (b) FDMNP samples incubated MCF-7 and L929 cell lines for 24 hours. (Results of MTT assays are expressed as the mean ± standard deviation (SD) Compared with non-treated controls).

At the lowest concentration value of DMNP, 10 µg/mL, the cell viability was 62.69% and 59.79% for MCF7 and L929, respectively which can imply their high toxicity. By increasing the concentrations from 10 to 500 µg/mL, the cell viabilities were reduced for DMNP, which means that DMNP is no longer biocompatible. Thus, for *in vivo* applications, one should coat them suitably to prevent the toxic, hence the adverse effects, for example, by coating them by Polyethylene Glycol (PEG). But the test results for FDMNP showed a less toxicity. As its concentration increased from 10 to 500 µg/mL the amount of viability was reduced from 70% to 66% and 99.88% to 87%, respectively for MCF7 and L929 cells. The IC50 and IC20 represent the corresponding concentrations at which 50% and 20% of cell viability was inhibited. The results are given in Table 13.3.

Table 13.3. Inhibitory concentrations determined for DMNPs and FDMNPs incubated both MCF-7 and L929 cell lines in MTT assay for 24 h.

The name of NP/cell	IC50 (µg/mL)	IC20 (µg/mL)	Max conc. Tested (µg/mL)
DMNP/MCF-7	201.88	> 10	500
DMNP/L929	139.22	> 10	500
FDMNP/MCF-7	GMC	> 10	500
FDMNP/L929	GMC	GMC	500

GMC: Greater than maximum concentration tested

The 50% inhibitory concentration (IC50) for DMNP incubated L929 and MCF-7 cell lines were 139.22 and 201.88 µg/mL respectively, while in case of FDMNPs, the cell viability did not decrease to 50%. However, FDMNP incubated MCF-7 cells at above concentrations were not completely biocompatible (IC20 < 10 µg/mL). The results show that the conjugation of FITC with DMNP significantly has reduced the toxicity in comparison to DMNP. Moreover, FDMNPs are biocompatible even when treated at higher concentrations using L929 cells. On the other hand, FDMNPs incubated L929 cells showed a cell viability of 87%, which means FDMNPs are completely biocompatible in the tested concentration. Thus, 66% is the amount of cell viability of FDMNPs incubated MCF-7 cells which is introduced as not completely biocompatible.

Discussion

MTT assay

Fe_3O_4 nanoparticles have great oxidation tendencies. It has been reported (Song et al. 2012) that magnetite (Fe_3O_4) can cause larger oxidative DNA lesions in cultured A549 cells (the human lung epithelial cell lines) in comparison to maghemite (Fe_2O_3). Nevertheless, further studies are required to clarify the molecular mechanisms involved in the genotoxicity of iron oxide nanoparticles. Therefore, we suggest that they should be coated by other structures such as dendrimers for safer and proper utilization. To explain the possible differences of biocompatibility of these nanocomposites, it is indispensable to consider the influential factors which have significant roles in inducing the cells toxicity. FDA has proved 17 physico-chemical parameters of nanoparticles which are responsible for these differences. Size (Tenzer et al. 2011, Shang et al. 2014), surface chemical (hydrophilicity or hydrophobicity) (Aggarwal et al. 2009), surface charge (Ekkapongpisit et al. 2012), morphological shape (Wang et al. 2007) chemical composition, dose (Gautam and van Veggel 2013), and free radical production (Barnett et al. 2013) of iron oxide nanoparticles are described in various publications as the most important factors. Regardless of the specific internalization mechanism, the cell-NP interactions are, on the one hand, modulated by cell-specific parameters such as cell type or cell cycle phase (Wilhelm et al. 2002). To assess the impact of each of these factors, characterization results were used in this study. In our case, after the conjugation of FITC with DMNPs, the size of a nanoparticle was increased due to linking molecular groups. This is effective, but it can also be undermined due to minor changes in increasing molecular size. The spherical shape of DMNP did not change after FITC conjugation and the amount of concentrations used in the experiment were equal for both FDMNP and DMNP MTT assays.

As it is known, the surface of PAMAM dendrimer is hydrophyl (Esfanda and Tomalia 2001) but FITC is considered as a hydrophobe dye, so FITC functionalization of DMNP results in the formation of hydrophobe groups on their surfaces. Hydrophobicity affects both opsonization and the nature of bonding proteins. Due to dependence of toxicity on the nature of interacting proteins, it is not easy to decisively conclude which of these hydrophobe or hydrophyl groups are responsible for inducing more cell death. Moreover, the proteins are both hydrophyl and hydrophobe, so in each culture media the dominant case will determine the hydrophilicity or hydrophobicity of products and the result will affect toxicity. It could be said that hydrophobe surfaces adsorb plasma proteins quickly, which then will form a protective layer on the nanoparticle's surface known as "protein corona" which protects it from direct cells contact (Legrand 1998). Therefore, with FITC on the surface of DMNP, the cytotoxicity effect due to direct contact of cell membrane with DMNP surface will be prevented. Another factor that makes DMNP more toxic versus FDMNP is their surface charge. It has been demonstrated that cell membranes are negatively charged and adsorb cationic nanoparticles (Zhang 2009). Thus, the DMNP adsorbed by cell membranes can cause the membrane damage which results in an increased toxicity. As previously was reported (Alanagh et al. 2014) with functionalization of FITC, the surface charge of nanocomposite was reduced from +10 mV to −22.3 mV providing a better cell viability. Previously, El-sayed et al. reported that the reduction in surface charge of poly (amidoamine) dendrimers due to FITC causes the decrease in toxicity and increased permeability of nanoparticles into the Caco-2 cell monolayers (El-Sayed et al. 2002). Most, or perhaps all, pathogenic particles generate free radicals in cell-free systems. This can cause oxidative stress, which triggers inflammation and hence the cellular damage and genotoxicity. Oxidative stress arises when there is an imbalance between damaging oxidants, also referred to as reactive oxygen species (ROS) such as hydrogen peroxide, hydroxyl radicals, and the protective antioxidants of which vitamin C and glutathione are such examples. ROS are primarily formed by the incomplete reduction of oxygen (Khaing et al. 2012). The iron ions released from certain nanoparticles have the possibility to cause the conversion of cellular oxygen metabolic products, such as H_2O_2 and superoxide anions, to hydroxyl radicals (•OH), which are one of the main DNA damaging species. Fe (II) can also evince the production of H_2O_2 from molecular O2, which can diffuse through cellular and nuclear membranes to react with Fe bound to DNA, resulting in the generation of •OH (Liu et al. 2007). Accordingly, the exposure of MCF-7 and L929 cell lines to both DMNP and FDMNP produces free radicals, but the analysis of the relationship between the amounts of free radicals and the toxicity produced by FDMNP and DMNP in the vicinity of cells requires further detailed cell experiments. For equal size of nanoparticles, an influential factor affecting their biocompatibility is the differences in surface charge. An important point to consider along with all the other significant effective physico-chemical features of nanomaterials, is the key role of cell type and its interaction which can have a direct effect on the toxicity of nanoparticles. In this study, MCF-7 cells showed a lower toxicity with DMNP compared with L929 cells, whereas FDMNP triggered more cell viability than MCF-7 in L929 cell lines. These results prove that the role of specific cell types and their interactions must be evaluated separately.

Optical and fluorescence microscopy evaluations

Optical microscope images of FDMNP incubated MCF7 after 24 hours is shown in Figure 13.21. The morphology of cells at low concentrations of FDMNP is very similar to the control sample. As it can be seen, in samples with higher concentrations (Fig. 13.20f and g) due to the accumulation of nanoparticles on the cell surface and probably internalization of nanoparticles, the cells tend to change into more round shape.

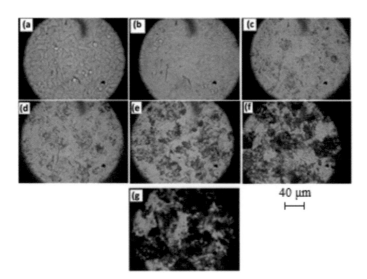

Figure 13.21. Bright-field microscopy of MCF-7 cell images with 400 × magnification after incubating with FDMNP at different exposure dosage (10–500 µg/mL) for 24 h. (a) Control group, (b) 10 µg/mL, (c) 25 µg/mL, (d) 50 µg/mL, (e) 100 µg/mL, (f) 250 µg/mL, and (g) 500 µg/mL.

Fluorescence microscopy

Figure 13.22 clearly illustrates the green emission light due to induced fluorescence excitation of FDMNPs by 495 nm light source of microscope.

The fluorescence is enhanced with increasing the concentration of FDMNPs. The images prove their capabilities for being used as molecular probes and provide a better detection and hence understanding of cellular mechanisms. The researchers who have used FITC conjugated nanoparticles to study the various cellular interactions have demonstrated their internalization and localization using stronger fluorescence

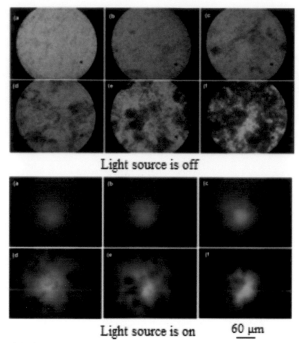

Figure 13.22. Comparison of the fluorescence microscope images of FDMNPs (incubated MCF7 cells after 24 h at different concentrations of (a) 10 µg/mL, (b) 25 µg/mL, (c) 50 µg/mL, (d) 100 µg/mL, (e) 250 µg/mL and (f) 500 µg/mL taken at 400 × magnification when light is on and off.

microscopes (Scutaru et al. 2010, Yu et al. 2009). The nanocomposites used here showed unique properties such as pH sensitive nature and the capability of fluorescence controlling with magnetic field which can be exploited in molecular imagining purposes (Alanagh et al. 2014). However, it is interesting to note in Figure 13.17, that the position of FDMNPs fluorescence is gradually shifted towards the peripheral of the dish. While the increase of fluorescence amplitude is justifiable with the concentration of NPs, the change in their position may be explained as follows. The distribution of dispersed NPs inside a static colloidal medium can be considered as Brownian motion using Lorentzian distribution, as normally is considered in soft matter physics. Therefore, one may assume that $\Psi(r') = d3r'\, ND(r')$, where $\Psi(r')$ is the probability of finding a NP at a distance, r' in a volume d3r' and ND (r') is a density distribution of NPs, a function which decays according to the spatially damped radial function. Thus, two possible sources could be sought, one the diffusion or mobility due to stronger Brownian motion within the dish which takes place radially, and secondly the extra eddy micro currents acting as non-uniform source of distribution when the NPs were added in the experiment.

MR relaxometry measurements

Fe_3O_4 NPs is known to be a T2 negative contrast agent, which decreases the MR signal by dephasing the transverse magnetization and reducing the value of transverse relaxation time T2. After calculating the amount of T2 from signal intensities using the values of TE, relaxation of spin–spin, R2 (1/T2) was also calculated. The effectiveness of each sample in image contrast improvement can be seen with plotting R values versus the concentration. FDMNPs can dramatically increase the MR contrast effects with shortening the T2 of water protons. Since T2 contrast effect is expressed with R2, so higher R2 will result in larger contrast effect. The transverse relaxation rate per mM of iron, standard index of contrast enhancement, r2 are obtained from the slope of R2 curve versus the concentration of samples. It is clear that under similar Fe concentration, uncoated Fe_3O_4 NPs show the most significant decrease of T2 signal intensity. DMNPs and FDMNPs also hampered the MRI signal but not so significantly, therefore the MR contrast effect is high enough to be used as a contrast agent in MRI. The plot of 1/T2 of MNPs, DMNPs, and FDMNPs as a function of Fe concentration is shown in Figure 13.23. It can be seen that the uncoated SPIONs have the highest r2 relaxivity (171.5 mM^{-1} S^{-1}) in the given Fe concentration range, whereas the r2 relaxivities of DMNP and FDMNPs are reduced to 105.47 and 103.67 mM^{-1} S^{-1}, respectively. This is because the PAMAM dendrimer coating on the Fe$_3$O$_4$ NPs shields water molecules from accessing their surfaces, hence causing r2 relaxivity of both DMNP and FDMNP to reduce (Zhang et al. 2007). Compared to DMNPs, the conjugation of FITC molecules onto the surface of DMNPs does not cause significant change in decreasing the T2 value. Therefore, DMNPs exhibit very similar r2 relaxivity to that of FDMNPs, with only 2 mM^{-1} S^{-1} difference.

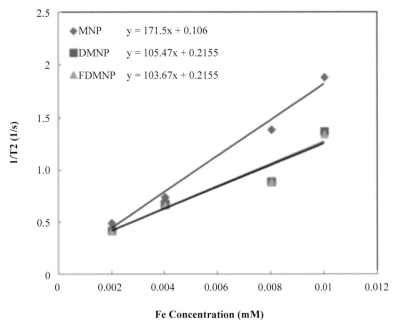

Figure 13.23. Linear fitting of inverse T2 relaxation times of uncoated Fe$_3$O$_4$ NPs, DMNPs and FDMNPs.

13.4.3 Characterization and cellular fluorescence microscopy of Fe$_3$O$_4$-functionalized third generation nano-molecular dendrimers: In vitro cytotoxicity and uptake study (Khosroshahi et al. 2016)

An optimal sample was selected as those synthesized at 70°C with particle size of about 10 nm << exchange length of 27 nm and a saturation magnetization of 67.8 emu/g. The samples were characterized with X-ray diffractometry (XRD), transmission electron microscopy (TEM), Fourier transform infrared (FTIR) spectroscopy, UV–vis spectroscopy, fluorescent spectroscopy (LIF), and magnetization measurements (VSM). The coated materials illustrated strong magnetic behaviour and XRD pattern like magnetite. The presence of Fe-O-Si bond in FTIR spectra confirmed the formation of thin APTS layer on the surface of magnetite nanoparticles. Thermogravimetric analysis (TGA) indicated that the modification of core synthesis technique can raise the efficiency of aminosilane coating reaction (as an initiator for PAMAM dendrimer) up to 98% with the production of about 610 dendritic arms. UV-vis spectrum of both SPIONs and ID-NPs was measured in the range of 340–380 nm with the maximum peak at about 350 nm. The fluorescence properties of ID-NPs distributed in a collagenous substrate and MCF 7 cells was studied by fluorescence microscopy. The results showed that the viability of L 929 and MCF 7 cells decreased from 100% and 90% to 53% and 23%, respectively between 10 μg/mL and 1 mg/mL. The rate of uptake increased with time and it was higher for ID-NPs than SPIONs.

Introduction

Magnetite, Fe_3O_4, is a common magnetic iron oxide that has a cubic inverse spinel structure with oxygen forming a fcc closed packing and Fe cations occupying interstitial tetrahedral sites and octahedral sites. They can have controllable sizes ranging from a few nanometers up to tens of nanometers, which is smaller or comparable to a cell (10–100 μm), a virus (20–450 nm) a protein (5–50 nm) (Pankhurst et al. 2003). When the size of these nanomagnets becomes so small (< 15 nm), they are considered as single magnetic domain where the magnetic moment of the particle as a whole is free to fluctuate in response to thermal energy. Under such a condition, the nanoparticle is said to be superparamagnetic iron oxide nanoparticle (SPION), which lacks a hysteresis loop and posses high field irreversibility, high saturation field and extra anisotropy contributions (Pankhurst et al. 2003, Gupta and Gupta 2005). Over the past decades SPIONs which possess extraordinary size and morphology dependent physical and chemical properties, have attracted world-wide research attention not only because of the unique properties, but also for their biocompatibility and remarkable magnetic properties, including chemical composition, granulometric uniformity, crystal structure, magnetic behaviour, surface structure, adsorption properties, solubility, and low toxicity (Yu et al. 2006, Jiang and Lang 2007, Pisanic et al. 2007, Khosroshahi and Ghazanfari 2012). Factors important for biomedical applications of nanoparticles mainly include: biocompatibility, particle size with overall narrow uniform size distribution (particles less than 100 nm have longer circulation time, larger effective surface areas, and low sedimentation rates), surface characteristics to provide easy encapsulation and protect them from degradation, stability, and good magnetic response.

Magnetite nanoparticles and have potential biomedical applications where they can be used as contrast agents for bioimaging (Corot et al. 2006). For example, recently Kim et al. (2013) could engineer fluorescent dendritic nanoprobes to contain multiple organic dyes and reactive groups for target-specific biomolecule labeling and other groups such as Linna et al. (2015) have suggested to employ dendrimers for visualization of their cellular entry and trafficking, cancer hyperthermia (Jordan et al. 1999), and targeted drug delivery (Sudeshna et al. 2011, Unterweger et al. 2014, Madaan et al. 2014), and photodynamic therapy (Narsireddy et al. 2015). Various synthetic methods have been used to produce magnetite nanoparticles including coprecipitation (Zhu and Wu 1999), microemulsion (Liu et al. 1999), laser pyrolysis (Hofmeister et al. 2001), and hydrothermal synthesis (Wu et al. 2005). Other investigators have reported the parameters affecting the production of magnetic nanoparticles such as pH, alkaline species (Vinod et al. 2010), reaction temperature (Dou et al. 2008). Functional groups play an important role in the production of organic shell around inorganic core to prepare uniform and stable suspension (Frankamp et al. 2005, Khosroshahi and Ghazanfari 2012). Dendrimers are a class of well-defined nanostructured macromolecules with a three-dimensional structure composed of three architectural components: a core (I), an interior of shells (generations) consisting of repeating branch-cell units (II), and terminal functional groups (the outer shell or periphery) (III) (Tomalia 2005, Peng et al. 2008). They are synthesized from a polyfunctional core by adding branched monomers that react with the functional groups of the core, in turn leaving end groups that can react again (Klajnart and Bryszewska 2002, Menjoge et al. 2010). One such example is poly (amidoamine) (PAMAM), which acts as a template or stabilizer for preparation of inorganic nanocomposites. Some important properties of these structures include a large number of end groups, the functionable cores, nanoporous nature of the interior at higher generations (Antharjanam et al. 2009). Also, their chemical structures, molecular weight, and molecular size can provide special type of functionality, which play a role in developing fields of materials science (Majoros et al. 2006, Syahir et al. 2009, Choi et al. 2012). Intrinsic fluorescence of dendrimer minimizes the difficulties associated with the synthesis and purification of dendrimer based drug carriers attached with conventional type fluorescent molecules. As this matter reduces steps required for production of fluorescent carrier, the final biocompatibility of delivery system will be improved. More importantly, this will result in the enhanced drug loading capacity for cases where drugs are attached to the periphery of dendrimers, as available free space will be more due to the absence of conventional fluorophores in the system (Jasmine et al. 2009, Yang et al. 2011, Biswal et al. 2009). In this study, we report the results of (i) Synthesis and characterization of SPION-PAMAM (ID-NPs), (ii) Evaluation of cytotoxicity and uptake of SPIONs and ID-NPs by MCF 7 breast cancer and L929 cell lines based on the UV-vis absorbance spectroscopy and intrinsic fluorescent properties of these nanocomposites.

Materials and methods

Synthesis of SPIONs

Solutions of ferric chloride hexahydrate (FeCl$_3$.6H$_2$O, 99%, Merck) and ferrous sulfate heptahydrate (FeSO$_4$.7H$_2$O, 99%, Merck) were prepared as iron source in double distilled water. The optimized value of 0.9 M of ammonia solution (NH4OH-Sigma Aldrich) as alkaline source was used according to our previous report (Tajabadi and Khosroshahi 2012) and vigorously stirred under N$_2$ bubbling at room temperature. The mixture of ferric and ferrous solutions was deoxygenated by bubbling N$_2$ gas following sonication for 30 minutes. This solution was added drop-wise to the stirring ammonia solution. The ferrofluid was prepared at two different temperatures. In the first group, the reaction temperature was kept constant at 25°C for 1 hour in a water bath before the mixture purified. The samples in the second group were mixed at the same condition (25°C for 1 hour) and then transferred to 70°C water bath under vigorous stirring for 30 minutes before purification. For both groups, the black precipitation was purified using magnetic separation five times and sedimented by centrifugation. The resultant material was dried by freeze dryer (Unicryo MC-4L) for 24 hours.

Functionalization of SPIONs by aminosilane (G0)

A solution of optimal iron oxide sample with concentration of 2.13 mM was prepared in ethanol (149 mL): double distilled water (1 mL) and sonicated for 30 minutes. An amount of 35 μL of aminopropyle triethoxysilane-H$_2$N (CH$_2$)$_3$Si(OC$_2$H$_5$)$_3$ (APTS, 99%, Sigma-Aldrich) was added to the mixture and stirred vigorously for 7 hours. It was then washed with ethanol five times using magnetic separation and finally sedimented by centrifugation. In order to remove the solvent, precipitated material was placed in freeze dryer for 24 hours.

Synthesis of dendrimer functionalized SPIONs (ID-NPs)

Formation of PAMAM dendrimer on the surface of amine-functionalized SPIONs was done according to the methods described by Pan et al. (2005) and Liu et al. (2008) with some modifications that we reported previously (Tajabadi et al. 2013). Dendritic polymer synthesis involves iteration of two main reactions which consist of two steps: Step one (Michael addition) alkylation of primary amines using MA (Methyl Acrylate, 99%, Aldrich), and Step two, amidation of the ester groups with Ethylene diamine (EDA, 99%, Sigma-Aldrich). Each Michael addition reaction produces a half generation of PAMAM dendrimer and amidation reaction creates the full generation.

Characterization

An X-ray diffractometer (Cu Kα, λ = 1.5406 Å, FK60-40) was used to determine the crystalline phase of nanoparticles. Magnetic properties of the samples were measured by vibrating sample magnetometer (VSM-PAR 155) at 300 K under magnetic field up to 8 KOe. The presence of silane and PAMAM typical bonds on the surface of SPIONs was proved by Fourier transform infrared (FTIR) spectroscopy (BOMEM, Canada). Particle size and morphology of the nanoparticles were determined by transmission electron microscopy (TEM, Philips CM-200-FEG microscope, 120 KV). The amount of APTS and PAMAM molecules covering the surface of SPIONs was estimated using Energy-dispersive X-ray spectroscopy (SEM-EDS: Oxford Instrument–UK) and Thermogravimetric analysis (TGA50, Shimadzu, Japan). The absorbance spectra of magnetite and different generations of nanodendrimers were observed using SpectroFluorophotometer (RF-1510, Shimadzu, Japan). The evaluation of fluorescence emission of ID-NPs (G3) nanoparticles at different excitation wavelengths was performed using an ion argon laser (Melles Griot-35MAP431). The fluorescence signals were detected by a 600 μm core diameter optical connected to spectrometer (UV-vis USB 4000, Ocean Optics). The excitation wavelengths covered a range between (454–514) nm. After obtaining the spectra of samples, they were smoothed by Gaussian model using

Findgraph software. The next set up was to evaluate the efficiency of these nanoparticles in coloring the polymeric substrate, using two kinds of natural polymers, i.e., cotton and collagen. After the injection of nanodendrimers solution to these substrates, fluorescence microscopy (Zeiss Axioshop-Germany) was used to study the materials fluorescence. The Fe content of cells after uptake in each well was measured using JENWAY 6305 UV/Vis Spectrometer.

In vitro cytotoxicity evaluation

MCF 7 (human breast cancer) and L929 (the primary mouse connective tissue cells) cell lines were obtained from the National Cell Bank of Iran (NCBI) Pasteur Institute. The cells were cultured in Dulbecco's modified Eagle's medium (DMEM) supplemented with 10% fetal bovine serum (FBS) and were seeded onto a glass cover-slips in a 96 well-plate at a density of 15,000 cells per well in 100 μL of medium at 37°C in a 5% CO_2 incubator for 24 h. Serial dilutions of ID-NPs (10 μg/mL–1000 μg/mL) were then added to each well. The control well represented the cells in culture medium without any nanoparticles. After 24 h of incubation of cells with ID-NP samples, all culture medium was replaced by 100 μl of MTT (3-(4,5-dimethylthiazol-2-yl)-2,5-diphenyltetrazolium bromide, Sigma-USA). After 4 h the formation of formazan crystals was checked by optical microscope and the supernatant was removed. In order to dissolve formazan crystals, 100 μl of isopropanol was added to each plate and they were placed inside an incubator (Memmert-GmbH) for 15 minutes. The absorbance of each well was read using microplate reader (stat fax-2100, AWARENESS, Palm City, USA) at 545 nm. The results were reported in the form of relative cell viability compared to control sample (which could be calculated by the following equation):

$$\% \text{ Viability} = \frac{A_{545(\text{magnetic sample})}}{A_{545(\text{Control})}} \tag{13.12}$$

Cell morphology and surface absorbed nanoparticles were detected by Scanning Electron Microscopy (SEM).

Uptake rate of ID-NPs

Nanoparticles play an important role in current cancer research, and the interaction of cells with nanoparticles is of particular interest. For this purpose, 10^5 L929 cells per mL of culture medium were seeded in 12 well-plate 24 hrs before addition of nanoparticles. 100 μL of ID-NPs with concentration of 100 μg/mL were added to each wells and samples were incubated for 4 and 10 hrs at 37°C in a 5% CO_2 incubator. The control sample represented the culture medium without any nanoparticles. After that, cells were washed twice with 100 μL fresh PBS and the resultant solution was placed in another fresh 12-well plate. The cell membranes were dissolved by addition of acetic acid 5% and the resultant absorption was recorded as up taken nanoparticles by the cells. The supernatant UV-Vis absorption of each samples were read at 3 major characteristics peaks of Fe_3O_4 (344, 354 and 373 nm) to evaluate the extent of Fe content of cells in each well. The absorption was read using JENWAY 6305 UV/Vis Spectrometer. The Fe content (%) was measured by following equation:

$$\text{Fe content } \% = \left(\frac{I_{\text{test}}}{I_{373\text{control}}} \right) \times 100 \tag{13.13}$$

Here, $I_{373 (\text{Control})}$ is the absorption regarding supernatant of control samples at 373 nm (Ghandoor et al. 2007, Shauo et al. 2007), I_{test} is the supernatant absorption of cells which contain magnetic nanoparticles after addition of acetic acid.

Cellular scanning electron microscopy

The L929 and MCF7 cells were cultured in 12 well-plate for 24 hours. Two different concentrations of 50 and 100 μg/mL of ID-NPs were added to each well and they were incubated for 8 and 24 hours. The cells were then fixed with 4% gluteraldehyde (Sigma, UK) buffered in PBS at room temperature for one hour. The cellular up take of nanoparticles at different concentrations and time were studied by SEM (XL30, Philips, USA).

Cellular fluorescence microscopy

Prior to this experiment, the fluorescent properties of the ID-NPs was studied using a concentration of 50 μg/mL in culture medium as a control sample. The same concentration was also suitably soaked in cotton and collagen substrates and the experiment was repeated. The fluorescence was observed using a fluorescence microscope (Axioscop, Zeiss, Germanny). Next, the L929 and MCF7 cells with concentration of 10^4 per test were seeded in FBS pretreated slides containing collagen as a substrate for the cells deposition purpose. The ID-NPs were then added to the cultured cells and after 24 hrs, the medium was removed and the cells were rinsed with phosphate buffer saline (PBS). The fluorescent emission of the samples was detected as before.

Results and discussion

SPIONs

It is known that the particles size and shape strongly depend, among other factors, on the balance of nucleation and growth rates (Jiang and Lang 2007, Ghazanfari and Khosroshahi 2015). When ingredients of reaction are added together, the nucleation phenomena occurs at supersaturation state. In our case, in order to produce tiny nuclei, the initial temperature of this study was set to 25°C and after 1 hour, group 1 was purified which resulted in particles with larger size (average diameter is about 14 nm). Figure 13.24 show respectively the slight decrease of particle size and increase of saturation magnetization of SPIONs at elevated temperature because of loss of surface defects. Given that the completeness of diffusion and growth processes of samples are influenced by the reaction time (Hosono et al. 2009, Nagy et al. 2009), in our case, this was achieved at an elevated temperature of 70°C and prolonged time where the samples with less crystal defects and smaller particle size (average diameter is about 10 nm) were produced. With increase of ingredient (alkaline media) concentration, more materials are available on the growth phase and thus particles with higher diameter could be obtained (Fig. 13.24b). With increase of alkaline media

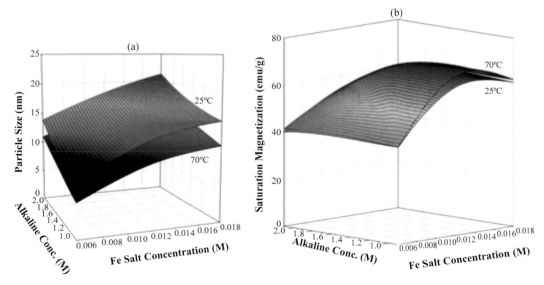

Figure 13.24. Variation of magnetite particle size (a) and saturation magnetization (b) with alkaline and salt concentration for different synthesizing temperatures.

concentration, the probability of non-magnetite layer production (magnetically dead layer) increases with decrease of saturation magnetization, which indicates there is a limit for positive effect of alkaline media on saturation magnetization (Fig. 13.24).

In magnetic materials the magnetic properties such as saturation magnetization, susceptibility, and coercivity are tremendously affected by particle size. Figure 13.25 illustrates the variation of coercivity of synthesized SPIONs with alkaline concentration at a given Fe concentration and temperature. It appears that at a lower temperature, the coercivity shows a little change whereas at a higher temperature the change is more significant.

Therefore, the results suggest that coercivity is strongly size-dependent and bulk samples with sizes greater than the domain wall width can cause magnetization reversal due to domain wall motion. As domain walls move through a sample, they can become pinned at grain boundaries and additional energy is needed for them to continue moving. Pinning is one of the main sources of the coercivity. The grain size dependence of coercivity and permeability (GSDCP) theory and its modified form for ultrafine particles are described in Eqs. (9.13) and (9.14), respectively.

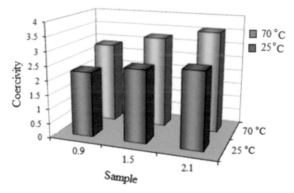

Figure 13.25. Dependence of coercivity of magnetite nanoparticles on alkaline media concentration.

SPION-PAMAM

XRD

Crystalline structure of SPIONs were analyzed by XRD, as shown in Figure 13.26. The results confirmed the formation of highly purified magnetite phase of iron oxide with inverse spinel structure (JCPDS file no. 19-0629) without any interference with other phases of Fe_xO_y. The XRD graph of APTS-coated SPIONs shows no significant change in crystalline structure except a slight decrease in the Bragg peak intensity at 511 and 440 Miller indices planes. However, a further decrease of peaks were noticed when the SPION-APTS nanoparticles were coated with PAMAM, likely due to the amorphous nature of dendrimer covering the surface of underlying layers. The corresponding particle sizes of magnetite, APTS-coated

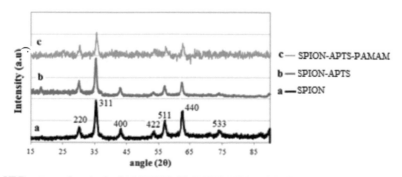

Figure 13.26. XRD pattern of synthesized (a) SPION, (b) SPION-APTS and (c) SPION-APTS-PAMAM nanodendrimers.

and PAMAM-grafted magnetite nanoparticles were found 9.98 nm, 11.2 nm, and 13.5 nm, respectively using the Scherrer equation, see Eq. (9.19).

TEM

Morphology and mean particle size of prepared SPIONs synthesized at elevated temperature are shown in Figure 13.27a, where the nanoparticles exhibited a quasi-sphere shape and have sizes ranging from 9.5 to 16 nm. As it is seen, magnetic nanoparticles are aggregated and form a cluster, which makes it hard to determine their geometrical shape. The aggregation results mainly from high surface-to-volume ratio, increased dipole-dipole interactions, the freeze-drying, and sample treatment procedures. Figure 13.27b indicates the particle size distribution from 5 to 16 nm with a normal distribution fit, where the mean particle size is about 10 ± 2.1 nm. However, the polydispersivity is much lower than those nanoparticles prepared at lower temperature because of reduced surface defects at higher temperature (Choi et al. 2012). There is a critical size which defines the superparamagnetic region approximately defined by $Vp \approx 25$ kT/K, where k is Boltzmann constant, K denotes anisotropy constant ($Fe_3O_4 = 1.35 \times 10$ J/m^3), and T is the absolute temperature (Yamaura et al. 2004). At room temperature, 300 K, the critical size is equal to 27 nm, hence confirming the results. Figure 13.27 (a–d) represent the SPION coated APTS and SPION-PAMAM respectively.

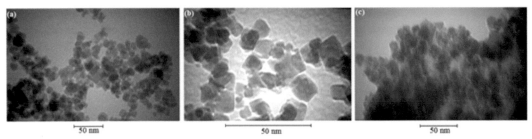

Figure 13.27. SEM of (a) SPION, (b) SPION-APTS and (c) SPION-APTS-PAMAM nanodendrimers.

VSM

Figure 13.28 indicates the VSM results determined for all the magnetic nanoparticles. It confirms the superparamagnetism behaviour of the materials and that the maximum Ms value of 68 emu/g for SPIONs

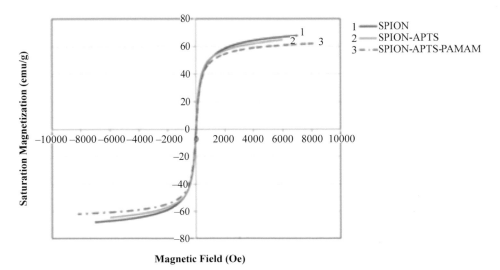

Figure 13.28. VSM of (1) SPION, (2) SPION-APTS and (3) SPION-APTS-PAMAM nanodendrimers.

gradually decreases to about 62 emu/g for PAMAM-grafted magnetite nanoparticles due to hindering effect of non-magnetic layers, cation distribution, and spin effects on the surface of core (Guang et al. 2007). To prove this assertion, FTIR spectroscopy was performed.

FTIR

Figure 13.29 shows the absorption bonds at 420 and 446 cm^{-1} and strong peaks around 581 and 629 cm^{-1}, which confirm the formation of magnetite nanoparticles (Feng et al. 2008, Hong et al. 2008). The peak at 993 cm^{-1} (G$_0$ curve) is related to Si-O-Fe bonds and the stretching vibration of C-N bond, which overlaps with stretching vibration of Si-O observed at 1048 cm^{-1} (Launer 1987, Dussán et al. 2007). The peak at 1151 cm^{-1} (PAMAM-SPION) indicates the presence of C = O bond in ester group (Zheng et al. 2009). In these spectra two intense peaks at 1570 cm^{-1} and 1631 cm^{-1} are observed that can be assigned to the N-H bending/C-N stretching (amide II) and C-O stretching (amide I) vibration of PAMAM dendrimer, respectively (Grabchev et al. 2003, Chou and Lien 2010, Li et al. 2010, Baykal et al. 2012).

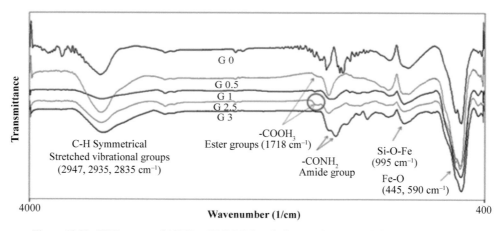

Figure 13.29. FTIR spectra of APTS and PAMAM-grafted magnetite nanoparticles at different stages.

TGA

One trustworthy way of quantifying the number of coated molecules on the surface of nanoparticles is thermographic analysis (TGA). Figure 13.30 presents TGA curve of magnetite nanoparticles modified with APTS and PAMAM dendrimer. As can be seen in this figure, the APTS-coated compound lost 8 percent of its weight at 700°C, while the weight loss began at about 300°C. This may be explained by vaporization of organic component. Since the mean diameter of the magnetite nanoparticles was known and there was no weight loss for unmodified magnetite nanoparticle, so the number of APTS molecules is calculated according to Eq. (9.111). Here N$_{APTS}$ is the APTS number on each particle, N$_a$ = 6.22 × 10^{23} is Avagadro's number, W$_l$ is the weight loss, ρ is the density of magnetite (5.17 g/cm^{-3}), and M$_{APTS}$ = 221.37 is the relative molecular weight of APTS. As a result, it can be estimated that 610 APTS molecules, i.e., amine groups are available on the surface of each coated Fe$_3$O$_4$ nanoparticle which effectively could participate in the reaction leading to the formation of dendritic arms for PAMAM dendrimer coating on the surface of SPION nanoparticles.

The TGA results are similar to previous studies related to synthesis of PAMAM dendrimer (Baykal et al. 2012, Shi et al. 2009). The percent of weight loss was increased with increasing the dendrimer generation number, which is expected due to the increase in chain length of C-backbone and molecular weight of dendrimers (compared to the lower generations). The remaining quantities may manifest the residual inorganic content due to the existence of iron oxide phase. Our findings are in good agreement with Niu et al. report (Niu et al. 2011), which declared ester terminated products (half generation) are thermally stable under 200°C. Clearly, the TGA curves of PAMAM dendrimer have two stages of weight loss which

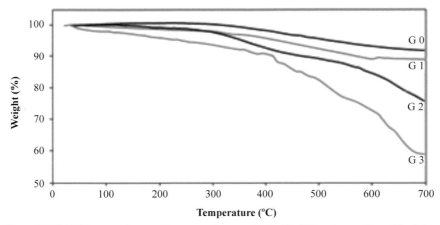

Figure 13.30. TGA curve of magnetite nanoparticles modified with different generation of dendrimer.

was observed and reported before (Zheng et al. 2009). At the first stage, the formation of hydrogen bonds between the amine groups leads to the increase in viscosity of G_1, G_2, and G_3 which made the complete removal of amine groups difficult at first stage. The second stage accounts for the decomposition of the dendrimer structure. TGA graphs show the average weight loss of about 8%, 11.5%, 24.3%, and 41% for different generations of dendrimer grafted magnetite nanoparticles (generation 0 to 3, respectively).

UV-vis and fluorescence spectroscopy

Figure 13.31 shows the absorption peaks for the UV-vis spectrum of magnetite nanoparticles in aqueous ammonia solution in the range of 340–380 nm, where the maximum occurs at about 350 nm. In general, the fluorescence behaviour in various solvents can reflect the interaction between the solvent and fluorophore. With formation of polymeric layer on the surface of Fe_3O_4 core, the intensity of the peaks correspondingly decreases at higher generation order. There are three types of electronic transitions: (1) Fe^{III} crystal or ligand field transitions, (2) interactions between magnetically coupled Fe^{II} ions, and (3) Oxygen-metal charge transfer excitations from the O(2P) non-bonding valence bands to the Fe(3d) (Cornell and Schwertmn 2003). The absorption band in the region of 330–450 nm originates primarily from the absorption and scattering of UV radiation by magnetic nanoparticles. The absorption band at about 320–370 nm indicates the formation of nanosized particles. The intensity of the light scattered depends on the polarizability and that, in turn, depends on the molecular weight. This property of light is a valuable tool for measuring

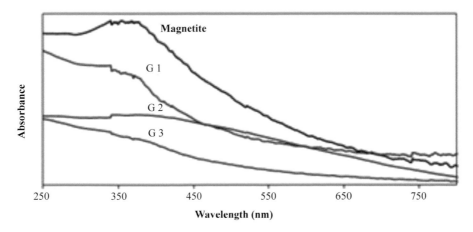

Figure 13.31. Absorbance spectroscopy of magnetite and PAMAM dendrimer nanoparticles (G1, G2, and G3).

molecular weight. Considering the significance of the mean cosine scattering angle θ (anisotropy factor), $g = \int_{4\pi} p(\theta)\cos(\theta)ds'$ where p is scattering phase function and ds' is scattered new direction, one can conclude that the bigger particles scatter light more isotropic than smaller ones. Rayleigh scattering explains the scattering for the centers with sizes smaller than wavelength, but for sizes larger than wavelength, Mie scattering provides a better description. The charge transfer transitions involving Fe^{II}-O or Fe^{II}-Fe^{III} are mainly responsible for absorption of visible light. They produce an absorption band centered in the near UV whose absorption edge extends into the visible region (550–900 nm). The inset in Figure 13.31 indicates the peaks of Fe and Si obtained from EDS where the atomic ratio of Fe/Si is calculated as 40.02/1.55 = 25.81. This shows that the atomic percent of Si is close to the expected value and confirms the formation of APTS molecular layer on the surface of SPIONs. For the magnetodendrimers experiment, ethanol was used as solvent. Alince PAMAM has fluorescent property due to $-NH_2$, $-OH$ and $-COO-$, therefore, it is an excellent way of recognizing the formation of the dendrimers moieties on the surface of the magnetic core. The concept of intrinsically fluorescing dendrimers which exhibit an unusual luminescence in the visible region, in the absence of conventional fluorophores, was initially reported for carboxylate terminated PAMAM dendrimers (Wang and Imae 2004). The results of laser-induced spectroscopy (LIF) are shown in Figure 13.32, where it is seen that the intensity amplitude of output emission signal increases with increasing the excitation wavelengths between (454–514) nm, as can be seen in Figure 13.32a. The corresponding fluorescence emission shown in Figure 13.32b covers a range between (490–550) nm with a significant bandwidth between 480–500 nm where 450 nm peak is assigned to carboxylic acid and 470 nm to $-NH_2$ bond. Clearly, there are three pronounced emitted peaks observed at 488, 495, and 550 nm. It is well known that the lower generation dendrimers are highly asymmetric and tend to exist in relatively open forms. As the generation number increases, their dendric conformations gradually approach towards a global shape and are covered by densely exterior groups. These changes in molecular conformation of higher generations favor a π-π interaction between phenyl rings, which leads to the formation of phenyl excimer. Thus, G3 displays an enhanced structures emission due to the excimer formation. Most of the densely packed phenyl form parallel arrangement due to the reduced distance between phenyl rings, leading to a stronger π-π interaction. It is interesting to note that with the generation increasing, functional groups attached to dendrimer surfaces can interact with one another and exhibit new functions (Wang et al. 2004). The fluorescence intensities differ across all emission wavelengths for each of the spectra shown and it is evident that the number of photons increase as the fluorescence wavelength increases (hence, decrease of photon energy). A close approximation of quantum yield can be obtained using,

Q.Y = No. of photons emitted/No. of photons absorbed   (13.14)

The photon energy for every wavelength is determined using, $E_p = h\nu = hc/\lambda$ where h is Planck's constant and c is velocity of light and λ is laser wavelength. The number of photons for each corresponding wavelength can be determined from (N_p = Laser power/photon energy). Using the data from Figure 13.33,

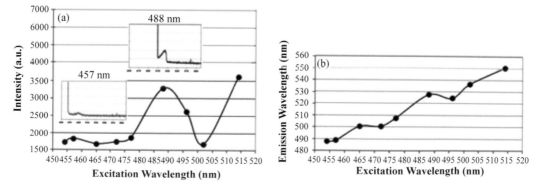

Figure 13.32. Laser-induced fluorescence spectroscopy of third generation PAMAM (G3). (a) Variation of intensity of emitted wavelengths with excitation wavelengths and (b) the emitted wavelengths with excitation wavelengths.

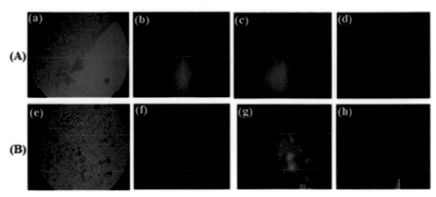

Figure 13.33. Fluorescence microscopy of (A) Collagen substrate embedded by ID-NPs, (B) MCF 7 cells seeded in collagen substrate containing ID-NPs. The samples (a,e), (b,f), (c,g) and (d,h) are control and excited samples at different wavelengths using Blue, Green, and Red filters, respectively.

a close approximation was obtained as 0.93. To explain such a wide spectrum, it is noteworthy that there are three kinds of functional groups existing in NH2-terminated PAMAM dendrimers: amides, internal tertiary amine groups, and terminal primary amines and normally they exhibit a photoluminescence spectra in a broad range increasing. The excitation wavelength results in red-shift of emission peaks, which can cover the entire visible region due to high structural heterogeneity and the broad molecular weight distribution of the hyperbranched PAMAMs (Tajabadi and Khosroshahi 2012) and also, electron-hole recombination processes involving correlated electron-hole exciton states between localized states of electrons and holes (Pastor-Pérez et al. 2007).

Prior to evaluation of cytotoxicity and cellular uptake of the nanocomposites, their fluorescence properties were tested using cotton and collagen fibers as substrates as explained above. Figure 13.33a illustrates the fluorescence of ID-NPs distributed in collagen substrate and Figure 13.33b shows the same experiment results with MCF 7 cells using blue, green, and red filters of fluorescence microscope. Considering the chemical structures of collagen and cotton, there is a possibility of hydrogen interaction between the hydroxyl group of the substrate and amine group of dendrimer nanocomposites, which produces a new fluorescent moieties with a time dependent behaviour. The longer the time, the more fluorescent moieties is produced hence, more intense fluorescence image could be obtained.

Cytotoxicity and uptake evaluation

The cytotoxicity of SPIONs and ID-NPs was determined by colorimetric MTT assay experiments. The interaction of mitochondrial dehydrogenase in living cells with MTT oxidizes tetrazolium salt, which results in formation of a dark blue formazan product. The dehydrogenase activity of damaged or dead cells is noticeably lower than the normal cells (Jevprasesphant et al. 2003, Sgouras and Duncan 1990). Figure 13.34 represents the histogram plot of two cell lines viability (L 929 and MCF7) cultured with different concentration of SPIONs (Fig. 13.34a) and ID-NPs (Fig. 13.34b). The cell viability was studied after 24 hours incubation at 37°C and the calculations are based on the absorbance of samples at 545 nm and normalized using the Eq. (13.12). In the first case (i.e., SPIONs), the viability of MCF 7 and L 929 cells remains above 100% at 10 µg/mL, respectively but for L 929, it decreases to about 78% at 1 mg/mL. As in the second case (i.e., ID-NPs), the viability decreased from (90 to 23)% and from (100 to 53)% at corresponding values of 10 µg/mL and 1 mg/mL for MCF 7 and L 929 cells, respectively. This clearly confirms the concentration and cell type dependence of cytotoxicity. These findings are in good agreement with those reported by Sgouras and Duncan (1990), Roberts et al. (1996), and Jevprasesphant et al. (2003) regarding the cytotoxicity of third generation of dendrimer in the absence of magnetite nanoparticles.

The decrease in cell viability with increase of nanoparticle concentration in the medium is more likely due to the enhanced uptake and the surface coverage of cells as a result of interaction between the cationic periphery of PAMAM-grafted magnetite nanoparticles and negatively charged cell surfaces (Pradhan et al.

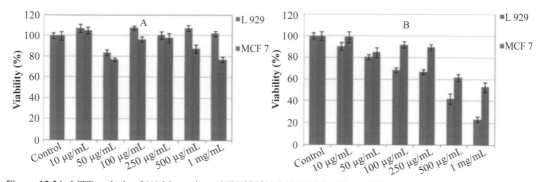

Figure 13.34. MTT analysis of (A) Magnetite and (B) SPION-PAMAM dendrimer (G3) nanoparticles in L 929 and MCF 7 cells at different concentrations.

2010). The lower compatibility of MCF 7 compared to L 929 is partly because of nanoparticles attachment on the surface as seen by SEM in Figure 13.35 and higher rate of internalization of nanoparticles by the endocytosis pathway, which is clearly observable form the fluorescent images shown in Figure 13.36. This is further discussed in the following section.

The last stage of the experiment was to evaluate the uptake of SPIONs and ID-NPs by MCF 7 cells by UV-vis absorbance spectroscopy at three main iron oxide absorption peaks as explained earlier. Clearly, Figure 13.37 illustrates the increase of uptake with time and that it is in order of ID-NPs > SPIONs for 344 nm > 354 nm > 373 nm, respectively. This finding can have an important impact on the cancer therapy in nanomedicine.

To explain and justify the mechanism behind the higher rate of ID-NPs uptake compared to SPIONs, one can use the concept of the Zeta potential ξ, quantitatively without going through the vigorous mathematical treatment. Basically, ξ is an electrostatic potential that exists at the shear plane of a particle and is related to both surface charge and the local environment of the particle. Zeta potential has been used in cell biology to study cell adhesion, activation, and agglutination based on cell-surface-charge properties (Veronesi et al. 2002, Fontes et al. 2006, Shi et al. 2007, Lin et al. 2006, Zhang et al. 2008). Nanoparticles' uptake by cells is considered a two-step process: (i) binding of nanoparticles to the cell surface, followed by (ii) the internalization of nanoparticles by the specific endocytosis pathway. The relative Zeta potential Zr of cells during the adsorption of nanoparticles is expressed as:

$$Z_r = \exp \left(m_{bin} \times \frac{\beta_{binding}}{2} + m_{int} \times \frac{\beta_{int}}{2} \right) \tag{13.15}$$

where m_{bin} is the total mass of nanoparticles binding to the cell surface, m_{int} is the total mass of nanoparticles internalized within the cell, and β measures how the presence of nanoparticle adsorption affect the free energy of the ions at a distance from the cell surface. Thus, when nanoparticles bind onto the negatively charged cell surface with the same sign of ξ, it increases the free energy of the ions at a distance from the

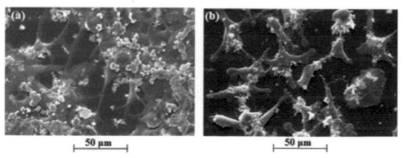

Figure 13.35. SEM micrograph of cellular distribution of SPION-PAMAM nanodendrimers in (a) MCF 7 and (b) L 929 cells using a concentration of 50 μg/mL.

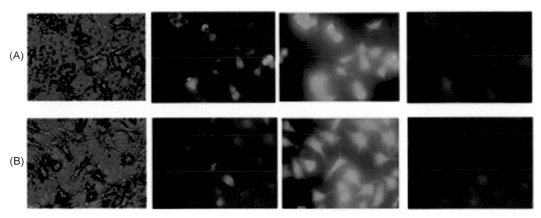

(A)

(B)

Figure 13.36. Fluorescence microscopy of cellular distribution of SPION-PAMAM nanodendrimers (50 μg/mL) in (A) L 929 and (B) MCF 7 cells using Blue, Green and Red filters respectively.

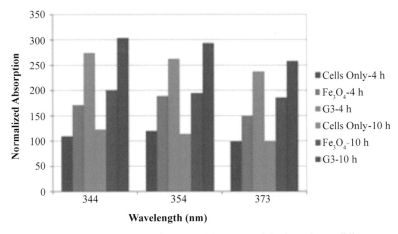

Figure 13.37. Uptake level of Fe_3O_4 and G3 nanoparticles by MCF 7 cell lines.

cell surface, so the β binding is positive, i.e., $Zr > 1$. However, in our case, the PAMAM functionalized SPIONs have measured positively charged ξ, which is opposite to ξ sign of the cells. Therefore, the free energy of the ions at a distance from the cell surface is decreased and $β_{binding}$ becomes negative, i.e., $Zr < 1$ and the internalization mechanism dominates. Since, during the internalization of nanoparticles by the endocytosis pathway βint is positive, i.e., $Zr > 1$, the position of the plane of shear is shifted and the negative surface charge is increased compared to the binding process. The binding and internalization processes could be modeled by Langmuir adsorption (Wilhelm et al. 2002, Zhang et al. 2008). In short, when the binding effect dominates, the cell's negative ξ will first increase with time and then decrease, but when the internalization effect dominates during the whole adsorption process, the cell's negative ξ will decrease to a stable stage.

13.5 Photoacoustic (PA) and thermoacoustic (TA) imaging

The generation of acoustic waves by absorption of optical radiation is known as the photoacoustic (PA). Briefly, when a laser radiation is absorbed in the surface of a material it causes heating and the thermal energy then propagates into the material as thermal waves. The heated region undergoes a rapid thermal expansion, generating thermoelastic stresses and subsequently elastic waves (i.e., ultrasound) which propagates deep within the material, as seen in Figure 13.38. The ultrasound is then detected by a wideband transducer that converts the mechanical acoustic waves to electric signals. The captured signals are then processed to form an image. The amplitude of the acoustic wave is linearly proportional to the absorbed

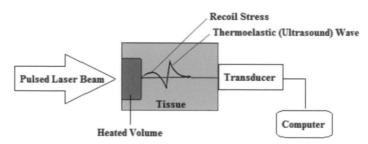

Figure 13.38. Schematic representation of photoacoustic thermoelastic (bipolar) signal.

energy density (i.e., fluence), while the shape of the wave is dependent on the absorption distribution, kaser parameters, and boundary condition. PA generation can be classified as: (a) direct and (b) indirect. In the former case, the acoustic wave is generated directly by absorption of laser energy, whereas in the latter, it is generated in a coupling medium adjacent to the sample. Also, PA can be classified according to the method of excitation modes: (a) pulsed mode and (b) continuous modulation mode. In the former mode, the duty cycle is very low, but very high peak power can be obtained. The signal is acquired and analyzed in the time domain thus, making gating techniques for noise suppression relatively easy. In the latter case, the beam is modulated almost at 50% of duty cycle and has a low peak power. The signal is analyzed in the frequency domain, amplitude, and phase of one or more Fourier components are measured and narrow-band filters can be used to suppress noise.

As discussed above, medical imaging is very important for medical diagnosis and research and each of imaging modality has its own strength and weakness. There are two techniques for non-invasive as well as non-destructive imaging—one is a hybrid biomedical imaging called (a) photoacoustic imaging (PAI) and (b) thermoacoustic imaging (TAI).

a) PAI: Energy in the optical (400–700 nm), NIR (700–1300) nm and RF region can be used for PA excitation in soft tissues because the waves in these range are non-ionizing, safe for humans, and can provide high contrast and sufficient penetration depths. The optical properties including absorption and scattering of biological tissues in the visible and NIR regions are related to the molecular constituents of tissues and their electronic and vibrational structures. The RF properties, however, are related to the physiological nature of their electrical properties described by complex permittivity and complex conductivity. Therefore, no ionizing radiation is used in PAI, implying the absence of potential hazard to human health. Optical scattering in soft tissues degrades spatial resolution significantly with depth, while ultrasonic waves have 2–3 orders of magnitude weaker than optical waves scattering in biological tissues. Thus, ultrasound can provide a better resolution than optical imaging at depths greater than about 1 mm. However, ultrasound imaging (USI) relies in the detection of mechanical properties in tissues, so it has weak contrasts and cannot reveal early stage of tumors. Ultrasound is unable to image either oxygen saturation or the concentration of hemoglobin, while optical absorption is very sensitive to these parameters. In short, PAI provides both structural and functional information. It has a high contrast and resolution due to combination of excellent selectivity of optical imaging and high penetration of USI. The image resolution and maximum imaging depth can be adjusted with the ultrasonic frequency and penetration of diffuse photons. PAI has a close relationship with optical, thermal, and acoustic properties of biological tissues. There two types of PAI systems:

   i) PA microscopy (PAI). It uses spherically focused ultrasonic transducers with 2-D point-by-point scanning to localize the PA sources in linear or sectors scans, then reconstruct the image directly from the measured data, so it requires reconstruction algorithm.

   ii) PA tomography (PAT), sometimes is called Thermoacoustic Tomography (TAT) or optoacoustic tomography (OAT). The system relies on the PA signals measured at various locations around the subject under study. It utilizes an unfocused (wideband) ultrasound detector to obtain the PA signals, normally in a circular or spherical fashion and then reconstructs the optical absorption distribution of the tissue. PAT can reach a depth of 1 cm at 580 nm with an axial resolution of less than 100 μm, and at 1.064 μm (i.e., Nd:YAG laser) it can detect 2 mm blood vessels at the depth of 7.5 cm with 0.4 mm depth resolution and 1 mm lateral resolution. A wide beam of pulsed light heats a layered medium, the light energy deposition profile throughout the depth will be replicated by the detected PA signal. Thus, one can determine the depth-related information of the sample, such as depth structure and properties from the temporal PA signal.

b) TAI: Unlike PAI, a TAI excitation source involves far-infrared light or microwaves. It involves longer imaging depth due to a different electromagnetic radiation. This system offers higher spatial resolution than microwave imaging and receives much deeper imaging than most optical imaging techniques (Qin et al. 2012). Since it is based on different absorption mechanism, TAI can capture information about dielectric properties (e.g., distribution of some polar molecules and ions) of the relevant physiology and pathology inside tissues.

13.5.1 PAI contrast agents

There are number of endogenous contrast agents with corresponding absorption coefficients available in tissue for PAI, mainly:

Hemoglobin: 400 nm > 570 nm > 750 nm ($10^3 \rightarrow 10^1$ cm^{-1})

Oxyhemoglobin: 400 nm > 570 nm > 920 nm ($10^3 \rightarrow 10^1$ cm^{-1})

Lipid: 900 nm < 1.04 μm < 1.21 μm ($10^{-1.69} \rightarrow 10^{0.23}$ cm^{-1})

Water: 970 nm < 1.18 μm < 1.45 μm < 1.95 μm < 2.94 μm ($10^0 \rightarrow 10^3$ cm^{-1})

In some situations where there are no, or very little, contrast agents available for imaging, one can utilize external agents to effectively solve the problem depending on depth of target and use of correct laser wavelength. Some contrast agents have passive-targeting ability, i.e., they can extravasate into tumor tissues because of impaired vasculature and the enhanced permeability and retention (EPR) effect in solid tumors. Other contrast agents have the active-targeting ability, i.e., conjugated with a molecular probe including antibodies, protein or receptors in target cells or tissues. Ligands, however, bind to a specific subset of receptors in target cells or tissues. See §13.3 for some of major contrast agents used in PAI.

13.5.2 TAI contrast agents

For TAI, contrast agents are the distributional difference of water content and ion's concentration. Though none of agents are approved for clinical applications, due to their promising potential such as strong magnetic field responses, efficient particle size distribution, and relatively easy preparation, some magnetic nanoparticles have been employed as powerful diagnostic tools in biomedical investigations, for example:

Carbonyle iron (Nie et al. 2010), Dextran-coated Fe_3O_4 (Qin et al. 2012), NMG2[Gd(DTPA)], which is a paramagnetic material with high relaxation and seven unpaired electrons in 4f orbital of the Gd3$^+$ ion. The charged ions and unpaired electrons can interact with a microwave field and transform the absorbed energy into heat. Fe_3O_4/polyaniline (PANI), is another superparamagnetic nanoparticles conjugated to folic acid. These NPs can bind specifically to the surface of the tumor receptor, i.e., folate receptor. Nie et al. (2010) have used a 6 GHz TAT system to study intravenous administration of the targeted NPs to mice tumor and showed a five-fold greater thermoacoustic signal than that of non-targeted NPs. Other agents are MBs and SWANTs, which were discussed as multimodal imaging agents. A well-documented tables and list of references are provided by Dan et al. (2014) which can be referred to for further details.

13.6 Photoacoustic monitoring

13.6.1 *Design and application of photoacoustic sensor for monitoring the laser generated stress waves in an optical fibre* (Khosroshahi 2004)

Measurements of stress transients generated by a 400 ns pulsed HF laser in an infrared fluoride glass fibre has been made using fast time–response piezoelectric film transducer. Acoustic signals of up to 12 mV with frequencies ranging in megahertz generated by 21 mJ laser pulse when passed along the fibre axis. It is shown that useful information such as onset of non-linear behaviour of the fibre can be achieved from such measurements, which in turn can be used as a means of monitoring the quality of fibre surface during an operation.

Introduction

The interaction between laser light and the material in general is of great interest. The efficient generation of ultrasonic waves promises to have a variety of practical applications (Chardon and Huard 1982, Dyer and Srinivasan 1989, Philip et al. 1993, Pushkarsky et al. 2002). The physical principle of the photoacoustic effect consists in the fact that, for a time-varying light beam propagating through a medium, the radiationless absorption causes differential heating and thermal expansion generation both stress and thermal waves. It should be noted that radiation not transformed into heat such as scattering, etc. is not detected photoacoustically (Burt and Ebeling 1980). A very high signal to- noise ratio is achieved with this method, since the measured signal depends directly on the absorbed beam energy. Photoacoustic generation can be classified as either direct or in direct. In direct generation, the acoustic wave is produced in the sample where the excitation beam is absorbed. In indirect generation, the acoustic wave is produced in a coupling medium adjacent to a sample, usually due to heat leakage and to acoustic transmission from the sample (Tam 1986). There is currently much interest in the development of fibre delivering system for tissue ablation (Dyer et al. 1993, Lemberg and Black 1996), imaging (Guadagni and Nadeau 1991, Ning et al. 1992), spectroscopy (Teng and Nishioka 1987, Baraga et al. 1990), thermometry (Kajanto and Friberg 1988, Drizlikh et al. 1991), and similar fields using IR and UV lasers. Here, the potential of a fluoride glass fibre for delivering multiline HF laser pulses is evaluated. Also, a diagnostic technique based on the use of a wideband width PVDF thin film piezoelectric transducer is developed to measure the stress waves generated in optical fibre as a means of monitoring the integrity of fibre surface during the operation.

Theoretical background

Stress waves are generated in laser irradiated media through a variety of mechanisms which depend on the local condition (Cleary 1977). Whenever photons are absorbed or reflected there is an associated radiation pressure which is directly proportional to the irradiance. In transparent media electrorestrictive forces are developed and, if the irradiance is high enough, dielectric breakdown can occur leading to the formation of a high pressure plasma and the production of large amplitude stress waves in the irradiated sample. In absorbing samples two additional mechanisms are encountered: thermoelastic effect and ablative recoil stress.

Thermoelastic effect

It is well known that most materials expand upon heating, as an increase in temperature leads, on average, to a larger equilibrium atomic spacing. The expansion is driven by internal forces, and if this is hindered, as in the case of a constrained body or by the material inertia under conditions of rapid heating, large stresses develop. This is known as the thermo elastic effect. The generation of stress waves by the thermoelastic effect in liquids and solids irradiated by pulsed lasers has been studied extensively since the early days of the lasers (Carome et al. 1964, Bushnell and McClosley 1968). The effect of rapid heating is to produce stress waves propagating away from the energy deposition site, as shown schematically in Figure 13.39.

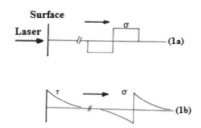

Figure 13.39. (a) Surface adjusted to new mechanical equilibrium position with bipolar stress wave propagating into sample, (b) stress wave form for exponential absorption, T and σ are step temperature and stress respectively.

Neglecting heat conduction, the temperature profile is rectangular and prior to the material adjusting to its new mechanical equilibrium position there will be a pressure rise associated with this higher temperature region. Here for a free surface (unconstrained) a rarefaction wave R_0 propagates into the material from the surface and a rarefaction (R_1) and compression (c_1) wave move away from the other pressure step. The leftward propagating rarefaction is inverted as it is reflected at the free surface and after a time $\tau = \dfrac{2d}{v_a}$, where v_a is the acoustic velocity, the surface has adjusted to its new mechanical equilibrium position. The resulting stress wave propagating into the material consists of a symmetric bipolar signal σ (compression followed by rarefaction) propagating at the sound speed (Fig. 13.39a). A stress wave detector located to the right of the surface thus registers a bipolar temporal signal. When laser absorption is replaced by the more realistic case of an exponential fall-off of absorbed energy with distance into the material, similar arguments apply, but the acoustic transient now mirrors the assumed exponential drop, as shown in Figure 13.39b. These qualitative arguments are substantiated by mathematical modelling based on the thermoelastic wave equation (Sigrist 1986). An important and valuable finding is that for exponential attenuation one dimensional wave propagation, the early portion of the stress waveform, σ, is exponential in time and of the form:

$$\sigma = Ae^{at'} \tag{13.16}$$

Here A is a constant, $a = \alpha v_a$ where α is the attenuation coefficient for radiation in the absorbing medium at $t' = t - 1/v_a$ where l is the distance from the surface to photoacoustic transducer. Thus, as first shown by Carome et al. (1964), the measured stress transient can provide information on the attenuation coefficient, provided v_α is known. This is particularly valuable under conditions where both absorption and scattering contribute to attenuation, as is often the case with tissue samples. Relatively simple forms for the thermoelastic transients can be derived for a laser pulse shape of the form:

$$I = I_0 (1 - e^{-kt})e^{-mt} \tag{13.17}$$

where I is the irradiance, k and m define the rates of rise and fall of the pulse respectively. I_0 is defined as:

$$I_0 = m(m+k)F/k \tag{13.18}$$

where F is the fluence. With an irradiance of the form described by Eq. (13.17) and assuming the instantaneous relaxation of absorbed energy to heating, no heat conduction and one-dimensional wave propagation, then the stress becomes (Cross et al. 1987, 1988):

$$\sigma = \frac{\Gamma}{2}\alpha\, I_0 \frac{ke^{at'}}{(m+a)(k+m+a)} \qquad t' \le 0 \tag{13.19a}$$

$$\sigma = \frac{\Gamma}{2}\alpha I_0 \left[\frac{2me^{-mt'}}{(m^2-a^2)} - \frac{2(m+k)_e^{-(m+k)t'}}{(m+k)^2-a^2} - \frac{k_e^{-at'}}{(m-a)(k+m-a)} \quad t' > 0 \right] \tag{13.19b}$$

where Γ is the Gruneisen constant

$$\Gamma = \gamma \, v_a^2 / C_v \tag{13.20}$$

where γ is the volume expansion coefficient, and c_v the specific heat capacity at constant volume.

Ablative stress

The ablative removal of material from a sample (e.g., optical fibre) can generate strong stress transients through the imparted recoil momentum (Dyer and Srinivasan 1986, Srinivasan et al. 1987). Photoacoustic monitoring of these transients can provide information on the inception time and duration of ablation in both gaseous and liquid environment (Cross et al. 1988, Srinivasan et al. 1987). Although usually only a small mass of material is involved, the short expulsion times and high ablation velocities can lead to large amplitude stress waves. It is assumed that the ablation commences once a threshold fluence, F_t is exceeded and the ablative stress, σ_A is approximately given by:

$$\sigma_A = V_a \rho \, \dot{x} \tag{13.21}$$

where ρ is the material density, and $\dot{x}$ the surface recession speed. The stress during the pulse is:

$$\sigma_A = 0, \qquad F < F_t$$

$$\sigma_A = V_b \, \rho \, I / \alpha \int_0^t I dt, \qquad F > F_t \tag{13.22}$$

where I is the laser irradiance. For a laser pulse with $I = \dfrac{F}{\tau_p}$ where τ_p the pulse duration, the peak stress is reached when

$$\int_0^t I dt = F_t$$

$$\sigma_{A \, max} = \frac{V_b \, \rho \, F}{\tau_p \, \alpha \, F_t} \tag{13.23}$$

Experimental set up

A home-built laser was used in these experiments operated on an SF_6-C_3H_8 gas mixture at low pressure (≈ 60 torr) and was excited by a fast, transverse, high voltage discharge between a pair of chang profile electrodes. Multiline output energies up to 380 mJ in a 400 ns full width half maximum (FWHM) pulse was obtained at a pulse repetition rate of ~ 0.2 Hz. Spectral measurements revealed 20 output transitions spanning between 2.67–2.96 μm with the dominant emission at 2.76, 2.78, 2.82, and 2.92 μm. The output beam from the laser was passed through a circular aperture to select a region of uniform fluence and this aperture was then suitably imaged on to the target zone using an NaCl lens of 50 mm focal length. A set of glass attenuators was used to vary the fluence, energy measurements being made using a Gen-Tech pyroelectric joulemeter. An IR grade quartz beam splitter after the aperture directed a small fraction of the output beam on to a InAs photodiode (Judson J12), allowing the relative laser output to be monitored on a shot-by-shot basis. A fluoride glass optical fibre supplied by Infrared Fibre Systems was used in experiments. The diameters of the core and core - plus - cladding were 500 and 600 μm, respectively, and the overall fibre diameter of 800 μm. The fibre ends were cleaved and polished using aerosol cutting polish (RS556-34) and then inspected under visible light illumination using an optical microscope (Fig. 13.40).

For this experiment, a short length of the fibre (~ 30 mm) was fitted with a simple photoacoustic sensor based on a polyvinylidene fluoride (PVDF) piezoelectric film (Metal Box Co), as seen in Figure 13.41. This sensor consisted of 9 μm thick single layer of PVDF film (10×20 mm^2) wrapped around a perspex cylinder, through which the fibre was placed. The 5 mm radius cylinder acted as impedence matching stub which minimized acoustic reflection at the interface, giving a rise time limited by the transit time of the longitudinal wave in the transducer, 4 ns in the present case. An intimate contact was maintained between the fibre and cylinder by means of silicone grease. A second cylinder of perspex was used to clamp the

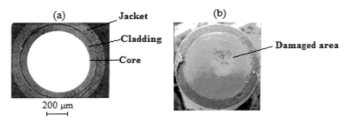

Figure 13.40. (a) Optical micrograph of polished fluoride glass fibre under white light transmission, (b) scanning electron micrograph of damaged input face of fibre by 1 pulse at 35 Jcm^{-2}.

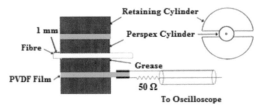

Figure 13.41. Schematic diagram of photoacoustic transducer used to investigate loss at the input surface of fibre. The PVDF film forms a partial wrap around the inner perspex cylinder.

film in place. Electrical contacts were made to the aluminized PVDF film using silver epoxy and the output leads taken to Tektronix amplifier in a Tektronix 7834 oscilloscope. The output voltage can be shown to be

$$V(t) = \frac{d_t\, f(t)}{c_D + c_L} \qquad (13.24)$$

where f(t) is the time-varying normal force at the transducer, ($C_D \sim 2.7$ nF) and C_L are the transducer and load capacitance, respectively, and $d_t \sim 20$ pC N^{-1} is the thickness mode strain constant for PVDF. The overall transducer display system has a rise time estimated to be ≤ 5 ns. In this way, the thermoelastic stress waves generated by heating as a result of laser absorption at the fibre face could be detected, following their propagation through the fibre and inner cylinder of the photoacoustic sensor. In addition, for some experiment a sensitive InAs detector (Judson J12) was employed to detect laser radiation scattered from the fibre at different positions along its length.

Experimental results

The presence of non-linear absorption at the entrance surface to the fibre was obtained from measurements using the photoacoustic sensor. With the fiber input surface located 1 mm away from the front face of the transducer as indicated in Figure 13.41, measurements of the voltage response were made as a function of the input fluence. The transient voltage response shown in Figure 13.42 (see inset) consisted of an initial step delayed by ~ 2 µs with respect to the HF laser pulse, and rising to produce a relatively large amplitude pulse peaking at ~ 4µs. The initial delay is consistent with the propagation time for an acoustic wave to travel through the fibre and the perspex cylinder, having originated at or near the fibre surface. The maximum signal amplitude, shown in Figure 13.42 as a function of the input fluence exhibited a linear increase up to 15 Jcm^{-2} but beyond this increased loss is non-linearly related to the fluence.

At high fluence where physical damage resulted at fibre input face, the response of the sensor exhibited a relatively complicated behaviour. The first laser pulse at 37 Jcm^{-2} caused a plasma formation as evidenced by a bright spark and audible noise and recorded photoacoustic signal was essentially unipolar, as shown in Figure 13.43. The second pulse produced a unipolar, compressive photoacoustic signal with brighter and louder plasma response. As the exposure continued, the plasma became progressively weaker and the signal decreased correspondingly. This is illustrated by the steady drop in the peak signal after the second pulse, shown in Figure 13.43.

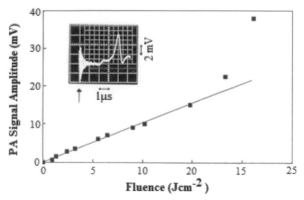

Figure 13.42. Peak amplitude of the photoacoustic transducer response as a function of fluence to fluoride glass fibre.

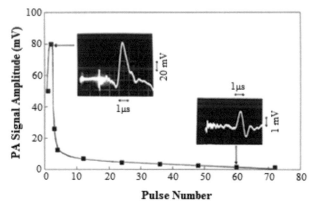

Figure 13.43. Peak amplitude of the photoacoustic transducer as a function of laser pulse number at 37 Jcm⁻².

At this stage, the origin of non-linear behaviour beginning at fluence ≥ 15 Jm⁻² was of interest to investigate. Measurements using the side viewing IR photodiode appeared to rule out any physical damage as a contributory factor to this loss. This is evidenced by the constancy of the scattered signal (Fig. 13.44) with number of laser pulses, even at fluences considerably above the value at which the photoacoustic response became non-linear. However, at higher fluences, e.g., ≥ 32 Jcm⁻² where catastrophic laser damage to the fibre input face occurred [Fig. (13.40b)], the scattered signal increased abruptly, as shown in Figure 13.44.

In this case, the input radiation is scattered out of the fibre core due to damaged surface. The fibre transmission can be conveniently summarized by plotting the output versus the input fluence for a fibre

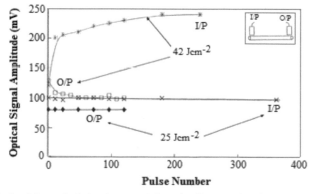

Figure 13.44. Amplitude of the optical signal scattered from the fibre as a function of number of pulses. The signal was detected using a side – viewing IR photodiode at the input and output end of the fibre.

length of l5 cm as shown in Figure 13.45. Here the output fluence from the fibre was calculated using the core area and the results are based on the transmission after exposure to 100 pulses at each fluence. For input above ~ 15 Jcm⁻², the transmission begins to fall due to increasing end losses and beyond ~ 32 Jcm⁻² catastrophic damage produced by the 400 ns duration HF laser pulse and the output fluence drops sharply.

Tests of the fibre lifetime could only be carried out over a relatively small number of pulses, because of the low pulse rate of the laser. However, the limited results obtained indicated that for input fluences 15 Jcm⁻², the fibre transmission remained constant for at least 700 pulses, as shown in Figure 13.46. At higher fluences not only was the initial transmission lower, but also continued to decrease with continued exposure as indicated, for example, for a fluence of 24 Jcm⁻².

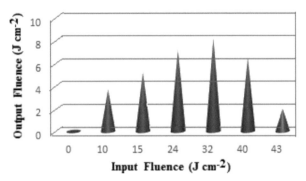

Figure 13.45. Variation of output fluence with input fluence for multiline HF laser transmission in a 15 cm long sample of fluoride glass fibre.

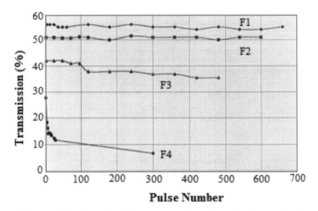

Figure 13.46. Fibre transmission as a function of number of laser pulses for pulses for various input fluences: F1 = 10 Jcm⁻², F2 = 15 Jcm⁻², F3 = 24 Jcm⁻², F4 = 43 Jcm⁻².

Discussion

It is demonstrated that relatively large diameter infrared fluoride glass fibre (~ 500 μm core) can be used to deliver the multiline HF laser at suitably high output fluence. Fast time responses provided by photoacoustic technique have been found to provide useful information on the interaction of short pulse laser with materials. A variety of relevant parameters can be measured from the detected stress waves including laser attenuation coefficient using the thermoelastic response in the subablation regime, ablation threshold and timescales, and the magnitude and nature of potentially disruptive stress transients. The observation of thermoelastic signals also provides evidence for fast thermalization of photoexcited states. The origin of the stress wave signal observed in these experiments assumed to be the thermoelastic effect produced by the local temperature rise associated with the absorption of laser radiation at fibre input surface and its subsequent decay to heat. The precise mechanism is not known, but it most likely relates to absorption at surface states at the fibre input (and possibly exit) faces. Optical signal measurements using the side

-viewing IR photodiode appeared to rule out physical damage as a contributory factor to loss at 15 Jcm^{-2} where non-linearity began. This is confirmed by the constancy of the signal (Fig. 13.46) with number of laser pulses, even at fluences considerably above the value at which the photoacoustic response became non-linear. At higher fluences where catastrophic laser damage to the input face of the fibre occurred, the scattered signal increased sharply. In this case input radiation is scattered out of the core because of the damage end face.

13.6.2 Combined photoacoustic ultrasound and beam deflection signal monitoring of gold nanoparticles agglomerate concentration in tissue phantoms using a pulsed Nd:YAG laser
(Khosroshahi and Mandelis 2015)

The purpose of this paper is to show and discuss the effects of gold nanoparticle (Au-NPs) concentration inside a tissue phantom using a combined system of PA and optical beam deflection and their applications particularly to photoacoustic imaging. We found that the PA signal from aggregated Au nanoparticles is significantly enhanced. The stock concentration of 100 nm Au-NPs was 3.8×10^9 particles/mL, from which three samples with 30%, 70%, and 90% concentration were prepared using polyvinyl chloride-plastisol. Each sample was then irradiated across a line scan using a 10-ns pulsed Q-switched Nd:YAG laser at 1 Hz repetition rate and 5 Wcm^{-2}, so that no physical ablation was observed. The corresponding photoacoustic pressure was found to approximately cover a range between 10 and 51 kPa. This corresponds to approximately 130–315 pJ of acoustic energy radiated by Au-NPs into the tissue. Maximal efficacy of transformation of optical energy into thermal energy was ~ 29%. Time-resolved photoacoustic deflection was also used to monitor the laser-interaction process. The results clearly indicated that: (i) The photoacoustic signal amplitude varies in a given sample as a result of the non-uniform concentration distribution of embedded Au-NPs; (ii) Increasing the concentration increased the signal amplitude linearly; and (iii) At higher nanoparticle concentrations, the probe deflection was found to increase due to a steeper thermoelastic gradient as a result of higher absorption by particle agglomerates and particles size-dependent dispersions.

Introduction

In recent years growing interest has been shown in developing new techniques for the non-invasive monitoring and imaging of biomedical structures and tissues. Optical scattering in soft tissue degrades resolution significantly with depth, while ultrasound can provide a better resolution than optical in depths greater than about 1 mm. Thus, the combination of high optical absorption contrast and the high ultrasonic spatial resolution (low scattering) makes it a very useful imaging technique. Basically, photoacoustics (PA) is a material probing modality in which the absorption of incident pulsed laser radiation leads to impulsive heating of the irradiated tissue volume, followed by rapid thermoelastic expansion and subsequent generation of broadband ultrasonic thermoelastic waves (Tam 1986). Equally, the photothermal deflection (PTD) is based on the localized heating of a sample by a focused laser source acting as "thermal piston". The rapid heating is then transferred to air molecules in the vicinity of surrounding gas, producing a temperature gradient field which effectively when the beam passing through this heated region is deflected by the thermally modulated index of refraction gradient. The amplitude and the phase of the deflected beam carry some information about optical and thermo-physical properties of the solid or liquid, thereby both techniques enabling a number of biomedical applications (Dyer 1988, Khosroshahi and Ghasemi 2004). In this manner, one can obtain a better contrast and spatial resolution of tissue images (O'Neal et al. 2004). Despite much valuable research work regarding PA imaging (Esenaliev et al. 1999, Beard 2002, Telenkov et al. 2009), further enhancement of photoacoustic (or optoacoustic) imaging contrast would be necessary for the early detection of cancer at deep subsurface locations. Gold nanoparticles (Au-NP) exhibit unique optical properties, namely strong localized surface plasmon resonance (LSPR) which is defined as a collective and coherent oscillation of conduction electrons when excited by an external source of electromagnetic field. As a consequence of the plasmon oscillation, a dipolar is generated with a huge enhancement of the local electric field at the nanoparticles surface. This electric field leads to strong light absorption and scattering at the SPR frequency by the particle (Pustovalov and Babenkov 2004, Govorov and Richardson 2007, Hasannejad and Khosroshahi 2013) and their major advantages are: biocompatibility due to their inert surface, nontoxicity, surface conjugation chemistry, lack of photobleaching, or blinking as with quantum dots (Weibo et al. 2008, Khosroshahi and Nourbakhsh 2011). Besides, Au-NP are relatively simple to synthesize, they are photostable and can be easily conjugated with proteins, antibodies, and specific cancer ligands (Sinha et al. 2012, Khosroshahi and Ghazanfari 2012). Thus, they have been chosen for bioimaging (Zhang et al. 2009, Sajjadi et al. 2012) mainly due their ability to convert absorbed light into heat (i.e., PA efficiency) (Pustovalov et al. 2010), drug delivery (Kuznetsov et al. 2001, Mahmoodi et al. 2011), cancer cell diagnosis and therapeutics (Welinsky and Grinstaff 2008, Patra et al. 2010), laser tissue welding and soldering (Gobin et al. 2005, Khosroshahi and Nourbakhsh 2011). Above all, since cellular uptake and endocytosis of particles results in their aggregation, it also has significant impact on the application of plasmonic metal nanoparticles for molecular imaging. The goal of this paper is to study the effects of gold NP concentration on PA signals using a Q-switched pulsed Nd:YAG laser and simultaneously monitoring the interaction process based on photoacoustic deflection signals.

Experimental

Materials

To study the effects of Au-NP concentration on photoacoustic signals, a tissue phantom made of polyvinyl chloride-plastisol (PVCP), synthesized from chloride monomers, non-toxic plastic and soluble in water was purchased from M-F Manufacturing Co., Fort Worth, TX, USA. PVCP is a viscoelastic material and its creep deformation is very low compared with other plastics due to limited molecular motion at ordinary temperature. For these type of materials the relationship between stress and strain depends on time and the stiffness will depend on the rate of rate of applied load. In addition, mechanical energy is dissipated by conversion of heat in the deformation of viscoelastic materials. The solution is an oil-based liquid and was uniformly heated and stirred continuously using a magnetic stirrer up to $\approx 200°C$, in order to avoid structural and optical inhomogeneities and then allowed to cool. It has no or very negligible optical absorption at 1.06 μm wavelength of Nd:YAG laser and has a similar speed of sound (1400 ms^{-1}) and density to tissue and makes a suitable candidate for modeling tissue biomedical applications (Spirou et al. 2005). A 25 mL gold nanoparticles (Au-NPs) source with 100 nm diameter and concentration of 3.8×10^9 particles/mL (i.e., 9.5×10^{10} particles) stabilized as suspension in citrate buffer was purchased from Sigma-Aldrich. Three samples were prepared by injecting 0.3 ml, 0.7 ml, and 0.9 ml of Au-NPs in 1 cm^3 of PVCP solution. Upon cooling, the solution solidified and was easily removed from the container.

Method

The experimental set-up is shown in Figure 13.47. Each sample was irradiated using a 10-ns pulsed Q-switched Nd:YAG laser (Continum-Surelite) at 1.064 μm wavelength with 1-mm collimated pulse at 1 Hz and 5 Wcm^{-2} intensity. The thermoelastic signals were detected by a 2.2-MHz focused transducer (V305, Olampus NDT Inc., Panametrics) with 18.8 mm diameter and 25 mm focal length, and were then recorded with a fast digital oscilloscope (Tektronix-DPO 7104-1 GHz).

A 2 mW He-Ne laser (632 nm) was used as a probe beam for photoacoustic deflection measurements. The beam was focused with a lens of 100-mm focal length to a diameter of about 0.5 mm. The dependence of the photodiode response ΔV on the beam deflection is (Diaci and Mozina 1992)

$$\Delta V = V_0 \, erf [\, 2^{1/2} \, \varphi/\theta]$$
(13.25)

with φ and θ being the beam angular deflection due to change in refraction and angular divergence, respectively. Also, the thermally or PA pressure-induced optical deflection, φ, is directly related to rate of change of refractive index and the temperature.

$$\varphi = 1/n \; \partial n/\partial T \; \partial T/\partial z \, L$$
(13.26)

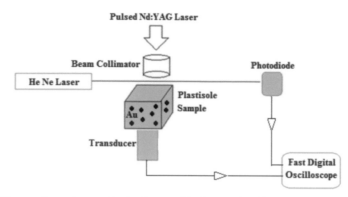

Figure 13.47. The experimental set-up for simultaneous PA ultrasound and laser beam deflection measurements.

where n is the refractive index, T is the temperature, and L is the probe beam path. It is interesting to notice that since pure plastisol (i.e., without impurities) acts as a weakly absorbing material at Nd:YAG laser, thus, the temperature in the relation (13.25) is mainly due to absorption by Au-NPs. The temperature of one single NP is given by Eq. (13.26), where it increases linearly with absorbed power, but inversely related to medium thermal conductivity, $K_p (= D_p \rho_p c_p)$ with ρ_p, c_p and D_p being the density, specific heat capacity, and the thermal diffusivity of the NP, respectively (Falsa et al. 2011).

$$\Delta T = \frac{P}{4\pi R_p K_p} \tag{13.27}$$

where P is the laser power and Rp is the NP radius. Thus, larger the sphere, the longer it takes for heat to diffuse or transfer to the surrounding medium (i.e., it cools slowly in longer time). In fact, both PA and PTD are observable with the same set up, except that PA deflections occur at much earlier time scale. The output signal was then registered using a Si-based photodiode (THORLABS-DET10A) with spectral sensitivity between 200–1100 nm. In combining PA ultrasound detection with a conventional transducer and PA beam deflection, some additional sample information can be obtained, such as sound velocity, elasticity, temperature, flow velocity, thermal diffusivity, and thickness. In the case of viscoelasticity, if we assume the tensile stress, σ and differentiating it with respect to x,

$$\sigma = E_y [\epsilon_0 - \beta T(x,t)]$$
$$\partial\sigma/\partial x = E_y [\partial\epsilon/\partial x - \beta \, \partial T/\partial t \, (x,t)] \tag{13.28}$$

where $E_y = \sigma/\epsilon_0$ is the Young's modulus, $\epsilon_0 = \partial u/\partial x$ is strain or the displacement of particle in x-direction, $\beta = \dfrac{\Delta P C_p}{c_a^2 \alpha F}$ represents the volumetric thermal expansion, ΔP is the pressure increase due to volume expansion, C_p is specific heat capacity, c_a is the acoustic velocity in the material, α the material absorption coefficient, and F is the laser fluence. Since $T(x,t) = \alpha \displaystyle\int_0^t \frac{I dt}{\rho C_p}$

$$\frac{dT}{dx} = \frac{\alpha}{\rho C_p} \frac{\partial \int_0^t I dT}{\partial x} = \frac{1}{C_p} \frac{\partial W}{\partial x} \tag{13.29}$$

where, $W = \dfrac{\alpha}{\rho C_p} \partial \displaystyle\int_0^t I dt$ is the absorbed energy per unit volume. Using the Newton's second law of motion, we obtain,

$$\frac{\partial^2 u}{\partial t^2} = \frac{1}{\rho} \frac{\partial\sigma}{\partial x} \tag{13.30}$$

Substituting the Eq. (13.28) and (13.29) in Eq. (13.30) and simplifying,

$$\frac{\partial^2 u}{\partial x^2} = \frac{1}{c_a} \frac{\partial^2 u}{\partial t^2} = \frac{\beta}{Cp} \frac{\partial W}{\partial x}$$

$$\frac{\partial^2 u}{\partial x^2} = \frac{1}{c_a} \frac{\partial^2 u}{\partial t^2} = \frac{\Delta P}{C_a^2} \frac{1}{\alpha F} \frac{\partial W}{\partial x} \qquad (13.31)$$

It can be seen from the relations (13.29) and (13.31) that the rate of change of temperature is directly related to absorption coefficient of material and the laser intensity and hence to optical deflection, φ. Secondly, for an unknown material the value of $(E_y/\rho)^{1/2}$ can be deduced using the experimental value of acoustic propagation velocity (i.e., $_{ca} = (E_y/\rho)^{1/2}$).

Results and discussion

The amplitude of bipolar thermoelastic signals increased approximately linearly with increasing Au-NP concentration, as expected from linear photoacoustic theory. Some examples of PA thermoelastic responses are shown in Figure 13.48a and b. The increasing trend of average PA amplitude with Au concentration at constant power density is illustrated in Figure 13.28c. The peak output voltage from the transducer can be converted to a corresponding normal force and hence to a pressure (= F/A, Pa) if the irradiated area, A, is known. From the known voltage amplitude, V, and other constants of the PZT transducer, the corresponding values of the average photoacoustic pressure can be found using $P = CV(t)/d_t A$ where, $C = (C_l + C_d \approx 10^{-9} \, F)$ is the sum of load and transducer capacitance and $d_t \approx 10^{-12} \, pC.N^{-1}$, is the strain constant. Thus, it was found from the measured amplitudes that the corresponding calculated acoustic pressure covered the range between 10 and 51 kPa.

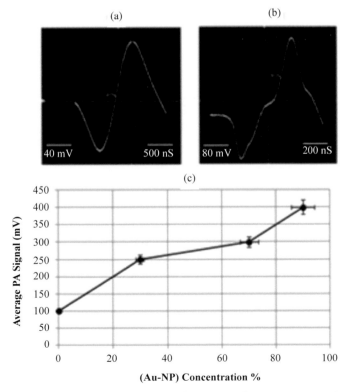

Figure 13.48. Examples of some typical thermoelastic signals for (a) 30% of Au-NP: 160 mV, 550 ns, (b) 70%: 400 mV, 160 ns (b) and (c) PA signal variation with NPs concentration.

458 *Applications of Biophotonics and Nanobiomaterials in Biomedical Engineering*

The narrowing of the pressure transient FWHM, Δt, with concentration at constant power density, Figure 13.48b, can be explained by considering the simple relation (1) below which relates the acoustic energy, ΔE_a, delivered to tissue to pulse peak pressure, P_0, and Δt through (Dyer et al. 1993):

$$\Delta E_a \approx P_0^2 A \, \Delta t / \rho c_a \tag{13.32}$$

Thus, the peak value of pressure (P_0) is directly proportional to $\Delta t^{-1/2}$ under conditions of fixed acoustic energy which, in practice, means a decrease in transient pulse duration is compensated by increasing the pressure. The pressure itself is, of course, directly proportional to laser fluence in the linear regime. Therefore, taking the value of PVCP density as close to soft tissue, $\rho \approx 1000$ kg m^{-3} and the acoustic velocity of about 1400 ms^{-1} using the ref. (Khosroshahi and Ghazanfari 2012), area of irradiation, $A \approx 7.85 \times 10^{-3}$ cm^2, and then by substituting the experimental values of acoustic pressure (10–51) kPa and the pressure pulse widths measured at full width half maximum in Eq. (13.32), the amount of acoustic energy delivered to the tissue without and with nanoparticles are approximately determined as 45 pJ and (130–315) pJ, respectively. Figure 13.49 shows the PA signal waveforms detected by transducer and Figure 13.49b indicates the PA-induced probe beam deflection detected by photodiode at the relatively high concentration of 70% of Au-NPs, equivalent to 26 μg/mL, where rapid heating as a result of absorption of laser radiation by the sample generates fast thermoelastic expansion followed by deep rarefaction due to various non-radiative excitation processes occurring inside the PVCP. Our results are similar and comparable with those of Sell et al. (1991) and they suggested that polarities of the deflection signal are consistent with the evolution of a shock wave from a sound wave. When this occurs, the negative leading edge tends to shorten and steepen, while the positive shock's wave edge broadens. Although there is no agreed upon value for safety threshold (it varies case by case), the concentration used in this experiment is almost half the amount (56 μg/mL) used by Bayer et al. (2013) and Sun et al. (2013) for PA imaging of drug release.

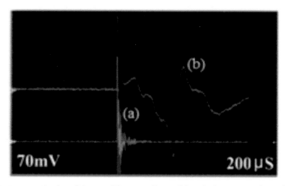

Figure 13.49. (a) Typical photoacoustic signal detected by transducer (b) and photoacoustic probe beam deflection waveforms detected from the surface of the tissue phantom.

Using the expression for the nanoparticle diameter $R_p = (D_p.\tau_p)^{1/2}$, τ_p is the laser pulse duration, we can assume all NP volume was heated during the laser pulse action because R_p (50 nm) $\ll X_T \approx (D_p.\tau_p)^{1/2} \approx 1$ μm, where X_T is the thermal diffusion length and for gold NP $D_p \approx 1.2 \times 10^{-4}$ m^{2}s^{-1} (Lopez-Munoz and Pescador-Rojas 2012). Similarly, the thermal diffusion length delivered by the NPs in tissue would be $(D_t.\tau_p)^{1/2} \approx 4$ μm, taking $D_t \approx 1.3 \times 10^{-3}$ cm^2 s^{-1} (Walsh and Cummings 1990). Now Eq. (13.33) below is used to determine the characteristic thermal relaxation time nanoparticles with radius, R

$$\tau_r = \rho_p.c_p R_p^2 / 3K_p \tag{13.33}$$

With $\rho_p \approx 19.3$ g/cm^{-3} and $c_p \approx 0.13$ J.g^{-1}.C^{-1}, Eq. (13.33) yields $\tau_r \approx 7$ ps $\ll \tau_p \approx 10$ ns (Pustovalov et al. 2010, 2005). Therefore, in our case, $\tau_p \gg \tau_r$, and we have a non-adiabatic situation where no thermal confinement is achieved within a nanoparticle and there is a heat exchange between NP and tissue. Our findings are in close agreement with Bayer et al. (2013) where PA signals from agglomeration were stronger than from monodisperse NPs. This is so because the PA signal is sensitive to the heat transfer properties of embedded nanoparticles relative to their surroundings, therefore, it is expected that changes to the temporal and spatial characteristics of heat transfer due to aggregation lead to signal increase which is linked to the thermal properties and thermodynamics of the nanoparticle-surroundings system (Bayer et al. 2013, Shah et al. 2008). In terms of energy, the PA signal is insensitive to the scattering effect because the PA signal is determined by the absorbed fraction of the incident optical energy that is converted to heat. However, the photon density distribution of light changes when it is scattered. This causes a change in the heated region and introduces a change in the shape of sound source.

While the optical absorption depends on the material type, the scattering is caused by inhomogeneity in the refractive index of a medium and spatial distribution of the scattering depends on the size and the shape of the inhomogeneity relative to source wavelength. It is known that for a turbid medium the reduced scattering coefficient, $\beta' = \beta (1-g)$ where β is the scattering coefficient and g is the anisotropy factor g or the mean cosine of the scattering which varies between -1 and 1. Since, in our case, $R_p \approx 50$ nm $\leq \lambda/20 \approx 53$ nm and $x = 2\pi R_p/\lambda \approx 0.3 < 1$, thus Rayleigh scattering can be assumed, where $g = 0$. However, when the particle size increases due to for example NPs clustering, the intensity distribution increases in the forward direction, $g = 1$, and the scattering phase function, $p(\hat{s}, \hat{s}')$ for small angles becomes much higher than for all other angles. The minimum value of $g = -1$ indicates the backward scattering $p(\hat{s}, \hat{s}')$ describes the fraction of light energy incident on scatterer from $\hat{s}'$ direction that gets scattered in the new direction $\hat{s}$.

However, it must be emphasized that the concept, and hence the effects of agglomeration or clustering under optical interaction irradiation, are different from the situation where high numbers of single particle dispersions exist within the medium. This can further be understood and clarified by noting that basically, the agglomeration process for colloidal particles results from the coupling between two main interactions: (1) particle-fluid interactions, which play a role in the motion of particles within a flow and govern the number of particle-particle encounters, and (2) particle-particle interactions, which control whether colliding particles will adhere (adhesion or attractive interaction) or simply bounce (repulsive interaction). The second process, as in this case, is described by the DLVO (Derjaguin, Landau, Verwey, and Overbeek) theory (Derjaguin and Landau 1941, Verwey and Overbeek 1948) which defines inter-particle forces as the sum of van der Waals and double-layer electrostatic contributions. Taking this idea into consideration, it then can be assumed that the number of spherical solid particles (N_{NP}) dispersed in a medium (analogous to the Gibbs energy) is proportional to the change of average particle diameter (D), equivalent to the coordination number, at any time

$$N_{NP} = P (D_{max} - D) \tag{13.34}$$

where D_{max} is the maximum diameter that particles can reach when a minimum number of particles remain in the dispersion and P is a proportionality constant that takes into account the shape factor of the particles. The variation of the number of particles with respect to time due to agglomeration is (Loria et al. 2011):

$$-dN_{NP}/dt = kN^n \tag{13.35}$$

Here k is the agglomeration rate coefficient, and n is the reaction order and deriving Eq. (13.34):

$$dN_{NP} = -Pd(D) \tag{13.36}$$

Substituting Eq. (13.34) in (13.36) in (13.35),

$$P\frac{d(D)}{dt} = k [P(D_{max} - D)]^n \tag{13.37}$$

Considering $n = 1$ (Thompson et al. 2008),

$$P\frac{d(D)}{dt} = k (D_{max} - D) \tag{13.38}$$

If at $t = 0$, $D = D_0$, then the Eq. (13.38) becomes,

$$D = (D_{max} - \exp (kt) (D_{max} - D_0) \tag{13.39}$$

where D_0 is the particle initial diameter at $t = 0$,

Dividing the equation by D_0 and rearranging we obtain,

$$d = d_{eq} - \exp(-kt)(d_{eq} - 1) \tag{13.40}$$

where $d = D/D_0$ and $d_{eq} = D_{max}/D_0$. Equation (13.40) represents the behaviour of the particle diameter as a function of time for $n = 1$. The agglomeration rate, k, is a function of temperature. The calculation of the activation energy is necessary to determine the nature of the agglomeration process. Now, it is well-known that quantitative PA imaging in the presence of nanoparticles is based on the linearity of the PA signal (maximum signal voltage, V_{max}), and on the number of nanoparticles (N_{NP}) with a wavelength-dependent optical absorption cross-section, $\sigma(\lambda)$, in the illuminated volume with fluence F, and on the deposited energy (σF). This relationship is given as:

$$V_{max}(F) - V_0(F) \propto \Gamma_{eff}\sigma(\lambda) N_{NP}F \tag{13.41}$$

where Γ_{eff} is the effective Grüneisen constant for a given NP in a non-absorbing solvent, and V_0 is the PA signal from any endogenous absorbers. This relation holds as long as the NP absorption cross-section and environment are constant, and particle-to-particle thermal and electromagnetic coupling can be neglected. If V_0 is negligible, then V_{max} results from the NPs only and $\Gamma_{eff}\sigma(\lambda)$ is a constant that can be measured independently. Based on Eq. (13.41), the PA signal was increased by increasing the Au-NP concentration.

13.7 Contrast-enhanced photoacoustic imaging

13.7.1 *Frequency-domain photothermoacoustic and ultrasonic imaging of blood and opto-thermal effects of plasmonic nanoparticle concentrations* (Khosroshahi et al. 2015)

We describe the use of combined ultrasonic imaging (USI) and photoacoustic radar imaging (PARI) with linear chirp laser modulation to provide visualization of blood with and without the use of gold nanoparticles. A blood vessel simulating sample (S1) containing pure sheep blood was shown to be an optically weak absorbing medium which satisfies thermal but not acoustic confinement. On the contrary, the blood-gold combinations (S2) using 10% and S3 (20%) Au concentrations behaved as optically strongly absorbing media. A heating efficiency of 0.54 to 8.60×10^3 Kcm^2 J^{-1} was determined for Au NPs. The optimal optical power modulation spectral density was determined to be in the range of 0.5 to 0.8 MHz and 0.3 to 1.0 MHz for USI and PARI, respectively. USI produced a better structural image, while PARI produced a better functional image of the simulated blood vessel in the order of S2 > S3 > S1 due to enhanced signal-to-noise ratio. Two-dimensional images of the simulated blood vessel were also obtained. In summary, the PA signal does not increase linearly with Au NP concentration and the change of blood osmolarity due to temperature increase can cause thermo-hemolysis of red blood cells, which in turn degrades the PA signal, and thus the blood imaging quality. On the other hand, USI produced the best structural image, S4, due to the strong US reflection response from Au NPs and its insensitivity to the presence of blood.

Introduction

There are a number of imaging modalities which can be employed to visualize tissue at cellular and molecular levels, including nuclear imaging (positron emission tomography), single photon emission computed tomography, x-ray computed tomography, magnetic resonance imaging, optical imaging, ultrasound imaging (USI), and photoacoustic imaging (PAI). It is well-known that growing cancer cells need an additional blood supply and gradually develop dense microvascular networks inside or around tumors. Angiogenesis appears to be a marker for breast cancer growth and may have clinical implications in diagnosis and treatment (Pan et al. 2011). The interaction of light and ultrasound (US) with blood plays an important role in diagnostics and therapeutics, for instance, for the noninvasive assessment of blood composition. It is equally important to emphasize that the interaction process and its bioeffects are governed by the biophysical properties of whole blood. The optical properties (absorption and scattering) of biological tissues in the visible (400 to 750 nm) and near-IR (750 to 1300 nm) spectral ranges are fundamentally related to the molecular constituents of tissues and their vibrational/electronic structures. Although optical methods are severely limited by their short penetration depth in tissue, their major benefit is their sensitivity to tissue composition. For example, optical absorption generates endogenous contrast by blood constituents such as deoxyhemoglobin (Hb), oxyhemoglobin (HbO_2), lipids, water, and intrinsic chromophores with distinct fluorescent properties. It is known that when a laser light interacts with a turbid medium such as biological tissue, photons can be both absorbed and scattered. Some of the scattered photons, which are called "ballistic" photons, travel a straight distance through the medium, while others deviate. It is the ballistic photons which define the degree of resolution, therefore, the higher the degree of scattering or deviation, the more the resolution degrades with depth. In other words, the efficiency of high coherent resolution medical imaging relies on the degree of detected ballistic photons. US can provide better resolution than optical probes at greater depths, but with much compromised contrast. Thus, the combination of high-optical absorption contrast and high-ultrasonic spatial resolution (low scattering), a feature of biomedical PAI, constitutes a very useful imaging technique. Briefly, the pulsed photoacoustic (PA) effect is based on the absorption of pulsed laser energy by a material creating transient, localized heating. The increase in temperature leads to rapid thermal expansion which, in turn, generates thermoelastic stress waves. In recent years, wide interest has been shown in PA imaging of blood vessels and cancer (Genina et al. 2000, Oraevsky et al. 2002, Wilson et al. 2013). Optical (Gussakovsky et al. 2012) and PA spectroscopic studies (Laufer et al. 2005, Fredrich et al. 2012) of blood containing structures in tissues can measure Hb and HbO_2 concentrations, mainly due to the fact that Hb and HbO_2 have different wavelength-dependent optical absorption properties which allow signal differentiation between arteries and veins. Normal whole blood consists of about 55 vol% plasma and 45 vol% cells. A normal red blood cell (RBC) is mainly characterized by a flat bioconcave shape with volume, surface area, and diameter ranging from 80 to 108 μm^3, 119 to 151 μm^2, and 7 to 8 μm, respectively (Yaroslavasky et al. 2002). The RBC membrane contains proteins and glycoproteins embedded in, or attached to, a fluid lipid bilayer that gives it a viscoelastic behaviour. RBCs are by far the most dominant absorbing element in blood in the wavelength range between 250 and 1100 nm, mainly due to the presence of hemoglobin, beyond which water becomes the main absorber (Friebel et al. 2009). This difference in light scattering between RBCs and other blood constituents arises from the different refractive indices between RBCs and the surrounding blood plasma (Meinke et al. 2007). Because RBCs are acoustically weak scatterers (impedance contrast between RBCs and plasma is only about 13%), multiple scattering can be neglected. Light scattering by a single RBC depends on its disk-type shape, volume, refractive index, and orientation. Blood vessels usually exhibit orders of magnitude larger absorption than surrounding tissues depending on the Vis to NIR range which implies a drastic blood/tissue change. However, there is enough contrast for PAI to visualize blood vessels or abnormal angiogenesis for imaging *in vivo* subcutaneous vasculature for a variety of applications. The use of a variety of nanostructures in medicine and biomedical engineering has also been growing in recent years. For example, plasmonic nanoparticles exhibit unique optical properties. Specifically, the major advantages due to the photophysical properties of gold nanoparticles are: strong localized surface plasmon resonance (SPR), surface-enhanced scattering, nonlinear optical properties, tunable resonance across the Vis-NIR due to adjustable nanoparticle size and shape (Pustovalov and Babenkov 2004, Hossain et al. 2009, Baffou and Quidant 2013, Hasannejad and Khosroshahi 2013) biocompatibility due to their inert surface, nontoxicity, surface conjugation chemistry, i.e., they can be linked to specific ligands for tumor targeting, imaging and therapies, lack of photobleaching or blinking as with quantum dots, and very low oxidation (Khlebtsov et al. 2006, Hung et al. 2007). As a result, Au nanoparticles have been extensively used in applications like bioimaging (Yang et al. 2008, Wang et al. 2010, Pustovalov et al. 2010, Luke et al. 2011, Zangandeh et al. 2013) mainly due to their ability to convert absorbed light into heat (i.e., photothermal efficiency), but also due to their drug delivery properties (Mahmoodi et al. 2011, Gormley et al. 2012, Hassannejad and Khosroshahi 2013), cancer cell diagnostics and therapeutics (Welinsky and Grinstaff 2008, Patra et al. 2010, Pattani and Tunnell 2012, Sadat et al. 2014), laser tissue welding and soldering (Gobin et al. 2005, Khosroshahi and Nourbakhsh 2011). In this work, we use linear frequency modulation waveforms and cross-correlation processing similar to radar technology [the photoacoustic radar (PAR)] with modulated or coded optical excitation to provide both high-axial resolution and signal-to noise ratio (SNR) by using a matched filter at the signal processing stage (Fan et al. 2004). The SNR of frequency domain photoacoustics (FDPA) can be similar or higher only in very specific cases, and that depends on the transducer bandwidth and other technical issues, such as maximum available laser power. The main advantages of FD-PA over pulsed-laser excitation besides being compact and less expensive are: its ability to control and manipulate instrumentation system parameters, no jitter noise, low fluence of the frequency-chirped laser modulation, depth profiling over a wide range of frequencies, high-spatial resolution, possible parallel multichannel lock-in-signal processing, and wide signal dynamic range using lock-in filtering, and much higher duty cycle ($\approx$ 50%) than pulsed-laser PAs ($\approx$ 10–4% to 10–6%) (Telenkov and Mandelis 2006). On the other hand, the main advantages of pulsed PAI include higher efficiency of PA signal generation due to high energy per pulse, hence, giving a strong SNR. But there is a trade-off between the amount of pulse energy, pulse repetition frequency, and a fast acquisition system. Other advantages include less accumulated thermal effect, which may occur with continuous wave (CW) and modulated laser source, providing axial resolution along the ultrasonic propagation direction and a difference in the time of flight of PA waves, which reduces signal cluttering (Telenkov et al. 2011). Also, in a theoretical study, it was shown that the SNR of PAI systems based on CW lasers with a chirped modulation frequency are about 20 to 30 dB worse than systems based on pulsed lasers. However, this was based on the assumptions of a top hat 1 to 5 MHz transducer and a matched filtering in the FD-PA. Following our previous work (Telenkov et al. 2009, Lashkari and Mandelis 2011), we employ frequency domain PAR (FD-PAR) imaging to extend our investigation to studies of the effects of Au NPs concentration on imaging blood vessels using a chirped diode laser and a US transducer.

Theory

Au NP properties

The importance of metallic nanostructures originates in their ability to absorb and scatter the incident light in both the visible and infrared regions. The interaction of an electromagnetic field $E(r,t) = [E_0(t)e^{i(kz-\omega t)}]$ of a laser with gold nanoparticles causes the dielectric polarization, μ, of surface charges as a result of which charges oscillate like simple dipole moment nanoparticles, where ω is the angular frequency of light traveling in the z-direction, and k is the wave number. The oscillating dipole radiates electromagnetic waves with a large enhancement of the local electric field at the NP surface and polarization proportional to the incident field. This electric field leads to strong absorption and scattering at the SPR frequency by the particle which consequently damps the oscillations, causing the displacement to become out of phase, φ, with the varying field and requiring an input of energy to sustain the oscillation. The SPR absorption in Au NPs is followed by energy relaxation through non-radiative decay channels. This results in an increase in kinetic energy, leading to overheating of the local environment around the light-absorbing species. The complex refractive index is defined as

$$\tilde{n} = n_b(\omega) + i\, k_e(\omega) \tag{13.42}$$

According to the principle of causality, the real and imaginary parts of the complex refractive index are connected through Kramers–Kronig relations. The real part, $n_b(\omega)$, is the refractive index of blood and the imaginary part, $k_e(\omega) = \lambda\mu_a/4\pi$ is the extinction coefficient, λ is the laser wavelength, and μ_a is the absorption coefficient. $\tilde{n}(\omega)$ of the metal (gold) nanoparticle is related to the frequency dependent NP complex dielectric permittivity $\varepsilon_g = \varepsilon_r + i\varepsilon_i$ through $\varepsilon_g - \tilde{n}^2 - (n_r + ik_e)^2$ where $n_r - k\lambda/2\pi$ is the real part of the refractive index indicating the phase velocity. Substituting $(n_r + ik_e)$ in the plane wave expression, it gives

$$E(z,t) = e^{-2\pi kz/\lambda}\, Re[E_0 e^{i(kz-\omega t)}] \tag{13.43}$$

The real part, $\varepsilon_r = (n_g^2 - k_e^2)$, determines the degree to which the metal polarizes in response to an applied external electric and it determines the SPR spectral peak position. The imaginary part, $i\varepsilon_i = 2n_g k_e$, quantifies the relative phase shift, $\Delta\varphi = \Delta[2\pi(n_r + ik_e)/\lambda]2R_g$ of the induced polarization with respect to the external field, i.e., it determines the bandwidth and includes losses such as ohmic heat loss. The extinction coefficient is maximum when $\varepsilon_g + 2\varepsilon_m = 0$, where ε_g represents the Au particle giving rise to the

SPR band (Khlebtsov et al. 2006). According to Mie theory, the absorption cross section, σ_{abs}, of a particle embedded in a medium, $\varepsilon_m \approx -\varepsilon_g/2$, is given by (Baffou and Quidant 2013).

$$\sigma_{abs} = \frac{8\pi^2}{\lambda} R_g^3 \left[\frac{\varepsilon_g(\omega) - \varepsilon_m}{\varepsilon_g(\omega) + 2\varepsilon_m} \right]$$

(13.44)

where R_g is the radius of a gold particle. Similarly the scattering cross section is

$$\sigma_{sca} = \frac{128\pi^5}{\lambda^4} R_g^6 \left[\frac{\varepsilon_g(\omega) - \varepsilon_m}{\varepsilon_g(\omega) + 2\varepsilon_m} \right] = \frac{8\pi k^4}{3} R_g^6 |\mu|^2$$

(13.45)

where μ is the polarizability of a metallic sphere. The extinction cross section, σ_{ext}, of a spherical particle is $\sigma_{ext} = \sigma_{abs} + \sigma_{sca}$. The extinction efficiency, η_{ext}, of a particle is the normalized extinction cross section of an area,

$$\eta_{ext} = \sigma_{ext}/\pi R_g^2$$

(13.46)

and η_{abs} is the particle absorption efficiency,

$$\eta_{abs} = \sigma_{abs}/\pi R_g^2$$

(13.47)

Using $\varepsilon_r = (n_g^2 - k_e^2) \approx -7.6$ and $\varepsilon_i = 2n_g k_e \approx 1.56$ yields $\varepsilon_g \approx -6$ and $\varepsilon_m = \varepsilon_g/2 \approx -3$. Now substituting these values in Eq. (13.42) yields $\sigma_{abs} \approx 1.35 \times 10^{-15}$ m^2 which is comparable with the values obtained by Jain et al. (2006) and Pustovalov and Babenkov (2004). Furthermore, using Eq. (13.45b) yields, $\eta_{abs} \approx 17 \times 10^{-2}$.

Optical and photoacoustic interaction with (B-Au NP) medium

A schematic diagram representing the interaction and propagation of a laser beam and US with a B-Au NP ensemble is illustrated in Figure 13.50, where the direction of the laser beam is perpendicular to the surface of the medium and the US incidence is oblique. It is seen that RBCs can be oriented in random directions with different number density causing different amount of backscattering, while agglomeration (e.g., in static mode) can change the spatial configuration of the cells which can also affect optical and US backscattering.

When light passes through a suspension of an absorbing medium such as blood, photons that do not encounter RBCs are not absorbed. This is called "absorption flattening effect" (Fribel et al. 2006). As a consequence, the transmitted light intensity is higher than it would be if all hemoglobin were uniformly dispersed in the solution. When a beam of light interacts with a blood volume element, the first event taking place between the plasma and the surrounding medium is Fresnel reflection, F, defined by

$$F = [(n_{pl} - n_b)/(n_{pl} + n_b)]^2$$

(13.48)

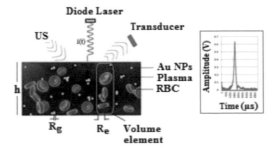

Figure 13.50. Schematic diagram of laser interaction with a B-AuNPs tube. The inset shows an example of a PA signal generated by a local B-AuNP volume when crossed by the laser beam.

where $n_{pl} = 1.33$ and $n_b = 1.42$ are the refractive indices of plasma and blood, respectively. If $\Sigma_c(\vec{X})$ represents the cross-sectional area of RBCs per unit volume, which in fact indicates the geometric attenuation coefficient in the beam direction $\vec{X}$, then this parameter can be resolved into two different components given as an integral over all possible orientations of the RBCs in the blood volume (Yim et al. 2012)

$$\Sigma_c(\vec{X}) = \int_u n(\vec{u}) \, \sigma_c(\vec{u}, \vec{X}) \, d\vec{u} \tag{13.49}$$

Here $n(\vec{u})$ indicates the number of RBCs per unit volume with orientation $\vec{u}$ and $\sigma_c(\vec{u}, \vec{X})$ corresponds to the cross–sectional area of an RBC with an orientation $\vec{u}$ when exposed to light in the $\vec{X}$ direction. The value of $\sigma_c(\vec{u}, \vec{X})$ mainly depends on the shape of the cells interacting with light, i.e., the shape or structure factor $S(\vec{q})$ which quantifies the effect of the spatial random organization of the scatterers on the back scattering coefficient where the scattering vector, $\vec{q} = -\vec{k}$. Here $|\vec{k}| = k = 2\pi f/c_a$ is the acoustic wavenumber, f is the acoustic frequency, and $c_a \approx 1570$ ms^{-1} is the speed of sound in blood (Lide 2002). The ability of a tissue to generate acoustic echoes is often quantified by the frequency-dependent backscattering coefficient, β', which for a heterogeneous material such as blood composed of weakly scattering particles is given as (Coussios 2002)

$$\beta' = n(\vec{u}) \, S(\vec{q}) \, \sigma_{\beta'} \tag{13.50}$$

where $\sigma_{\beta'}$ is the backscattering cross-section of a single scatterer. In addition, there is a refractive index mismatch between the cell membrane and the surrounding plasma medium, which results in light scattering by RBCs. Also, RBC is an orientation-dependent structure and the scattering intensity distribution will, therefore, depend on the angle of incidence. For large particle sizes (i.e., $2\pi r_p/\lambda > 1$) where r_p is the radius of particle, the intensity distribution of light increases in the forward direction and the cosine of scattering phase function for small angles is much higher than for all other angles. However, the optical mean free path $< d >$ within the medium is limited by the scatterer density, Φ_s and by the effective scattering cross section, σ_s, i.e., $< d > = 1/ \Phi_s \, \sigma_s$.

The PAR technique involves light that is intensity modulated at high frequencies which, when propagating through a scattering medium, exhibits amplitude and phase variations. However, if the distance between NPs is larger than their size, the NPs act as discrete thermal point sources and the temperature should be a sum over all the sources provided there is no clustering. Then, the heat source becomes (Govorov et al. 2006)

$$Q(r,t) = \Sigma_n q_n(t)\delta(r - r_n) \tag{13.51}$$

where the coefficients $q_n(t)$ describe heat produced by the n-th Au NP. The sinusoidally varying irradiance at modulation angular frequency, ω_m, which illuminates the cross-sectional area of the sample is:

$$I(\omega_m) = 1/2 \, I_0(\omega)\left[1 + e^{i\omega t}\right] \tag{13.52}$$

The spectral component $Q_s(z,\omega_m)$ at any value of ω_m is given by:

$$Q_s = (z,\omega_m) = \mu_a I_0 e^{-\mu_a(h + z) + i\omega t} \tag{13.53}$$

where h is the thickness of the B-Au NP container, and z is depth, so that $-h \leq z \leq 0$.

Materials and methods

Preparation

A 25 mL 100-nm diameter gold nanoparticle source with concentration of 3.8×10^9 particles/mL stabilized as suspension in citrate buffer was purchased from Sigma-Aldrich. Sheep blood was kept in a refrigerator before each experiment. Prior to each test the blood was anti-coagulated with ethylene diamine tetraacetic acid (EDTA). Initially, 30 mL of blood was mixed with 3 mL of EDTA (i.e., 10:1) giving a total blood source volume of 33 mL. For a sample labeled S2 (10% ratio of 0.05:0.5 mL of NPs:blood) was used and for a sample labeled S3 (20%) the amount of NPs was doubled. The number of NPs and the corresponding concentration for S2 using 0.05 mL of Au were calculated as 196×10^6 and 345×10^6 mL^{-1}, respectively. Similarly for S3 using 0.55 mL of B-Au, the values of 380×10^6 and 633×10^6 mL^{-1} were obtained. A total of four samples were prepared using the aforementioned labeling: S1 (blood only), S2 (blood + 10% (3.8 μg/mL) Au NPs), S3 (blood + 20% (7.6 μg/mL) Au NPs), S4(Au NPs only). All samples were safely mounted next to each other with 5-mm separation inside a saline solution container 50 mm below the water surface and irradiated with laser light in transverse and longitudinal directions. In the former (latter) case, the direction of scanning was perpendicular (parallel) to the sample surface.

Experimental setup

As shown in Figure 13.51, the intensity modulated output of a CW 800-nm diode laser (Jenoptik AG, Germany) with a chirp duration, τ_c, of 1 ms was used as an excitation source for PA generation at 1.6 W peak power.

The laser driver was controlled by a software function generator to sweep the laser power modulation frequency range between 0.3 and 2.6 MHz. A collimator was used to produce a collimated laser beam with 2–3 mm spot size on the sample. A focused ultrasonic transducer (V382, Olympus NDT Inc., Panametrics) with a center frequency at 3.95 MHz, 12.5 mm diameter, a focal length of 25 mm, and an estimated lateral resolution of 0.87 mm was used for transmitting the US signal. The sensitivity of this transducer was measured to be 31.8 μV/Pa using a calibrated hydrophone. The back scattered pressure waves were detected by a focused transducer (V305, Olympus NDT Inc., Panametrics) with a center frequency at 2.25 MHz, 18.8 mm diameter, a focal length of 25 mm, and beam width of approximately 0.9 mm. The distance between the samples and the transducer immersed in water was kept at about 25 mm. The setup was designed for backscattering mode operation, and the angle between the laser beam and the center axis of each transducer was about 27°. A 3-mm diameter silicone rubber tube was used to simulate a blood vessel in a physiological saline container. The tube was linearly scanned with 0.5-mm step. The scanned distance was shorter than the tube length. In the NIR ($\geq$ 700 nm) region, blood has an absorption coefficient $\mu_a \approx 7$ cm^{-1} corresponding to an optical penetration depth of about 1.4 mm. Depending on the type of silicone rubber, the acoustic impedance, Z, ranges between $(1.1–1.5) \times 10^6$ kg m^{-2} s^{-1}. Blood has an acoustic impedance of about 1.60×10^6 kg m^{-2} s^{-1}. Therefore, the amplitude reflection at the tube wall-blood interface varies between 0.1 and 3.4%. Data acquisition and signal processing were performed using Lab View software. Linear frequency modulation and matched filtering were used to generate A-scans with the PAR system. The similarity between two waveforms as a function of delay time is defined by the cross-correlation function, where time delay is equivalent to a phase shift in the frequency domain. In our experiments over 80 detected signals of 16 trains of 1-ms long chirps (i.e., 44) with 1-s delay between them were averaged by software processing the collected data at each point, thereby giving a total of 1280 chirps. The chirp bandwidth was adjusted to maximize the PAR and US SNRs simultaneously.

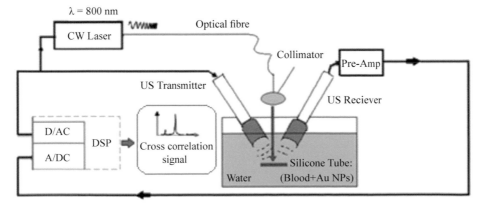

Figure 13.51. The experimental setup.

Results

The results are based on the backscattered signals using a volume fraction,V_f, in calculations related to S1 and S2

$$V_f = \frac{\left(F_g \times V_g \right) + \left(F_b \times V_b \right)}{V_g + V_b}$$ (13.54)

where F_g and F_b represent the corresponding applied parameters for Au NP and blood, respectively, and V_g and V_b are the corresponding volumes of a gold solution and blood, respectively. The acoustic parameters for all different cases are given in Table 13.4.

An example of a PA pulsed signal is shown in the inset of Figure 13.50, which indicates how the signal amplitude changes when the laser interacts with a B-Au N medium during the scanning process. In other words, time represents the coordinate location of NPs. This is an important example because the imaging contrast depends on physical processes, such as the scattering mechanism which is also a size-dependent factor, the particle distribution density, orientation, and the shape factor of RBCs, as described by Eq. (13.47). One such situation is the mismatch between the hemoglobin solution inside the cell and the surrounding plasma. Figure 13.52 indicates the US and PA cross correlations for 10% Au NPs (a) and 20% (b), respectively, generated by a 3.95 MHz transducer. The PA signals are very similar. The oscillations are mainly due to reflections of ultrasonic waves from the walls of the silicone rubber tube and transducer. The cross-correlation peak position on the PA delay time axis is related to the depth of the signal source (e.g., RBC or NPs).

Figure 13.53a shows the envelope for the US cross correlation where the amplitudes decrease in the order S4 (Au only) > S3 (20%) > S2 (10%) > S1 (blood only). The area under the curve of each envelope represents the total output energy of the matched filter at constant input energy. The profile amplitude provides a better SNR than the in-phase correlation alone. Although the US cross correlation produces

Table 13.4. Acoustic characteristics of blood, Au and B-Au NPs for S2 (10%) and S3 (20%).

	C_a (ms^{-1})	λ_a (mm)	Reflection amplitude %
Blood	1570	0.590–3.4(ω_1) 5.200.590(ω_2)	0.1–3
Au	3200	1.2–0.612 10–0.612	34.70
(Au+Blood)	1718 S2(10%)	0.645–0.328 5.7–0.645	1.38
	1842 S3(20%)		4.40

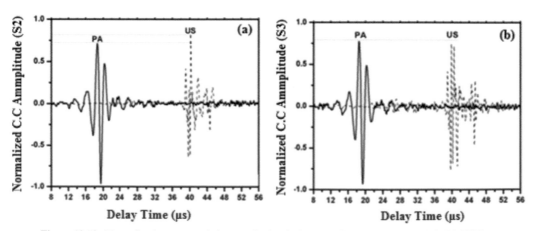

Figure 13.52. Normalized cross-correlation amplitude of US and PA for (a) S2 (10%) and (b) S3 (20%).

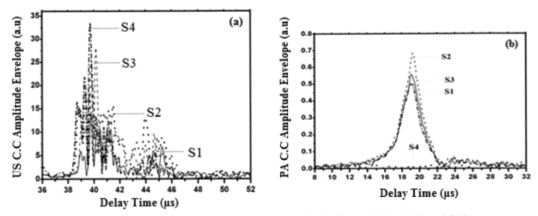

Figure 13.53. Cross-correlation amplitude envelope for S1, S2, S3, and S4 for (a) US and (b) PA.

better SNR, its absorption is insensitive to material composition but the degree of reflection depends on the acoustic impedance of the medium. Since S4 contains Au NPs only, it exhibits the highest reflection, in other words, by decreasing the NPs concentration in S3, S2, and S1, blood plays a more effective role in producing the frictional forces, which consequently reduces the amplitude of acoustic reflection. On the contrary, the PA correlation amplitudes, Figure 13.53b, decrease in the order S2 > S3 > S1 > S4. Despite its lower SNR, the PAR response is superior to US due to its specificity, as the results are based on the NP material optical absorption, concentration, and also on the blood absorption coefficient. The fact that RBCs are very deformable and their shapes vary in response to thermal and mechanical stresses (Rogan et al. 1999) which may damage their membrane may be a reason for S2 > S3.

Acoustic attenuation in whole blood can be attributed to a number of different mechanisms: (i) at the cellular level due to cell membrane separating different intracellular and extracellular fluids; and at the molecular level within the (ii) intracellular and (iii) extracellular fluids. Molecular level absorption mechanisms include viscosity, thermal relaxation time, and structural processes. The longer the relaxation time of a medium, the higher the absorption of ultrasound is. Another factor to be considered in US interaction with RBC cells is the attenuation linearity where the scattering component is mainly due to mismatch acoustic impedance between the encapsulated proteins by RBC membrane and the surrounding fluid. However, according to Zinin (1992), for suspended erythrocytes the contribution of scattering to attenuation in the frequency range of 0.2–10 MHz may be neglected. By far the most dominant contribution of ultrasound absorption by biological tissues is due to relaxation processes among potential, chemical, and structural forms of energy. There are frequency ranges over which some energy can transform to another state during ultrasonic compression, but with insufficient time for the process to completely reverse itself during rarefaction. Therefore, there will be a net energy transfer and hence absorption. As a result, quantitative US techniques are based on the frequency analysis of backscattered signals by biological tissues. Power spectral density (PSD) is the frequency response of a random or periodic signal x (t) indicating the average power distribution as a function of frequency:

$$<P> = \lim_{T \to \infty} 1/2T \int_{-T}^{T} x(t)^2 dt \tag{13.55}$$

Figure 13.54a shows the corresponding US-PSD for S1 with a peak maximum at about 500 kHz followed by decreasing amplitudes due to higher attenuation in the B-Au NP medium. However, when 10% Au NPs were added (S2), Figure 13.54b, the amplitude increased significantly between 300 and 800 kHz. In addition, an increased distribution between 1.4–3.0 MHz was observed, indicating that a possible effect of Au NP agglomeration is the result of modification in spatial configuration of the cells, producing increased ultrasound backscattering. At 20%, Figure 13.54c, the power spectrum amplitude decreased by almost 37% compared to Figure 13.54b in the same frequency range, leading to lower SNR and indicating a non-linear behaviour possibly due to additional structural and thermal relaxation processes at the cellular level. Again, there is an increased frequency distribution between 1.5–2.5 MHz. This will

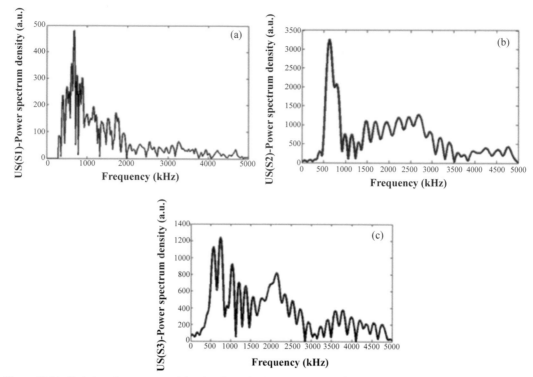

Figure 13.54. Variation of power spectral density of US with frequency for (a) S1(blood only), (b) S2 (10%), and (c) S3 (20%).

be discussed in detail in the next section. The US response exhibits more peaks with relatively higher side lobes which may be due to its stronger interaction with medium followed by more pronounced reflections from the tube walls and the blood. Secondary features like oscillations at higher frequencies are likely due to reflections of signals from particles closer to the surface of the tube.

Figure 13.55 shows the corresponding PAR-PSD results for S1(a), S2(b), and S3(c), respectively. Inspection of the spectra of two signals (Fig. 13.55 (b) and (c)), shows that the PA signal is dominated by low frequency components with the amplitudes in the order S2 > S3 > S1. In the low frequency range, the PA response is affected only by the mixture of blood and NPs, so it does not reflect the signature of each individual component. The higher resolution of the US cross-correlation signals is mainly due to the thermoelastic energy conversion effect of the PA phenomenon which affects the spectrum like a low-pass filter, thereby limiting spatial resolution.

Furthermore, the PAR-PSD exhibits a non-linear behaviour consistent with the US results, which can be related to the thermal effects of Au NPs on the RBC biomechanical properties and structure (Gershfeld and Murayama 1988). The main feature in the case of PAR, unlike US, is that there is little frequency content above the main peak frequency and the information is completely concentrated within the 300–800 kHz range, particularly for S2, which exhibits the strongest power spectrum. Physically, this implies that light does not penetrate as much as US, as expected, and thus does not interact with the Au NPs which are situated deeper than the optical penetration depth in the blood sample. A 2-D image (scan direction vs. depth) was produced by plotting all 1D-depth images (time traces) next to each other. Figure 13.56 illustrates the images obtained by scanning along the length of each tube using US (a) and PAR (b). Clearly, the best images correspond to S2 for PAR and S4 for US, which is consistent with Fig. 13.53 (a) and 13.53 (b), and is further discussed in the next section. This confirms the well-known fact that the US reflection amplitude, $[(Z_2–Z_1)/(Z_1+Z_2)]^2$, increases with concentration of Au NP whereas in the PAR case, it is the absorption coefficient of the medium which is the determining parameter. Transversely scanned (cross-sectional) PAR images of S2 and S3 artificial blood vessel tubes are illustrated in Figure 13.57. They, too, are indicative of the higher intensity distribution produced by 10% than with 20% Au NPs.

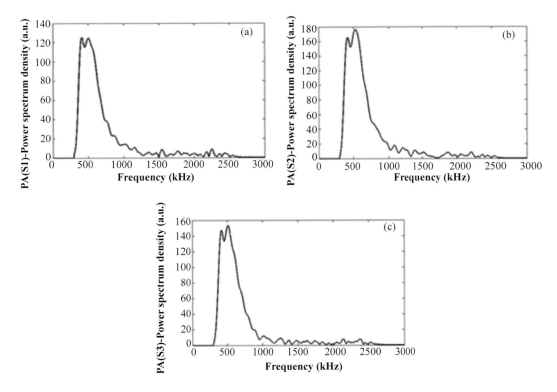

Figure 13.55. Variation of power spectral density of PA with frequency for (a) S1 (blood only), (b) S2 (10%), and (c) S3 (20%).

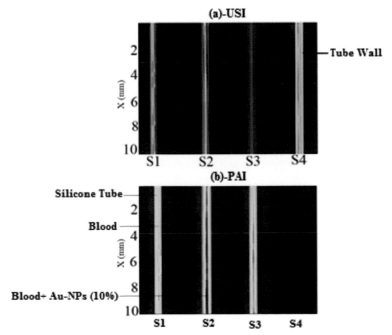

Figure 13.56. 2-D longitudinal image of the blood vessel simulating tube.

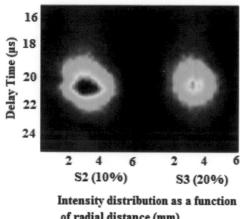

Intensity distribution as a function of radial distance (mm)

Figure 13.57. 2-D transverse images along a cross-section of the blood vessel.

Discussion

i) Heat generation and transfer by Au NPs

Initially, the absorption of pulsed or modulated laser energy by NPs produces a heating effect which is quickly equilibrated within the NP ensemble. Subsequently, the heat is transferred from the NPs to the surrounding medium or matrix (blood) via non-radiative relaxation within a few ps. In the absence of phase transformations, heat transfer in a system with NP thermal sources is described by the heat conduction equation:

$$\rho_g(r)\, c_g(r)\, \frac{\partial T(r,t)}{\partial t} = K_m \nabla^2 T(r,t) + Q(r,t) \tag{13.56}$$

where $T(r,t)$ is temperature, Q is the heating source, $\rho_g(r)$ $c_g(r)$ are density, and specific heat of a Au NP, respectively, and K_m is the thermal conductivity of the surrounding medium. The total amount of heat produced is $Q_T = Q_b + Q_g$, where Q_b and Q_g represent the components produced by blood and gold NPs, respectively. In our case, the approximation $2\pi R_g/\lambda$ (≈ 0.4) < 1 holds, so it is assumed that each NP is quasi-transparent to the incident light and Q_g is constant across each nanoparticle. For a single Au NP exposed to a laser beam the generated power is $P = I_0 \sigma_{abs}$ (W) where σ_{abs} is defined by Eq. (13.43) and $Q_g = P/V_g$ [Wcm^{-3}] where V_g is the volume of the NP. The heat source is derived from the heat power density $h_\rho(r) = \int_v h_\rho(r)\, d^3r$, where the integral is over the NP volume V_g. To calculate $Q_g(r,t)$, we assume the size of a Au NP is smaller than the laser wavelength so that electrons inside the NPs respond collectively to the applied electric field of the laser radiation, $E(r,t) = [3\varepsilon_b/2\varepsilon_g + \varepsilon_g]\, E_0$, where ε_b is the blood permittivity. It is found that (Baffou and Quidant 2013)

$$Q_g(r,t) = <j(r,t)\,.\, E(r,t)> = \frac{\omega_m}{8\pi} \left| E(r,t) \right|^2 \operatorname{Im} \varepsilon_g \tag{13.57}$$

where $j(r,t)$ is the current density inside the metallic NP. The heat generated is thus directly proportional to the square modulus of the NP electric field (Govorov et al. 2006). The temperature field induced by chirped-laser heating can be modeled via conductive heat transfer, assuming that the laser energy absorption in the B-Au medium is quantified by the volumetric heat generation which decays exponentially from the point of absorption defined by Eq. (13.53). Since the laser beam spot size, $\varphi_b \approx 2$ mm is larger than both the optical penetration depth, $\delta_o \approx 1.4$ mm and the thermal diffusion length, X_T, the temperature field $T(r,t)$ of a single nanoparticle can be obtained using the 1-D heat conduction equation. If all the absorbed optical energy is converted to nanoparticle heating, the temperature increase can be evaluated using Eq. (13.58) where F is the laser fluence and m_g is the mass of a gold particle (Cox et al. 2009)

$$\Delta T_{1max} = \frac{F\sigma_{abs}}{C_g m_g} \tag{13.58}$$

The maximum temperature change of blood volume element, $\Delta T_{max/e}$, is

$$\Delta T_{max/e} = N_{g/e} \frac{R_g}{R_e} \Delta T_{1max} \tag{13.59}$$

where $N_{g/e}$ is the number of Au NPs per unit element and R_e is the radius of the irradiated element. The maximum temperature occurs at the surface of the NP, $r = R_g$. Thus, the larger the NP sphere, the longer it takes for heat to diffuse or transfer to the surrounding medium (i.e., it cools down more slowly). On the microscale it can be assumed that NPs are totally embedded within the blood matrix and are small enough to have a uniform steady-state temperature equal to the surrounding blood temperature, T_b, owing to fast heat transfer and thermalization time. However, on a larger scale, for example after some agglomeration, the blood temperature of a spatially localized element may be different due to possible thermal overlapping of a larger fraction of NPs and clustering at that element. It is interesting to note that because NPs are dispersed inside a static colloidal medium, their distribution within the tube can be considered as Brownian motion. Normally, in soft matter physics the Brownian motion of colloidal dispersions (as in this case) results in a Lorentzian distribution. Therefore, assuming, $\Psi(r') = d^3r' \, N_D(r')$ where $\Psi(r')$ is the probability of finding a NP at a distance r' in a volume d^3r', and $N_D(r')$ is the density distribution of NPs, a function which decays according to the spatially damped radial function (Baba-ahmad et al. 1987).

$$N_D(r) = \frac{N_g R_g}{R_v} \frac{1}{4\pi R_v^2} \frac{e^{-r/R}}{r} \tag{13.60}$$

where R_v is the blood vessel radius.

ii) PA generation and its transfer by B-Au NP

While PA signal generation is mainly based on the illuminated material optical absorption properties, the subsequent ultrasound propagation within the medium is directly conditioned by the properties of the surrounding medium such as the acoustic matching impedance, the absorption coefficient which is affected by the viscosity, and the relaxation time of the medium, the scattering coefficient which depends on the particle number density, and the size and level of the spatial distribution of the scatterers. The transducer properties and the signal processing instrumentation also contribute sensitively to the PA signal. The interaction of a laser pulse with a relatively weakly absorbing heterogeneous medium, such as blood containing a suspension of strongly absorbing nanoparticles, generates a PA signal enhancement effect. While the absorbers are the NPs, the signal propagates in the surrounding fluid and heat transfer defines the signal generation process. Therefore, the produced acoustic signal is proportional to the amount of energy deposited into the NPs and the thermoelastic properties of the surrounding environment. Absorption of optical chirp energy by the medium results in the generation of similar-frequency-modulated acoustic waves propagating within the medium. Quantitative PAI in the presence of nanoparticles is a function of the PA response signal (maximum signal voltage, V_{max}). The amplitude is given as a function of independent responses from single particles, the wavelength-dependent optical σ_{abs}, the number of nanoparticles (N_{NP}), and the deposited energy ($\sigma_{abs} F$). The PA signal is given as (Cook et al. 2013)

$$V_{max} - V_0 \propto \Gamma_{eff} \sigma_{abs} N_{NP} F \tag{13.61}$$

where $\Gamma_{eff} = \frac{\beta c_a^2}{C_p}$ is the effective Grüneisen constant for a given NP type, β is the volume thermal expansion, C_p is the specific heat of the surrounding medium, and V_0 is the PA signal from any endogenous absorbers, such as whole blood defined by the product of the blood absorption coefficient, μ_{ab}, and the optical fluence, F (Cox et al. 2009)

$$V_0 = \Gamma_{eff} \mu_{ab} F \exp\left[-(\mu_{ab} c_a t)\right] \tag{13.62}$$

Here $\mu_{ab} = \varepsilon_{Hb}(\lambda)[Hb] + \varepsilon_{HbO2}(\lambda)[HbO_2]$, Hb and HbO_2 are the relative hemoglobin and oxyhemoglobin concentrations, ε_{Hb} and ε_{HbO} are the corresponding molar extinction coefficients (Hu and Wang 2010). If, however, V_0 is negligible, then V_{max} is due to NPs only. Relation (13.59) holds as long as the NP absorption cross-section and environment are constant, and particle-to-particle thermal and electromagnetic coupling can be neglected. The propagating spherical pressure field detected by a transducer at a distance, r_d has spatial profile (Maslov and Wang 2008)

$$P(r,t) = \frac{\left|\tilde{P}(r_s,\omega)\right|}{4\pi \left|r_d - r_s\right|} e^{i\left[\omega(t - \left|r_d - r_s\right| / c_a) + \phi\right]} \tag{13.63}$$

where r_s is the distance from the laser to the object or heat source within the tissue, $|\tilde{P}(r,\omega)|$ is the pressure amplitude and ϕ is a phase constant due to thermoelastic conversion. At low frequencies (a few MHz), and for weakly scattering NPs, the relation between the backscattering cross section and the RBC acoustic properties is simple and is described by Rayleigh scattering. In the case of RBCs with radius $R_b \approx 3$ μm this is valid up to ≈ 27 MHz (Savery and Clouteir 2007), that is, within the range $kR_b \ll 1$. Although the PA signal is produced by the absorbed fraction of the incident optical energy that is converted to heat, the photon density distribution in a turbid medium changes when it scatters. This causes a change in the heated region and in the shape of the PA sound source. Since the optical penetration depth in blood, δ_0 (1.4 mm at 800 nm) $\approx \varphi_r$ where $\varphi_r = 1$ mm is the beam radius, and $X_T \ll 2\varphi_r$, where X_T is the thermal diffusion length in blood, $X_T \approx (4D_b \tau_c)^{1/2}$, where τ_c is the chirp duration and D_b is the thermal diffusivity of blood, it follows that the PA source in blood can be assumed to be spherical and a 1-D model can be used. Using Duck (1990), $D_b \approx 1.38 \times 10^{-3}$ cm² s⁻¹, one finds $X_T \approx 23$ μm and ≈ 47 μm for $\tau_c = 1$ and 4 ms, respectively. The latter is the minimum irradiation time followed by 1-s delay time before the next 4 ms chirp. Also, the values for blood thermal relaxation time are $\tau_r \approx \delta_0^2/4D_b \approx 3.6$ s and for acoustic transient time $\tau_a = \delta_0/c_a \approx 890$ ns, respectively. Based on the results shown in Table 13.5, since $\mu_a c_a \ll \omega_{im}$ and ω_{fm}, $\mu_a X_T \ll 1$ and $\tau_c < \tau_r$, and $\tau_c \gg \tau_a$ where ω_{im} and ω_{fm} are initial and final angular modulation frequencies, it can be deduced that S1 is effectively weakly absorbing (i.e., a thermally thick and optically transparent medium, $X_T \ll \mu_a^{-1}$) which satisfies thermal but not acoustic confinement. However, when Au NPs are added to blood, the situation begins to reverse and the medium becomes strongly absorbing (i.e., $\mu_a c_a \gg \omega_{im}$ and ω_{fm}, $\mu_a X_T \gg 1$, a thermally thin and optically opaque medium). The relation $\varepsilon_i = 2n_g k_e \approx 1.56$, gives a value of $k_e \approx 2.78$ for gold at 800 nm, which is comparable with that obtained by (Etchegoin et al. 2006). Also, one obtains $\mu_a = 4\pi k_e/\lambda \approx 4.3 \times 10^5$ cm⁻¹ for gold. By substituting the values of μ_a (blood) and μ_a (Au) for F_b and F_g in Eq. (13.52), the corresponding value of volume fraction absorption coefficient can be determined. Despite the fact that the B-Au NP medium is a stronger absorber than pure blood, nevertheless, $\tau_c \gg \tau_r$ and $\tau_c \gg \tau_a$ and neither the thermal nor the acoustic confinement condition is met.

Figure 13.58 shows the $X_T(f)$ values for a 0.3–2.6-MHz chirp using $X_T \approx (2D_c/\omega_m)^{1/2}$, where D_c is the combined, or volume fraction, value of thermal diffusivity of the B-Au NP medium. One key result is that almost 75% of the total thermal-wave penetrates the medium within 0.3–1 MHz and correspondingly 19% between 1–2 MHz and 6% between 2–3 MHz. Figure 13.59 indicates that not only does X_T increase with chirp duration, but also after 8 ms the curves show a sub-linear increase. Two biophysical reasons can be invoked for interpreting this finding. First, the depth of diffusive laser-induced heating occurs within a given time and possible implications regarding the breakdown of blood tissue integrity within that depth must be considered. Next, the laser-tissue interaction process may be non-linear. Therefore, identifying that process might be crucial in further understanding its bioclinical consequences.

Table 13.5. Calculated thermo-acoustic properties of B-Au NPs for S2 (10%) and S3 (20%).

(Blood+Au)	ρ_c (kg m⁻³)	C_c (JKg⁻¹C⁻¹)	D_c (m²s⁻¹)	K_c (W m⁻¹K⁻¹)	τ_r (ns)	τ_a (ps)	αc_a	αX_T (μm)
S2 (10%)	2.66×10^6	3830	1.1×10^{-4}	27.8	7.60	58	69×10^6	26.5–150
S3 (20%)	4×10^6	3520	2×10^{-4}	50.20	4.20	54	133×10^6	64–374

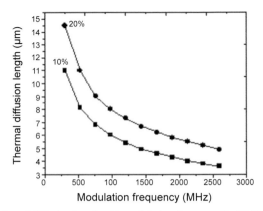

Figure 13.58. Variation of diffusion length with modulation frequency for S2 (10%) and S3 (20%).

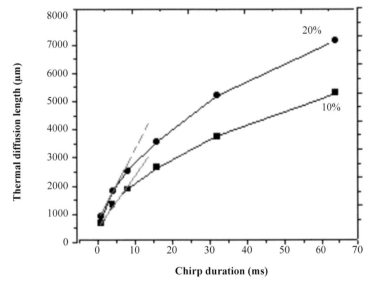

Figure 13.59. Variation of diffusion length with chirp duration for S2 (10%) and S3 (20%).

Figure 13.60 shows further analysis of thermal diffusion length distribution for different frequency ranges during a given chirp duration, i.e., a thermal diffusion length breakdown in terms of frequency. It is interesting to note that not only does the thermal diffusion length increase with chirp duration as expected from photothermal-wave behaviour, but also, the energy content of thermal diffusion for a given chirp duration takes place at lower frequencies as expected from the low-pass filtering nature of photoacoustic signal (Lashkari and Mandelis 2011).

It can be seen from Eq. (13.55) that the amount of heat generated is directly proportional to modulation angular frequency and Eq. (13.57) states that the larger the number of NPs and the higher the laser fluence, the higher the temperature in each volume element of a blood-vessel simulating tube during irradiation. Consequently, for contrast-enhanced PAI of a given blood containing tissue volume, not only the laser parameters, but also the NP concentration should be carefully optimized. Furthermore, according to Eq. 13.58, it is expected that temperature changes for each volume element with the density distribution function of NPs. This is then followed by a corresponding PA signal voltage generation according to relation (13.59). This PA pressure increase is described by Eq. (13.61). Therefore, it appears that both the temperature increase due to higher number of NPs and their density variation within each volume element and on the entire volume can increase the PA signal and the imaging SNR. It is well known that any modification of

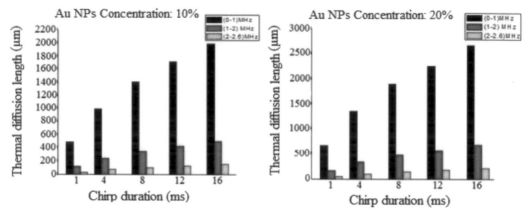

Figure 13.60. Distribution of thermal length as a function of chirp duration for S2 (10%) and S3 (20%).

cellular plasma membrane or even the cytoplasm contents including proteins will affect the absorption and scattering behaviour of RBC. Therefore, it is expected that a better image contrast should be obtained with S2 compared with S3, as observed in Figures 13.57 and 13.53b. In fact, it has been suggested (Gershfeld and Murayama 1988) that change of the optothermal properties of blood due to decrease of osmolarity changes the shape of the erythrocytes due to higher optical absorption. Based on this fact and on the fact that the cross–sectional area of an RBC, $\sigma_c(\bar{u}, \bar{X})$, depends on the shape of the cells interacting with light and the shape factor $S(\bar{q})$, see Eq. (13.48), the lower PA amplitude of S3 than S2, Figure 13.53b, can be better understood, i.e., higher rates of optical absorption and heat transfer to the surrounding medium may have a direct impact on the structural integrity and the optical properties of RBCs. The basis of this fact goes back to 1865 when Schultz reported for the first time the morphological changes induced by heating cells when microspherocytosis and fragmentation were observed. Since then much research has confirmed this thermo-biological effect. One related issue of interest is the deformation of RBCs irradiated with laser power and the consequences of laser irradiation in biomedical applications (Karle 1969, Sarj et al. 2010). Thus, the amount of Au NPs which can be used to enhance the PA signal is a decisive factor and must be optimized. In our case, this is clearly shown by the higher Au NP concentration (S3) which generated a lower PA signal due to probably irreversible cellular thermal damage. The heating efficiency of Au NPs is defined as (Pustovalov et al. 2010)

$$\xi_H = \Delta T_0/F \tag{13.64}$$

where $\Delta T_0 = T_{max} - T_i$ and $T_{max} \approx P/4\pi R_g K_m$. In fact, ξ_H determines the increase of particle temperature under the action of laser irradiation and depends on NP density, the thermal properties of the surrounding medium (in this case, blood), and chirp duration. Using the laser power, $P = 1.6$ W in our experiment, Eq. (13.62) yields, $\xi_H \approx 4.39 \times 10^6/I\tau_c \approx 8.78/\tau_c$ where $I \approx 500$ kWcm^{-2} for a 2-mm laser spot size. Figure 13.61 shows the variation of heating efficiency with chirp duration which is found to decrease rapidly for chirp durations longer than 1 ms. For durations $\tau_c > \tau_r (\approx R_g^2 c_g \rho_g/3K_m)$ the heat loss from NPs via heat conduction during the time τ_c is rate limiting to the attainment of maximum temperature in the blood-NP mixture.

The maximum efficiency of heat transformation into acoustic pressure is given by (Zangandeh et al. 2013)

$$\xi_a = P(t)/F = (\eta_{abs} R_g^2 \rho_m \beta_g/4r\rho_g c_g \tau_p) \tag{13.65}$$

where ρ_m is the density of the surrounding medium, β_g is the effective thermal expansion coefficient of the Au NP material, r is the distance of the observation point from the source and $f(t)$ is a function defining the time dependence of the laser radiation intensity. Equation (13.60) shows that the pulsed PA signal at the onset $t = 0$ will increase by increasing the Au NP concentration, but it is also possible that agglomeration and cluster formation affects the interaction which effectively increases the attenuation at later times

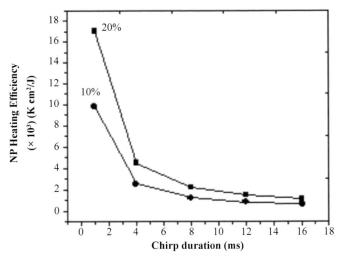

Figure 13.61. Change of Au NPs thermal efficiency with chirp duration for S2 (10%) and S3 (20%).

t > 0. Indeed, it has been shown that the PA signal increase with NP concentration may be explained in terms of clustering due to thermal overlapping, which is greater than when the NPs are monodispersed or are less clustered (Bayer et al. 2013, Khosroshahi et al. 2014). However, Roper et al. (2007) have shown that modulating the incident laser irradiation increases NP efficiency of acoustic transduction in an aqueous solution more than two orders of magnitude compared with an unmodulated cw argon laser, and that modulation can decrease NP-NP aggregation: decreasing the chopping frequency lowers the efficiency ξ_a. Therefore, the rate of modulation should be much higher than the NP-NP interaction frequency in order to increase the efficiency, ξ_a. Bearing in mind that the diffusion time constant for coagulative interactions between neighboring Au NPs using the Stokes-Einstein diffusivity, is ≈ 0.35 ms (i.e., ≈ 2.8 kHz). Between consecutive chopped pulses, NP temperatures relax rapidly within ≈ 27–79 ps. Therefore, when laser light is chopped, NP-NP interactions are less likely to cause aggregation. As a result, decreasing the chopping frequency decreases the transduction efficiency.

13.7.2 The effect of laser power on photothermoacoustic imaging of blood containing gold nanoparticles and deoxygenation using a frequency-domain phased array probe: An in vitro assay (Khosroshahi et al. 2015)

Imaging modality has a significant impact on clinical applications such as cancer diagnosis and therapy. We describe the *in vitro* results of imaging of different samples of blood only (S1), blood containing gold nanoparticles (Au NPs, S2) and deoxygenated blood (S5) using radar-based photoacoustic imaging (PARI) technique. The results showed that lower concentration Au NPs (S2) produces higher PA signals compared with the higher concentration sample (S3). After the optimization of concentration, three samples of S1, S2, and S5 were selected for the imaging experiment. The PA signal amplitudes in all samples increased linearly up to 2.5 W in the order of S5 > S2 > S1 from there onwards the signals decreased sharply. The cellular deformation time of S1 was found to be faster than S2 and S5, but from 2.5 W afterwards S1 and S2 showed the same rate of decrease. The increase of signals in S1, S2, and S5 are thought to be due to hemoglobin, surface plasmon resonance (SPR)-induced heating effect and release of choleoglobin and carboxyhemoglobin like oxidation products, respectively. The consistent decrease in the signal amplitudes, however, at higher power levels is mainly attributed to the change of the thermo-optical properties of blood leading to decrease of the blood osmolarity due to temperature increase and hence causing irreversible deformability resulting in thermo-hemolysis of red blood cells (RBCs) which eventually degraded the photoacoustic signals.

Materials and methods

Materials preparation

The preparation method is as described in § 13.7.1 above, except that in this case, a total of five samples were prepared as follows: S1(blood only), S2 (blood + 10% (3.8 µg/mL) Au NPs), S3 (blood + 20% (7.6 µg/mL) Au NPs), S4 (Au NPs only), and S5 (de-oxygenated blood). For sample S2 (10%) a ratio of 0.5:0.05 mL of blood: NPs was used and for sample S3 (20%) the amount of NPs was doubled giving a total volume of 0.6 mL. The number of NPs (volume × concentration) and the corresponding concentration, S2 (10%), using 0.05 mL of Au were calculated as 196×10^6 and 345×10^6 (N/mL), respectively. Similarly for S3 (20%) using 0.1 mL of Au, the values of 380×10^6 and 633×10^6 (N/mL) were obtained. All samples were safely mounted next to each other with 5 mm separation inside a saline solution container 50 mm below the water surface and irradiated with laser light. The experiment consisted of two parts: (i) optimization of Au NPs concentration, and (ii) to study the effect of laser power on imaging using S1, S2 (optimized Au NP sample) and S5. To prepare the sample S5, sodium dithionate ($Na_2S_2O_4$) crystalline powder with a weak sulfurous odor which is most common and convenient reagent for the deoxygenation was used. The sample was prepared according to Oraevsky et al. (2002) by adding $Na_2S_2O_4$ to blood sample (S1) with the ratio of 0.02 mg/mL which corresponds to $\approx 80\%$ of O_2 (i.e., 20% deoxygenation) and the final product appeared darker compared to S1 and S2.

Experimental

The experimental setup is similar to that shown in Figure 13.51. Here, a 3 mm diameter silicone rubber tube was used to mimic a blood vessel in the physiological saline container. For the first part of the experiment, where the tube was linearly scanned with 0.5 mm step and the back scattered pressure waves were detected by a focused transducer (V305, Olympus NDT Inc., Panametrics) with a center frequency at 2.25 MHz, 18.8 mm element diameter, a focal length of 25 mm, and beam width of approximately 0.9 mm. For the second part, the imaging was performed using a 64-elements plane phase array (Ultrasonics) with a central frequency of 3 MHz and a sampling rate of 60 MHz/s with high lateral resolution. The returning PA signals were received by the various elements or groups of elements and then processed by the instrument software. Each received signal represents the reflection from a particular angular component of the beam or from a particular focal depth. The distance between the samples and the transducer immersed in water was kept at about 25 mm. In the NIR (≈ 700 nm) region, blood has an absorption coefficient $\alpha_b \approx 7$ cm^{-1} corresponding to an optical penetration depth of about 1.4 mm. Depending on the type of silicone rubber, the acoustic impedance, Z, ranges between $(1.1–1.5) \times 10^6$ kg m^{-2} s^{-1}. Blood has an acoustic impedance of about 1.60×10^6 kg m^{-2} s^{-1}. Therefore, the amplitude reflection at the tube wall-blood interface varies between (0.1–3.4)%. Data acquisition and signal processing were performed using Lab View software.

Results

Based on the results given in Figure 13.53, the sample S2 was chosen as an optimized gold containing blood sample. The spectrum decomposes the content of a stochastic process into different frequencies present in that process, and helps identify periodicities. The corresponding PAR-PSD for S2 is shown in Figure 13.55a, where it can be seen that the PA signal is dominated by low frequency components. In the low frequency range, the PA response is affected only by the mixture of blood and NPs, so it does not reflect the individual signature of each component. The main feature in the case of PAR is that there is no frequency content above the main peak frequency and the information is completely concentrated within the 300–800 kHz which exhibits the strongest power signal. The next stage was to perform PAI of S1, S2, and S5 and to compare the results. As it is seen from Figure 13.62, S1 showed a very weak acoustic response at 1.5 W, but at higher power a relatively weak signal was detected and the image was barely visualized, as we can see from the encircled region.

In the case of S2 (Blood + Au NPs) in Figure 13.63, however, the PA signals were clearly enhanced which corresponds to a better image of blood tube containing Au NPs. As it is observable, the image

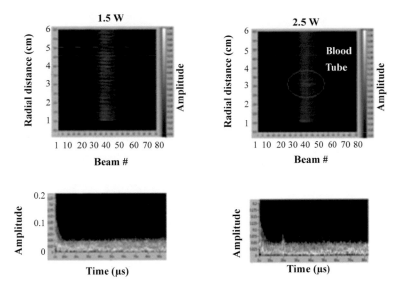

Figure 13.62. Phase array PA images of S1 at different powers with the corresponding acoustic signal amplitudes.

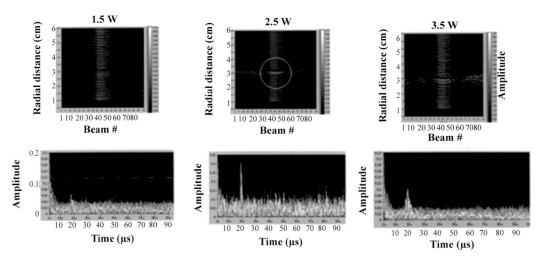

Figure 13.63. Phase array PA images of S2 at different powers with the corresponding acoustic signal amplitudes.

quality or the resolution improved by increasing the power up to 2.5 W but beyond this power level, the signal decreased and hence the quality of image was correspondingly degraded.

As Figure 13.64 shows, a similar trend to S2 was also observed in the case of S5 (blood + $Na_2S_2O_4$) but at higher signal levels. This is in agreement with the fact that deoxygenated hemoglobin has a local maximum about 10 cm^{-1} at around 760 nm (Briley and Bjornerud 2000). Again, a non-linear behaviour was repeated after 2.5 W which will be discussed later.

Figure 13.65 illustrates the change of PA signal amplitude with increase of laser power for different blood samples in the order of S5 > S2> S1. Clearly, all samples demonstrated a consistent behaviour where the PA signal maximizes at 2.5 W and beyond that it gradually decreases. The increase is almost negligible for S1 as it is expected from blood as a relatively weak absorbing medium at 800 nm. However, it is significant for S2 and S5. There are number of significant observations regarding Fig. 13.65 in that the trend of curves appears to be a Gaussian-type shape with almost similar symmetrical distribution with a peak representing the maximum signal amplitude. Also, all curves exhibited a maximum point at the same laser power (2.5 W) which statistically implies that the probability density function of such occurrence

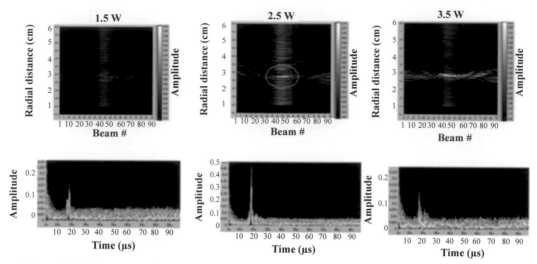

Figure 13.64. Phase array PA images of S5 at different powers with the corresponding acoustic signal amplitudes.

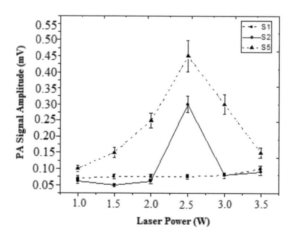

Figure 13.65. Variation of PA signal amplitudes with laser power for S1, S2, and S5.

is meaningful. The full width half maximum is correlated to standard deviation and narrower the width the closer it is to the central point. In our case, S2 is narrower than S5 with corresponding lower standard deviation, σ, (i.e., $\sigma_{S2} \approx 9.5\% \ll \sigma_{S5} \approx 13\%$).

Discussion

The first and foremost important issue to be emphasized is the interaction process of nanoparticles with RBCs. In a biological medium, NPs; particularly colloidal NPs; can undergo an interaction process with biomolecules such as proteins, nucleic acids, lipids due to their nano-size and significant surface-to volume ratio. Among these, the adsorption of proteins to NP surface is particularly important, since it results in the formation of NP-protein complex which is known as "NP-protein corona". Proteins as polypeptides with a defined conformation have a net surface charge which depends on the pH of the surrounding medium. The pH value is a key environmental factor, especially in chemical and biomedical systems. Any value above 7.0 is considered as alkaline and below that is acidic. A healthy blood pH without cancer has acid + alkaline balance almost equal. It affects the dissociation of functional groups on the surface of self-assembled monolayers, consequently changes in the pH will result in changes of gold particle coverage.

In fact it has been shown that the nanoparticle surface coverage and the spectral position of LSPR are both highly dependent on pH, i.e., it was red shifted by increasing the pH (Park et al. 2006, Saptarshi et al. 2013).

Adsorption of proteins at nano-bio level occurs mainly by forces such as hydrogen bonds and Van der Waals interactions. Physical interactions of Au NPs with physiological fluids, e.g., blood plasma can change their physiochemical properties such as size, aggregation, and surface charge area. High ionic strength solutions are known to cause Au NPs aggregation due to electrostatic screening (Zhu et al. 2014). The longetivity of the NP-protein interaction depends on the rate of association or dissociation of proteins from the surface. Equally, it is important to note that NP-protein interaction process is subject to change even in a given medium due to changing rate of adsorption and desorption of proteins from the NP surface. Thus, such a process is dynamic where proteins with higher binding affinity for the surface can occupy the surface more than those with lower affinity. Regardless of different types of endocytosis mechanism, NPs may also enter cells by passive penetration of the cell membrane. Since RBCs lack endocytosis mechanism hence a passive transport or diffusion takes place after NPs are built at the surface of cell membrane.

Photoacoustic imaging contrast which is based on optical absorption properties of tissue and the underlying molecular composition is a suitable modality for molecular imaging. In this paper, the use of linearly frequency modulated diode laser and a plane FD-phase array was used for imaging blood tubes at different conditions. The analysis shows that since, the optical penetration depth in blood, δ_0 (1.4 mm at 800 nm) $\approx \varphi_r$, where $\varphi_r = 1$ mm is the beam radius, and $X_T \ll 2\varphi_r$, where X_T is the thermal diffusion length in blood, $X_T \approx (4D_b\tau_p)^{1/2}$, and D_b is the thermal diffusivity of blood then the PA source in blood can be assumed to be spherical and 1-D model can be used. Using $D_b \approx 1.38 \times 10^{-3}$ cm^{2}s^{-1} (Duck 1990), $X_T \approx 23$ μm and ≈ 47 μm for $\tau_p = 1$ and 4 ms, respectively. Also, the values for blood thermal relaxation time, $\tau_r \approx \delta_0^2/4D_b \approx 3.6$ s and the acoustic transient time, $\tau_c = \delta_0/c_a \approx 890$ ns. Since in our case, $\alpha_b c_a \ll \omega_{im}$ and ω_{fm}, $\alpha_b X_T \ll 1$ and $\tau_c \ll \tau_r$, and $\tau_c \gg \tau_a$ where ω_{im} and ω_{fm} are initial and final angular modulation frequencies, α_b is blood absorption coefficient, it can be deduced that S1 is effectively a weakly absorbing medium which satisfies thermal but not acoustic confinement. However, when Au NPs are added to blood, the situation begins to reverse and the medium becomes strongly absorbing, i.e., $\alpha_c c_a \gg \omega_{im}$ and ω_{fm}, $\alpha_c X_T \gg 1$. Figure 13.66 indicates the X_T values for a 0.3–2.6-MHz chirps using $X_T \approx (2D_c/\omega_m)^{1/2}$, where Dc is thermal diffusivity of the combined volume fraction (blood and Au NPs). As it is seen, the thermal length decreases with increasing the modulation frequency and it increases with chirp duration. The analysis showed that almost 75% of thermal diffusion takes place between 0.3–1 MHz.

Initially, the interaction of a laser pulse with a relatively weakly absorbing heterogeneous medium, such as blood, containing a suspension of strongly absorbing nanoparticles generates a heating effect which is quickly equilibrated within the NP ensemble. Subsequently, the heat generated is transferred from the NPs to the surrounding medium or matrix (blood) via non-radiative relaxation within a few ps. In the absence of phase transformations, heat transfer in a system with NP thermal sources is described by Eq. (13.56). Thus, the interaction of a laser pulse with a relatively weakly absorbing heterogeneous medium, such as blood, containing a suspension of strongly absorbing nanoparticles generates a PA signal

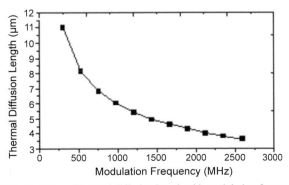

Figure 13.66. Variation of thermal diffusion length with modulation frequency for S2.

enhancement effect. While the absorber is the NPs, the signal propagates in by the surrounding fluid and heat transfer defines the signal generation process. Therefore, the produced acoustic signal is proportional to the amount of energy deposited into the NPs and the thermoelastic properties of the environment. According to Eq. (13.68), the absorption of optical chirp energy by the medium results in the generation of similar-frequency-modulated acoustic waves propagating within the medium. The quantitative PAI in the presence of nanoparticles is a function of the response of the PA signal (maximum signal voltage, V_{max}) amplitude given as a function of independent responses from single particles, the wavelength-dependent optical σ_{abs}, the number of nanoparticles (N_{NP}), and the deposited energy ($\sigma_{abs}F$). The PA signal dependence relationship is given as (Cook et al. 2013)

$$V_{max} - V_0 \; \Gamma_{eff} \sigma_{abs} N_{NP} F \tag{13.66}$$

where $\Gamma_{eff} = \dfrac{\beta c_a^2}{C_p}$ is the effective Grüneisen constant for a given NP type, β is the volume thermal expansion,

C_p is the specific heat, and V_0 is the PA signal from any endogenous absorbers such as whole blood defined by product of, α_b, and optical fluence, F (Cox et al. 2009).

$$V_0 = \Gamma_t \alpha_b F \exp -\left(\alpha_b c_a t\right) \tag{13.67}$$

Here $\alpha_b = \varepsilon_{Hb}(\lambda)[Hb] + \varepsilon_{HbO2}(\lambda)[HbO_2]$, Hb and HbO_2 are the relative hemoglobin and oxyhemoglobin concentrations, ε_{Hb} and ε_{HbO} are the corresponding molar extinction coefficients (Hu and Wang 2010). If, however, V_0 is negligible then V_{max} is due to NPs only. As for the role of sodium dithionate, it is used to dissociate dioxygen from HbO_2 in erythrocytes by removing the external O_2 rather than diffusion into the RBCs (Dalziel and O'Brian 1954). The RBC color depends on the state of the hemoglobin: when combined with oxygen the resulting oxyhemoglobin is scarlet, and when oxygen has been released the resulting deoxyhemoglobin is dark red in color, and can appear bluish through the vessel wall and skin. It has been known that the action of oxygen on the Hb in $Na_2S_2O_4$ solution results in the formation of choleglobin-like oxidation products with increased light absorption in red and decreased absorption at shorter wavelengths (Lemberg et al. 1941). An unstable oxidation product of $Na_2S_2O_4$ is hydrogen peroxide which reacts with several haem pigments. If HbO_2 is reduced by $Na_2S_2O_4$ and then converted into carboxyhemoglobin the absorption spectrum of the product shows greater absorption in the red (Dalziel and O'Brian 1954). This may explain the reason for the higher PA signal produced by absorption of 800 nm photons by S5 in Figure 13.67. In fact, the rate of dissociation of HbO_2 in the presence of $Na_2S_2O_4$ may indicate that it has a direct effect on the pigment and modifies the kinetics of the dissociation. In any case, it is important to note that the extinction coefficient of $Na_2S_2O_4$ is strongly dependent on time and it has been shown that the deoxygenation takes place less than one minute and then extinction coefficient rapidly increases (Dalziel and O'Brian 1957). The maximum efficacy of heat transformation into acoustic pressure is given by (Pustovalov et al. 2010).

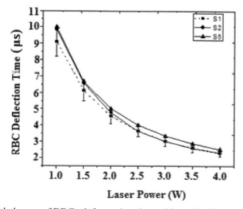

Figure 13.67. Calculated change of RBCs deformation time with applied laser power for S1, S2, and S5.

$$\xi_a = P(t) / I_0 = (C_T/d_t.A) V/I_0 \tag{13.68}$$

$$\xi_a \propto V/I_0 \tag{13.69}$$

where P(t) is the pressure amplitude, I_0 is the intensity, C_T is the element total capacitance, d_t is the strain constant, A is the irradiated area and V is the measured voltage. Using the corresponding values of the signal amplitudes at peak value of 2.5 W in each case, see Figure 13.67, the relation (13.69) yields the approximate values of 0.9×10^{-6}, 3.8×10^{-6} and 5.6×10^{-6} V cm^2 W^{-1} for S1, S2, and S5, respectively. From practical clinical point of view it is however, important to consider when and why the PA signal amplitude decreases which subsequently affects the imaging quality. There could be number of reasons for such a behaviour namely thermal damage of erythrocytes. It is well known that any modification of cellular plasma membrane or even the cytoplasm contents including the proteins will affect the absorption and scattering behaviour of RBC. One of the main channels through which the PA signal can be influenced is temperature which directly affects the biomechanical and thermal properties of RBCs and their integrity. An increase in the temperature weakens the structure of the cell membrane. When the temperature reaches to a critical point where an irreversible thermal damage is unavoidable, hemolysis occurs where the cell membrane ruptures by the phospholipids breaking down to produce pores in the membrane through which the contents are released. However, it is also suggested (Greshfeld 1986) that even at moderate temperatures a mechanism based on the concept of the critical bilayer assembly temperature of the cell membrane accounts for hemolysis. Echinocytosis, which is an indicator for morphological change, is a characteristic of RBC thermal damage frequently used for this purpose. It was shown that one of the earliest morphological manifestation of RBC following heat injury is their transformation from disc to spherical shape (Barr and Arrwsmith 1970). Other approach of analysis is the ray optics which deals with the deformability of cells. This approach is valid only when the size of a biological object is much larger than the laser wavelength, i.e., $2\pi r_c/\lambda \approx 27.5 >> 1$ where $r_c \approx 3.5 \times 10^{-6}$ m is RBC radius such as in our case.

When the RBCs are at rest or at very small shear rates, they tend to aggregate and stack together in an energetically favorable manner. The attraction is attributed to charged groups on the surface of cells and to the presence of fibrinogen and globulins (Pirkl and Bonder 2010). Based on the fact light carries momentum, so whenever a ray of light is reflected or refracted at an interface between media with different refractive indices, changing direction or velocity, its momentum is transferred from the light to the interface and by Newton's law a force is exerted on the interface. As a result a transient cell deformation occurs until elastic forces balance the applied optical forces unless the applied load exceeds and the cell membrane ruptures. The characteristic time, t_c, for cellular deformation is defined as (Lubarda and Manzani 2009)

$$t_c = \mu_c c\, r_c^2 / n_m QP \tag{13.70}$$

where, $F_o = n_m\, PQ/c \tag{13.71}$

Here μ_b, F_o, n_m, Q, c are respectively, the viscosity of blood $\approx (3-4) \times 10^{-3}$ Pa.s (Ihab et al. 2010), optical force, refractive index of medium; for blood only $n_b = 1.42$, for $n_{b+Au} = 1.32$ and $n_{b+Na2} = 1.29$ determined as volume fraction, the factor that describes the amount of momentum transferred (Q = 1 for absorbing medium), and the speed of light in vacuum (3×10^8 m s^{-1}).

Figure 13.67 indicates, as it is expected, that by increasing the laser power, the deformation time decreases, implying that the RBC will be damaged faster and is found in the order of S5 > S2 > S1, i.e., in our case, S1 reaches the damage point first at the peak value of 2.5 W. In general, the exact temperature for the onset of cell necrosis is rather difficult to determine not only the temperature achieved, but also the temporal duration of this temperature, which plays a significant role for the induction of irreversible damage. However, for a quantitative approximation of remaining active molecules or cells at a certain temperature level, one can use the well known Arrhenius equation:

$$\ln \frac{C(t)}{C(0)} = -A \int_0^t \exp (\Delta E/RT\, (t')\, dt' \equiv 0 \tag{13.72}$$

where C_0 is the initial concentration of cells, $C(t)$ is the concentration at a time t, A is Arrhenius constant, R is the universal gas constant and $\Delta E \approx kT/h \exp \Delta S/R$ is the activation energy and Ω is specific tissue property, ΔS is the activation entropy, k is Boltzmann's constant, and h is Planck's constant. The local degree of damage defined by the damage integral given in Eq. 10 is the fraction of deactivated cells

$$C_d(t) = \frac{C_0 - C(t)}{C_0} = 1 - \exp(\Omega) \qquad (13.73)$$

Thus, by inserting an appropriate value of the tissue constant, one is able to calculate the probable damage degree $C_d(t)$ as a function of time. Since there are different mechanisms which can cause the cellular damage namely: photochemical, photothermal, photoablation, and photodisruption; it thus requires a further investigation to determine carefully the nature of damage and independently in each given case. However, considering our experimental conditions and optical parameters, it is suggested that the decrease in PA signal observed in Figure 13.67 after the peak point is probably due to opto-thermal irreversible damage or thermohemolysis. In other words, increasing the temperature can decrease the blood osmolarity, hence causing thermo-hemolysis of erythrocytes, which in effect, degrades the photoacoustic signals.

Keywords: Bioimaging, Multimodal imaging, Multifunctional agents, SPION, PAMAM dendrimers, Fluorescence, Fluorescence microscopy, Fluorescence spectroscopy, Cytotoxicity, Uptake, Therapy, Hybrid nanostructure, MTT assay, MRI contrast agent, Photothermoacoustic, Ultrasound, Diode laser, Frequency-domain, Gold nanoparticles, Blood, Thermo-hemostasis, Blood osmolarity.

Reference

Aggarwal, P., J. Hall, C. McLeland, M. Dobrovolskaia and S. McNeil. 2009. Nanoparticle interaction with plasma proteins as it relates to particle biodistribution, biocompatibility and therapeutic efficacy. Adv. Drug Del. Rev. 61: 428–437.

Akers, W., C. Kim and M. Berezin. 2010. Non-invasive photoacoustic fluorescent sentinel lymph node identification using dye-loaded perfluorocarbon nanoparticles. ACS Nano 5: 173–182.

Alanagh, H., M.E. Khosroshahi, M. Tajabadi and H. Keshvari. 2014. The Effect of pH and magnetic field on the fluorescence spectra of fluorescein isothiocyanate conjugated SPION-dendrimer nanocomposites. J. Supercond. Nov. Magn. 27: 2337–2345.

Antharjanam, P., M. Jaseer, K.K. Ragi and E. Prasad. 2009. Intrinsic luminescence properties of ionic liquid crystals based on PAMAM and PPI dendrimers. J. Photoch. Photobio. A 203: 50–55.

Arias, J., V. Gallardo, S. Gómez-Lopera, R. Plaza and A. Delgado. 2001. Synthesis and characterization of poly(ethyl-2-cyanoacrylate) nanoparticles with a magnetic core. J. Cont. Rel. 77: 309–321.

Baba-ahmad, L., M. Benmouna and M. Grimson. 1987. Elastic scattering from charged colloidal dispersions. J. Phys. Chem. 16: 235–238.

Bao, G., S. Mitragotri and Sh. Tong. 2013. Multifunctional Nanoparticles for Drug Delivery and Molecular Imaging. 15: 253–282.

Baffou, G., R. Quidant and C. Girard. 2009. Heat generation in plasmonic nanostructures: influence of morphology. Appl. Phy. Lett. 94: 153109.

Baffou, G., R. Quidant and F. García de Abajo. 2010. Nanoscale control of optical heating in complex plasmonic systems. ACS Nano 4: 709–716.

Baffou, G. and H. Rigneault. 2011. Femtosecond-pulsed optical heating of gold nanoparticles. Physical Rev. B. 84: 035415.

Baffou, G. and R. Quidant. 2013. Thermo-plasmonics: using metallic nanostructures as nano-sources of heat. Laser Photonics Rev. 7: 171–187.

Balogh, L., R. Valluzzi, K. Laverdure, S. Gido, G. Hagnauer and D. Tomalia. 1999. Formation of silver and gold dendrimer nanocomposites. J. Nanopart. Res. 1. 353–368.

Baraga, J., R. Rava and P. Taroni. 1990. Laser induced fluorescence spectroscopy of normal and atherosclerotic human aorta using 306–310 nm excitation. Lasers Surg. Med. 10: 245–261.

Barnett, C., M. Gueorguieva and M. Lees. 2013. Physical stability, biocompatibility and potential use of hybrid iron oxide-gold nanoparticles as drug carriers. J. Nanopart. Res. 15: 1706–1720.

Barr, S. and D. Arrwsmith. 1970. Thermal damage of red cells. J. Clin. Path. 23: 572–576.

Bayer, C., S. Nam, Y. Chen and S. Emelianov. 2013. Photoacoustic signal amplification through plasmonic nanoparticle aggregation. J. Biomed. Opt. 18: 016001.

Baykal, A., M. Toprak, Z. Durmus, M. Senel, H. Sozeri and A. Demir. 2012. Synthesis and characterization of dendrimer-encapsulated iron and iron-oxide nanoparticles. J. of Superconductivity and Novel Mag. 25: 1541–1549.

Beard, P. 2002. Photoacoustic imaging of blood vessel equivalent phantoms. SPIE Proc. 4618: 54–64.

Berer, T., E. Holzinger and A. Hochreiner. 2015. Multimodal noncontact photoacoustic and optical coherence tomography imaging using wavelength-division multiplexing. J. Biomed. Opt. 046013–1.

Berry, C. and A. Curties. 2003. Functionalization of magnetic nanoparticles for applications in biomedicine. J. Phys. D: Appl. Phys. 36: 198–206.

Biswal, B., M. Kavitha, R. Verma and E. Prasad. 2009. Tumor cell imaging using the intrinsic emission from PAMAM dendrimer: a case study with HeLa cells. Cytotechnology 61: 17–24.

Briley, K. and A. Bjornerud. 2000. Accurate de-oxygenation of *ex vivo* whole blood using sodium dithionate. Proc. Int. Soc. Mag. Reson. Med. 8: 2025–2026.

Brindle, K. 2003. Molecular imaging using magnetic resonance: new tools for the development of tumour therapy. British J. Radiolog. 76: S111–S117.

Brindle, K. 2008. New approaches to imaging tumour responses to treatment. Nature Rev. Cancer. 8: 94–107.

Bronstein, L. and L. Shifrina. 2011. Dendrimers as encapsulating, stabilizing, or direction agents for inorganic nanoparticles. Chem. Rev. 111: 5301–5344.

Burt, J. and K. Ebeling. 1980. Observation of the optoacoustic effect in an optical fibre. Optics Communications. 32: 159–162.

Bushnell, J. and D. Mc Closley. 1968. Thermoelastic stress production in solids. J. Appl. Phys. 39: 5541–5546.

Carome, E., N. Clark and C. Moeller. 1964. Generation of acoustic signal in liquids by ruby-induced thermal stress transients. Appl. Phys. Lett. 4: 95–497.

Cha, E., E. Jang and I. Sun. 2011. Development of MRI/NIR fluorescence activable multimodal imaging probe based on iron oxide nanoparticles. J. Cont. Rel. 155: 152–158.

Caminade, A., R. Laurent and J. Mjoral. 2005. Characterization of dendrimers. Adv. Drug Del. Rev. 57: 2130–2146.

Cleary, S.F. 1977. Laser pulses and the generation of acoustic transients in biological material laser. pp. 175–219. *In*: M.L. Wolbarsht (ed.). Applications in Medicine and Biology. Plenum Press, New York, USA.

Chardon, D. and S. Huard. 1982. Thermal diffusivity of optical fibre measured by photoacoustics. Appl. Phys. Lett. 41: 341–342.

Cherry, S. 2009. Multimodality imaging: beyond PET/CT and SPECT/CT. Semin. Nucl. Med. 39: 348–353.

Choi, S., A. Myc, J. Silpe, M. Sumit, P. Wong and K. McCarthy. 2012. Dendrimer-based multivalent vancomycin nanoplatform for targeting the drug-resistant bacterial surface. ACS Nano 7: 214–228.

Cook, J., W. Frey and S. Emeilanov. 2013. Quantitative photoacoustic imaging of nanoparticles in cells and tissues. ACSN nano 7: 1272–1280.

Chou, C. and H. Lien. 2011. Dendrimer-conjugated magnetic nanoparticles for removal of zinc (II) from aqueous solutions. J. Nanopart. Res. 13: 2099–2107.

Corot, C., P. Robert, J. Idee and M. Port. 2006. Recent advances in iron oxide nanocrystal technology for medical imaging. Adv. Drug Del. 58: 1471–1504.

Cornell, R. and U. Schwertmn. 2003. The Iron Oxides: Structure, Properties, Reactions, Occurences and Uses. Wiley-VCH.

Coussios, C. 2002. The significance of shape and orientation in single-particle weak-scattering Models. J. Acoust. Soc. Am. 112: 906–915.

Cox, B., J. Laufer and P. Beard. 2009. The challenges for quantitative photoacoustic imaging. Proc. SPIE. 177: 717713.

Cross, F.W., R. Al-Dhahir, P.E. Dyer and A. Mac Robert. 1987. Time resolved photoacoustic studies of vascular tissue ablation at three laser wavelengths. Appl. Phys. Lett. 50: 1019–1021.

Cross, F.W., R. Al-Dhahir and P.E. Dyer. 1988. Ablative and acoustic response of a pulsed UV laser irradiated vascular tissue in a liquid environment. J. Appl. Phys. 64: 2194–2200.

Dalziel, K. and J. O'Brian. 1954. Spectrophotometric studies of the reaction of methaemoglobin with hydrogen peroxide. 1. The formation of methaemoglobin-hydrogen peroxide. Biochem. J. 56: 648–659.

Dalziel, K. and J. O'Brian. 1957. Side reactions in the deoxygenation of dilute oxyghaemoglobin solution by sodium dithionate. Biochem. J. 67: 119–125.

Dan, W., L. Huang, M. Jiang and H. Jiang. 2014. Contrast agents for photoacoustic and thermoacoustic imaging: a review. Mol. Sci. 15: 23616–23639.

Denora, N., V. Laquintana and A. Lopalco. 2013. *In vitro* targeting and imaging the translocator protein TSPO 18-kDa through G(4)-PAMAM-FITC labeled dendrimer. J. Cont. Rel. 172: 1111–1125.

Derjaguin, B. and L. Landau. 1941. Theory of the stability of strongly charged lyophobic sols and of the adhesion of strongly charged particles in solution of electrolytes. Acta Physicochim. URSS 14: 633–662.

Diaci, J. and J. Mozina. 1992. A study of blast wave forms detected simultaneously by microphone and a laser probe during laser ablation. Appl. Phys. A 55: 84–93.

Divsar, F., A. Nomani, M. Chaloosi and I. Haririan. 2009. Synthesis and characterization of gold nanocomposites with modified and intact polyamidoamine dendrimers. Microchimica Acta. 165: 421–426.

Dolvoich, M. and R. Labiris. 2004. Imaging drug delivery and drug responses in the lung. Proc. Am. Thorac. 1: 329–337.

Dou, H., H. Tao and K. Sun. 2008. Interfacial coprecipitation to prepare magnetite nanoparticles: concentration and temperature dependence. Colloids Surf. A 320: 115–122.

Drizlikh, S., A. Zur and F. Moser. 1991. Microwave warming of biological tissue and its control by IR fibre thermometry. Optical Fibres in Medicine VI SPIE. 142: 53–63.

Duck, F. 1990. Physical Properties of Tissue: A Comprehensive Reference Book. Academic Press Inc., San Diago.

Dussán, K., O. Giraldo and C. Cardona. 2007. Application of magnetic nanostructures in biotechnological processes: biodiesel production using lipase immobilized on magnetic carriers. Eur. Cong. Chem. Eng. (ECCE-6), Copenhagen.

Dyer, P.E. and R. Srinivasan. 1986. Nanosecond photoacoustic studies on ultraviolet laser ablation of organic polymers. Appl. Phys. Lett. 48: 445–447.

Dyer, P.E. 1988. Nanosecond photoacoustic studies of UV laser ablation of polymers and biological materials. pp. 164–174. *In*: P. Hess and P. Pezel (eds.). Photoacoustic and Photothermal Phenomena. Springer Verlag, Heidelberg.

Dyer, P.E. and R. Srinivasan. 1989. Nanosecond photoacoustic studies an ultraviolet laser ablation of organic polymer. Appl. Phys. Lett. 48: 445–447.

Dyer, P.E., M.E. Khosroshahi and S. Tuft. 1993. Studies of laser-induced cavitation and tissue ablation in saline using a fibre delivered pulsed HF laser. Appl. B. 56: 84–93.

Ekkapongpisit, M., A. Giovia, C. Follo, G. Caputo and C. Isidoro. 2012. Biocompatibility, endocytosis, and intracellular trafficking of mesoporous silica and polystyrene nanoparticles in ovarian cancer cells: effects of size and surface charge groups. Int. J. Nanomed. 7: 4147–4158.

El-Sayed, M., M. Ginski, C. Rhodes and H. Ghandehari. 2002. Transepithelial transport of poly (amidoamine) dendrimers across Caco-2 cell monolayers. J. Cont. Rel. 81: 355–365.

Esenaliev, R., A. Karabutov and A. Oraevsky. 1999. Sensitivity of laser opto-acoustic imaging in detection of small deeply embedded tumors. IEEE J. Quan. Elect. 5: 981–988.

Esfanda, R. and D. Tomalia. 2001. Poly (amidoamine) (PAMAM) dendrimers: from biomimicry to drug delivery and biomedical applications. Drug Discovery Today 6: 427–436.

Esumi, K., A. Suzuki, A. Yamahira and K. Torigoe. 2000. Role of poly(amidoamine) dendrimers for preparing nanoparticles of gold, platinum, and silver. Langmuir. 16: 2604–2608.

Esumi, K., H. Houdatsu and T. Yoshimur. 2004. Antioxidant action by gold-PAMAM dendrimer nanocomposites. Langmuir. 20: 2536–2538.

Esumi, K., T. Matsumoto, Y. Seto and T. Yoshimura. 2005. Preparation of gold-gold/silver-dendrimer nanocomposites in the presence of benzoin in ethanol by UV irradiation. J. Colloid Interf. Sci. 284: 199–203.

Etchegoin, P., E. Le Ru and M. Meyer. 2006. An analytic model for the optical properties of gold. J. Chem. Phys. 125: 164705.

Falsa, B., A. Rachida, A. Boussaid, M. Benmouna and R. Benmouna. 2011. Heating of biological tissues by gold nanoparticles: effects of particle size and distribution. J. Biomat. Nanotech. 2: 49–54.

Falanga, A., R. Tarallo, E. Galdiero, M. Cantisani and J. Nanophot. 2013. Review of a Viral Peptide Nanosystem for Intracellular Delivery 7: 071599.

Faiyas, A., E. Vinod, J. Joseph, R. Ganesan and R. Pandey. 2009. Dependence of pH and surfactant effect in the synthesis of magnetite (Fe_3O_4) nanoparticles and its properties. J. Mag. Mag. Mat. 322: 400–404.

Fan, Y., A. Mandelis, G. Spiro and A. Vitkin. 2004. Development of a laser photothermoacoustic frequency-swept system for subsurface imaging: theory and experiment. J. Acoust. Soc. Am. 116: 3523–3533.

Feme, C. 2005. Role of imaging to choose treatment. Cancer Imaging. 5: S113–S119.

Feng, B., R. Hong, L. Wangm, L. Guo and H. Li. 2008. Synthesis of Fe_3O_4/APTES/PEG diacid functionalized magnetic nanoparticles for MR imaging. Colloids Surf. A 328: 52–59.

Fontes, A., H. Fernandes, A. Thomaz, L. Barbosa and M. Barjas Castro. 2006. Studying the red blood cells agglutination by measuring electrical and mechanical properties with a double optical tweezers. Micros. Microanal. 12: 1758–1759.

Fontes, A., H. Fernandes, A. de Thomaz and L. Barbosa. 2007. Studying red blood cell agglutination by measuring electrical and mechanical properties with a double optical tweezers. European Conf. Biomed. Opt. Int. Soc. Opt. Photo, 2007 66330R.

Fontes, A., H. Fernandes, A. de Thomaz and L. Barbosa. 2008. Measuring electrical and mechanical properties of red blood cells with double optical tweezers. J. Biomed. Opt. 13: 014001.

Frankamp, B., A. Boal and T. Mark. 2005. Direct control of magnetic interaction between iron oxide nanoparticles through dendrimer-mediated self-assembly. J. Am. Chem. Soc. 127: 9731–9735.

Fribel, M., A. Roggen and G. Muller. 2006. Determination of optical properties of human blood in the spectral range 250–1100 nm using Monte Carlo simulations with hematocrite-dependent effective scattering phase functions. J. Biomed. Opt. 11: 03402.

Friebel, M., J. Helfmann, U. Netz and M. Meink. 2009. Influences of oxygen saturation on the optical scattering properties of human red blood cells in the spectral range 250 to 2000 nm. J. Biomed. Opt. 14: 034001.

Fredrich, C., M. Mienkina, C. Brenner, N. Gerhardt and M. Jorger. 2012. Photoacoustic blood oxygenation imaging based on semiconductor lasers. Photonics and Optoelect. 1: 48–54.

Fu, L., V. Dravid and D. Johnson. 2001. Self-assembled bilayer molecular coating on magnetic nanoparticles. Appl. Surf. Sci. 181: 173 178.

Garcia, M. and L. Baker. 1998. Crooks preparation and characterization of dendrimer–gold colloid nanocomposites. Analy. Chem. 71: 256–258.

Gautam, A. and F. van Veggel. 2013. Synthesis of nanoparticles, their biocompatibility, and toxicity behavior for biomedical applications. J. Mater. Chem. B1: 5186–5200.

Genina, E., S. Lapin, V. Petrov and V. Tuchin. 2000. Optoacoustic visualization of blood vessels *in vitro*. Proc. SPIE. 3916: 84–86.

Gershfeld, N. and M. Murayama. 1988. Thermal instability of red blood cell membrane bilayers: Temperature dependence of hemolysis. J. Membr. Biol. 101: 67–72.

Ghandoor, H., H. Zidan, M. Khali and M. Ismail. 2007. Synthesis and some physical properties of magnetic properties. Int. J. Electrochem. Sci. 7: 5734–5745.

Ghazanfari, L. and M.E. Khosroshahi. 2014. Simulation and experimental results of optical and thermal modeling of gold nanoshells. Mat. Sci. Eng. C. 42: 185–191.

Ghazanfari, L. and M.E. Khosroshahi. 2015. Superparamagnetic iron oxide nanoparticles size and magnetic characteristics. IJRSET 4: 6659–6666.

Gioux, S., H. Choi and J. Frangioni. 2010. Image-guided surgery using invisible NIR light: fundamentals of clinical translation. Mol. Imaging. 9: 237–255.

Gobin, A., D. Patrik, O. Neil, D. Watkins, N. Halas, R. Drezek and J. West. 2005. Near infrared laser-tissue welding using nanoshells as an exogenous absorber. Lasers Surg. Med. 37: 123–129.

Gormley, A., N. Larson, Sh. Sadekar, R. Robinson, A. Ray and H. Ghandehari. 2012. Guided delivery of polymer therapeutics using plasmonics photothermal therapy. Nano Today 7: 158–167.

Govorov, A., W. Zhang, T. Skeini and H. Richardson. 2006. Gold Nanoparticles as heaters and actuators: Melting and collective plasmon resonances. Nanoscale Res. Lett. 1: 84–90.

Govorov, O. and H. Richardson. 2007. Generating heat with metal nanoparticles. Nano Today 1: 30–38.

Grabchev, I., V. Bojinov and J. Chovelon. 2003. Synthesis, photophysical and photochemical properties of fluorescent poly(amidoamine) dendrimers. Polymer 44: 4421–4428.

Greshfeld, N. 1986. Phospholipid surface bilayers at the air-water interface. III. Relation between surface bilayer formation and lipid bilayer assembly in cell membranes. Biophys. J. 50: 457–461.

Gupta, A. and M. Gupta. 2005. Synthesis and surface engineering of iron-oxide nanoparticles for biomedical applications. Biomaterials. 26: 3995–4021.

Guang, Y., T. Zhang, X. Qiao, J. Zhang and L. Yang. 2007. Effects of synthetical conditions on octahedral magnetite nanoparticles. Mater. Sci. Eng. B. 136: 101–105.

Guadagni, S. and T. Nadeau. 1991. Imaging in digestive video endoscopy. SPIE. 1420: 1420–1426.

Gussakovsky, E., Y. Yang, J. Rendell and O. Jilkina. 2012. NIR spectroscopic imaging to map Hemoglobin + myoglobin oxygenation, their concentration and optical path length across a beating pig heart during surgery. J. Biophotonics 5: 128–139.

Hannah, A., D. Vander Laan and Y. Chen. 2014. Photoacoustic and ultrasound imaging using contrast perfluorcarbone nanodroplets triggered by laser pulses at 1064 nm. Biomed. Opt. Exp. 5: 3042–3052.

Hassannejad, Z. and M.E. Khosroshahi. 2013. Synthesis and evaluation of time dependent optical properties of plasmonic–magnetic nanoparticles. Opt. Mat. 35: 644–651.

Hassannejad, Z., M.E. Khosroshahi and M. Firouzi. 2014. Fabrication and characterization of magnetoplasmonic liposome carriers. Nanosci. Tech. 1: 1–9.

He, J., R. Valluzzi, K. Yang, T. Dolukhanyan, C. Sung, J. Kumar and J. Tripathy. 1999. Electrostatic multilayer deposition of a gold-dendrimer nanocomposite. Chem. Mat. 11: 3268–3274.

Hoffman, L., G. Andersson, A. Sharma, S. Clarke and N. Voelcker. 2011. New insight into the structure of PAMAM dendrimer/gold nanoparticle nanocomposites. Langmuir 27: 6759–6767.

Hofmeister, H., J. Huisken, B. Kohn, R. Alexandrescu and S. Cojocaru. 2001. Filamentary iron nanostructures from laser-induced pyrolysis of iron pentacarbonyl and ethylene mixtures. Appl. Phys. A 72: 7–11.

Hong, R., J. Li, H. Li, J. Ding and Y. Zheng. 2008. Synthesis of Fe_3O_4 nanoparticles without inert gas protection used as precursors of magnetic fluids. J. Mag. Mag. Mater. 320: 1605–1614.

Hosono, T., H. Takahashi, A. Fujita, R. Joseyphus and K. Tohji. 2009. Synthesis of magnetite nanoparticles for AC magnetic heating. J. Mag. Mag. Mater. 321: 3019–3023.

Hossain, M., Y. Kitahma, G. Hung, X. Hun and Y. Ozaki. 2009. Surface-enhanced Raman scattering: Realization of localized surface plasmon resonance using unique substrates and methods. Ana. Bioanal. Chem. 394: 1747–1760.

Hu, S. 2010. Wang. Photoacoustic imaging and characterization of the microvasculature. J. Biomed. Opt. 15: 011101–1.

Huang, X., P. Jain, I. El-Sayed and M. El-Sayed. 2008. Plasmonic photothermal therapy (PPTT) using gold nanoparticles. Lasers Medical Sci. 23: 217–228.

Huang, J., X. Zhuang, L. Teng, D. Li and X. Chen. 2010. The promotion of human malignant melanoma growth by mesoporous silica nanoparticles through decreased reactive oxygen species. Biomaterials 31: 6142–6153.

Hung, X., P. Jain, I. El-Sayed and M. El-Sayed. 2007. Gold nanoparticles: interesting optical properties and recent applications in cancer diagnostics and therapy. Nanomed. 2: 681–693.

Ihab, S., W. David, M. Marr and C. Eggleton. 2010. Linear diode laser bar optical stretchers for cell deformation. Biomed. Opt. Exp. 482–488.

Jain, P., K. Lee, I. El-Sayed and M. El-Sayed. 2006. Calculated absorption and scattering properties of gold nanoparticles of different size, shape, and composition: applications in biological imaging and biomedicine. J. Phys. Chem. B 110: 7238–7248.

Jang, B., S. Park and Se. Kang. 2012. Gold nanorods for targeted selective SPECT/CT imaging and photothermal therapy *in vivo*. Quant. Imag. Med. Surg. 1–15.

Jasmine, M., M. Kavtha, E. Prasad and J. Lumin. 2009. Effect of solvent-controlled aggregation on the intrinsic emission properties of PAMAM dendrimers. 129: 506–513.

Jevprasesphant, R., J. Penny, R. Jalal, D. Attwood and N. McKeown. 2003. The influence of surface modification on the cytotoxicity of PAMAM dendrimers. Int. J. Pharm. 252: 263–266.

Jiang, Q. and X. Lang. 2007. Size dependence of structures and properties of materials. Open Nanosci. J. 1: 32–59.

Jiang, G., Y. Wang and X. Sun. 2010. Fluence on fluorescence properties of hyperbranched poly(amidoamine)s by nano golds. J. of Polymer Sci. Polymer Phy. 48: 2386–2391.

Jin, Y., C. Jia, S. Huang and X. Gao. 2010. Multifunctional nanoparticles as coupled contrast agents. Nat. Commun. 1: 1 8.

Jordan, A., R. Scholz, P. Wust, H. Fähling, F. Roland and R. Felix. 1999. Magnetic fluid hyperthermia (MFH): cancer treatment with AC magnetic field induced excitation of biocompatible superparamagnetic nanoparticles. J. Mag. Mag. Mat. 201: 413–419.

Josephson, L., M. Kircher, U. Mahmood and Y. Tang. 2002. NIR fluorescent nanoparticles as combined MR/optical imaging probes. Bioconjugate Chem. 13: 554–560.

Kajanto, I. and A. Friberg. 1988. A silicon based fibre optic temperature sensor. J. Phys. E: Sci: Inst. 21: 652–656.

Karaoglu, E. 2011. Effect of hydrolyzing agents on the properties of poly(ethylene glycol) - Fe_3O_4 nanocomposite Nano-Micro Lett. 3: 79–85.

Karle, H. 1969. Effect on red blood cells of a small rise in temperature: *in vitro* studies. Brit. J. Haemat. 16: 409–419.

Kent, M., J. Port and N. Altorki. 2004. Current state of imaging for lung cancer staging. Thoractic Surg. Clinc. 14: 1–13.

Kim, D., S. Park, J. Lee and Y. Jeong. 2007. Antibiofouling Polymer-coated gold nanoparticles as a contrast agent for *in vivo* X-ray computed Tomography imaging. J. Am. Chem. Soc. 129: 7661–7665.

Kim, D., M. Yu and T. Lee. 2011. Amphiphilic polymer-coated hybrid nanoparticles as CT/MRI dual contrast agents. Nanotechnology 22: 155101.

Kim, Y., S. Oh and R. Crooks. 2003. Preparation and characterization of 1–2 nm dendrimer-encapsulated gold nanoparticles having very narrow size distributions. Chem. Mater. 16: 167–172.

Kim, Y., S.H. Kim, M. Tanyeri, J. Katzenellenbogen and C. Schroeder. 2013. Dendrimer probes for enhanced photostability and localization in fluorescence imaging. Biophys. J. 2: 1566–1575.

Kimura, Y., R. Kamisugi and M. Narazaki. 2012. Size-controlled and biocompatible Gd_2O_3 nanoparticles for dual photoacoustic and MRI imaging. Adv. Healthc. Mater. 1: 657–660.

Khaing, M., Y. Yang, Y. Hu, M. Gomez and H. Du. 2012. Gold nanoparticle-enhanced and size-dependent generation of reactive oxygen species from protoporphyrin IX. ACS Nano 6: 1939–1947.

Khlebtsov, B., V. Zharov, A. Melikov, V. Tuchin and N. Khlebtsov. 2006. Optical amplification of photothermal therapy with gold nanoparticles and nanoshells. Nanotechnology 17: 5167–5179.

Khlebtsov, B. and N. Khlebtsov. 2007. Biosensing potential of silica/gold nanoshells: sensitivity of plasmon resonance to the local dielectric environment. J. Quant. Spect. 106: 154–169.

Khodadust, R., G. Unsoy, S. Yalcın, G. Gunduz and U. Gunduz. 2013. PAMAM dendrimer-coated iron oxide nanoparticles: synthesis and characterization of different generations. J. Nanopart. Res. 15: 1488–1494.

Khosroshahi, M.E. and A. Ghasemi. 2004. Interaction studies of multimode pulsed HF laser with enamel tissue using photothermal deflection and spectroscopy. Lasers Med. Sci. 18: 196–203.

Khosroshahi, M.E. 2004. Design and application of photoacoustic sensor for monitoring the laser generated stress waves in optical fibre. Int. J. Eng. Transaction B: Applications 17: 1–6.

Khosroshahi, M.E. and M. Nourbakhsh. 2010. Preparation and characterization of self-assembled gold nanoparticles on amino functionalized SiO_2 dielectric core. World Academy of Sci., Eng. and Technol. 64: 353–356.

Khosroshahi, M.E. and M. Nourbakhsh. 2011. *In vitro* skin wound soldering using SiO_2/Au nanoshells and a diode laser. Med. Laser Appl. 26: 35–42.

Khosroshahi, M.E. and M. Nourbakhsh. 2011. Enhanced laser tissue soldering using indocyanine Green chromophore and gold nanoshells combination. J. Biomed. Opt. 16: 088002.

Khosroshahi, M.E. and L. Ghazanfari. 2011. Amino surface modification of Fe_3O_4/SiO_2 nanoparticles for bioengineering applications. Surf. Eng. 27: 573–580.

Khosroshahi, M.E. and L. Ghazanfari. 2012. Synthesis and functionalization of SiO_2 coated Fe_3O_4 nanoparticles with amine groups based on self-assembly. Mat. Sci. Eng. C. 32: 1043–1049.

Khosroshahi, M.E. and L. Ghazanfari. 2012. Physicochemical characterization of Fe_3O_4/SiO_2/Au multilayer nanostructure. Mat. Chem. Phys. 133: 55–62.

Khosroshahi, M.E., M. Tajabadi and Sh. Bonakdar. 2013. An efficient method of SPION synthesis coated with third generation PAMAM dendrimer. Colloids Surf. A: Physicochem. Eng. Aspects. 431: 18–26.

Khosroshahi, M.E. and A. Mandelis. 2014. Combined photoacoustic ultrasound and beam deflection signal monitoring of gold nanoparticle agglomerate concentrations in tissue phantoms using a pulsed Nd:YAG Laser. Int. J. Thermophys. 36: 880–890.

Khosroshahi, M.E., A. Mandelis and B. Lashkari. 2014. Combined photoacoustic ultrasound and beam deflection signal monitoring of gold nanoparticle agglomerate concentrations in tissue phantoms using a pulsed Nd:YAG laser. J. Int. Therm. Phys. 06: 1773–3.

Khosroshahi, M.E., M. Tajabadi, Sh. Bonakdar and V. Asgari. 2015. Synthesis and characterization of SPION functionalized third generation dendrimer conjugated by gold nanoparticles and folic acid for targeted breast cancer laser hyperthermia: An *in vivo* assay. World Cong. Med. Phys. & Biomed. Eng. 823–826.

Khosroshahi, M.E., A. Mandelis and B. Lashkari. 2015. Frequency-domain thermo-photoacoustics and ultrasonic imaging of blood vessel using different plasmonics nanoparticles concentration. J. Biomed. Opt. 20: 076009–1.

Khosroshahi, M.E., R. Alanagh, H. Keshvari, Sh. Bonakdar and M. Tajabadi. 2016. Effect of SPION and fluorescin conjugated PAMAM dendrimers on biomolecular imaging cell viability and T2 relaxity. Mat. Sci. Eng. C 62: 544–552.

Khosroshahi, M.E., M. Tajabadi and Sh. Bonakdar. 2016. Characterization and cellular fluorescence microscopy of Fe_3O_4 functionalized third generation nano-molecular dendrimers: *In vitro* cytotoxity and uptake study. J. Nanomat. Mol. Nanotech. 5: 1: 2016.

Klajnart, B. and M. Bryszewska. 2002. Fluorescence studies on PAMAM dendrimers interactions with bovine serum albumin. Bioelectrochem. 55: 33–35.

Kripfgans, O., J. Fowlkes and D. Miller. 2000. Acoustic droplet vaporization for therapeutic and diagnostic applications. Ultr. Med. Biolo. 26: 1177–1189.

Kumar, S. 2006. Biomarkers in cancer screening, research and detection: present and future: A review. Biomarkers 11: 385–405.

Kuznetsov, A., V. Filippov, R. Alyautdin and N. Torshina. 2001. Application of magnetic liposomes for magnetically guided transport of muscle relaxants and anti-cancer photodynamic drugs. J. Mag. Mag. Mat. 225: 95–100.

Lashkari, B. and A. Mandelis. 2011. Comparison between pulsed laser and frequency-domain photoacoustic modalities: Signal-to-noise ratio, contrast, resolution, and maximum depth detectivity. Rev. Sci. Inst. 82: 094903.

Lashkari, B. and A. Mandelis. 2014. Coregistered photoacoustic and ultrasonic signatures of early bone density variations. J. Biomed. Opt. 3: 36015.

Laufer, J., C. Elwell, D. Delpy and P. Beard. 2005. *In vitro* measurements of absolute blood oxygen saturation using pulsed near-infrared photoacoustic spectroscopy: Accuracy and resolution. Phys. Med. Biol. 50: 4409–4428.

Launer, P. 1987. Infrared analysis of organosilicon compounds: spectra structure correlations. In laboratory for materials, Inc., Burnt Hills: New York.

Lee, K., Y. Jeong and J. Han. 2004. T1 non-small cell lung cancer: imaging and histopathologic findings and their prognostic implications. Radiogrph. 24: 1617–1636.

Lee, C. and J. MacKay. 2005. Designing dendrimers for biological applications. J. Nat. Biotechnol. 23: 1517–1526.

Lee, K. and M. El-Sayed. 2005. Dependence of the enhanced optical scattering efficiency relative to that of absorption for gold metal nanorods on aspect ratio, size, end-cap shape, and medium refractive index. J. Phys. Chem. B 109: 20331–20338.

Lee, H., Z. Li and K. Chan. 2008. PET/MRI dual modality tumor imaging using arginine-glycine-asparic red-conjugated radiolabelled iron oxide nanoparticles. J. Nuclear Med. 49: 1371–1379.

Legrand, A. 1998. The Surface Properties of Silicas. John Wiley New York.

Lehman, C. 2007. Cancer yield of mammography, MR, and US in high risk women: prospective multi-institution breast cancer screening study. Radiology. 244: 381–388.

Lemberg, R., J. Legge and W. Lockwood. 1941. Coupled oxidation of ascorbic acid and haemoglobin: quantitative studies on choleglobin formation. Estimation of haemoglobin and ascorbic acid oxidations. Biochem. J. 35: 339–352.

Lemberg, V. and M. Black. 1996. Variable focus side firing endoscopic device. Optical fibres in Medicine VI SPIE. 2671: 178–183.

Lerner, R., S. Huang and S. Parker. 1990. Sonoelasticity images derived from ultrasound signals in mechanically vibrated tissues. Ultrasound in Med. & Biolog. 16: 231–239.

Li, Z., P. Huang, X. Zhang, J. Lin, S. Yang and B. Liu. 2009. RGD-conjugated dendrimer-modified gold nanorods for *in vivo* tumor targeting and photothermal therapy. Mol. Pharmaceutics 7: 94–104.

Li, J., Q. Chen and L. Yang. 2010. The synthesis of dendrimer based on the dielectric barrier discharge plasma grafting amino group film. Surface Coating Tech. 205: S257–S260.

Li, L., W. Jiang, K. Luo, H. Song and F. Lan. 2013. Superparamagnetic iron oxide nanoparticles as MRI contrast agents for non-invasive stem cell labeling and tracking. Theranostics 3: 595–615.

Lide, D.R. 2002. CRC Handbook of Chemistry and Physics, 7first Edition (1990-1991).

Lin, D., L. Zhong and S. Yao. 2006. Zeta potential as a diagnostic tool to evaluate the biomass electrostatic adhesion during ion-exchange expanded bed application. Biotechnol. Bioeng. 95: 185–191.

Linna, W., Y. Li, P. Li, R. Naveen and X. Liang. 2015. Time-resolved proteomic visualization of dendrimer cellular entry and trafficking. J. Am. Chem. Soc. 137: 12772–1277.

Liu, R., Y. Ren, Y. Shi, F. Zhang, L. Zhang, B. Tu and D. Zhao. 2007. Controlled synthesis of ordered mesoporous $C-TiO_2$ nanocomposites with crystalline titania frameworks from organic–inorganic–amphiphilic coassembly. Chem. Mater. 20: 1140–1146.

Liu, Z., X. Wang, K. Yao, G. Du and Q. Lu. 1999. Synthesis of magnetite nanoparticles in W/O Microemulsion. J. Mater. Sci. 39: 2633–2636.

Liu, H., J. Guo, L. Jin, W. Yang and C. Wang. 2008. Fabrication and functionalization of dendritic poly(amidoamine)-immobilized magnetic polymer composite microspheres. J. Phys. Chem. B. 112: 3315–3321.

Liu, R., Y. Ren, Y. Shi, F. Zhang and L. Zhang. 2008. Controlled synthesis of ordered mesoporous $C-TiO_2$ nanocomposites with crystalline titania frameworks from organic-inorganic amphilhilic coassembly. Chem. Mater. 20: 1140–1146.

Lopez-Munoz, G. and J. Pescador-Rojas. 2012. Thermal diffusivity measurement of spherical gold nanofluids of different sizes/concentrations. Nanoscale Res. Lett. 7: 423–427.

Loria, H., P. Pereira-Almao and C. Scott. 2011. Determination of agglomeration kinetics in nanoparticle dispersions. Indust. Eng. Chem. Res. 50: 8529–8535.

Lubarda, V. and A. Manzani. 2009. Viscoelastic response of thin membranes with application to red blood cells. Acta Mechanica. 202: 1–16.

Luke, G., D. Eager and S. Emelianov. 2011. Biomedical applications of photoacoustic imaging with exogenous contrast agents. Annl. Biomed. Eng. 40: 422–437.

Ma, L., M. Feldman, J. Tam and A. Paranjape. 2009. Small multifunctional nanoclusters (nanoroses) for targeted cellular imaging and therapy. ACS Nano 3: 2686–2696.

Madaan, K., S. Kumar, N. Poonia, V. Lather and D. Pandita. 2014. Dendrimers in drug delivery and targeting: drug-dendrimer interactions and toxicity issues. J. Pharm. Bioallied. Sci. 6: 139–150.

Madru, R., P. Kjellman and P. Olsson. 2012. 99mct-labeled SPIONs for multimodality SPECT/MRI of sential lymph nodes. J. Nucl. Med. 53: 459463.

Mahmoodi, M., M.E. Khosroshahi and F. Atyabi. 2011. Dynamic study of PLGA/CS nanoparticles delivery containing drug model into phantom tissue using CO_2 laser for clinical applications. J. Biophotonics 6: 403–411.

Majoros, I., A. Myc, T. Thomas, C. Mehta and J. Baker. 2006. PAMAM dendrimer-based multifunctional conjugate for cancer therapy: synthesis, characterization, and functionality. Biomacromolecules 7: 572–579.

Maeda, A., B. Jiachuan, J. Chan, G. Zheng and R. DaCosta. 2014. Dual *in vivo* photoacoustic and fluorescence imaging of HER2 expression in breast tumour for diagnosis, margin assessment and surgical guidance. Mol. Imag. 43: 1–9.

Maslov, K. and L. Wang. 2008. Photoacoustic imaging of biological tissue with intensity-modulated continuous-wave laser, J. Biomed. Opt. 13: 024006.

Menjoge, A., R. Kannan and D. Tomalia. 2010. Dendrimer-based drug and imaging conjugates: design considerations for nanomedical applications. Drug Discov. Today 15: 171–185.

Meinke, M., G. Muller, J. Helfmann and M. Friebel. 2007. Properties of platelets and blood plasma and their influence on the optical behavior of whole blood in the visible to NIR wavelength Range. J. Biomed. Opt. 12: 014024.

Mody, V., A. Cox, S. Shah, A. Singh and W. Bevins. 2014. Magnetic nanoparticle drug delivery systems for targeting tumor. Appl. Nanosci. 4: 385–392.

Mosseri, S., A. Henglein and E. Janata. 1989. Reduction of dicyanoaurate (I) in aqueous solution: formation of nanometallic clusters and colloidal gold. J. Phys. Chem. 93: 6791–6795.

Nagy, D., I. Nyirokosa and M. Posfai. 2009. Size and shape control of precipitated magnetite nanoparticles. Eur. J. Mineral 21: 293–302.

Narsireddy, A., K. Vijayashree, M. Adimoolam and S. Manorama. 2015. Photosensitizer and peptide-conjugated PAMAM dendrimer for targeted *in vivo* photodynamic therapy. Int. J. Nanomed. 10: 6865–6878.

Neuberger, T. 2005. Superparamagnetic nanoparticles for biomedical applications: possibilities and limitations of a new drug delivery system. J. Mag. and Mag. Mat. 293: 483–496.

Nie, L., Z. Ou, S. Yang and D. Xing. 2010. Thermoacoustic molecular tomography with magnetic nanoparticle contrast agents for targeted tumour detection. Med. Phys. 37: 4193–4200.

Ning, Y., T. Grattan and A. Palmer. 1992. Fibre optic interferometric systems using low coherence light sources. Sensors and Actuators. A. 30: 181–192.

Niu, Y., H. Lu, D. Wang, Y. Yue and S. Feng. 2011. Synthesis of siloxane based PAMAM dendrimers and luminescent properties of their lanthanide complexes. J. Organomet. Chem. 696: 544–550.

Okugaichi, A., K. Torigoe, T. Yoshimura and K. Esumi. 2006. Interaction of cationic gold nanoparticles and carboxylate-terminated poly(amidoamine) dendrimers. Colloids and Surf. A: Physicochem. Eng. Aspects. 273: 154–160.

O'Neal, D., L. Hirch and N.J. Halas. 2004. Photothermal tumor ablation in mice using near infrared-absorbing nanoparticles. Cancer Lett. 209: 171–176.

Oraevsky, A., E. Savateeva, S. Solomatin, A. Karabutov and V. Andreev. 2002. Optoacoustic imaging of blood for visualization and diagnostics of breast cancer. Proc. SPIE. 4618: 81–94.

Pallwein, L., M. Mitterberger and P. Struve. 2007. Real-time elastography for detecting prostate cancer: preliminary experience. British J. Ult. Int. 100: 42–46.

Pan, B., F. Gao and H. Gu. 2005. Dendrimer modified magnetite nanoparticles for protein immobilization. J. Colloid Inter. Sci. 284: 1–6.

Pan, D., M. Pramanik, A. Senpan, J. Allen and H. Zhang. 2011. Molecular photoacoustic imaging of angiogenesis with integrin-targeted gold nanobeacons. The FASEB J. 25: 875–882.

Pastor-Pérez, L., Y. Chen, Z. Shen, A. lahoz and S. Stiriba. 2007. Unprecedented blue intrinsic photoluminescence from hyperbranched and linear polyethylenimines: polymer architectures and pH-effects. Macromol. Rapid Commun. 28: 1404–1409.

Patra, Ch., R. Bhttacharya, D. Mukhopadhyay and P. Mukhejjee. 2010. Fabrication of gold nanoparticles for targeted therapy in pancreatic cancer. Adv. Drug. Del. Rev. 62: 346–361.

Peng, X., Q. Pan and G. Rempel. 2008. Bimetallic dendrimer-encapsulated nanoparticles as catalysts: a review of the research advances. Chem. Soc. Rev. 37: 1619–1628.

Paeng, J. and D. Lee. 2010. Multimodal molecular imaging *in vivo*. The Open Nucl. Med. J. 145: 145–152.

Pankhurst, Q., J. Connolly, S. Jones and J. Dobson. 2003. Applications of magnetic nanoparticles in bio medicine. J. Phys. D: Appl. Phys. 36: 167–181.

Park, S., M. Park, K. Han and S. Lee. 2006. The effect of pH-adjusted gold colloids on the formation of gold clusters over APTMS-coated silica cores. Bull. Korean Chem. Soc. 27: 1341–1345.

Park, C., Y. Rhee and F. Vogt. 2012. Advances in microscopy and complementary imaging techniques to assess the fate of drugs *ex vivo* in respiratory drug delivery: an invited paper. Adv. Drug Deliv. Rev. 64: 344–356.

Patra, Ch., R. Bhttacharya, D. Mukhopadhyay and P. Mukhejjee. 2010. Fabrication of gold nanoparticles for targeted therapy in pancreatic cancer. Adv. Drug. Del. Rev. 62: 346–361.

Pattani, V. and J. Tunnell. 2012. Nanoparticle-mediated photothermal therapy: a comparative study of heating for different particle types. Lasers Surg. Med. 44: 675–684.

Philip, A., P. Radhakrishnan and K. Nampoori. 1993. Photoacoustic studies on multilayer dielectric coatings. J. Phys. D: Appl. Phys. 26: 836–838.

Pirkl, L. and T. Bonder. 2010. Numerical simulation of blood flow using generated oldroyed-B model blood. European Conf. on Computational Fluid Dynamic.

Pisanic, T., J. Blackwell, V. Shubayev, R. Fiñones and S. Jin. 2007. Nanotoxicity of iron oxide nanoparticle internalization in growing neurons. Biomaterials 28: 2572–2581.

Pradhan, P., J. Giri, F. Rieken, C. Koch and O. Mykhaylyk. 2010. Targeted temperature sensitive magnetic liposomes for thermo chemotherapy. J. Control Release 142: 108–121.

Pushkarsky, M., O. Webber, A.R. Baghdassarian, C. and K. Narasimhan. 2002. Laser-based photoacoustic ammonia sensors for industrial applications. Appl. Phys. B. 75: 391–396.

Pustovalov, V. and V. Babenkov. 2004. Optical properties of gold nanoparticles at laser radiation wavelengths for laser applications in nanotechnology and medicine. Laser Phys. Let. 10: 516–520.

Pustovalov, V. and V. Babenkov. 2005. Computer modeling of optical properties of gold ellipsoidal nanoparticles at laser radiation wavelengths. Laser Phys. Lett. 2: 84–89.

Pustovalov, V. 2005. Theoretical study of heating of spherical nanoparticle in media by short laser pulses. Chem. Phys. 308: 103–108.

Pustovalov, V., L. Astafyeva, E. Galanzha and V.P. Zharov. 2010. Thermo-optical analysis and selection of the properties of absorbing nanoparticles for laser applications in cancer nanotechnology. Cancer Nano 1: 35–46.

Qin, H., S. Yang and D. Xing. 2012. Microwave-induced thermoacoustic computed tomography with a clinical contrast agent of $NMG_2[Gd(DTPA)]$. Appl. Phys. Lett. 100: 033701.

Rezvani, H., M.E. Khosroshahi, M. Tajabadi and H. Keshvari. 2014. Effect of pH and magnetic field on the fluorescence spectra of fluorescein isothiocyanate conjugated SPION-dendrimers nanocomposites. J. Supercond. Nov. Mag. 27: 2337–2345.

Roberts, J., M. Bhalgat and R. Zera. 1996. Preliminary biological evaluation of polyamidoamine (PAMAM) Starburst dendrimers. J. Biomed. Mat. Res. 30: 53–65.

Rogan, A., M. Friebel, K. Dorschel and A. Hahn. 1999. Optical properties of circulating blood in the wavelength range 400–2500 nm. J. Biomed. Opt. 4: 36–46.

Roper, D., W. Ahn and M. Hoepfner. 2007. Microscale heat transfer transduced plasmon resonant gold nanoparticles. J. Phys. Chem. C 111: 3636–3641.

Sadat, M., R. Patel, J. Sookoor, S. Budko, R. Ewing and J. Zhang. 2014. Effect of spatial confinement on magnetic hyperthermia via dipolar interaction in Fe_3O_4 nanoparticles for biomedical applications. Mat. Sci. Eng. C 42: 52–63.

Sajjadi, A., A. Suratkar and K. Mitra. 2012. Short-pulse laser-based system for detection of tumors: administration of gold nanoparticles enhances contrast. J. Nanotech. Eng. Med. 3: 021002(1-6).

Saptarshi, Sh., A. Duschl and A. Lpata. 2013. Interaction of nanoparticles with proteins: relation to bio-reactivity of the nanoparticle. J. Nanobiotech. 11: 1–12.

Sardar, R., A. Funston, P. Mulvaney and R. Murray. 2009. Gold nanoparticles: past, present, future. Langmuir. 25: 13840–13851.

Sarj, I., J. Chichester and E. Hoover. 2010. Cell deformation cytometry using diode-bar optical stretchers. J. Biomed. Opt. 15: 047010, 1–7.

Sassaroli, E., K. Li and B. Neill. 2009. Numerical investigation of heating of a gold nanoparticle and the surrounding microenvironment by nanosecond laser pulses for nanomedicine applications. Phys. in Med. and Biol. 54: 5541.

Satoh, K., T. Yoshimura and K. Esumi. 2002. Effects of various thiol molecules added on morphology of dendrimer–gold nanocomposites. J. of Colloid Int. Sci. 255: 312–322.

Satija, J., V. Gupta and N. Jain. 2007. Therapeutic drug carrier systems. Crit. Rev. 24: 257–306.

Savery, D. and G. Clouteir. 2007. High-frequency ultrasound backscattering by blood: analytical and semi analytical models of the erythrocyte cross section. J. Acoust. Soc. Am. 121: 3963–3971.

Scultz, M. 1865. Ein heizbarer objektisch und sein ver-wendung bei untersuchung des blutes. Arch. Mickro. Anat. 1: 1–42.

Scutaru, A., M. Krger, M. Wenzel, J. Richter and R. Gust. 2010. Investigations on the use of fluorescence dyes for labeling dendrimers: cytotoxicity, accumulation kinetics, and intracellular distribution. Bioconjug. Chem. 21: 2222–2226.

Sell, J., D. Heffelfinger, P. Ventzek and R. Gilgenbach. 1991. Photoacoustic and photothermal beam deflection as a probe of laser ablation of materials. J. Appl. Phys. 69: 1330–1336.

Sgouras, D. and R. Duncan. 1990. Methods for the evaluation of biocompatibility of soluble synthetic polymers which have potential for biomedical use: 1-Use of the tetrazolium-based colorimetric assay (MTT) as a preliminary screen for evaluation of *in vivo* cytotoxicity. J. Mat. Sci. Med. 1: 67–78.

Shah, J., Park, S. Aglyamov and T. Larson. 2008. Photoacoustic and ultrasound imaging to guide photothermal therapy: *ex vivo* study. SPIE 6856: 68560U-1.

Shang, L., K. Nienhaus and G. Nienhaus. 2014. Engineered nanoparticles interacting with cells: size matters. J. Nanobiotech. 12: 5–8.

Shauo, Ch., Ch. Chao, T. Wu and H. Shy. 2007. Magnetic and optical properties of isolated magnetic nanocrystals. Mat. Tran. 48: 1143–1148.

Shen, M. and X. Shi. 2010. Dendrimer-based on organic/inorganic hybrid nanoparticles in biomedical applications. Nanoscale. 2: 1596–1610.

Shi, X., T. Ganser and K. Sun. 2006. Characterization of crystalline dendrimer-stabilized gold nanoparticles. Nanotechnology 17: 1072–1078.

Shi, X., S. Wang, H. Sun and J. Baker. 2007. Improved biocompatibility of surface functionalized dendrimer-entrapped gold nanoparticles. Soft Matter 3: 71–74.

Shi, X., Su Wang, S. Swanson and S. Ge. 2008. Dendrimer-functionalized Shell-crosslinked Iron Oxide Nanoparticles for *in vivo* Magnetic Resonance Imaging of Tumors 20: 1671–1678.

Shi, D., H. Cho, Y. Chen and H. Xu. 2009. Fluorescent polystyrene–Fe3O4 composite nanospheres for *in vivo* imaging and hyperthermia. Adv. Mat. 21: 2170–2173.

Shi, X., S. Wang, M. Shen, M. Antwerp and X. Chen. 2009. Multifunctional dendrimer-modified multi-walled carbon nanotubes: synthesis, characterization, and *in vitro* cancer cell targeting and imaging. Biomacromolecules 10: 1744–1750.

Shi, X. and K. Sun. 2009. Spontaneous formation of functionalized dendrimer-stabilized gold nanoparticles. J. Phys. Chem. C. Nanomat. Inter. 112: 8251–8258.

Sigrist, M. 1986. Laser generated acoustic waves in liquids and solids. J. Appl. Phys. 60: 83–121.

Sinha, R., G. Kim and Sh. Nie. 2012. Nanotechnology in cancer therapeutics: bioconjugated nanoparticles for drug delivery. Mol. Cancer Ther. 7: 1909–1917.

Soenen, S., U. Himmelreich, N. Nuytten and M. De Cuyper. 2011. Cytotoxic effects of iron oxide nanoparticles and implications for safety in cell labelling. Biomaterials. 32: 195–205.

Song, M., Y. Li, H. Kasai and K. Kawai. 2012. Metal nanoparticle-induced micronuclei and oxidative DNA damage in mice. J. Clin. Biochem. Nutr. 50: 211–216.

Spirou, G., A. Oraevsky, I. Vitkin and W. Whelan. 2005. Optical and acoustic properties at 1064 nm of polyvinyl chloride-plastisol for use as a tissue phantom in biomedical optoacoustics. Phys. Med. Biol. 50: N1 41–53.

Srinivasan, R., P.E. Dyer and B. Braren. 1987. Far ultraviolet laser ablation of the cornea: photoacoustic studies. Lasers Surg. Med. 6: 514–519.

Streszewski, B., W. Jaworski, K. Paclawski, E. Csapó, I. Dékány and K. Fitzner. 2012. Gold nanoparticles formation in the aqueous system of gold(III) chloride complex Ions and hydrazine sulfate-kinetic studies. Colloids Surf. A: Physicochemical Eng. Aspects 397: 63–72.

Strohm, E., M. Rui, M. Kolios and I. Gorelikov. 2010. Optical droplet vaporization photoacoustic characterization of perflurocarbon droplets. IEEE Int. Ult. Symp. 449–498.

Strijkers, G., M. Mulder, J. Willem, F. van Tilborg and A. Geralda. 2007. MRI contrast agents: current status and future perspectives. Anti-Cancer Agents in Med. Chem. 7: 291–305.

Sudeshna, C., D. Sascha, L. Heinrich and D. Bahadur. 2011. Dendrimer-doxorubicin conjugate for enhanced therapeutic effects for cancer. J. Mater. Chem. 21: 5729–5737.

Sun, Y., C. King and B. O'Neal. 2013. Photoacoustic imaging in the evaluation of laser controlled drug release using gold nanostructure agents. SPIE 8581: 85813F-1.

Syahir, A., K. Tomizaki, K. Kajikawa and H. Mihara. 2009. Poly(amidoamine)-dendrimer modified gold surfaces for anomalous reflection of gold to detect biomolecular interactions. Langmuir. 25: 3667–3674.

Tam, A. 1986. Applications of photoacoustic sensing techniques. Rev. Mod. Phys. 58: 381–395.

Teng, P. and R. Nishioka. 1987. Acoustic studies of the role of immersion in plasma mediated laser ablation IEEE. J. QE. 23: 1845–1852.

Telenkov, S. and A. Mandelis. 2006. Fourier-domain biophotoacoustic subsurface depth selection amplitude and phase image of turbid phantoms and biological tissue. J. Biomed. Opt. 11: 044006(1-10).

Telenkov, S., A. Mandelis, B. Lashkari and M. Forcht. 2009. Frequency-domain photothermoacoustics: Alternative imaging modality of biological tissues. J. Appl. Phys. 105: 102029(1-8).

Tenzer, S., D. Docter, S. Rosfa, A. Wlodarski, J. Kuharev and A. Rekik. 2011. Nanoparticle size is a critical physicochemical determinant of the human blood plasma corona: a comprehensive quantitative proteomic analysis. ACS Nano 5: 7155–7162.

Tajabadi, M. and M.E. Khosroshahi. 2012. Effect of alkaline media concentration and modification of temperature on magnetite synthesis method using FeSO$_4$/NH$_4$OH. Int. J. Chem. Eng. Appl. 3: 206–211.

Tajabadi, M., M.E. Khosroshahi and Sh. Bonakdar. 2013. An efficient method of SPION synthesis coated with third generation PAMAM dendrimer. Colloids Surf. A Physicochem. Eng. Aspects. 431: 18–26.

Tajabadi, M., M.E. Khosroshahi and Sh. Bonakdar. 2015. Imaging and therapeutic applications of optical and thermal response of SPION-based third generation plasmonic nanodendrimers. Opt. Phot. J. 5: 212–226.

Telenkov, S. and A. Mandelis. 2009. Photothermoacoustic imaging of biological tissues: maximum depth characterization comparison of time and frequency-domain measurements. J. Biomed. Opt. 14: 044025.

Thompson, J., J. Vasquez, J. Hill and P. Pereira-Almao. 2008. The synthesis and evaluation of up-scalable molybdenum based ultra dispersed catalysts: Effect of temperature on particle size indust. Eng. Chem. Fund. 123: 16–23.

Thompson, D., J. Hermes, A. Quinn and M. Mayor. 2012. Scanning the potential energy surface for synthesis of dendrimer-wrapped gold clusters: design rules for true single-molecule nanostructures. ACS Nano 6: 3007–3017.

Tomalia, D. 2005. Birth of a new macromolecular architecture: dendrimers as quantized building blocks for nanoscale synthetic polymer chemistry. Prog. Polym. Sci. 30: 294–324.

Torigoe, K., A. Suzuki and K. Esumi. 2001. Au (III)-PAMAM Interaction and formation of Au-PAMAM nanocomposites in ethyl acetate. J. Colloid Int. Sci. 241: 346–356.

Unterweger, H., R. Tietze, C. Janko, J. Zaloga and St. Lyer. 2014. Development and characterization of magnetic iron oxide nanoparticle with a cisplatin-bearing polymer coating for targeted drug delivery. Int. J. Nanomed. 9: 3659–3676.

Uzun, K. 2010. Covalent immobilization of invertase on PAMAM-dendrimer modified superparamagnetic iron oxide nanoparticles. J. Nanopart. Res. 12: 3057–3067.

Vahrmeijer, A., H. Merlijn and R. Joost. 2013. Image-guided cancer surgery using NIR fluorescence. Rev. 10: 507–518.

Venditto, V., C. Regino and M. Brechbiel. 2005. PAMAM dendrimer-based macromolecules as improved contrast agents. Mol. Pharm. 2: 302–311.

Veronesi, B., C. de Haar, L. Lee and M. Oortgiesen. 2002. The surface charge of visible particulate matter predicts biological activation in human bronchial epithelial cells. Toxicol. Appl. Pharmacol. 178: 144–154.

Verwey, E. and J. Overbeek. 1948. Theory of Stability of Lyophobic Colloides. Elsevier Press, Amesterdam.

Vinod, E., A. Faiyas, J. Joseph, R. Ganesan and R. Pandey. 2010. Dependence of pH and surfactant effect in the synthesis of magnetite (Fe_3O_4) nanoparticles and its properties. J. Mag. Mag. Mater. 322: 400–404.

Walsh, J.T. and J. Cummings. 1990. Tissue tearing caused by laser pressure. pp. 12–21. *In*: S.L. Jacques (ed.). Laser Tissue Interactions. SPIE Proc. 1202.

Wang, S., X. Shi, M. Van Antwerp and Z. Ca. 2007. Dendrimer-functionalized iron oxide nanoparticles for specific targeting and imaging of cancer cells. Adv. Funct. Mat. 17: 3043–3050.

Wang, D., T. Imae and M. Miki. 2007. Fluorescence emission from PAMAM and PPI dendrimers. J. Colloid Inter. Sci. 306: 222–227.

Wang, Y., A. Liao and J. Chen. 2012. Photoacoustic/ultrasound dual-modality contrast agent and its application to thermotherapy. J. Biomed. Opt. 17: 0450011–0450018.

Wang, Y., Strohm, Y. Sun and N. Chengcheng. 2014. PLGA/PFC particles loaded with gold nanoparticles as dual contrast agents formphotoacoustic and ultrasound imaging. Proc. SPIE. 8943: 89433M-1.

Wang, Y., Sh. Haung, Z. Shan and W. Yang. 2009. Preparation of Fe_3O_4@Au nano-composites by self-assembly technique for immobilization of glucose oxidase. Chinese Sci. Bull. 54: 1176–1181.

Wang, B., P. Joshi, V. Sapozhnikova, J. Amirian and S. Litovosky. 2010. Intravascular photoacoustic imaging of macrophages using molecularly targeted gold nanoparticles. Proc. SPIE 7564.

Welinsky, J. and M. Grinstaff. 2008. Therapeutic and diagnostic applications of dendrimers for cancer treatment. Adv. Drug Del. 60: 1037–1055.

Weibo, C., G. Ting, H. Hao and S. Jiangto. 2008. Applications of gold nanoparticles in cancer nanotechnology. Nanotech. Sci. Tech. 1: 17–32.

Westcott, S., S. Oldenburg, T. Lee and N. Halas. 1998. Formation and adsorption of clusters of gold nanoparticles onto functionalized silica nanoparticle surfaces. Langmuir. 14: 5396–5401.

Wilhelm, C., F. Gazeau and J. Roger. 2002. Interaction of anionic superparamagnetic nanoparticles with cells: kinetic analyses of membrane adsorption and subsequent internalization. Langmuir. 18: 8148–8155.

Wilson, K., T. Wang and J. Willmann. 2013. Acoustic and photoacoustic molecular imaging of Cancer. Focus on Mol. Imaging. 54: 1851–1854.

Wolinsky, J. and M. Grinstaff. 2008. Therapeutic and diagnostic applications of dendrimers for cancer treatment. Adv. Drug Del. Rev. 60: 1037–1055.

Wu, M., Y. Xing, Y. Jia, H. Niu, H. Qi et al. 2005. Magnetic field-assisted hydrothermal growth of chain-like nanostructure of magnetite. Chem. Phys. Lett. 401: 374–378.

Wu, C., C. Yu and M. Chu. 2011. A gold nanoshell with a silica inner shell synthesized using liposome templates for doxorubicin loading and near-infrared photothermal therapy. Int. J. Nanomedicine 6: 807–813.

Wang, D. and T. Imae. 2004. Fluorescence emission from dendrimers and its pH dependence. J. Am. Chem. Soc. 126: 13204–13205.

Wang, B., X. Zhang, X. Jia, Y. Luo and Z. Sun. 2004. Poly(amidoamine) dendrimers with phenyl shells: fluorescence and aggregation behaviour. Polymer. 45: 8395–8402.

Wang, Y., X. Xie and T. Goodson. 2005. Enhanced third-order nonlinear optical properties in dendrimer-metal nanocomposites. Nano Letter 5: 2379–2384.

Wang, C., D. Baer and J. Amonette. 2007. Morphology and oxide shell structure of iron nanoparticles grown by sputter-gas-aggregation. Nanotechnology 18: 255603.

Weinmann, H., M. Laniado and W. Mutzel. 1984. Pharmacokinetics of GdDTPA/dimeglumine after intravenous injection into healthy volunteers. Physiol. Chem. Phys. Med. Nmr. 16: 167–172.E.

Werner, E., A. Datta, J. Jocher and K. Raymond. 2008. High-relaxivity MRI contrast agents: where coordination chemistry meets medical imaging. Angwandte Chemie. Int. Edition 47: 8568–8580.

Xie, J., K. Chen and J. Huang. 2010. PET/MRI/NIR fluorescence triple functional iron oxide nanoparticles. Biomaterials 31: 3016–3022.

Xing, Z., J. Wang and K. Hengte. 2010. The fabrication of novel nanobubble ultrasound contrast agent for potential tumour imaging. Nanotech. 21: 1–8.

Yamaura, M., R. Camilo, L. Sampaio, M. Macedo and M. Nakamura. 2004. Preparation and characterization of (3aminopropyl) triethoxysilane-coated magnetite nanoparticles. J. Mag. Mag. Mater. 279: 210–217.

Yang, X., S. Skrabalak, E. Stein, B. Wu and X. Wei. 2008. Photoacoustic tomography with novel contrast agent based on gold nanocages or nanoparticles containing NIR dyes. Proc. SPIE. 685601: 1–10.

Yang, W. and C. Pan. 2009. Synthesis and fluorescent properties of biodegradable hyperbranched poly(amido amine)s. Macromol. Rapid Commun. 30: 2096–2101.

Yang, X., H. Hong and H. Grailer. 2011. cRGD-functionalized, dox-conjugated and (6)(4)cu-labelled SPIONs for targeted anticancer drug delivery and PET/MR imaging. Biomaterials 32: 4151–4160.

Yaroslavsky, A., A. Priezzhev, A. Rodriquez, I. Yaroslavsky and H. Battarbee. 2002. Optics of blood. pp. 169–216. *In*: Handbook of Optical Biomedical Diagnostics. Press, Bellingham, SPIE.

Yim, D., G. Baranoski, B. Kimmel and T. Miranda. 2012. A cell-based light interaction model for human blood. Eurographics. 31: 845–854.

Yokosawa, K., R. Shinomura and S. Sano. 1996. A 120-MHz ultrasound probe for tissue imaging. Ult. Imaging. 18: 231–239.

Yu, W., T. Zhan, J. Zhang, X. Qiao and L. Yang. 2006. The synthesis of octahedral nanoparticles of magnetite. Mat. Lett. 60: 2998–3001.

Yu, J., H. Zhao, L. Ye, L. Yang, S. Ku and N. Yang. 2009. Effect of surface functionality of magnetic silica nanoparticles on the cellular uptake by glioma cells *in vitro*. J. Mat. Chem. 19: 1265–1270.

Zangandeh, S., H. Li, P. Kumavor, O. Alqasmi, A. Aguirre and I. Mohammad. 2013. Photoacoustic imaging enhanced by indocynine green-conjugated single-wall carbon Nanotubes. J. Biomed. Opt. 18: 096006 (1-10).

Zerda, A., M. Kircher, J. Jokerst and C. Zalvaeta. 2013. A brain tumour molecular imaging strategy using a new triple-modality MRI-photoacoustic-Raman nanoparticle. Proc. SPIE. 8581: 85810G-1.

Zhao, M., L. Sun and R. Crooks. 1998. Preparation of Cu nanoclusters within dendrimer templates. J. Am. Chem. Soc. 120: 4877–4878.

Zhang, C., B. Wängler, B. Morgenstern, H. Zentgraf and M. Eisenhut. 2007. Specific targeting of tumour angiogenesis by RGD-conjugated ultrasmall superparamagnetic iron oxide particles using a clinical 1.5-T magnetic resonance scanner. Langmuir 23: 1427–1434.

Zhang, Y., M. Yang, N. Portney, D. Cui and G. Budak. 2008. Zeta potential: a surface electrical characteristic to probe the interaction of nanoparticles with normal and cancer human breast epithelial cells. Biomed. Microdevices 10: 321–328.

Zhang, Y. 2009. Magnetic nanocomposites of Fe_3O_4/SiO_2 FITC with pH-dependent fluorescence emission. Chin. Chem. Lett. 20: 969–972.

Zhang, Q., N. Iwakuma, B. Moudgil and C. Wu. 2009. Gold nanoparticles as a contrast agent for *in vivo* tumor imaging with photoacoustic tomography. Nanotechnology 20: 1–8.

Zhang, Yu. and S. Ahmad. 2009. Soft template synthesis of super paramagnetic Fe_3O_4 nanoparticles a novel technique. Polym. Mat. 19: 355–360.

Zhang, Z., F. Rong, S. Niu, Y. Xie, Y. Wang, H. Yang and D. Fu. 2010. Investigation the effects of nano golds on the fluorescence properties of the sectorial poly(amidoamine) (PAMAM) dendrimers. Appl. Surf. Sci. 256: 7194–7199.

Zhang, M., J. Li, G. Xing, R. He, W. Li, Y. Song and H. Guo. 2011. Variation in the internalization of differently sized nanoparticles induces different DNA-damaging effects on a macrophage cell line. Arch. Toxicology 85: 1575–1588.

Zheng, J., J. Petty and R. Dickson. 2003. High quantum yield blue emission from water-soluble au-nanodots. J. Am. Chem. Society 125: 7780–7781.

Zheng, P., L.Gao, X. Sun and Sh. Mei. 2009. The thermolysis behaviours of the first generation dendritic polyamidoamine. Iran Polym. J. 18: 257–264.

Zhu, Y. and Q. Wu. 1999. Synthesis of magnetite nanoparticles by precipitation with forced mixing. J. Nanopart. Res. 1: 393–396.

Zhu, J., W. Li, M. Zhu, W. Zhang, W. Niu and G. Liua. 2014. Influence of the pH value of a colloidal gold solution on the absorption spectra of an LSPR-assisted sensor. AIP Advances 4: 031338-6.

Zinin, P. 1992. Theoretical analysis of sound attenuation mechanisms in blood and in erythrocyte suspensions. Ultrasonics 30: 26–34.

Index